AF449152

CMV: PATHOGENESIS AND PREVENTION OF HUMAN INFECTION

March of Dimes Birth Defects Foundation
Birth Defects: Original Article Series, Volume 20, Number 1, 1984

CMV: PATHOGENESIS AND PREVENTION OF HUMAN INFECTION

**International Workshop Held April 20–22, 1983
at The Children's Hospital of Philadelphia, PA
Sponsored by
The March of Dimes Birth Defects Foundation
The National Institutes of Health (Grant #AI-19773)
Federal Drug Administration
Foundation for Microbiology**

Editors:

Stanley A. Plotkin, MD
The Children's Hospital of Philadelphia
The Wistar Institute
The University of Pennsylvania
Philadelphia, PA

Susan Michelson, PhD
Institut Pasteur
Paris, France

Joseph S. Pagano, MD
University of North Carolina
Chapel Hill, NC

Fred Rapp, PhD
Milton S. Hershey Medical Center
Hershey, PA

Associate Editor: **Natalie Paul**
March of Dimes Birth Defects Foundation

Assistant Editors: **Florence Dickman**
Elizabeth O'Brien Eakin
Sue Conde Greene
March of Dimes Birth Defects Foundation

ALAN R. LISS, INC., NEW YORK

To enhance medical communication in the birth defects field, the March of Dimes Birth Defects Foundation publishes the *Birth Defects Compendium (Second Edition)*, an *Original Article Series*, *Syndrome Identification*, a *Reprint Series*, and provides a series of films and related brochures.

Further information can be obtained from:

Professional Education Department
March of Dimes Birth Defects Foundation
1275 Mamaroneck Avenue
White Plains, New York 10605

Published by:
Alan R. Liss, Inc.
150 Fifth Avenue
New York, New York 10011

Library of Congress Cataloging in Publication Data
Main entry under title:

CMV, pathogenesis and prevention of human infection.

   (Birth defects : original article series ; v. 20,
no. 1, 1984)
   Papers from the International Workshop on
Cytomegalovirus.
   Bibliography: p.
   Includes index.
   1. Cytomegalic inclusion disease—Congresses.
2. Cytomegaloviruses—Congresses. 3. Cytomegalic
inclusion disease—Preventive inoculation—Congresses.
I. Plotkin, Stanley A. II. March of Dimes Birth Defects
Foundation. III. International Workshop on
Cytomegalovirus (1983 : Children's Hospital of Philadel-
phia) IV. Title: C.M.V., pathogenesis and prevention
of human infection. V. Series: Birth defects original
article series ; v. 20, no. 1. [DNLM: 1. Cytomegalo-
viruses—Congresses. 2. Cytomegaloviruses—Pathogenicity
—Congresses. 3. Cytomegalic inclusion disease—
Prevention and control—Congresses. W1 BI966 v.20 no.1 /
QW 165.5.H3 C649 1983]
RG626.B63 vol. 20, no. 1   616.043s [616'.0194]   83-23894
[RC136.8]
ISBN 0-8451-1057-8

Contents

Contributors   xi

Preface
Stanley A. Plotkin, Susan Michelson, Joseph S. Pagano, and
Fred Rapp   xv

List of Abbreviations   xvii

Adventures in Vaccine Research
A.J. Beale   1

**SECTION 1: THE HUMAN CYTOMEGALOVIRUS:
INTRODUCTION, DNA AND PROTEINS**

Perspective on Cytomegalovirus
Joseph S. Pagano   9

Isolation of the Human Cytomegaloviruses
Thomas H. Weller   15

Cellular Responses to Human Cytomegalovirus Infection
Thomas Albrecht, Jui-Lien Li, Dan Speelman, Rebecca Ball,
Mostafa Nokta, Michael Fons, Chan Hee Lee, Odd Steinsland,
William C. Thompson, and Darrell H. Carney   21

**The Physical and Transcriptional Organization of the Human
Cytomegalovirus Genome**
Jean M. DeMarchi   35

The Proteins of Human Cytomegalovirus
Mark F. Stinski   49

SECTION 2: NATURAL HISTORY OF CYTOMEGALOVIRUS

**Congenital and Perinatal Cytomegalovirus Infections: Clinical
Characteristics and Pathogenic Factors**
Sergio Stagno, Robert F. Pass, Meyer E. Dworsky,
William J. Britt, and Charles A. Alford   65

viii / Contents

The Relationship of Epidemiology and Treatment Factors to Infection and Allograft Survival in Renal Transplantation
Robert F. Betts 87

Cytomegalovirus Infection Following Marrow Transplantation: Risk, Treatment, and Prevention
Joel D. Meyers 101

SECTION 3: PATHOGENESIS OF CYTOMEGALOVIRUS

Sexual Transmission of CMV and Its Relationship to Kaposi Sarcoma in Homosexual Men
W. Lawrence Drew 121

Immunology of Cytomegalovirus: Immunosuppressive Effects During Infections
Monto Ho 131

Immune Balance in the Cytomegalovirus-Infected Host: In Vitro Studies of Virus-Lymphocyte Interactions and the Effects on Specific Lymphocyte Function
Paolo Casali, George P.A. Rice, and Michael B.A. Oldstone . . . 149

Cytomegalovirus–Leukocyte Interactions
Martin S. Hirsch 161

Cytomegalovirus and Human Cancer
Fred Rapp and Deanna Robbins 175

The Oncogenicity of Human Cytomegalovirus
Eng-Shang Huang, Eng-Chun Mar, Istvan Boldogh, and
John Baskar 193

Equine Cytomegalovirus: Genomic Structure, Protein Composition and Role in Oncogenic Transformation and Persistent Infection
John Staczek, Gretchen B. Caughman, and
Dennis J. O'Callaghan 213

The Guinea Pig Cytomegalovirus Model of Congenital Human Cytomegalovirus Infection
Frank J. Bia, Scott A. Miller, and Kathy H. Davidson 233

SECTION 4: VACCINATION AGAINST CYTOMEGALOVIRUS

The Importance of Cytotoxic Cellular Immunity in the Protection From Cytomegalovirus Infection
Gerald V. Quinnan, Jr. and Alain H. Rook 245

Live Cytomegalovirus Vaccination of Healthy Volunteers: Eight-Year Follow-up Studies
Harold Stern 263

Prevention of Cytomegalovirus Disease by Towne Strain Live Attenuated Vaccine
Stanley A. Plotkin, M. Lynn Smiley, Harvey M. Friedman, Stuart E. Starr, Gary R. Fleisher, Cliff Wlodaver, Donald C. Dafoe, Allan D. Friedman, Robert A. Grossman, and Clyde F. Barker 271

Cytomegalovirus Vaccine in Renal Transplant Candidates: Progress Report of a Randomized, Placebo-Controlled, Double-Blind Trial
Henry H. Balfour, Jr., Gregory W. Sachs, Patricia Welo, Richard C. Gehrz, Richard L. Simmons, and John S. Najarian . . 289

Selection of Particles and Proteins for Use as Human Cytomegalovirus Subunit Vaccines
Wade Gibson and Alice Irmiere 305

SECTION 5: PASSIVE IMMUNIZATION AND ANTIVIRALS

Prevention of Cytomegalovirus Infection in Bone Marrow Transplant Recipients by Prophylaxis With an Intravenous, Hyperimmune Cytomegalovirus Globulin
Richard M. Condie and Richard J. O'Reilly 327

Therapeutic Approaches to the Control of Cytomegalovirus Infections
Meyer Dworsky, Robert F. Pass, Sergio Stagno, and Richard J. Whitley 345

Abstracts 355

Index 501

Contributors

Thomas Albrecht, PhD, Department of Microbiology, University of Texas Medical Branch, Galveston, TX 77550 **[21]**

Charles A. Alford, MD, Departments of Pediatrics and Microbiology, The University of Alabama in Birmingham, School of Medicine, Birmingham, AL 35294 **[65]**

Henry H. Balfour, Jr., MD, Departments of Laboratory Medicine and Pathology, and Pediatrics, University of Minnesota Health Sciences Center, Minneapolis, MN 55455 **[289]**

Rebecca Ball, BS, Department of Microbiology, University of Texas Medical Branch, Galveston, TX 77550 **[21]**

Clyde F. Barker, MD, Department of Surgery, University of Pennsylvania, Philadelphia, PA 19104 **[271]**

John Baskar, ScD, Cancer Research Center, The University of North Carolina at Chapel Hill, Chapel Hill, NC 27514 **[193]**

A.J. Beale, Department of Biological Products, The Wellcome Research Laboratories, Beckenham Kent BR3 3BS, England **[1]**

Robert F. Betts, MD, Infectious Diseases Unit, Department of Medicine, University of Rochester School of Medicine, Rochester, NY 14642 **[87]**

Frank J. Bia, MD, MPH, Departments of Medicine and Laboratory Medicine, Virology 151/B, West Haven VA Medical Center, West Haven, CT 06516 **[233]**

Istvan Boldogh, PhD, Cancer Research Center, The University of North Carolina at Chapel Hill, Chapel Hill, NC 27514 **[193]**

William J. Britt, MD, Departments of Pediatrics and Microbiology, The University of Alabama in Birmingham, School of Medicine, Birmingham, AL 35294 **[65]**

Darrell H. Carney, PhD, Department of Human Biological Chemistry and Genetics, University of Texas Medical Branch, Galveston, TX 77550 **[21]**

Paolo Casali, MD, Department of Immunology, Scripps Clinic and Research Foundation, La Jolla, CA 92037 **[149]**

Gretchen B. Caughman, PhD, Department of Microbiology, University of Mississippi Medical Center, Jackson, MS 39216 **[213]**

The boldface number in brackets following each contributor's affiliation is the opening page number of that author's article.

Richard M. Condie, PhD, Department of Surgery, University of Minnesota School of Medicine, Minneapolis, MN 55455 [327]

Donald C. Dafoe, MD, Department of Surgery, University of Pennsylvania, Philadelphia, PA 19104 [271]

Kathy H. Davidson, Virology 151/B, West Haven VA Medical Center, West Haven, CT 06516 [233]

Jean M. DeMarchi, PhD, Department of Microbiology, Vanderbilt University School of Medicine, Nashville, TN 37232 [35]

W. Lawrence Drew, MD, PhD, Clinical Laboratory and Infectious Diseases, Mount Zion Hospital and Medical Center, San Francisco, CA 94120 [121]

Meyer E. Dworsky, MD, Department of Pediatrics, The University of Alabama in Birmingham, School of Medicine, Birmingham, AL 35294 [65, 345]

Gary R. Fleisher, MD, The Children's Hospital of Philadelphia, Philadelphia, PA 19104 [271]

Michael Fons, BA, Department of Microbiology, University of Texas Medical Branch, Galveston, TX 77550 [21]

Allan D. Friedman, MD, The Children's Hospital of Philadelphia and Department of Pediatrics, University of Pennsylvania, Philadelphia, PA 19104 [271]

Harvey M. Friedman, MD, Children's Hospital of Philadelphia, and Hospital of the University of Pennsylvania, Philadelphia, PA 19104 [271]

Richard C. Gehrz, MD, Department of Pediatrics, St. Paul Children's Hospital, St. Paul, MN 55102 [289]

Wade Gibson, Department of Pharmacology and Experimental Therapeutics, The Johns Hopkins University School of Medicine, Baltimore, MD 21205 [305]

Robert A. Grossman, MD, Department of Medicine, University of Pennsylvania, Philadelphia, PA 19104 [271]

Martin S. Hirsch, MD, Infectious Disease Unit, Department of Medicine, Massachusetts General Hospital, Harvard Medical School, Boston, MA 02114 [161]

Monto Ho, MD, Departments of Infectious Diseases and Microbiology, Graduate School of Public Health and Division of Infectious Diseases, Department of Medicine, School of Medicine, University of Pittsburgh, Pittsburgh, PA 15261 [131]

Eng-Shang Huang, PhD, Cancer Research Center, Department of Medicine, Department of Microbiology and Immunology, The University of North Carolina at Chapel Hill, Chapel Hill, NC 27514 [193]

Alice Irmiere, Department of Pharmacology and Experimental Therapeutics, The Johns Hopkins University School of Medicine, Baltimore, MD 21205 [305]

Chan Hee Lee, BS, Department of Microbiology, University of Texas Medical Branch, Galveston, TX 77550 [21]

Jui-Lien Li, PhD, Department of Microbiology, University of Texas Medical Branch, Galveston, TX 77550 [21]

Eng-Chun Mar, PhD, Cancer Research Center, The University of North Carolina at Chapel Hill, Chapel Hill, NC 27514 [193]

Joel D. Meyers, MD, Program in Infectious Diseases and Clinical Virology, Fred Hutchinson Cancer Research Center, and the University of Washington School of Medicine, Seattle, WA 98104 **[101]**

Susan Michelson, PhD, Virologie Medicale, Institut Pasteur, 25 Rue du Docteur Roux, Paris 75724 Cedex 15, France **[xv]**

Scott A. Miller, MD, Norfolk Diagnostic Clinic, 850 Kempsville Rd., Norfolk, VA 23502 **[233]**

John S. Najarian, MD, Department of Surgery, University of Minnesota Health Sciences Center, Minneapolis, MN 55455 **[289]**

Mostafa Nokta, MD, Department of Microbiology, University of Texas Medical Branch, Galveston, TX 77550 **[21]**

Dennis J. O'Callaghan, PhD, Department of Microbiology, University of Mississippi Medical Center, Jackson, MS 39216 **[213]**

Michael B.A. Oldstone, MD, Department of Immunology, Scripps Clinic and Research Foundation, La Jolla, CA 92037 **[149]**

Richard J. O'Reilly, MD, The Memorial Sloan-Kettering Cancer Center, New York, NY 10021 **[327]**

Joseph S. Pagano, MD, Departments of Medicine and Microbiology and Immunology, and Cancer Research Center, University of North Carolina at Chapel Hill, Chapel Hill, NC 27514 **[xv, 9]**

Robert F. Pass, MD, Departments of Pediatrics and Microbiology, The University of Alabama in Birmingham, School of Medicine, Birmingham, AL 35294 **[65, 345]**

Stanley A. Plotkin, MD, Children's Hospital of Philadelphia, The Wistar Institute and the University of Pennsylvania, Philadelphia, PA 19104 **[xv, 271]**

Gerald V. Quinnan, Jr., MD, The Division of Virology, Office of Biologics, National Center for Drugs and Biologics, Food and Drug Administration, Bethesda, MD 20205 **[245]**

Fred Rapp, PhD, Department of Microbiology and Cancer Research Center, The Pennsylvania State University College of Medicine, Hershey, PA 17033 **[xv, 175]**

George P.A. Rice, MD, Department of Immunology, Scripps Clinic and Research Foundation, La Jolla, CA 92037 **[149]**

Deanna Robbins, PhD, Department of Microbiology and Cancer Research Center, The Pennsylvania State University College of Medicine, Hershey, PA 17033 **[175]**

Alain H. Rook, MD, The Division of Virology, Office of Biologics, National Center for Drugs and Biologics, Food and Drug Administration, Bethesda, MD 20205 **[245]**

Gregory W. Sachs, MS, Departments of Laboratory Medicine and Pathology, and Pediatrics, University of Minnesota Health Sciences Center, Minneapolis, MN 55455 **[289]**

Richard L. Simmons, MD, Department of Surgery, University of Minnesota Health Sciences Center, Minneapolis, MN 55455 **[289]**

M. Lynn Smiley, MD, Department of Medicine, University of Pennsylvania, Philadelphia, PA 19104 **[271]**

xiv / Contributors

Dan Speelman, MA, Department of
Microbiology, University of Texas
Medical Branch, Galveston, TX 77550
[21]

John Staczek, PhD, Department of
Microbiology, University of Mississippi
Medical Center, Jackson, MS 39216
[213]

Sergio Stagno, MD, Departments of
Pediatrics and Microbiology, The
University of Alabama in Birmingham,
School of Medicine, Birmingham, AL
35294 **[65, 345]**

Stuart E. Starr, MD, The Children's
Hospital of Philadelphia, The Wistar
Institute and the University of
Pennsylvania, Philadelphia, PA 19104
[271]

Odd Steinsland, PhD, Department of
Pharmacology, University of Texas
Medical Branch, Galveston, TX 77550
[21]

Harold Stern, MB, ChB, PhD, FRCPath,
Department of Virology, St. George's
Hospital Medical School, London
SW17 0RE, England **[263]**

Mark F. Stinski, PhD, Department of
Microbiology, College of Medicine,
University of Iowa, Iowa City, IA
52242 **[49]**

William C. Thompson, PhD,
Department of Human Biological
Chemistry and Genetics, University of
Texas Medical Branch, Galveston, TX
77550 **[21]**

Thomas H. Weller, MD, Department of
Tropical Public Health, Harvard School
of Public Health, Boston, MA 02115
[15]

Patricia Welo, BSN, Departments of
Laboratory Medicine and Pathology, and
Pediatrics, University of Minnesota
Health Sciences Center, Minneapolis,
MN 55455 **[289]**

Richard J. Whitley, MD, The
Department of Pediatrics, The
University of Alabama in Birmingham,
School of Medicine, Birmingham, AL
35294 **[345]**

Cliff Wlodaver, MD, Department of
Medicine, University of Pennsylvania,
Philadelphia, PA 19104 **[271]**

Preface

The meeting which forms the basis of this book was held at the Children's Hospital of Philadelphia on April 20–22, 1983, and was organized for three reasons.

First, the human cytomegalovirus has become a focus of research in different areas of medicine: congenital infection, oncology, blood transfusion, organ transplantation, and immunology. While infections can be acquired in various ways, the virus can play a significant role in causing or potentiating human disease in each of these situations.

Second, a number of strategies for prevention of CMV disease have been proposed and even put into clinical trial, but there has been little opportunity to review the data and to compare the results.

Third, the only previous meetings devoted solely to CMV were held in 1970 and 1975. Otherwise CMV has been appended onto other meetings, with inadequate individual treatment.

The meeting in Philadelphia was attended by over 200 scientists from 11 countries. Included in this volume are the texts of the keynote presentations plus abstracts of other papers. The enthusiastic participation of the community of cytomegalovirologists was gratifying to us, as it confirmed the need for this conference.

The interest of non-scientists in CMV was illustrated by the message of support we received from His Holiness John Paul II, who himself was the victim of CMV disease following blood transfusion.

Of course, the conference could not have been held without financial support, notably by the March of Dimes, which provided initial funds, supplemented later by the Federal Drug Administration, the NIH, and the Foundation for Microbiology. Funds were also made available by Atlantic Richfield Company, Burroughs Wellcome USA, Burroughs Wellcome UK, Institut Meriuex, Merck, Sharp and Dohme, Ross Laboratories, Schering Corporation, Smith Kline Beckman, Syva Corporation, Upjohn Company, and Wyeth Laboratories. The Children's Hospital of Philadelphia and the Wistar Institute provided key logistic support. We are grateful to all of the above for helping us surmount the difficult problems of organizing a conference of this size. To Jeanne Cole, the Meeting Coordinator, no ordinary accolade is sufficient to the labors she performed.

The papers published in this book show that we heard a great deal of new information about the virus, its genome and proteins, about its pathogenesis and possible relationship to cancer, about vaccines and antivirals, and other facets of the problem. Thus, the book represents our most advanced knowledge of CMV as of April 1983, and publication enables this knowledge to be disseminated far beyond Philadelphia.

We did not, of course, resolve all the issues concerning CMV at this meeting, but a dialogue between basic and clinical virologists was initiated. We hope this dialogue will continue and eventually yield means to control this complex agent.

THE ORGANIZING COMMITTEE
Stanley A. Plotkin, MD
Susan Michelson, PhD
Joseph S. Pagano, MD
Fred Rapp, PhD

List of Abbreviations

Ab–antibody
ACIF–anticomplement
    immunofluorescence
ADCC–antibody-dependent cell-mediated
    cytotoxicity
AIDS–acquired immunodeficiency
    syndrome
ara-C–cytosine arabinoside
ATG–antithymocyte globulin

BMT–bone marrow transplant(ation)

CF–complement fixing (fixation)
CH–cycloheximide
CI–cytoplasmic inclusion
CMI–cell-mediated immunity
CMV–cytomegalovirus
CNS–central nervous system
Con A–concanavalin A
CPM–counts per minute
CTL–cytotoxic T-lymphocyte

DTH–delayed type hypersensitivity

EBV–Epstein-Barr virus
EBVNA–Epstein-Barr virus nuclear
    antigen
ECMV–equine CMV
EHV–equine herpesvirus
ELISA–enzyme-linked immunosorbent
    assay
EMEM–Eagle's minimal essential medium
ERV–equine rhinopneumonitis

FBS–fetal bovine serum
FN–filament network

GP CMV–guinea pig CMV
GP CMV-SG–guinea pig CMV salivary
    gland
GVH(D)–graft-versus-host (disease)

HBsAG–hepatitis B surface antigen
HCMV–human cytomegalovirus
HEL–human embryonic lung
HLA–human lymphocyte antigen
HPBL–human peripheral blood leukocyte
HSV–herpes simplex virus

ICSGP–infected cell specific
    glycopolypeptides
ICSP–infected cell specific polypeptides
IE–immediate early
IEA–immediate early antigen
IFN–interferon
Ig–immunoglobulin
IHA–indirect hemagglutination assay
IL–interleukin
IM–intramuscular(ly)
ISG–immune serum globulin
IV–intravenous(ly)

KS–Kaposi sarcoma

LGL–large granular lymphocyte
LP–lymphocyte proliferation

MCMV–murine cytomegalovirus
MHC–major histocompatibility complex
MLC–mixed leukocyte culture
MLR–mixed leukocyte reaction
MNC–mononuclear cell
MOI–multiplicity of infection
MW–molecular weight

NA–nuclear antigen
N-Ab–neutralizing antibody
NDV–Newcastle disease virus
NI–nuclear inclusion
NK–natural killer

PAA–phosphonoacetic acid
PBL–peripheral blood lymphocyte
PBMC–peripheral blood mononuclear cell
PBML–peripheral blood mononuclear
    lymphocyte
PFU–plaque-forming unit

PHA–phytohemagglutinin
PI–postinfection
PMNL–polymorphonuclear leukocyte
PNEA–prenuclear early antigen
PPD–purified protein derivative
PWM–pokeweed mitogen

RIA–radioimmunoassay
RTC–renal transplant candidate

SC–subcutaneous(ly)
SI–stimulation index
SM–skin and muscle

URI–upper respiratory infection

VP–virus polypeptide
VP1–viral protein 1
VZV–varicella zoster virus

Adventures in Vaccine Research

Dr. A.J. Beale

The Wellcome Research Laboratories, Beckenham Kent BR3 3BS, England

It is a sign of age and, one hopes, the wisdom born of experience when one is asked to write about a philosophic or personal aspect of vaccines. It is a recognition by one's colleagues, if not by oneself, that the brain is softening and is unable to cope with the hard cutting edge of science. That is not a comfortable thought when the science is still so exciting, and advances in molecular biology are opening up new vistas for those of us interested in vaccine development. To predict the direction of any research is hazardous and to see it in perspective, difficult. When I first started studying virology, I remember being told by Dr. Leslie Hoyle, a pioneer in influenza virus research alongside Dr. Henle of this city, that when he went into medical microbiology in the early 1930s his chief told him medical bacteriology was finished as a subject. The Medical Research Council had just commissioned a mammoth multivolume treatise on the subject to document the record of a completed subject. You will understand, therefore, that I have a lively sense of the impossible nature of the task you have set for me, which was to talk about perspective, and, hence, I have substituted the word "adventures." I have seen a great many advances in virus vaccine research and virology since I first started to study the subject, and perhaps I can look at my experience to see what lessons it teaches.

The first lesson is that we are observing a dynamic interaction between microbe and host, and the study of the changing epidemiology is of key importance. The emergence of epidemic poliomyelitis and the urge to do something about it was the starting point for some of us. We now know that the toll of poliomyelitis in developing countries where it is endemic is as great as it was during the epidemics in the USA and elsewhere before vaccines were developed. There are many other examples; in Philadelphia,

Birth Defects: Original Article Series, Volume 20, Number 1, pages 1–6
© **1984 March of Dimes Birth Defects Foundation**

one thinks of the emergence of Legionnaire's disease. More relevant to us is the changing pattern of infection due to smaller families and improved hygiene so that infection is postponed to later life. For example, primary infection with herpes simplex used to be mainly with type 1 in infancy by the oral route. Now, it is often a primary infection with type 2 by the genital route and this has much to do with the impact of genital herpes in recent years. Similarly, the emergence of AIDS illustrates the new challenges the medical microbiologist has to face.

A second lesson I have learned is the slowness of the advance in terms of application of discoveries in vaccine research to human medicine. Jenner discovered smallpox vaccination in 1796 and the disease was finally controlled on a global scale in 1978. Also, the importance of CMV as a cause of mental retardation and other symptoms became apparent in the 1960s, but we are still doing nothing practical about the prevention of the disease.

We have meetings like this one to discuss the latest work, but except for a few pioneers like Harold Stern and Stanley Plotkin, who have done excellent and courageous work on the development of vaccines, our efforts at prevention seem to me to be not commensurate with the size of the problem. To take a third example, during the early 1970s, John Bauer and Peter Collins at The Wellcome Research Laboratories in Beckenham discovered the antiviral action of a range of acyclic nucleosides prepared by Howard Schaeffer at Burroughs Wellcome in North Carolina against herpesviruses. It was not until 1981 that any drug from that research was launched on the market and made available for the benefit of patients, and it will not be until this year that the major impact of this discovery is made in medicine. Acyclovir is an interesting and important drug, indeed, a landmark in the development of antiviral chemotherapy, and another member of the series is even more active in vivo and also active against CMV. We know this as BW759 and you will learn something about it later in this volume. We make exciting medical scientific advances but their application is slow; perhaps this is a British disease, or a more particular British disease; I do not think this is quite true, although the story of prevention of diphtheria might lead one to that conclusion. By the late 1920s, Mr. A.T. Gleeny, at Wellcome, had laid the basis for immunization against diphtheria. He had discovered the difference between a primary and a secondary immune response to an antigen; uncovered, albeit by accident, the fact that formalin destroyed the toxicity but preserved the immunogenicity of diphtheria toxin and that aluminium salts acted as an adjuvant for antibody production. Everything was in place to prevent diphtheria, then causing more than a thousand deaths a week in England. However, nothing effective was done until a decade later when World War II galvanized the authorities into action, and a successful campaign was launched. By contrast, in Toronto the discovery was taken up immediately, and in that city the disease was controlled in the early 1930s.

Similarly, the efforts that have been made in the USA to eradicate measles are wholly commendable, and make a dismal contrast for us in the United Kingdom, where, despite the fact that we appointed the first Medical Officer of Health, and the fact that we have an all-embracing National Health Service, we can barely achieve an immunization rate for measles of 50%.

I think the slow pace should be changed, and there are some signs that it is changing. A requirement for this change is a confident, determined group of public health professionals, able and willing to undertake the daunting task of educating our masters—the public at large and the politicians they elect— of the benefits of preventive medicine. Lewis Thomas has rightly observed that vaccines represent the true, high technology medicine. This involves a basic understanding of the root causes of the problem and opens up the way to prevention and, possibly, eradication of disease. Iron lungs for poliomye- litis victims, dialysis for renal failure, transplants and machines for heart failure are all magnificent ingenious solutions, but they represent only half- way technology to a medical scientist.

Vaccines are, of course, either living or dead. Dead ones may contain a whole organism or a part of it. Until recently, vaccinology has been an empiric branch of medical science, but suddenly advances in molecular biology, genetics, and immunology are ushering in a new revolution with prospects of a new advance for both sorts of vaccine. First has come advances in immunology so that the role of circulating antibody, of local antibody at the portal of entry, or various aspects of cell-mediated immunity (CMI), particularly cytotoxic T cells and delayed type hypersensitivity, are beginning to be clarified for different infections. For example, work in our laboratories, and in others, has shown conclusively in mice that secretory IgA is the most important determinant of prophylactic immunity to influenza virus, especially within a drift series. Specific cytotoxic T cells are important for cure but not prevention, and delayed type hypersensitivity (DTH) seems positively harm- ful. By contrast, work by Drs. Howard and Liew in The Wellcome Research Laboratories at Beckenham has shown DTH to be the essential requirement for protection in leishmaniasis. On the other hand, for many diseases, for example, malaria, circulating antibody is the crucially important response, as it is for some virus diseases, such as poliomyelitis, measles, and hepatitis. High titer CMV immunoglobulin also seems valuable prophylactically for mitigating the consequences of infection with cytomegalovirus.

Even when circulating antibody is necessary, the antibody must be against the right antigen. The importance of this was first identified by Boulter and

Appleyard working with rabbit poxvirus as a model for smallpox which is preventable by vaccinia virus. They found that killed vaccinia gave rise to serum neutralizing antibody titers manyfold higher than titers obtained in rabbits convalescent from infection. Paradoxically, the relatively low titer convalescent serum was found to be much more effective in preventing disease and was even effective in curing rabbit pox. The reason was that the vaccinia virus for the killed vaccine was derived by disruption of infected cells and thus contained mainly intracellular virus released from infected cells. A similar story has been elucidated for measles and paramyxoviruses; the essential immunogenic component for these viruses is the fusion protein.

A key question for the vaccine developer is to identify the right antigen and to find a means of measuring it. This task has been much simplified by the advent of monoclonal antibodies. The immunogen has then to be presented to the immune system so that the appropriate clinically protective immune response is made. In earlier times, modified live or attenuated viral vaccines were always preferred because it was either impossible or very difficult to produce viral antigens in adequate quantities to make an effective killed vaccine. Now this objection is rapidly disappearing because viral antigens can be obtained in quantity by means of cell culture and, increasingly, by means of genetic manipulation or synthesis of immunogens. As a result, they can be produced, not only in quantity, but, also, essentially pure.

There are problems for killed vaccines made by new technology; first, there are teething problems in producing sufficient amounts of antigen, as, for example, the problems of producing HBsAg in *E coli*. Another problem experienced with foot and mouth disease and polio virus has been the identification of the immunogen. Thus, one of the capsid proteins of the foot and mouth disease virion, viral protein 1 (VP1), will raise antibodies, but they are poorly protective. This problem has been solved in principle by the discovery that isolated peptide sequences of VP1 had different effects. Thus, although many stretches were immunogenic in the sense of producing antibodies, these were not neutralizing antibodies. Two sequences of amino acids, 141–160 and 200–213, did produce neutralizing antibodies, the former to much higher titers than the latter. Moreover, the 141–160 region generated a protective immune response in animal challenge experiments. Intact VP1 produced only antibodies to the 200–213 region in the immunized animals; whereas intact virions produce antibodies to both regions. Another feature of pure antigens, illustrated most clearly for synthetic peptides, is the problem of adequate immunogenicity. They commonly require an adjuvant to enhance immunogenicity to levels produced by intact virus; also the isolated peptides need to be attached to a carrier protein to confer immunogenicity. Moreover, our knowledge of adjuvants and the basis of immunogenicity is so rudimentary that although reasonable enhancement of circulating antibodies can be achieved, our weapons are still blunderbusses. The methods for specific stimulation of T-cell subsets or for local immunity are not yet available.

It is for these reasons that many workers still favor living attenuated vaccines as the means to control virus diseases. They will contain the right antigens; they will multiply and stimulate the whole range of immune responses. Although derived empirically as host range mutants, they have an impressive record of safety and effectiveness. The considerable knowledge that is being developed about the virulence factors may enable attenuated strains to be engineered in the future rather than derived empirically. This, however, remains to be achieved, although for some viruses, eg, poliovirus, it may well prove possible because there are very few nucleotide changes between the virulent parent of the Sabin type 3 strain, the attenuated strain, and a revertant virus. However, if this section were deleted from the genome, would the first polypeptide product be cleaved properly? At present we do not know, but soon we will.

The solution of immunologic problems by different techniques of presentation of immunogens seems, to me at least, very attractive; it opens up the possibility of using defined chemicals as immunogens. It also opens up the possibility of doing better than nature with our vaccines. A hint of this possibility is seen in the work on leishmaniasis already mentioned. The reason for failure of immunity in some mouse strains is generation of specific suppressor T cells, but, when an immunization schedule is used that prevents the appearance of suppressor T cells, clinical immunity is conferred. This result is encouraging for the future. However, in the meanwhile, we should use the tools at hand. In my view, that means using the living CMV vaccines now available in more extended trials, as well as trying to develop killed vaccines. We should not be too fearful of conjectural dangers, but use our best endeavors to move cautiously but determinedly forward. The past gives cause for some hope. I can remember the problems when poliovaccines were introduced, for example, the fears about rhesus antigen from monkey kidney cells, the simian viruses; virus B had been recognized as a potential hazard but not the veritable Pandora's box of viruses from monkey kidney cells discovered by all of us who were working on poliovaccines in the 1950s, and first documented by Robert Hull. We survived these problems, and, indeed, the more serious one of living poliovirus in killed vaccines, because of the good surveillance, and our confidence that changes to improve the situation could be made. Another example is vaccinia. This vaccine was being called into question in the United States and Britain when WHO launched their eradication scheme because it was too dangerous;

yet, with this imperfect tool the disease was eliminated from the globe. This really is a triumph for courage and nerve to use the tools available now. My final example is measles where there were fears that the vaccine was too reactogenic, especially in Britain, and that encephalitis and subacute sclerosis panencephalitis might be increased by immunization. Another fear was that the immunity might not be lifelong. In the United States the vaccine has been adapted and improved, and used in a way which has been imaginative and effective to control the disease. I think we should gain great confidence from these experiences to take active interventionist policies in immunization, with careful feedback from surveillance of immunized populations. In this way, herpesviruses, especially CMV, may be added to our success stories in the control of virus diseases.

SECTION 1:
THE HUMAN CYTOMEGALOVIRUS: INTRODUCTION, DNA AND PROTEINS

Perspective on Cytomegalovirus

Joseph S. Pagano, MD

University of North Carolina at Chapel Hill, Chapel Hill, NC 27514

Cytomegalovirus is one of that remarkable group of viruses, the herpesviruses, that infect human beings universally and stay with us for life. Typically, CMV infects us harmlessly, persists for the rest of our lives quietly in a perfectly adapted latent infection, and reactivates without a tremor. Yet, the same virus may infect others with catastrophic results or reactivate with a panoply of disease, mild to fatal, including, perhaps, even cancer.

The purpose of this conference is to think about how to prevent infection with this virus. Serving this objective is the conviction in the minds of the organizers that basic knowledge about the virus is essential for intelligent design of vaccines and their rational application to control infection and disease.

Toward these ends pathogenetic studies are of the utmost importance, rivaled only by lucid epidemiology. Both require the deep knowledge that comes from molecular biology, now available, but for the most part still standing in the wings, to add light and technology to our purpose.

CMV is a common virus, but it is not any the less challenging through its ubiquity.

Infection with this virus is a worthy objective for prevention. Prevention will remain necessary even as therapy becomes available—and promising drugs are about to break on the scene.

Our objective—prevention—is not new for viruses, but CMV poses new problems for vaccines and novel decisions, and it opens uncharted paths for virologists, physicians, and for preventive medicine.

THE VIRUS AND ITS BIOLOGY

Indistinguishable morphologically from the other herpesviruses, CMV has one feature that sets it apart, the extraordinary size of its genome, 150×10^6

Birth Defects: Original Article Series, Volume 20, Number 1, pages 9–13
© **1984 March of Dimes Birth Defects Foundation**

daltons, discovered by Kilpatrick and Huang. The genome has a general structural organization that unites it with the other herpesviruses: unique and internally repeated sequences, isomeric forms, and terminal homology as first deduced from denaturation analyses of the human cytomegalovirus (HCMV) genome. These features have not yet been related to the biology of CMV. The coding capacity of this genome, relatively immense, is largely, if not entirely, untracked. The regulation of CMV genome expression is expected to follow the herpes simplex virus (HSV) model of temporal and abundance controls, but it would be a mistake to force CMV prematurely into herpes simplex modes of cascading transcription and translation with sequential ordering.

Key features of the virus are its worldwide distribution, multimodal transmission, tissue pleiotropism and oncogenic potential, which make the goal of prevention both formidable and worthy of our effort.

Hallmarks of the biology of CMV are silent primary infection, persistence, latency, and reactivation of the virus—hallmarks of all the herpesviruses that add to the complexity of evaluation of vaccine results.

The diseases of CMV cover a multitude of phenotypes, some probably as ancient as humanity, others, diseases of modern therapy. Striking are the differences between the symptoms of primary infection and those of reactivated infection. Striking also is the age-relatedness of disease phenotype—more so than for any of the other herpesviruses.

Finally, the immunologic determinants of CMV diseases and the immunologic consequences of infection with the virus are probably greater than for the other herpesviruses. HSV and varicella zoster virus (VZV) reactivation occur most usually without obvious immunodeficiency, but CMV seems to require considerable disturbance of immunoregulation for symptomatic reactivation—as does Epstein-Barr virus (EBV), which may require even greater disturbances for disease.

Furthermore, the effects of CMV on T-cell subset interplay seem to be greater than those produced by any other known human virus. Only infection with the virus of AIDS produces larger and more lasting reversals of helper-to-suppressor T-lymphocyte ratios.

OBJECTIVES

What are the major specific objectives for prevention of CMV infection? The most obvious is symptomatic congenital infection with the virus. Not obvious are more subtle possible effects of CMV infection in utero, and perhaps perinatal infection that may be even more important objectives. Nor do we know whether this major problem of congenital CMV infection, especially in some countries and some groups, is increasing. We look to our epidemiologic colleagues for new studies on these important questions relevant to vaccine development.

Finally, crucial to prevention of congenital infections is an understanding of how they come about. Is systemic infection needed, or is local infection sufficient? These questions of pathogenesis have remained unanswered too long. The remarkable demonstrations of CMV in human sperm may provide the missing link in the pathogenetic chain.

Allograft recipients are the most immediate target for immunization. In these patients, CMV infection may be a nuisance, or it may be fatal. The inevitability of infection with CMV in this risk group eases the ethical problem of experimental vaccine administration. However, it does not simplify the scientific questions, inasmuch as many of these patients are already infected with CMV. This fact raises the question of whether it will do any good to administer vaccine to someone already infected; and the further question, what are the consequences of infection in someone now immunized with vaccine? We already know that even in nature second exogenous infections with CMV and HSV (but not with EBV or VZV) occur with ease because of the ability of these two members of the herpes group to bypass humoral immune mechanisms by infecting locally.

The information, based on excellent data, that a second congenitally infected infant born of the same infected mother is likely to be asymptomatic, is a crucial concern for this conference, as is the notion that a reactivated CMV infection in an allograft recipient has less consequences than primary infection in the same setting. Here the data have been somewhat conflicting, but they appear to be moving toward resolution.

Disease in other high-risk groups not now predictable is likely to become identified in time, as exemplified in patients with AIDS, and add to our objectives.

VACCINES

Going back to the beginning of the making of vaccines up to the present day, we have two divergent avenues to choose in making vaccines: the avenue leading to an inactivated product, and the other leading to an attenuated living virus. New, however, are the diverse possibilities for inactivated products that have suddenly come upon us.

Attenuated virus vaccines against other virus infections have a history of success, but not unmitigated success. The major problem in making attenuated CMV is one that is not unprecedented, namely, the lack of markers of attenuation. The other major problem is unprecedented in the history of vaccines—a problem occasioned by the fact that herpesviruses persist in a viable form in the organism for life. This fact is likely to be true for attenuated viruses as well. The third problem comes from the primacy of asymptomatic infection with wild-type virus. Many, many people may need to be infected with attenuated CMV before we would ever know whether vaccine virus causes disease directly. A fourth problem comes out of one of the biologic hallmarks of herpesviruses, namely, reactivation. Viruses that initially infect silently may reactivate with disease. All of these considerations center on documentation of latency, which is difficult at best. Latent infection is surmised only in retrospect, when the infection is reactivated. We do not know whether latent attenuated virus, being well adapted to its host, may withstand moderate immunosuppression and reactivate only upon more severe provocation, and then unpredictably.

A final problem comes from the concern that in the absence of markers for either attenuation or oncogenicity, let alone markers that can distinguish between the two biologic effects, selection for qualities of attenuation may not eliminate oncogenic properties and could conceivably co-select for both properties.

The overriding problem for HSV, as well as CMV, vaccines applies equally to attenuated live virus vaccines and to inactivated virus vaccines, namely, the unlikelihood, and probably the impossibility, of either type of vaccine being able to prevent exogenous reinfection in the sequestered sites where CMV gains access to the body.

The possibilities for vaccines composed of inactivated virus preparations or virus constituents are being revolutionized through the application of contemporary molecular biology. Conventional inactivated virus vaccines are unlikely ever to be practicable, for the yield of virus from even the most efficient in vitro cell systems is relatively small. Similarly, so-called subunit vaccines in which the protein constituents of the virus are separated from the genomic DNA will probably remain impracticable. However, prospects for the use of recombinant DNA techniques to produce CMV proteins in *E coli,* or in yeast, or even via vectors in human cells are excellent. The difficulty of such approaches is tied to the elusiveness of the identity of the protective antigens of CMV. Finally, the ability to synthesize in vitro selected immunogenic CMV peptides is already within our grasp, did we but know which peptides to synthesize! Eventually we can imagine a shrewd selection of apposite peptides making up a vaccine that evokes an excellent immune response, at the same time threading its way past undesirable responses such as sensitizing reactions and deleterious effects on T lymphocytes—an elegant concept! For these high goals we need the biologists and protein chemists working on CMV more than we need further recombinant DNA know-how. Our knowledge about the detailed protein composition of CMV is still meager.

CONCLUSIONS

Unanswered questions exceed those for which we have answers on all sides, not only the molecular biologic, but also especially the pathogenetic and the epidemiologic. What could be more fascinating than to delve into the subtle and complex steps of generation of disease on a molecular and cellular level? What epidemiologist could resist the challenges of understanding how CMV is transmitted from one person to another, from one site to another, in necessary but inconstant linkage to specific disease? The opportunities for research are great, and if pursued, are very likely to yield unexpected dividends. CMV poses new problems for vaccines and the decisions needed to address these problems.

Human beings are interventionists. We do not seem to believe in letting nature take its course even though most of the time the balance of nature works to cause disease in only a few of those infected. This is the central dogma of preventive medicine, essential to its strategies. Indeed, the infrequency of disease in the face of frequent infection is a lasting mystery of infectious disease and probably of cancer as well.

These reflections should be our companions on the uncharted paths ahead in this task. As always, we improvise as we break new ground. We look to rational design, but settle for the pragmatic—an approach less than satisfactory for contemporary science—yet a way honored by achievement.

My guess is that the work will be vexatious and challenging, but our need to go ahead with less-than-perfect knowledge is nothing new.

Isolation of the Human Cytomegaloviruses

Thomas H. Weller, MD

Department of Tropical Public Health, Harvard School of Public Health, Boston, MA 02115

In retrospect, the Second International Conference on the Cytomegaloviruses (CMV) held at the Children's Hospital of Philadelphia in April 1983, will be a highly significant milestone in the evolution of our knowledge of a group of viruses ever increasing in social significance. This volume provides a comprehensive summary of the remarkable advances in knowledge that have occurred since 1970 when the first conference was held in St. Gallen, Switzerland. At that conference, I detailed the circumstances surrounding the isolation of the human CMV (HCMV) some 15 years earlier [1]. Knowledge of the CMV at that time was fragmentary; lacunae were identified and our immaturity of understanding of the then 15-year-old virologic offspring was likened to the difficult years of adolescence. The HCMVs now are vigorous 28-year-old entities. Reference to standard strains such as "AD169" and "Davis" are frequent in this volume. The organizing committee has asked that I again briefly summarize the events surrounding their recognition.

By 1950, the viral etiology of "salivary gland virus disease" of rodents had been demonstrated by passage of filtrates in animals; the agents were host-specific. Morphologic evidence had documented the frequent occurrence of enlarged, inclusion-containing cells in the salivary glands of infants, and postmortem studies had revealed a disseminated process referred to as "generalized cytomegalic inclusion disease." However, serial propagation of the etiologic agents had not been achieved. The relationship of the focal and disseminated processes observed in infants was obscure.

In 1948, we prepared suspended fragment cultures of human embryonic skin-muscle tissue in an effort to grow varicella virus. While tissue fragments in cultures inoculated with vesicle fluid became infected as evidenced by the

Birth Defects: Original Article Series, Volume 20, Number 1, pages 15–19
© **1984 March of Dimes Birth Defects Foundation**

appearance of intranuclear inclusion bodies [2], serial propagation of the virus was not achieved until a culture system was used that promoted growth of confluent sheets of cells [3]. However, in the interim it was demonstrated that the simple culture system would support growth of poliomyelitis virus [4,5]. This development brought many visitors to our laboratory. In May 1951, Dr. Margaret Smith of St. Louis visited our laboratory, desirous of applying the new methodology to the isolation of the salivary gland viruses; she successfully pursued her plan first to explore the mouse model [6], and then to move to the study of the human agent. Indeed, as indicated in a personal communication [1], Dr. Smith had by 1954 cultured a human strain from parotid tissues, although this finding was not recorded until 1956 [7].

In contrast to the targeted efforts of Dr. Smith, the isolation of CMV in Boston and in Bethesda involved an element of the serendipitous. In Boston, Dr. Eli Chernin and I had demonstrated that the protozoan, *Toxoplasma gondii*, could be grown serially in cultures of mouse and human tissues [8]. In January 1955, a 3-month-old infant exhibiting the then "classical triad" of congenital toxoplasmosis, ie, hepatosplenomegaly, cerebral calcification, and chorioretinitis, was admitted to the Children's Hospital. We sought to isolate *Toxoplasma* from liver biopsy material; 12 days later the inoculated cultures of human embryonic skin-muscle tissue developed focal collections of swollen cells, that, when stained, contained intranuclear inclusions. Subculture was readily accomplished by transfer of infected tissue; termed the Davis strain, this isolate from liver tissue was the first strain of CMV recovered from a living patient [9]. The focal cytopathology observed in the first subculture, and the typical changes in a stained preparation of the third Davis subculture are depicted in Figures 1 and 2.

As previously summarized [1], evidence was then accumulating that cytomegalic inclusion disease might be diagnosed during life by demonstration of inclusion-bearing cells in the urine. This led us to attempt to isolate virus from the urine of infants with suggestive clinical presentations; in May 1956, the Kerr strain, and in August 1956, the Esp. strain were recovered from urine specimens from infants with typical signs and symptoms [9]. The persistence of urinary viral excretion was established, the obvious term "viruria" was introduced, and usefulness of urine as a diagnostic source suggested.

Isolation of the AD169 strain of CMV in Bethesda derived from an unplanned observation. In 1955, Rowe and co-workers were defining a new group of viruses—the adenoviruses—by culturing uninoculated human adenoidal tissues [10]. Focal cytopathic changes developed in the fibroblastic

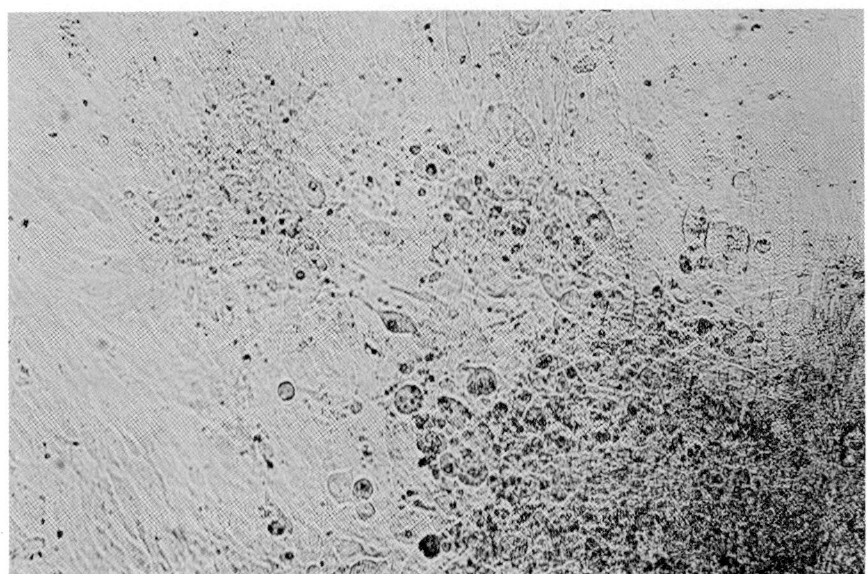

Fig. 1. Edge of focal lesion. First subculture of Davis strain in roller culture of foreskin tissue on 15th day, February 23, 1955 (×135).

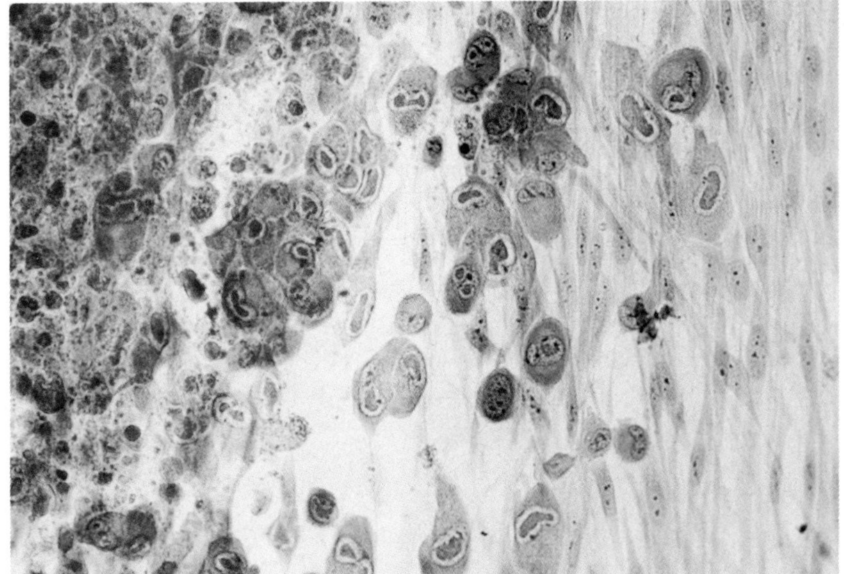

Fig. 2. Edge of focal lesion. Third subculture of Davis strain in roller culture of foreskin tissue. Fixed on 20th day, April 26, 1955 (H and E × 300).

outgrowth of cultures of adenoidal tissues from three children; the cytopathology and associated intranuclear inclusion bodies resembled changes we had described for varicella virus [3]. Therefore, in May 1955, Rowe brought primary cultures of AD169, prepared on February 28, 1955, to our laboratory for study. The focal lesions were not those of varicella but appeared identical to those we were obtaining with the Davis agent. As the result of Dr. Rowe's visit, the similarity of the agents recovered in St. Louis, Bethesda, and in Boston was established prior to publication. These events were briefly reported in November 1955 [11]. It was then assumed that prolonged cultivation of adenoidal tissue had unmasked AD169; in the light of current knowledge a salivary source of the virus deserves consideration.

As emphasis shifted from involvement of the salivary glands to the concept of a generalized viral process, the term "salivary gland virus" became inappropriate; in addition, an unrelated virus from bats had been so named. Likewise, as evidence accrued indicating that asymptomatic disseminated infection could occur, the term "cytomegalic inclusion disease virus" had inaccurate connotations. We therefore proposed that the agents of man and animals be referred to as the CMV group [12].

Prior to 1960, the HCMVs were considered to constitute an antigenically homogeneous group. At that time, as antisera prepared in animals were not available, we examined the neutralizing capacity of sera from congenitally infected infants against four homologous and heterologous strains of CMV [12]. The results with the Davis and AD169 agents indicated considerable dissimilarity, and tentatively these viruses were termed types 1 and 2. In the interim, as additional strains have been examined by various procedures, the concept of discrete types has been supplanted as evidence was developed that we are dealing with a group of agents that possess a spectral mosaic of antigens, varying in amount and perhaps in number. It is of interest that Davis and AD169 have a polar relationship on analysis by kinetic neutralization tests [13].

While the antigenic heterogeneity of HCMV strains is established, the practical implications of these differences need elucidation. This information will be available at the next international conference on CMV as investigators consider that strains of CMV may differ in pathogenic and immunogenic potential, and that these inherent attributes may alter on prolonged propagation in vitro.

REFERENCES

1. Weller TH: Cytomegaloviruses: The difficult years. J Infect Dis 122:532–539, 1970.

2. Weller TH, Stoddard MB: Intranuclear inclusion bodies in cultures of human tissue inoculated with varicella vesicle fluid. J Immunol 68:311–319, 1952.
3. Weller TH: Serial propagation in vitro of agents producing inclusion bodies derived from varicella and herpes zoster. Proc Soc Exp Biol Med 83:340–346, 1953.
4. Enders JF, Weller TH, Robbins FC: Cultivation of the Lansing strain of poliomyelitis virus in cultures of various human embryonic tissues. Science 109:85–87, 1949.
5. Weller TH, Robbins FC, Enders JF: Cultivation of poliomyelitis virus in cultures of human foreskin and embryonic tissues. Proc Soc Exp Biol Med 72:153–155, 1949.
6. Smith MG: Propagation of salivary gland virus of the mouse in tissue cultures. Proc Soc Exp Biol Med 86:435–440, 1954.
7. Smith MG: Propagation in tissue cultures of cytopathogenic virus from human salivary gland virus (SGV) disease. Proc Soc Exp Biol Med 92:424–430, 1956.
8. Chernin E, Weller TH: Serial propagation of *Toxoplasma gondii* in roller tube cultures of mouse and of human tissues. Proc Soc Exp Biol Med 85:68–72, 1954.
9. Weller TH, Macaulay JC, Craig JM, Wirth P: Isolation of intranuclear inclusion producing agents from infants with illnesses resembling cytomegalic inclusion disease. Proc Soc Exp Biol Med 94:4–12, 1957.
10. Rowe WP, Huebner RJ, Gilmore LK, Parrot RH, Ward TG: Isolation of a cytopathogenic agent from human adenoids undergoing spontaneous degeneration in tissue culture. Proc Soc Exp Biol Med 84:570–573, 1953.
11. Weller TH: Problems revealed by the expanding use of tissue culture procedures in studies of infectious agents. Am J Trop Med Hyg 5:422–429, 1956.
12. Weller TH, Hanshaw JB, Scott DM: Serologic differentiation of viruses responsible for cytomegalic inclusion disease. Virology 12:130–132, 1960.
13. Waner JL, Weller TH: Analysis of antigenic diversity among human cytomegaloviruses by kinetic neutralization tests with high-titered rabbit antisera. Infect Immun 21:151–157, 1978.

Cellular Responses to Human Cytomegalovirus Infection

Thomas Albrecht, PhD, Jui-Lien Li, PhD, Dan Speelman, MA, Rebecca Ball, BS, Mostafa Nokta, MD, Michael Fons, BA, Chan Hee Lee, BS, Odd Steinsland, PhD, William C. Thompson, PhD, and Darrell H. Carney, PhD

Departments of Microbiology (T.A., J.-L.L., D.S., R.B., M.N., M.F., C.H.L.), Pharmacology (O.S.), and Human Biological Chemistry and Genetics (W.C.T., D.H.C.), University of Texas Medical Branch, Galveston, TX 77550

CMV disease was first recognized by the unique cytopathologies, particularly enlarged cells with prominent nuclear inclusions (NI), observed at autopsy [1]. These unique cytopathic effects were confirmed when these viruses were isolated and examined in cell cultures derived from various human tissues [2–4]. Distinctive features in the cellular response to HCMV infection include formation of cytoplasmic (CI) and nuclear inclusions and enlargement of cells [2–4]. CMVs also induce cytopathic effects which, at least to some extent, are common to other viruses (eg, rounding cells [5–7]). Since the cellular responses to CMV may indicate fundamental changes in cell physiology essential for efficient replication of these viruses, we have focused our research on determining the molecular and cellular mechanisms involved in these responses and in the establishment of acute and persistent CMV infections. An understanding of these cellular responses may be particularly important in circumstances where CMV does not induce the complete cascade of physiologic and morphologic changes observed in productive infection, resulting in restriction of CMV replication and possibly leading to the formation of persistent infections and/or neoplasia.

In response to CMV infection, human embryo skin muscle (SM) cells undergo a characteristic sequence of morphologic changes in vitro (Table 1). The sequence of these cellular responses is rounding, "contraction," "relax-

Birth Defects: Original Article Series, Volume 20, Number 1, pages 21–34
© **1984 March of Dimes Birth Defects Foundation**

TABLE 1. Cellular Responses to HCMV*

Response	Time First Detected Hr (PI)	Comments	References
Cell rounding	5†		[5–7]
Depolymerization of microtubules	3–8	Time based on taxol inhibition studies.	[8]
CI	5	Extensive morphogenesis of the CI takes place during the ensuing 140 hr.	[4, 6, 9]
Alterations of mitochondria	5		(Albrecht et al, unpublished observations)
Filamentous projections on the plasma membrane	5		[6]
Early NI	5		[6, 7]
Clumping and margination of chromatin	5		[3, 4, 6, 10]
Condensation of the nucleoli	5		[6]
"Contraction"	5–24	While similarities are shared with smooth muscle contraction, the process may not be identical [12].	[6, 7, 11, 12]
Initiation of CMV DNA synthesis	12–16		[13, 14]
Stimulation of cell DNA synthesis	12–30		[8, 15, 16]
Disruption of cytoplasmic intermediate filaments (IF)	24		[17]
Alteration of Golgi apparatus	24		[18]
Polykaryocytes	24		[6]
Detection of IF associated protein in the nucleus	24		[17]
"Relaxation"	24–48‡		(see text)
Cell enlargement	48‡		[2–4, 6]
Late NI and development of cellulae	48	Extensive morphogenesis follows through 144 hr or later.	[6, 7]
Detection of IF associated protein in the NI	24–48		[17]
Progeny nucleocapsids	48		[7]
Virions in cytoplasm	72		[7]
Nuclear dense bodies	72		[6, 7]
Cytoplasmic dense bodies	96		[6]

*Timing of most of these events is dependent on the multiplicity of infection (MOI) and for some responses on the virus strain [6].
†Although 5 hr is the earliest reported time, unpublished observations indicate that cell rounding begins earlier.
‡As described in the text, studies with CH and papaverine suggest "relaxation" begins between 12 and 24 hr PI and that enlargement may begin by 24 hr.

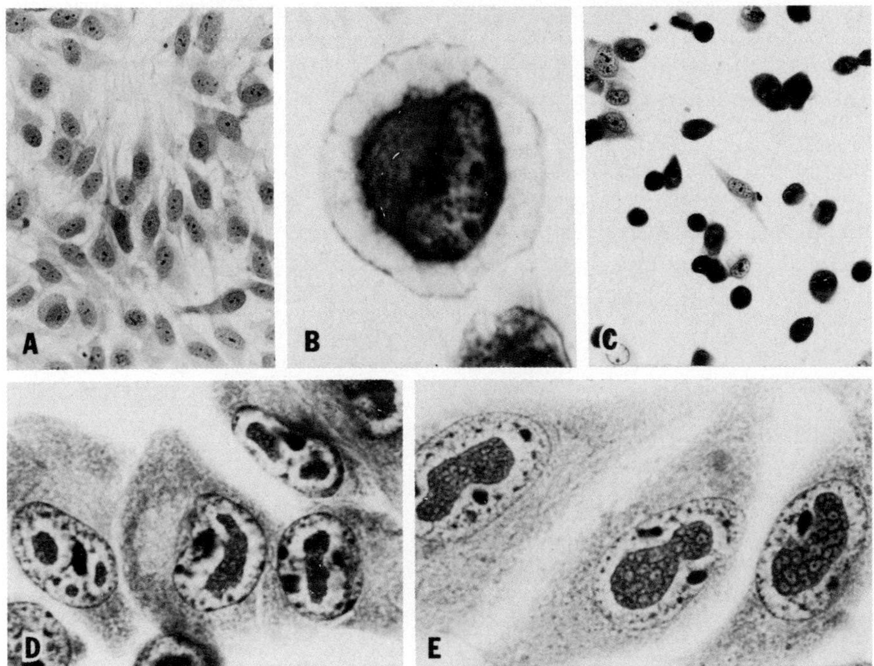

Fig. 1.   Human embryo SM cells infected with CMV (strain AD169) and fixed with Bouin's fluid. A) At 0 hr PI, there are no distinct cytopathic effects seen. B) At 5 hr PI, cell rounding and cytoplasmic inclusions are evident. A cell with thin peripheral cytoplasm in an intermediate stage of cell rounding is seen. C) At 24 hr PI, cell rounding is prominent. D) By 48 hr, cells are "relaxed" and are beginning to enlarge. E) At 96 hr PI, the cells are much enlarged and contain prominent NI consisting of cellulae. (H & E; A, × 216; B, × 1492; C, × 216; D and E, × 864.)

ation," and enlargement (Fig. 1) [6,7,11,12]. Rounding of cells begins before 5 hr PI when cells in intermediate stages of rounding are observed [6], and continues through 12 to 24 hr PI, at which time the population of these rounded cells with the smallest size is similar in diameter to that of the nucleus of uninfected cells (Fig. 1) [12]. By 48 hr PI most infected cells have "relaxed," partially flattened, and begun to enlarge. At later times, CMV-infected cells are observed to be much enlarged (Fig. 1).

We have investigated the mechanisms by which these morphologic and physiologic cellular responses occur. Three early observations suggested that the process of cell rounding shared some mechanistic features in common with smooth muscle contraction. First, images of cells in intermediate stages of rounding may be consistent with a contractile-like mechanism (Fig. 1).

Second, these cells round and diminish in size until their diameter appears to be considerably reduced (Fig. 1). Third, electron micrographs of these rounded cells reveal convoluted nuclear membrane profiles [7] similar to those observed by Majno [19] in contracting cells.

If in fact the mechanism of cell rounding were similar to smooth muscle contraction, then it is possible that smooth muscle-relaxing drugs could inhibit CMV-induced cell rounding. As shown in Figure 2, papaverine, sodium nitroprusside, hydralazine, and diazoxide at doses of about 1×10^{-4} M inhibited cell rounding. Measurement of the number of rounded cells relative to the number of fibroblastic cells indicated that the various drugs blocked rounding by about 85% to 95% (Table 2). Since numerous cellular responses consistent with a rise in intracellular free $[Ca^{++}]$ [20] were observed (see below), it seemed possible that cell rounding and these other responses could be related to a change in plasma membrane permeability and a concomitant

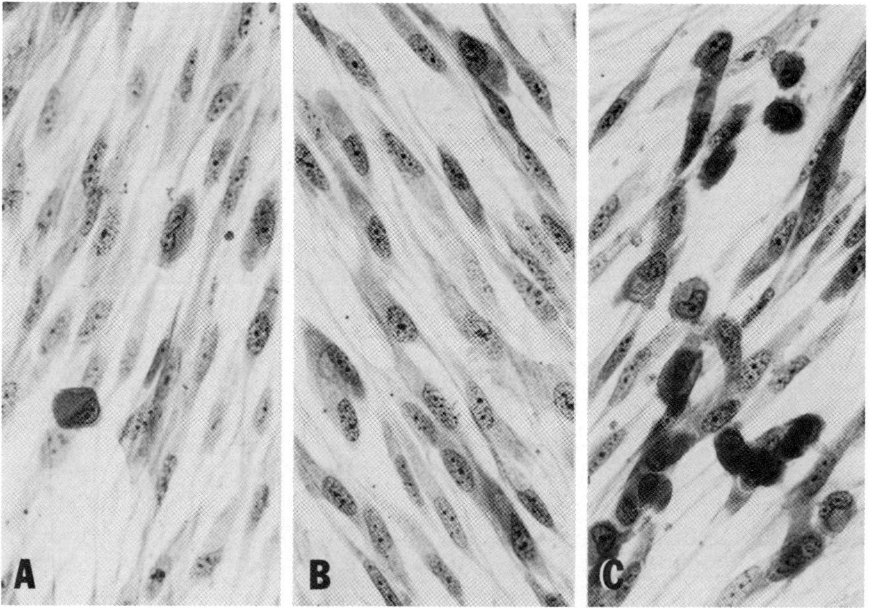

Fig. 2. Inhibition of CMV-induced cell rounding at 6 hr PI by smooth muscle-relaxing agents. A) Treated with hydralazine (1.9×10^{-4} M); B) treated with diazoxide (1.3×10^{-4} M); C) not treated. Papaverine, sodium nitroprusside, and verapamil (not illustrated) caused effects similar to hydralazine and diazoxide. Drugs were added at 0 hr PI. (Bouin's fixative, H & E, $\times$ 373.)

TABLE 2. Inhibition of HCMV*-Induced Cell Rounding by Smooth Muscle-Relaxing Agents

Treatment		Cell Morphology†		% Cells	% Inhibition of
Drug	Dose	Fibroblast	Rounded	Rounded	Cell Rounding
None		774	346	30.9	
Papaverine	8.8×10^{-5}M	1110	49	4.2	86.3
Nitroprusside	1.0×10^{-4}M	1098	95	8.0	74.2
Hydralazine	1.9×10^{-4}M	1114	47	4.0	86.9
Diazoxide	1.3×10^{-4}M	1000	32	3.1	90.0

*MOI = 4.1 PFU/ml.
†Mitotic cells were excluded from quantitation.

TABLE 3. Inhibition of HCMV*-Induced Cell Rounding by a Ca^{++} Influx Blocker

Treatment		Cell Morphology†		% Cells	% Inhibition of Cell
Drug	Dose	Fibroblast	Rounded	Rounded	Rounding
None		579	460	44.3	
Verapamil	2.0×10^{-4}M	1049	61	5.5	87.6
Verapamil	6.1×10^{-5}M	757	205	21.3	51.9

*MOI = 7.1 PFU/cell.
†Mitotic cells were excluded from quantitation.

Ca^{++} influx. If this were the case, then verapamil, a Ca^{++} influx blocker and smooth muscle-relaxing agent, might inhibit CMV-induced cell rounding. As we reported previously [11,12] verapamil at doses of 6.1×10^{-5} M or greater inhibited CMV-induced cell rounding (Table 3), confirming that a Ca^{++} influx was involved in the rounding process. Thus, it appears that CMV-induced cell rounding shares some features in common with contraction of smooth muscle cells.

Rounding and "contraction" of CMV-infected cells are early events occurring before the onset of CMV DNA synthesis [6]. "Relaxation" and enlargement, which occur after the time of onset of CMV DNA synthesis, at first hand, might be considered late events. When CMV DNA synthesis was blocked by cytosine-arabinoside (ara-C) (50 μg/ml), however, "relaxation" and enlargement occurred at the same time as in untreated cells (Fig. 3). Thus, enlargement, although ostensibly a late event, results from an early CMV function.

To examine more precisely the time at which enlargement began, CMV-infected cells were treated with cycloheximide (CH) at various times, and the cellular response was measured at 48 hr. Addition of CH (10 μg/ml) at 12 hr PI failed to prevent rounding, but blocked the cells in a "contracted"

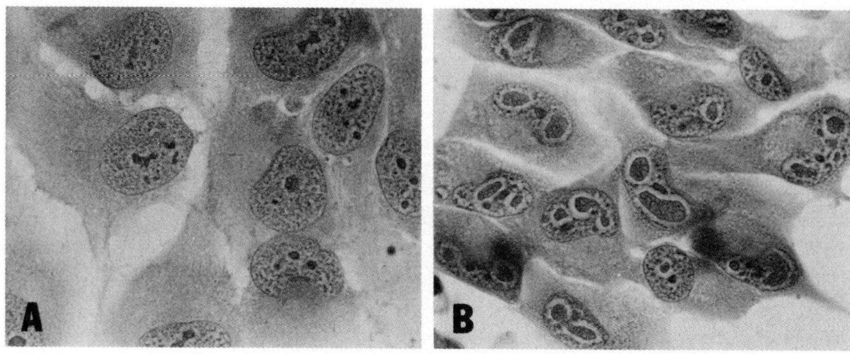

Fig. 3. The effect of ara-C on CMV-induced cell enlargement (cytomegaly) at 72 hr PI. Although ara-C added at 0 hr PI blocked the formation of NI, ara-C failed to inhibit cell rounding, "contraction," "relaxation," and enlargement, even though the latter two cellular responses occur after the time of onset of CMV DNA synthesis. Thus, although cytomegaly is a late event, it results from an early CMV function. A) treated with ara-C (50 μg/ml); B) not treated (A and B, $\times$ 544.)

or occasionally partially "relaxed" state (Fig. 4). When CH was added at 24 hr PI, the cells were observed to be blocked in a "relaxed," partially enlarged state, confirming that "relaxation" and enlargement begin between 12 to 24 hr PI. Addition of CH at 36 hr resulted in cells which were enlarged at 48 hr, although not to the extent observed in cultures of untreated cells. Thus, even though "relaxation" and enlargement occur at a time which follows the onset of CMV DNA synthesis, these events occur in the absence of CMV DNA synthesis, indicating that they are initiated by early CMV functions.

Since "relaxation" and enlargement were dependent on early CMV functions, it seemed possible that these late cellular responses might result from events related to the Ca^{++} influx. To test this possibility, SM were infected with CMV, and, at various times thereafter, were treated with either papaverine (8.8×10^{-5} M) or verapamil (6.1×10^{-5} M). Addition of papaverine at 5 hr resulted in cells which, for the most part, were still "contracted" at 48 hr (Fig. 5). When papaverine was added at 12 hr, "relaxation" occurred and the cells were found to be partially enlarged at 48 hr (Fig. 5). Addition of papaverine at 24 hr did not result in a substantial difference in the size of the treated cells from untreated, infected cell controls. Results with verapamil were essentially the same, except that this dose of verapamil was not as effective as a similar dose of papaverine in blocking enlargement; although, dose-response curves suggested that lower doses of either papaverine or verapamil could be used to block cell enlargement than to block cell rounding. Accordingly, "relaxation" and enlargement in CMV-infected cells are

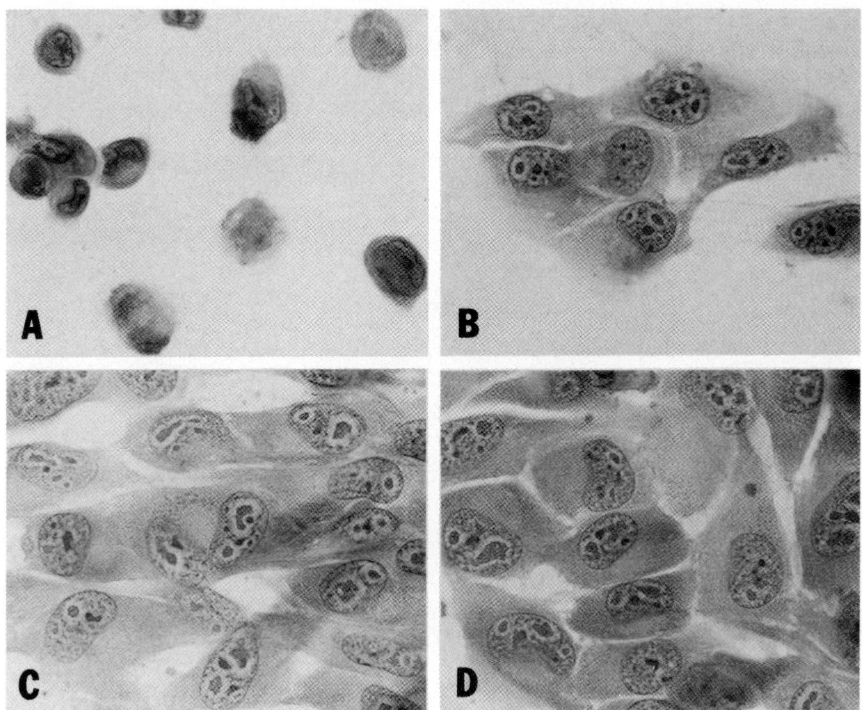

Fig. 4.   The effect of CH on "relaxation" and enlargement of CMV-induced rounded cells at 48 hr PI. CH (10 μg/ml) when added at A) 12, B) 24, or C) 36 hr PI failed to inhibit rounding and "contraction" of CMV-infected cells, but did inhibit "relaxation" (when added at 12 hr, but not 24 hr PI) and enlargement (only partially, when added at 24 hr) relative to D) CMV-infected cell controls. (Bouin's fixative, H & E, A–D, × 544.)

apparently, at least in part, dependent on a Ca^{++} influx and possibly other events inhibited by rising levels of cAMP and/or cGMP, since papaverine was more inhibitory than verapamil.

An unanticipated finding of the above series of experiments was the absence of NIs in cells treated with papaverine or verapamil. In most cells, NIs were not detected and, in the few cells where they were found, their size was much reduced (Fig. 5). These observations seemed to be of potential interest in light of the hypothesis [7] we have previously proposed to correlate the unique structures of the early (bead-like) and late (composed of cellulae, Fig. 6) CMV-induced NIs and their separate development with the apparent two phases of CMV DNA synthesis [13]. While this hypothesis provides an explanation for our morphologic and biochemic observations, it certainly

does not provide an understanding as to the underlying molecular mechanisms leading to the phasing of CMV DNA synthesis. It may be more than
coincidental, however, that the timing of the "contracted" and enlarged cell
states, the two phases of CMV DNA synthesis, and the development of early

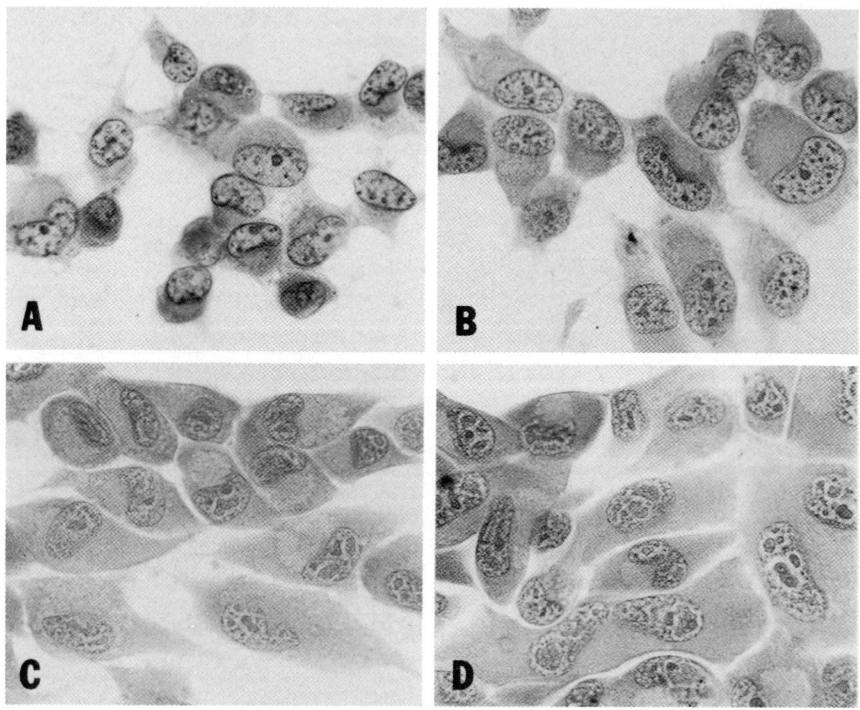

Fig. 5. The effect of a smooth muscle-relaxing agent on "relaxation" and enlargement of
CMV-induced rounded cells. Papaverine (8.8×10^{-5}M) when added at A) 5, B) 12, or C) 24
hr PI failed to inhibit rounding and "contraction" of CMV-infected cells (not illustrated), but
did inhibit "relaxation" (when added at 5 hr PI) and enlargement (when added at 5 or 12 hr
as measured at 48 hr PI relative to D) the CMV-infected cell controls. However, papaverine
had little effect on enlargement when added at 24 hr PI (C). (Bouin's fixative, H & E, A–D,
× 544.)

Fig. 6. The CMV (strain AD169)-induced NI at 96 hr. The electron dense fibrillar network
(FN) is packed with capsids and nucleocapsids. The center of each cellulae contains numerous
granules. At the interface of the fibrillar network and the electron-lucent area of the cellulae
fusiform, elongated dark structures (arrows), are incorporated within virus particles [7]
(× 16,980).

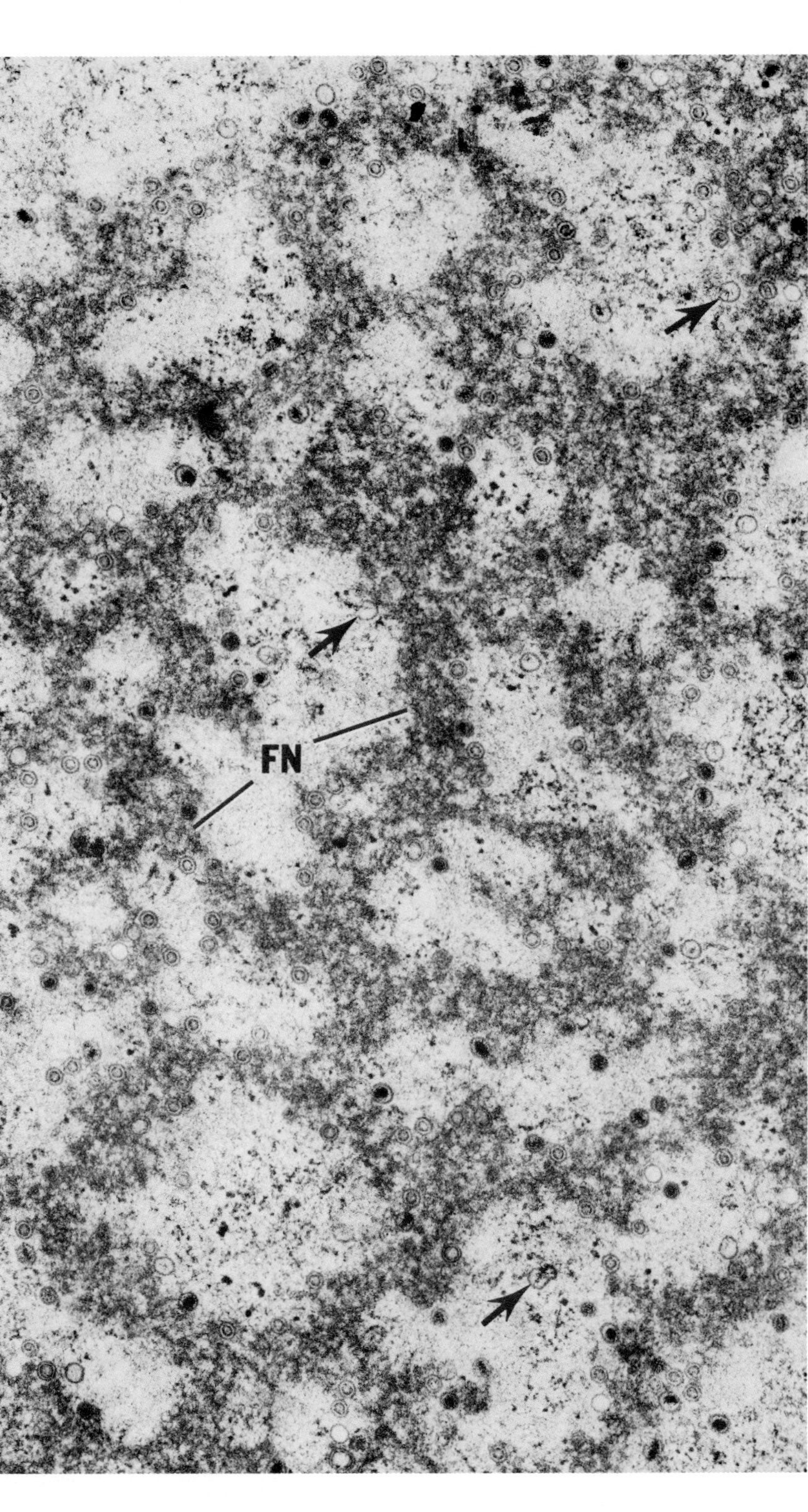

FN

and late NIs are similar. These observations suggest that CMV DNA synthesis and the formation of the NIs may be dependent on the physiologic changes evoking the cellular responses described earlier. Accordingly, drugs blocking the cellular response to CMV might be expected to adversely affect CMV replication. As shown in Table 4, papaverine, sodium nitroprusside, and verapamil inhibited CMV replication, although with various levels of efficiency. Papaverine was clearly the most effective of these drugs with a dose of 8.8×10^{-5} M inhibiting 99.999% of the CMV yield. Nitroprusside, while less effective than papaverine, still inhibited 99.8% of the yield. Verapamil was the least effective of the drugs, inhibiting only 90.6% of the yield. Since papaverine and nitroprusside were much more potent antiviral agents for CMV than verapamil, these data suggest that physiologic changes secondary to the Ca^{++} influx may also be important for productive CMV replication. Furthermore, the data for papaverine suggest that much smaller doses of this drug may be effective in inhibiting CMV replication. Dose-response curves were generated for papaverine and verapamil, indicating that a 2.9×10^{-6} M dose of papaverine gave about the same level of inhibition as a 6.1×10^{-5} M dose of verapamil. Whether or not these drugs will be useful in control of HCMV infection will require very cautious examination, since these smooth muscle-relaxing agents have potent pharmacologic activities. The concept that virus infections may be treated by controlling the cellular response, however, may be useful for other viruses, and in the selection and development of other drugs.

In the observations described above, we have considered the data primarily with regard to productive CMV replication. Yet CMV has been reported to produce abortive [16,21,22], persistent [23,24] and transforming infections [25,26]. While each of these reports has its unique features with regard to cellular responses, these infections, for the most part, involve restriction of CMV replication and expression of early CMV functions. It might be

TABLE 4. Inhibition of HCMV Replication by Smooth Muscle-Relaxing Agents

Treatment		Yield* (PFU/ml) at		% Inhibition
Drug	Dose	72 hr	120 hr	of Virus Yield†
None		1.0×10^6	8.0×10^6	—
Verapamil	6.1×10^{-5}M	3.0×10^4	7.5×10^5	90.6
Sodium nitroprusside	1.0×10^{-4}M	5.5×10^3	1.8×10^4	99.8
Papaverine	8.8×10^{-5}M	$<5.0 \times 10^1$	$<5.0 \times 10^1$	>99.999

*Determined using an initial MOI of 9.0 PFU/cell.
†Determined at 120 hr PI.

anticipated that under these conditions cellular responses could be measured that might be obscured in a productive infection. We have previously shown that CMV stimulates cellular DNA synthesis in cells capable of supporting productive or abortive infections [15,16]. In addition, we have shown that stimulation of cellular DNA synthesis involves expression of early CMV genes and primarily from defective CMV particles [16].

Identification of taxol as a microtubule stabilizing agent [27] has permitted studies examining the relationship between microtubule depolymerization and initiation of cell DNA synthesis. When taxol (10 μg/ml) was added at 3 hr PI, it inhibited the stimulation of cell DNA synthesis by CMV by up to 100% (Table 5) [8]. The effect of taxol on CMV-initiated cell DNA synthesis seems to be related specifically to this drug's stabilizing effect on microtubules, since both dose-response and time-course studies are similar to those obtained with taxol inhibition of colchicine- or growth factor-initiated DNA synthesis [8]. In addition, pretreatment of CMV with taxol has no effect on the stimulation of cellular DNA synthesis. Micromolar concentrations of Ca^{++} have been shown to induce depolymerization of microtubules in vitro [28], but whether or not CMV-induced stimulation of cellular DNA synthesis is related to changes in $[Ca^{++}]$ following CMV infection remains to be demonstrated. When considered together, these results suggest that CMV initiates cellular DNA synthesis through microtubule related events which may be a consequence of yet other physiologic responses to CMV infection.

Early cellular responses to CMV infection include not only effects on the actin network and the microtubules, but also the network of intermediate filaments. We have developed a hybridoma-secreting monoclonal antibody, apparently specific for an intermediate filament associated antigen. Reaction of this antibody with uninfected SM cells reveals a brightly fluorescent cytoplasmic filamentous network (Fig. 7). Nuclear fluorescence was not observed with this antibody preparation suggesting the absence of this antigen

TABLE 5. Effect of Taxol on CMV Initiation of Cellular DNA Synthesis

Treatment	Mean ^{3}H-Thymidine Incorporation (CPM)*	% Stimulation of DNA Synthesis†	% Inhibition by Taxol
CMV	34,400 ± 2160	151	—
CMV + taxol‡	18,880 ± 1640	41	73
Cell lysate	13,360 ± 480	—	—
Cell lysate + taxol‡	13,680 ± 2120	—	—

*24–30 hr PI.
†Relative to cell lysate controls.
‡10 μg/ml, added 3 hr PI.

TABLE 6. Effect of CMV on Intermediate Filaments (IF) as Detected by a Monoclonal Antibody to an IF-Associated Protein*

	Intermediate Filament Associated Antigen	
Hr PI	Cytoplasm	Nucleus
0	+ FN	−
5	+ FN	−
24	−	± NI
48	±	+ NI
72	+ FN	+ NI
96	+ FN	+ NI
120	+ FN	+ NI
Control	+ FN	−

*By Western transfer analysis and two dimensional gel electrophoresis the specificity of this antibody is to a protein of 47 to 50 kd.

FN = filament network.

NI = nuclear inclusion.

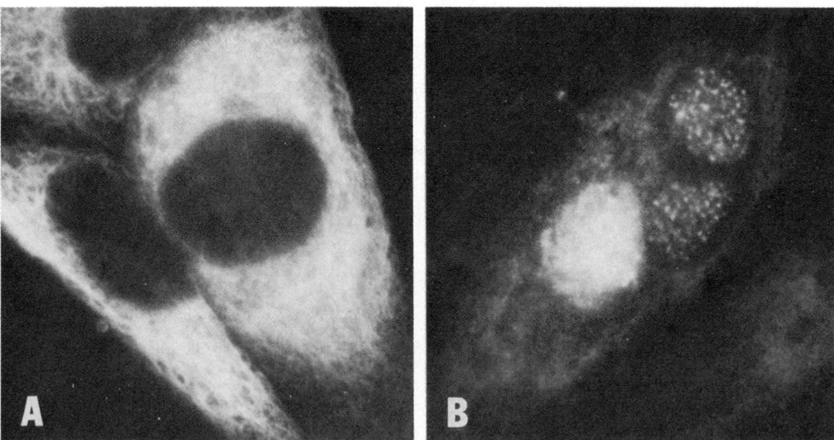

Fig. 7. Redistribution of an intermediate filament associated antigen (IFA) following CMV infection. A) Uninfected SM cells stained by indirect immunofluorescence procedures with monoclonal antibody IFA-1. B) CMV-infected SM cells at 72 hr PI stained with the same antibody. Note that much of the filamentous network has broken down and partially reformed with much of the antigen found in the nuclear and cytoplasmic inclusions (A and B, × 829).

from the nucleus. Following CMV infection, the cytoplasmic filamentous network appeared to break down and, surprisingly, after 24 hr PI, this intermediate filament associated antigen was observed in the nucleus (Table 6). By 48 hr PI, the fluorescent images observed in the nucleus were indistinguishable from the CMV NI, as detected by phase contrast or H & E staining (Fig. 7). Since the accumulation of the intermediate filament associated antigen in the nucleus is specific to the NI, the redistribution of this protein may be important for the efficient replication of CMV.

It is evident from the above descriptions that the cellular response to CMV infection may be more extensive than first reported. In fact, there appears to be a cascade of cellular responses to CMV infection. These cellular responses involve most cellular organelles and may result in stimulation of some cellular functions in contrast to the cellular response to most viruses. It is highly likely that these responses reflect underlying physiologic changes selected for the efficient replication of CMV. An understanding of these physiologic changes may ultimately permit the control of CMV infections. It is quite possible that the extensive array of early cellular responses also reflects selection of physiologic changes which facilitate the formation of persistent infections in appropriate circumstances.

REFERENCES

1. Jesionek A, Kiolemenglou B: Uber einen Befund von protozoenartigen Gebilden in den Organen eines hereditar leutischen Folus. Munch Med Wochenschr 51:1905, 1904.
2. Smith MG: Propagation in tissue cultures of a cytopathogenic virus from human salivary gland virus (SGV) disease. Proc Soc Exp Biol Med 92:424, 1956.
3. Rowe WP, Hartley JW, Waterman S, Turner HC, Huebner RJ: Cytopathic agent resembling human salivary gland virus recovered from tissue cultures of human adenoids. Proc Soc Exp Biol Med 92:418, 1956.
4. Weller TH, Macauley JC, Craig JM, Wirth P: Isolation of intranuclear inclusion producing agents from infants with illnesses resembling cytomegalic inclusion disease. Proc Soc Exp Biol Med 94:4, 1957.
5. Furukawa T, Fioretti A, Plotkin SA: Growth characteristics of cytomegalovirus in human fibroblasts with demonstration of protein synthesis early in viral replication. J Virol 11:991, 1973.
6. Albrecht T, Cavallo T, Cole NL, Graves K: Cytomegalovirus: Development and progression of cytopathic effects in human cell culture. Lab Invest 42:1, 1980.
7. Cavallo T, Graves K, Cole NL, Albrecht T: Cytomegalovirus: An ultrastructural study of the morphogenesis of nuclear inclusions in human cell culture. J Gen Virol 56:97, 1981.
8. Ball R, Albrecht T, Carney DH: Microtubule stabilization by taxol inhibits stimulation of cellular DNA synthesis by human cytomegalovirus. (Submitted for publication)
9. Kanich RE, Craighead JE: Human cytomegalovirus infection of cultured fibroblasts. I. Cytopathologic effects induced by an adapted and a wild strain. Lab Invest 27:263, 1972.

10. Ruebner BH, Hirano T, Slusser RJ, Medearis DN Jr: Human cytomegalovirus infection: Electron microscopic and histochemical changes in cultures of human fibroblasts. Am J Pathol 46:477, 1965.
11. Albrecht T, Speelman DJ, Steinsland O: Similarities between human cytomegalovirus-induced cell rounding and contraction of myofibroblasts or smooth muscle cells. Abstracts Int Workshop on Herpesviruses, July 27-31, 1981, Bologna, Italy, p 71.
12. Albrecht T, Speelman DJ, Steinsland OS: Similarities between cytomegalovirus-induced cell rounding and contraction of smooth muscle cells. Life Sci 32:2273, 1983.
13. Albrecht TB: Studies on the oncogenic potential of human cytomegalovirus, Ph.D. thesis. The Pennsylvania State University, University Park, Pennsylvania, 1973.
14. Stinski MF: Sequence of protein synthesis in cells infected by human cytomegalovirus: Early and late virus-induced polypeptides. J Virol 26:686, 1978.
15. St. Jeor SC, Albrecht T, Funk FD, Rapp F: Stimulation of cellular DNA synthesis by human cytomegalovirus. J Virol 13:353, 1974.
16. Albrecht T, Nachtigal M, St. Jeor SC, Rapp F: Induction of cellular DNA synthesis and increased mitotic activity in syrian hamster embryo cells abortively infected with human cytomegalovirus. J Gen Virol 30:167, 1976.
17. Li J-LH, Thompson WC, Albrecht T: Response of intermediate filaments and an associated protein to human cytomegalovirus infection. (In preparation)
18. Smith JD, de Harven E: Herpes simplex virus and human cytomegalovirus replication in WI-38 cells. I. Sequence of viral replication. J Virol 12:919, 1973.
19. Majno G: The story of the myofibroblasts. Am J Surg Pathol 3:535, 1979.
20. Garnett HM: Changes in enzymes following infection of human embryonic fibroblasts with HCMV. 3rd International Cong. of Virology, Madrid, 1975.
21. Fioretti A, Furukawa T, Santoli D, Plotkin SA: Nonproductive infection of guinea pig cells with human cytomegalovirus. J Virol 11:998, 1973.
22. Waner JL, Weller TH: Behavior of human cytomegaloviruses in cell cultures of bovine and simian origin. Proc Soc Exp Biol Med 145:379, 1974.
23. Rapp F, Geder L, Murasko D, Lausch R, Ladda R, Huang E-S, Webber MM: Long-term persistence of cytomegalovirus genome in cultured human cells of prostatic origin. J Virol 16:982, 1975.
24. Li J-LH, Albrecht T: Characterization of human cells persistently infected with cytomegalovirus and exposed to a chemical carcinogen. Int J Cancer 29:49, 1982.
25. Albrecht T, Rapp F: Malignant transformation of hamster embryo fibroblasts following exposure to ultraviolet-irradiated human cytomegalovirus. Virology 55:53, 1973.
26. Geder L, Lausch R, O'Neill F, Rapp F: Oncogenic transformation of human embryo lung cells by human cytomegalovirus. Science 192:1134, 1976.
27. Schiff PB, Fant J, Horwitz SB: Promotion of microtubule assembly in vitro by taxol. Nature 277:665, 1979.
28. Schliwa M, Euteneuer U, Bulinski JC, Izant JG: Calcium lability of cytoplasmic microtubules and its modulation by microtubule-associated proteins. Proc Natl Acad Sci USA 78:1037, 1981.

The Physical and Transcriptional Organization of the Human Cytomegalovirus Genome

Jean M. DeMarchi, PhD

Department of Microbiology, Vanderbilt University School of Medicine, Nashville, TN 37232

STRUCTURAL FEATURES OF THE HCMV GENOME
Size

It has been known for two decades that the genome of HCMV consisted of DNA [1], but not until recently has information on the structure and organization of the DNA become available. The HCMV genome is a linear duplex with a buoyant density of 1.716 gm/ml and an average G + C content of 56% [2,3]. The size of HCMV DNA (approximately 150 to 160 $\times$ 10^6 d or 230 kb pairs) has been determined by several methods, including velocity sedimentation [4–6], measurements of contour length [4,5,7], electrophoretic migration [7], and restriction enzyme digestion [8–11]. Furthermore, as shown by partial denaturation mapping [3] and renaturation kinetics [5,7], the DNA has nearly the same sequence complexity. Thus, HCMV has one of the largest virus genomes known, considerably larger than that of other herpesviruses, and is potentially capable of encoding a large number of proteins.

Structure

The structural organization of the HCMV genome is complex. That the DNA molecule contains inverted repetitions was demonstrated by self-annealing of denatured DNA strands (P. Sheldrick, personal communication). However, partial denaturation mapping [3] provided the first indication that

Birth Defects: Original Article Series, Volume 20, Number 1, pages 35–47
© 1984 March of Dimes Birth Defects Foundation

the DNA may exist in more than one sequence arrangement. Subsequent analyses with restriction endonucleases confirmed these findings and showed that DNA molecules extracted from virions consisted of four isomeric populations present in approximately equimolar amounts [8,9,12]. Thus, the HCMV DNA has a structural organization similar to that of HSV [13], consisting of two segments, L and S, bracketed by inverted repeat sequences that invert relative to one another (Fig. 1). The L and S segments comprise approximately 82% and 18% of the genome, respectively, the same proportions reported for HSV DNA [13]. As reported for all HCMV strains studied to date, one or both of the ends of the L and S segments are heterogeneous, and a given end fragment may consist of two or more species which differ in size by about 750 bps [8–12]. The nature of this heterogeneity is at present unknown.

INTERSTRAIN DIFFERENCES IN HCMV DNA

Little or no homology is shared between HCMV and the nonhuman CMVs, or with other herpesviruses [2]. The different HCMV strains, however, share about 80% sequence homology as determined by renaturation kinetics. The restriction patterns produced by digestion of different HCMV strains with a given restriction enzyme tend to be similar, but not identical [14]; consequently, the cleavage maps obtained for the various strains differ [8–12]. From analysis of the restriction fragments produced by digestion of the Towne, Davis, and AD169 strains, however, it appears that many fragments from the unique sequences of both the L and S segments are the same in both size and map position.

The most notable interstrain differences appear to occur around the region of the repeat sequences bracketing the L segment. The size of the L repeats has been shown to vary, from 12 kb pairs for the AD169 strain [11] to less than 4 kb pairs for the Davis strain [9]. The size of the repeats bracketing the S segment are, however, reported to be the same (2 to 3 kb pairs). Furthermore, it had been shown by cross-hybridization studies between the Towne and AD169 strains [15], and the Towne and Davis strains [10], that considerable homology is shared within the unique sequences, but a certain amount of variation is noted among sequences that occur at the regions of the joint and ends of the molecule.

The differences in cleavage sites and restriction enzyme patterns present in the DNA of different HCMV strains can be exploited as a powerful tool in epidemiologic studies [16,17].

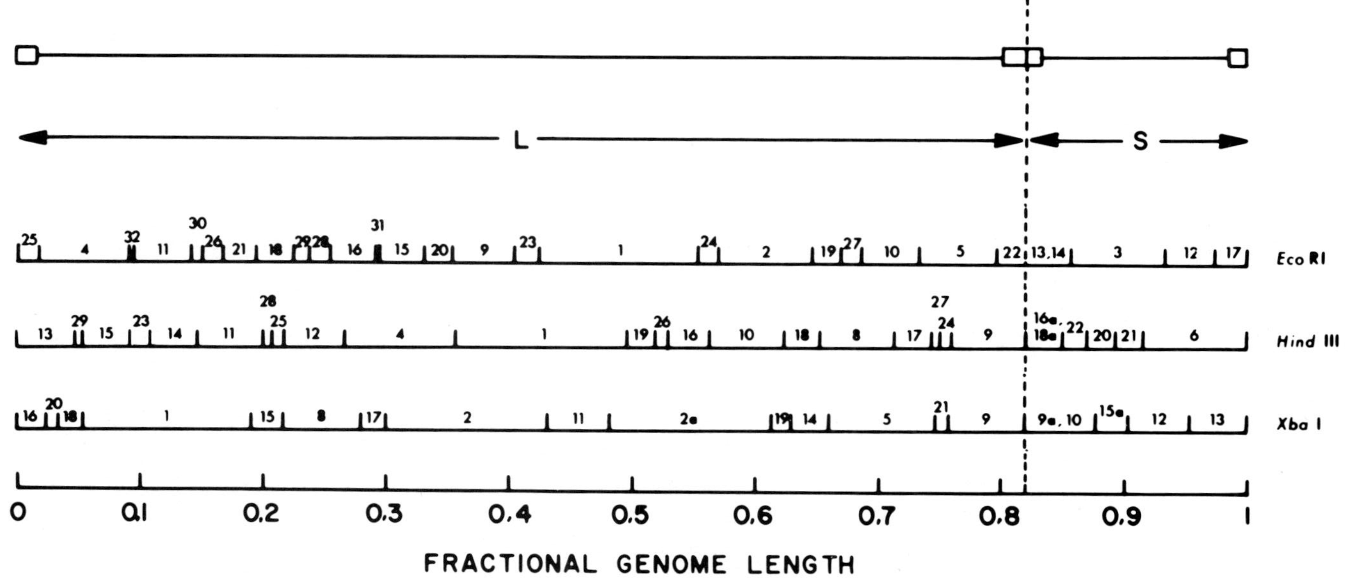

Fig. 1. Organization of the HCMV genome. Diagram of the linear duplex is shown at the top; rectangles indicate positions of the repeated sequences. Dotted lines indicate the point (termed the L-S junction or "joint") at which the L and S segments invert relative to one another. Physical maps of HCMV Davis for three different restriction enzymes [9] are shown in one prototypical orientation. In addition to the fragments indicated on the maps, four additional joint fragments for each digest arise from inversion of the L and S segments but are not indicated on the Figure.

TRANSCRIPTIONAL ORGANIZATION OF THE HCMV GENOME
Transcript Accumulation in Permissively Infected Cells

The transcription program of HCMV, like that of other herpesviruses, has been defined in terms of three temporal phases: 1) immediate early (IE) RNA, transcribed in the absence of de novo protein synthesis and in the presence of inhibitors of protein synthesis such as cycloheximide; 2) early RNA, transcribed before the onset of virus DNA synthesis and in the presence of inhibitors of virus DNA synthesis such as phosphonoacetic acid (PAA); and 3) late RNA, transcribed after the onset of virus DNA synthesis [9,18–21] (Fig. 2). Division of the transcription program into these three broad classes is obviously an oversimplification; subtle changes in transcript accumulation patterns exist within any one of these steps. Furthermore, as will be discussed below, transcription during the early phase probably involves the expression of subsets of early genes which are expressed sequentially and are possibly subject to host cell control.

Transcription during the IE phase (in cells infected in the presence of cycloheximide) is limited to only relatively few sequences and involves only about 20% of the genome [21–23] (Fig. 2). The major mRNA to appear on polysomes in Davis strain infected cells is a 2.2 kb RNA originating from the L segment (map positions 0.713-0.733, Fig. 3). Several other RNAs are also synthesized, two of which become polysome associated. Others remain associated with the nucleus during the IE phase of transcription [22] (Fig. 3). As expected, the major 2.2 kb transcript synthesized in cycloheximide-treated cells is also the first major transcript synthesized during the earliest stages of infection [22].

In general, for all the strains which have been tested, the major IE RNA originates from approximately the same area on the L segment [21–23], in striking contrast to either HSV or pseudorabies virus in which the major IE RNAs are encoded within repeated sequences near the L-S junction and termini of the genome [24–27].

Once the IE RNAs are translated, the transcription program moves into the early phase, during which stable transcripts accumulate from most regions of the genome (approximately 75% of the sequences, Figs. 2 and 4). One region in particular (map positions 0-0.033) produces abundant stable transcripts. This appears to be a characteristic of the early-phase transcription pattern for three different strains [9,20,21]. Sequences from which stable transcript accumulation cannot be detected include several regions on the L segment, as well as the region encompassing the joint and the right-hand end of the prototypical arrangement of the genome shown in Figures 1 and 4.

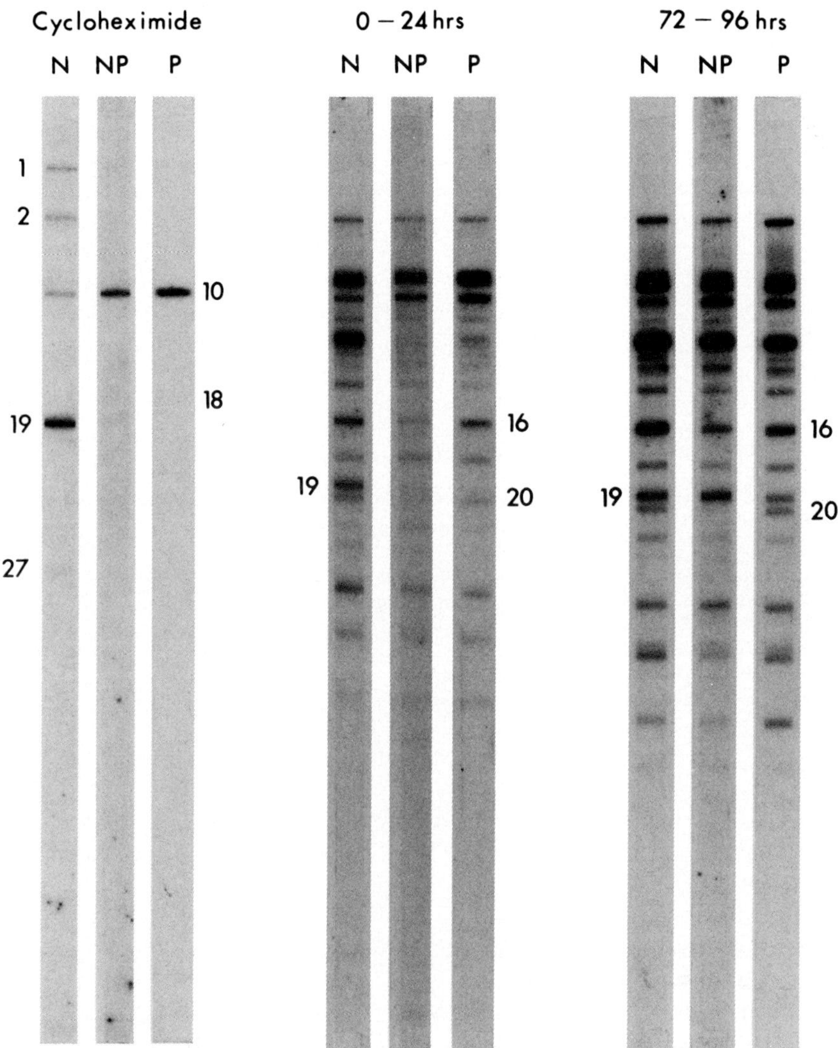

Fig. 2. Summary of the patterns obtained by hybridizing IE, early, and late RNA to filters containing electrophoretically separated fragments of *Eco* RI digested HCMV DNA. HCMV infected HEL cells were labeled with ^{32}P for 12 hr after infection in the presence of cycloheximide (IE RNA) and between 0–24 hr (early RNA) and 72–96 hr (late RNA) after infection without drug. The nuclear fraction (N) of the infected cells was isolated, the cytoplasm was separated into nonpolysomal (NP) and polysomal (P) fractions, and the RNA was extracted and hybridized to Southern filters of *Eco* RI digested HCMV Davis DNA. Different sets of filters were used for each phase of infection represented.

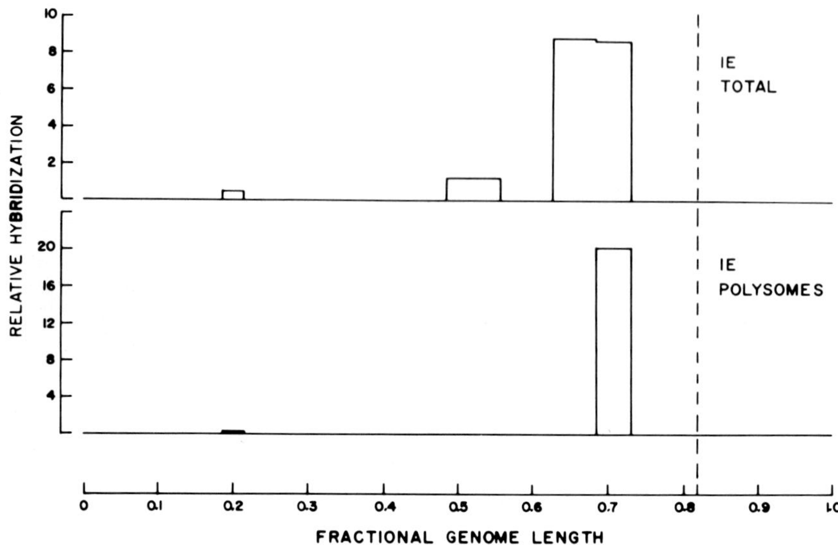

Fig. 3. Map positions of total and polysome-associated transcripts synthesized during the IE phase of infection. ^{32}P-labeled IE RNA was prepared and extracted according to the legend in Figure 2.

Most, but not all, of the stable transcripts which accumulate before the onset of virus DNA synthesis are also found on polysomes. It is noteworthy, however, that not all transcripts accumulating in the infected cells are similarly processed into mRNA. Some transcripts (map positions 0.630-0.687) remain associated with the nucleus during the early phase [22]. Furthermore, there appears to be preferential association with polysomes of some other transcripts (Figs. 2 and 4).

After the onset of DNA synthesis (approximately 24 hr after infection in this system), the transcription program moves into late phase. In general, most regions of the HCMV DNA genome (> 90%) appear to produce stable transcripts with the notable exception of sequences within the region of the joint and ends of the S segment. Most of the sequences produce stable transcripts which are also found on polysomes. However, as with early-phase transcripts, late-phase transcripts are not equally associated with polysomes; transcripts originating from certain areas of the L segment appear to be represented on polysomes in higher abundance than others (see Figs. 2 and 4).

Thus, during the IE, early, and late phases of infection, controls in the transcription program appear to exist at several levels: transcript accumulation, transport to the cytoplasm, and preferential association of transcripts

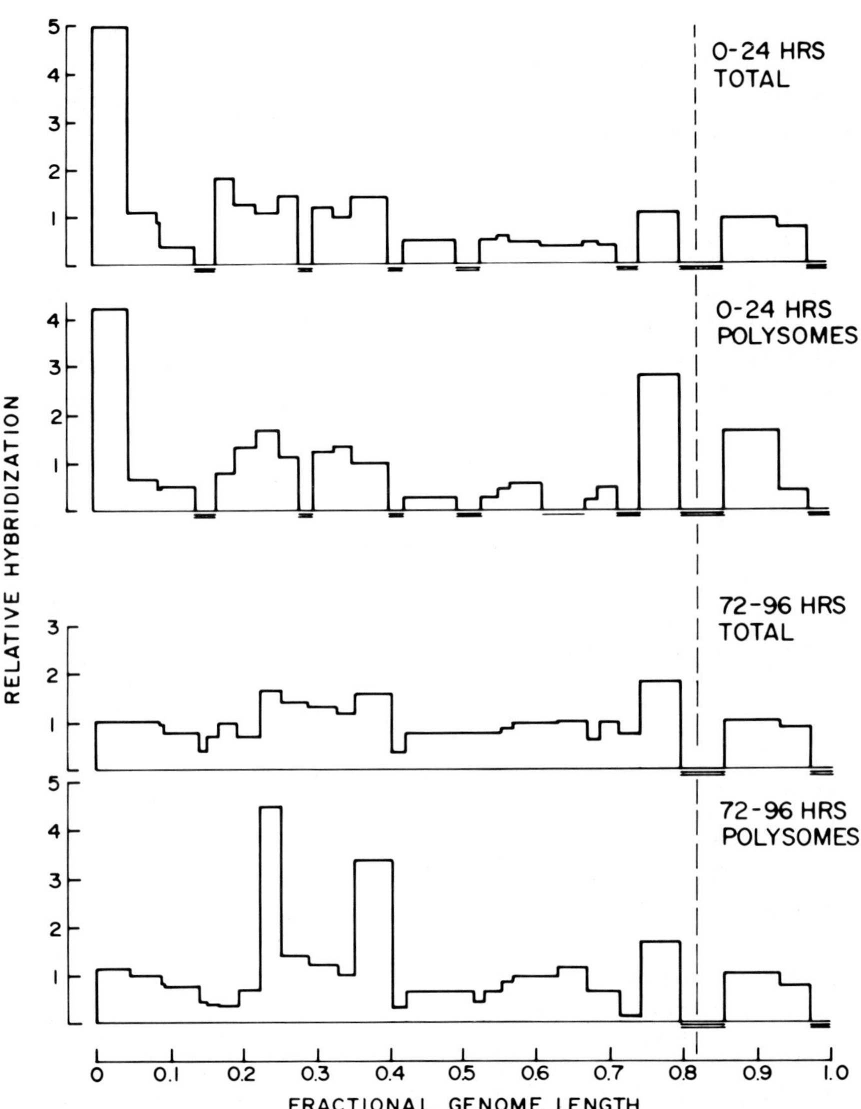

Fig. 4. Map positions of total and polysome-associated transcripts synthesized during the early and late phases of infection. See Fig. 2 for details.

with polysomes. Now that libraries of cloned subgenomic fragments are available for several HCMV strains [12,22,28–30], substantial progress should be made within the next few years toward elucidating the nature of the controls which operate during HCMV replication.

Accumulation of a Subset of Early Transcripts in Various Nonpermissively Infected Cells

As mentioned above, segregation of the transcription program into three discrete phases is actually an oversimplification of the complex and orderly series of controls that appear to govern the progression of HCMV expression. In fact, the available evidence suggests that the transcription program is blocked under certain conditions at different levels during the early phase, resulting in expression of "subsets" of early virus genes. For example, we and others [31–33] have found that certain functions which may be classified as "early" are expressed during replication in permissive human embryonic lung (HEL) cells, but not expressed in nonpermissive nonhuman cells (specifically, this includes the virus-specific DNA polymerase and shutdown of host cell DNA synthesis which are normally expressed during the early phase of productive infection). These nonpermissive cells do, however, allow the HCMV transcription program to progress from the IE into the early phase [34] (Fig. 5). That the infection is prevented from entering into late phase in nonhuman cells has been shown by the lack of inclusion formation, virus DNA, and infectious virus production [35].

We have infected various nonpermissive cell lines (rabbit kidney, RK; baby mouse kidney, BMK; and African green monkey kidney, Vero) with HCMV to investigate the levels of transcription which occur in these cells. The main points to emerge are as follows: In each of the cell lines tested, the transcription program progressed from the IE to early phase (Fig. 5). However, the level of accumulation of transcripts differed in each of the cell lines (Fig. 6). For example, transcription (or transcript accumulation) appeared to be least restrictive in BMK cells. In these infected cells the transcription pattern most resembled that seen in permissively infected HEL cells. Transcription was very restricted, however, in Vero cells, and the pattern of transcript accumulation appeared to be intermediate between early and IE phase (Fig. 6). At present, it is not known whether the differences in transcript accumulation reflect differences at the level of transcription, or transcript stability. However, it is clear that depending on the cell type used, the infection proceeds to different points within the early phase. This suggests that various host cell factors are involved in the processes leading to transcript accumulation in the HCMV infected cells.

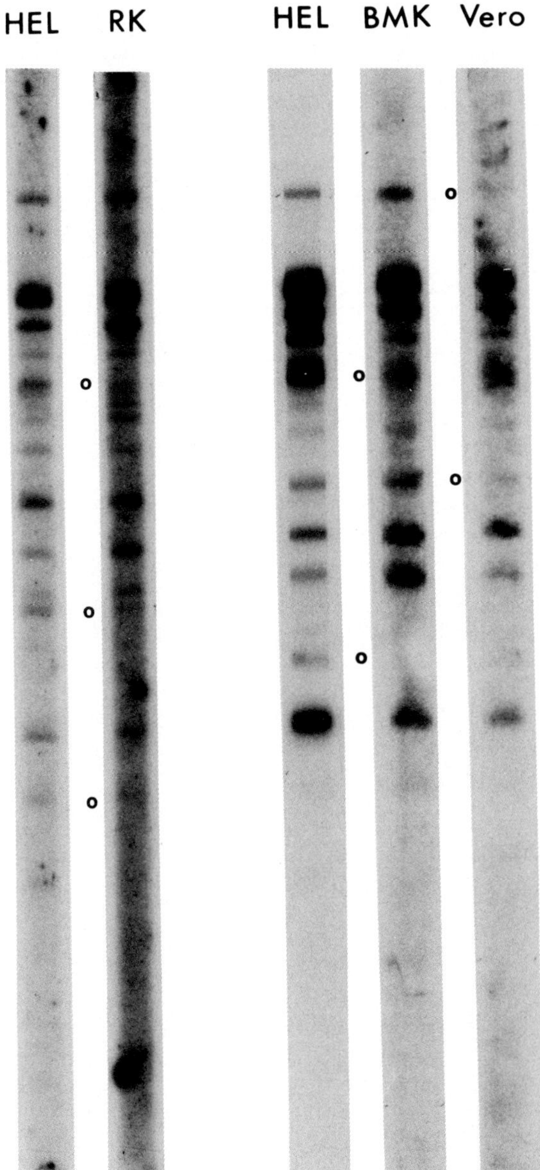

Fig. 5. Hybridization patterns of HCMV transcripts synthesized in nonpermissive cell lines. ^{32}P-labeled RNA was extracted 36 hr after HCMV infection in permissive HEL cells treated with 100 μg/ml PAA, and in nonpermissive BMK, RK, and Vero cells. The RNA was hybridized to Southern filters of *Eco* RI digested HCMV DNA.

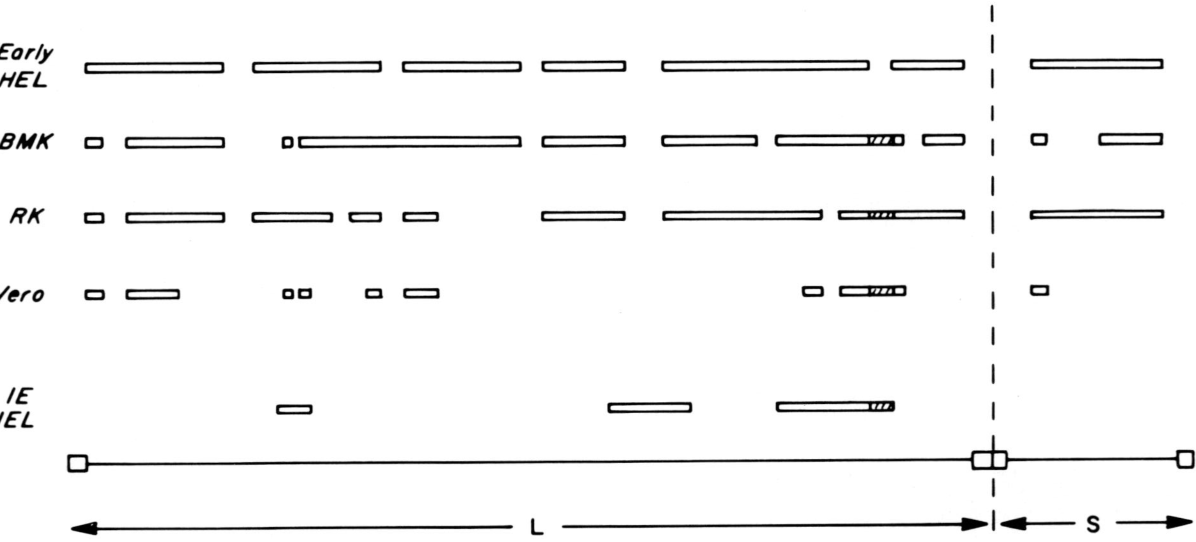

Fig. 6.   Schematic representation of different regions of the genome from which HCMV transcripts originate in different cell lines. Hatched bars indicate region from which the major IE RNA originates.

CONCLUSIONS

Despite the fact that HCMV has a large genome with a sequence complexity to match, and in principle can code for a large number of proteins, it reproduces slowly and inefficiently in permissive cells in vitro. Productive infection is limited primarily to human fibroblasts and does not appear to occur in cells of nonhuman origin. Thus, despite the relatively large size of the genome, HCMV growth appears to depend to a large extent on factors other than those which are virus encoded. Evidence is beginning to accumulate which indicates that the processes controlling the orderly transcript accumulation of the genome, at least in part, may be dependent on various cellular factors. For example, expression of the genome is arrested at different stages of the early phase in different nonpermissively infected cells. Thus, the presence (or absence) of these factors in different cells appears to modulate the transcript accumulation of the viral genome and thereby determines whether or not the cell is permissive for virus growth.

REFERENCES

1. Goodheart CR, Filbert JE, McAllister RM: Human cytomegalovirus: Effect of 5-fluoro-2-deoxyuridine (FUdR) on viral synthesis and cytopathology. Virology 21:530–532, 1963.
2. Huang E-S, Chen S-T, Pagano JS: Human cytomegalovirus. I. Purification and characterization of viral DNA. J Virol 12: 1473–1481, 1973.
3. Kilpatrick BA, Huang E-S: Human cytomegalovirus genome: Partial denaturation map and organization of genome sequences. J Virol 24: 261–276, 1977.
4. Geelen JLMC, Walig C, Wertheim P, Van der Noordaa J: Human cytomegalovirus DNA. I. Molecular weight and infectivity. J Virol 26:813–816, 1978.
5. DeMarchi JM, Blankenship ML, Brown GD, Kaplan AS: Size and complexity of human cytomegalovirus DNA. Virology 89:643–646, 1978.
6. Lakeman AD, Osborn JE: Size of infectious DNA from human and murine cytomegaloviruses. J Virol 30:414–416, 1979.
7. Stinski MF, Mocarski ES, Thomsen DR: DNA of human cytomegalovirus: Size heterogeneity and defectiveness resulting from serial undiluted passage. J Virol 31:231–239, 1979.
8. Westrate MW, Geelen JLMC, Van der Noordaa J: Human cytomegalovirus DNA: Physical maps for the restriction endonucleases Bgl II, Hind III, and Xba I. J Gen Virol 49:1–21, 1980.
9. DeMarchi JM: Human cytomegalovirus DNA: Restriction enzyme cleavage maps and map locations for immediate-early, early, and late RNAs. Virology 114:23–38, 1981.
10. LaFemina RL, Hayward GS: Structural organization of the DNA molecules from human cytomegalovirus. In Fields BN, Jaenisch R (eds): "Animal Virus Genetics." New York: Academic Press, 1980, pp 39–55.
11. Spector DH, Hock L, Tamashiro JC: Cleavage maps for human cytomegalovirus DNA strain AD169 for restriction endonucleases Eco RI, Bgl II, and Hind III. J Virol 42:558–582, 1982.

12. Oram JD, Downing RG, Akrigg A, Dollery AA, Duggleby CJ, Wilkinson GWG, Greenaway PJ: Use of recombinant plasmids to investigate the structure of the human cytomegalovirus genome. J Gen Virol 59:111–129, 1982.

13. Hayward GS, Jacob RJ, Wadsworth SC, Roizman B: Anatomy of herpes simplex virus DNA. Evidence for 4 populations of molecules that differ in relative orientations of their long and short components. Proc Natl Acad Sci USA 72:4243–4247, 1975.

14. Kilpatrick BA, Huang E-S, Pagano JS: Analysis of cytomegalovirus genomes with restriction endonucleases Hind III and Eco RI. J Virol 18:1095–1105, 1976.

15. Pritchett RF: DNA nucleotide sequence heterogeneity between the Towne and AD-169 strains of cytomegalovirus. J Virol 36:152–161, 1980.

16. Huang E-S, Alford CA, Reynolds DW, Stagno S, Pass RF: Molecular epidemiology of cytomegalovirus infections in women and their infants. N Engl J Med 303:958–962, 1980.

17. Yow MD, Lakeman AD, Stagno S, Reynolds RB, Plavidal FJ: Use of restriction enzymes to investigate the source of primary cytomegalovirus infection in a pediatric nurse. Pediatrics 70:713–716, 1982.

18. DeMarchi JM, Schmidt CA, Kaplan AS: Patterns of transcription of human cytomegalovirus in permissively infected cells. J Virol 35:277–286, 1980.

19. Wathen MW, Thomsen DR, Stinski MF: Temporal regulation of human cytomegalovirus transcription at immediate early and early times after infection. J Virol 38:446–459, 1981.

20. Wathen MW, Stinski MF: Temporal patterns of human cytomegalovirus transcription: Mapping of the viral RNAs synthesized at immediate early, early, and late times after infection. J Virol 41:462–477, 1982.

21. McDonough SH, Spector DH: Transcription in human fibroblasts permissively infected by human cytomegalovirus strain AD-169. Virology 125:31–46, 1983.

22. DeMarchi JM: Post-transcriptional control of human cytomegalovirus gene expression. Virology 124:390–402, 1983.

23. Stinski MF, Thomsen DR, Stenberg RM, Goldstein LC: Organization and expression of the immediate-early genes of human cytomegalovirus. J Virol 46:1–14, 1983.

24. Jones PC, Hayward GS, Roizman B: Anatomy of herpes simplex virus DNA. VII. αRNA is homologous to noncontinuous sites in both the L and S components of viral DNA. J Virol 21:268–276, 1977.

25. Clements JB, Watson RJ, Wilkie NM: Temporal regulation of herpes simplex virus type 1 transcription: Location of transcripts on the viral genome. Cell 12:275–285, 1977.

26. Feldman L, Rixon FJ, Jean J-H, Ben-Porat T, Kaplan AS: Transcription of the genome of pseudorabies virus (a herpesvirus) is strictly controlled. Virology 97:316–327, 1979.

27. Anderson KP, Costa RH, Holland LE, Wagner EK: Characterization of herpes simplex virus type 1 RNA present in the absence of de novo protein synthesis. J Virol 34:9–27, 1980.

28. Thomsen DR, Stinski MF: Cloning of the human cytomegalovirus genome as endonuclease Xba I fragments. Gene 16:207–216, 1981.

29. Fleckenstein B, Muller I, Collins J: Cloning of the complete human cytomegalovirus genome in cosmids. Gene 18:39–46, 1982.

30. Tamashiro JC, Hock LJ, Spector DH: Construction of a cloned library of the Eco RI fragments from the human cytomegalovirus genome (strain AD-169). J Virol 42:547–557, 1982.

31. DeMarchi JM: Correlation between stimulation of host cell DNA synthesis by human cytomegalovirus and lack of expression of a subset of early virus genes. Virology 129:224–286, 1983.

32. Hirai K, Furukawa T, Plotkin SA: Induction of DNA polymerase in WI-38 and guinea pig cells infected with human cytomegalovirus (HCMV). Virology 70:251–255, 1976.
33. Yamanishi K, Rapp F: Induction of host DNA synthesis and DNA polymerase by DNA-negative temperature-sensitive mutants of human cytomegalovirus. Virology 94:237–241, 1979.
34. DeMarchi JM: Nature of the block in the expression of some early virus genes in cells abortively infected with human cytomegalovirus. Virology 129:287–297, 1983.
35. Fioretti A, Furukawa T, Santoli D, Plotkin SA: Nonproductive infection of guinea pig cells with human cytomegalovirus. J Virol 11:998–1003, 1973.

The Proteins of Human Cytomegalovirus

Mark F. Stinski, PhD

Department of Microbiology, College of Medicine, University of Iowa, Iowa City, IA 52242

INTRODUCTION

The HCMV proteins necessary for replication of the virus or for maturation of the virion also play a key role in the diagnosis and control of the viral infection. This chapter will review current knowledge of the virus-specified proteins of HCMV, and will speculate on areas for potential early diagnosis or control of CMV infection.

HCMV replicates slowly in the human host as well as in cells cultured in vitro. In infected human fibroblast cells infectious virus production is slow, requiring days to reach maximum titers. Likewise, in the human host CMV is associated with slow and persistent infections. During replication of the virus, there are several crucial stages that determine whether or not infectious virus will be produced. With the exception of the first viral proteins expressed in the infected cell, each stage in the replication cycle requires a protracted period of time relative to other herpesviruses such as HSV. A perturbation or suppression in the synthesis of crucial viral proteins will either inhibit or delay the production of infectious virus. Because crucial stages in the replication of the virus occur slowly, it seems reasonable that medical scientists could devise an effective means of controlling CMV infections. Nevertheless, effective methods for the early diagnosis and control of CMV infections have been unavailable. However, the development of sensitive and specific reagents such as monoclonal antibodies and viral nucleic acid probes should contribute greatly to early diagnosis. The potential

Birth Defects: Original Article Series, Volume 20, Number 1, pages 49–62

for recombinant DNA technology may lead to new methods to stimulate immunologic control of CMV replication.

In the human host, CMV can potentially enter both nonproductive (non-permissive) and productive (permissive) cells. The nonproductive cell presumably does not succumb to infection by the virus because only early viral genes are expressed. Current knowledge suggests that viral DNA synthesis is blocked in the nonproductive cell. However, these cells also play an important role because they may harbor the virus in a latent stage. Therefore, the virus remains in the host in a nonreplicating state but as a potentially infectious agent.

In the productive cell, both early and late viral genes are expressed, and the cytopathology of the infectious process usually leads to the death of the cell. The viral genes are expressed sequentially and therefore, the genes have been grouped into three broad categories referred to as immediate early, early, and late. The IE genes are transcribed in the absence of prior viral protein synthesis and, consequently, these are the first virus-specified proteins to appear in the infected cell within one hour after infection. Early genes require the de novo synthesis of the IE proteins. They appear in the cell within four to six hours after infection prior to synthesis of the viral DNA. The IE, and at least some of the early proteins, are detectable in nonpermissive cells. However, the late viral proteins are not detectable in cells unable to permit CMV DNA synthesis.

In the productive cell, CMV DNA synthesis begins around 12 hours after high multiplicity infection. However, newly synthesized viral DNA accumulates in the cell very slowly, and, consequently, the late viral proteins also accumulate very slowly. In vitro, maximum late viral protein synthesis requires three to four days when the cells are infected at a multiplicity of one PFU per cell. It is assumed that the newly synthesized viral DNA also accumulates slowly in the infected cells of the human host and, consequently, late viral proteins and infectious virus are not produced rapidly. During the early stages of infection, CMV replication is presumably confined and therefore, subject to control by humoral or cellular immunity, IFN, or viral chemotherapy.

Progress in investigating HCMV pathogenesis and control has been slow because animal models for investigation are not possible. HCMV is a species-specific virus and, therefore, human cells are permissive and cells of animal origin are nonpermissive. Medical scientists have had to use viruses with similarities to HCMV that normally infect animals. These animal CMVs are also species-specific and consequently, one is forced to extrapolate observations using viruses that are not genetically related. Two useful and widely studied systems are murine CMV and guinea pig (GP) CMV. The properties of these CMVs and the potential of the animal model systems are reviewed in other chapters. In addition, simian and equine CMV (ECMV) have been useful models for studying the CMV-cell interaction in vitro. However, this chapter is restricted to reviewing only the proteins specified by HCMV. The molecular biology of HCMV and the virus-cell interaction has been reviewed recently [1,2]. This chapter will not attempt to review the methods and details used to investigate viral mRNAs or viral proteins associated with the infected cell. However, reference will be made to the relevant contributions from which one can obtain the details of experimentation.

IMMEDIATE EARLY PROTEINS

The first genes expressed after reactivation, or after primary infection, presumably code for a viral regulatory protein(s) that controls subsequent viral gene expression. These genes are hypothesized to be the IE viral genes, which are expressed independently of any preceding viral protein synthesis. Although IE RNA originates from a region (0.660 to 0.770 map units for Towne strain) in the large unique component of the viral genome, only the viral RNA originating between 0.709 and 0.751 map units (Towne strain) is mRNA that can be translated in a rabbit reticulocyte lysate [3]. We have failed to translate the viral IE RNA originating from approximately 0.660 to 0.709 map units. With the Davis strain [4], IE RNA from the above region remains associated primarily with the nucleus. Although some of the above RNA is detectable in the cytoplasm after a long 12-hr inhibition of protein synthesis with cycloheximide [5], this RNA may not have been fully processed to mRNA. In the region of 0.709 to 0.751 map units (Towne strain), there are three IE coding regions that have been designated regions 1, 2, and 3 [3]. Region one has been referred to as the major IE gene because this region is highly transcribed relative to regions two and three. The latter regions have been referred to as minor IE genes. The major IE gene (0.739 to 0.751 map units) codes for an abundant 1.95 kb mRNA that can be translated in vitro. In the infected cell an abundant 72,000 dalton IE protein is detectable within one hr after infection, or after the removal of an inhibitor of protein synthesis [3,6,7]. The 72,000 dalton IE viral protein synthesized in vitro is immunoprecipitated by the same monoclonal antibody that immunoprecipitates the abundant IE protein synthesized in vivo [3].

Other IE proteins are not detectable by pulse-labeling with [^{35}S]methionine unless viral mRNA is allowed to accumulate in the infected cell by treating the cell with cycloheximide. These viral mRNAs can also be isolated from the infected cell by selective hybridization and then translated in vitro [3,6]. Five different size classes of viral RNAs originated from the region of 0.732 to 0.739 map units and they ranged in size from 2.25 kb to 1.10 kb, but 1.75 and 1.40 kb viral RNAs were more abundant [3]. These viral mRNAs code for viral proteins found in the cell at relatively low concentrations.

Another IE gene is located between 0.709 and 0.728 map units. This viral gene codes for a single size class of mRNA of 1.95 kb that translates to a protein of 68,000 daltons [3]. The viral mRNA is detected in the infected cell under IE conditions at extremely low concentrations.

The viral mRNA for the abundant IE protein of 72,000 daltons is detectable in the cytoplasm as polyadenylated RNA within one hr after infection. The viral mRNA reaches its highest relative concentration by approximately 4 hr after infection (Stinski, to be published).

The abundant IE protein has a broad banding pattern ranging from 75,000 to 68,000 daltons. These proteins were initially identified as three distinct polypeptides of 75, 72, and 68,000 daltons [6]. However, the three different sizes represent different posttranslational modifications of the same protein. Gibson [8] has suggested that the modifications could be due to intermolecular or intramolecular interactions such as disulfide bonding or posttranslational modifications. The only modification established to date is phosphorylation [8]. In addition to size variation of the abundant IE protein within a strain, this protein varies in size among different strains of CMV such as Towne, AD169 and Davis [8,9]. Therefore, the mRNAs of the various strains must differ in the open reading frames for translation of the viral protein.

Several groups [10-12] identified the abundant IE proteins as virus-specific by immunoprecipitation with human covalescent serum specific for CMV antigens. Analysis of these immunoprecipitates by denaturing polyacrylamide gel electrophoresis identified polypeptides with apparent molecular weights that approximate those detected by in vitro translation or by pulse-labeling with [^{35}S]methionine.

Expression of the major IE gene at extremely high levels relative to the minor IE genes may be due to secondary structure and enhancer sequences. Upstream of the promoter of the major IE gene we have found four relatively stable putative cruciform structures with a repeat sequence always located to the top right-hand side of the unpaired region. Within the repeat sequence are eight nucleotides, $^{5'}$GGGNNTTTCC$^{3'}$, repeated with a 100% fidelity [13]. This sequence has similarities to enhancer sequences found in retroviruses [14] or papovaviruses [15-17]. Transcription of the major IE gene is at least tenfold higher than the minor IE genes. This phenomenon is presumably due to the regulatory sequences upstream of the major IE gene. In vitro, these regulatory sequences compete for RNA polymerase II more efficiently than the adjacent minor IE gene. This competition for RNA polymerase II by the regulatory region of the major IE gene is hypothesized to be due to the four hairpin structures with repeat sequences at the top of the cruciform structure. The minor IE gene between 0.732 and 0.739 map units has only two cruciform structures in the regulatory region that are relatively unstable. The direct repeat sequence has approximately a 44% to 60% similarity to the repeat sequence upstream of the major IE gene [13].

The IE antigens of CMV accumulate in the nucleus [18]. The viral proteins are presumably responsible for the stimulation of chromatin template activity as measured by the incorporation of [^{3}H]UMP in the presence of *E coli* RNA polymerase [19].

If the synthesis of the IE proteins is blocked by treatment with cycloheximide [5,7,20,21] or IFN [22], a switch from restricted to extensive transcription of the CMV genome does not occur. Therefore, the synthesis of the IE proteins is absolutely essential for the successful replication of the virus. After the synthesis of the abundant 72,000 dalton IE protein and possibly other IE proteins, changes occur in the relative abundance of the virus mRNA size classes associated with polyribosomes [5,7]. These mRNAs code for polypeptides also found in the cell at early times and are discussed in more detail below.

In conclusion, HCMV expresses primarily one gene immediately after infection. It is hypothesized that this protein is the major regulatory protein influencing the switch from restricted to extensive transcription. Presently, the function of this IE protein is not known. It could interact with host cell RNA polymerase II allowing the enzyme to more efficiently recognize early and late viral gene promoters. Alternatively, the protein could interact with viral or even cellular chromatin. Interaction with viral chromatin might play a role in activation of early or late viral gene promoters.

Since interference with the synthesis of this protein affects subsequent viral gene expression, a chemotherapeutic agent that would interfere with the function of the predominant IE viral protein would inhibit viral replication.

Since the major IE protein currently represents the most abundant known protein in the infected cell prior to viral DNA synthesis, the possibility exists that a sensitive test for the detection of this viral antigen might serve as an early diagnostic test for HCMV infection.

EARLY PROTEINS

The early proteins of HCMV have been defined as those viral proteins synthesized after the IE proteins but before viral DNA replication. Even though extensive transcription of the CMV genome occurs after the synthesis of the IE viral proteins, only the viral RNA originating from the large repeat and adjacent sequences in the large unique component of the viral genome is efficiently transported to the cytoplasm as polyadenylated RNA [5]. Other regions of the viral genome are also highly transcribed but the viral RNA is preferentially retained in the nucleus [4,5]. Therefore, important early genes of HCMV reside in the large repeat and adjacent sequences in the large unique component of the viral genome. Unique viral mRNAs and polypeptides appear in the infected cell within four to six hours after infection, ie, these viral RNAs differ in size and in translation product from the IE mRNAs [7]. However, this profile of viral mRNAs and proteins remains the same for 24 hr or more. Therefore, HCMV has a prolonged phase of early viral gene expression. This relatively prolonged expression of early genes may be related to the relatively slow rate of viral DNA synthesis [6,23] and infectious virus production [24]. The relationship between early viral protein synthesis and the propensity for HCMV to cause chronic or latent infections is speculative. If early viral gene expression is affected by the physiologic state of the cells, early viral proteins may be synthesized at relatively low molar ratios and, consequently, replication of the genome will proceed at a slow rate.

The size of the early viral polypeptides has been identified by denaturing gel electrophoresis of in vitro translation products or pulse-labeled infected cells [7]. Many of these virus-specified proteins are synthesized in infected cells at relatively low concentrations and, therefore they are difficult to identify by pulse-labeling with [^{35}S]methionine. There is presently no correlation between early viral polypeptides and functional viral proteins. Although the functions of the majority of the early CMV proteins remain unknown, they have been implicated in the induction of cytopathic effects [25] and host-cell macromolecular synthesis [26-29].

The synthesis of the early proteins of HCMV has been correlated with the time of stimulation of host-cell macromolecular synthesis, which is detectable at approximately 15 hr after infection [26-30]. HCMV replicates as cellular macromolecular synthesis continues [29]. This virus differs from HSV in that the latter inhibits cellular macromolecular synthesis. Productive infection by HSV demonstrates independence from host-cell functions to the point of even providing enzymes to ensure the presence of deoxynucleotide triphosphates for viral DNA replication. In contrast, HCMV either depends on, or prefers, an actively metabolizing cell.

Many of the early proteins of HCMV are presumably involved in viral DNA synthesis. Functionally intact proteins must be synthesized at early times (6 to 36 hr) because the presence of as little as 50 μg/ml of canavanine, an analog of arginine, significantly suppresses viral DNA synthesis [29].

One of the important early viral proteins is the virus-specific DNA polymerase. This viral enzyme can be distinguished from host-cell DNA polymerase by its different behavior in phosphocellulose chromatography, template specificity, salt sensitivity, and sedimentation property [31]. The virus-specified DNA polymerase also can be distinguished easily from host-cell DNA polymerase by its enhanced activity in high salt such as NaCl or $(NH_4)SO_4$ [31-34]. In addition, the virus-specified DNA polymerase is very sensitive to PAA [35]. As little as 50 μg PAA/ml can completely inhibit viral DNA replication, whereas this concentration has little or no effect on the host-cell DNA polymerase [35]. The HCMV DNA polymerase is also inhibited by aphidicolin, ara-ATP, and N-ethylmaleimide but it is resistant to 2', 3' dideoxyTTP [34]. Associated with the viral DNA polymerase is a 3'-5' exonuclease activity [34].

Even though HCMV stimulates host-cell DNA polymerase activity, it has evolved to ensure the synthesis of its DNA genome by coding for a viral DNA polymerase. The early stage in the viral replication cycle is a potential area for viral chemotherapy. Antiviral agents such as adenine arabinoside have been employed to control CMV infections [36–38], but the agents only temporarily suppress virus replication. Virus frequently reappears after the treatment is discontinued. HCMV does not code for the synthesis of a virus-specified thymidine kinase and, consequently, acycloguanosine, which effectively inhibits HSV DNA synthesis, has little effect on CMV DNA synthesis.

LATE PROTEINS

The late proteins specified by HCMV have been defined as those viral proteins that are detectable after viral DNA synthesis. Therefore, these viral proteins are not detectable in nonproductive cells of human or animal origin that do not allow for viral DNA synthesis [6,29]. They are also not detectable in productive human cells treated with an inhibitor of viral DNA synthesis [29]. Approximately 70% of the cells persistently infected with CMV in vitro have IE or early viral proteins, but late viral proteins are not detectable [39]. The absence of late viral proteins is presumably due to a delay or temporary suppression of viral DNA replication. In approximately 30% of the persistently infected cells, viral DNA replication occurs and late viral gene products are detectable.

Newly synthesized viral DNA accumulates in the infected cell very slowly. After a high multiplicity of infection of 10 to 20 PFUs per cell, newly synthesized viral DNA is detectable by 12 to 15 hr but it does not reach maximum levels until 72 to 96 hr after infection [6,23]. The relative amount of the late viral proteins in the cell correlates directly with the relative amount of viral DNA synthesis. Therefore, the relative rate of synthesis of late viral proteins increases linearly with time and simultaneously with the accumulation of newly synthesized viral DNA [6].

The presence of late viral proteins or glycoproteins has been studied by pulse-labeling with [^{35}S]methionine or [^{3}H]glucosamine. These viral proteins were referred to as infected cell-specific polypeptides (ICSP) or glycopolypeptides (ICSGP) when their relative molar ratios or electrophoretic mobilities differed from host-cell polypeptides or glycopolypeptides. However, the late proteins or glycoproteins were identified as virus-specified when they were either immunoprecipitated from infected cell lysates with HCMV specific antisera or by their association with purified virions.

When infected cells were pulse-labeled with ^{3}H-glucosamine, there were two phases of glycopolypeptide synthesis. At least two ICSGP were found at early times reaching their highest relative rates of synthesis at approximately 24 hr after infection. A different set of ICSGP was detectable at late times reaching their highest relative rates of synthesis at approximately 96 hr after infection [29]. The ICSGP synthesized at early times were also synthesized in the presence of an inhibitor of viral DNA replication, but the late ICSGP were not synthesized. It was possible to immunoprecipitate the late ICSGP with an antiserum to the glycoproteins associated with purified virions, but immunoprecipitation of the early ICSGP was unsuccessful. Therefore, it was uncertain whether or not the early ICSGP were virus-induced host cell-specified glycoproteins or virus-specified glycoproteins.

Early after infection of cells with HCMV, the membranes are modified with respect to both glycoprotein composition and immunologic specificity [40,41]. However, it remains uncertain which proteins or glycoproteins are responsible for this early modification. Therefore, virus-specified antigens are inserted into the plasma membrane at 24 hr after infection, as much as two days before virion and dense body maturation. Unique virus-induced glycoproteins are synthesized and bound to the plasma and microsomal membranes, but virus-specified antigen accumulates primarily on the plasma membrane [40]. In contrast, at late times after infection virus-specified antigen is very prominent on the plasma, endoplasmic reticulum, and nuclear membranes [40]. The appearance of virus-specified antigen on internal membranes coincides with the commencement of virion and dense body envelopment. Recognition of viral antigens on the plasma membrane by cytotoxic T cells presumably plays a key role in controlling HCMV infections. An impairment of cell-mediated immunity (CMI) by disease or immunosuppression is frequently associated with a CMV infection in the human host.

The late viral proteins of CMV reach their highest relative rate of synthesis by approximately 48 hr after infection. This rate of protein synthesis continues at a relatively constant rate for days. Approximately 50% to 60% of the total protein synthesis is viral and approximately 40% to 50% is host [29]. There is a sustained synthesis of host proteins even when 10^7 PFU/ml is produced by the infected cell culture [29]. Although approximately 35 structural proteins are found to be associated with purified virions and dense bodies, the continued synthesis of host-cell proteins complicated their identification in infected cells.

Some of the late proteins of CMV are synthesized at high molar ratios and, consequently, they are easily detectable by pulse-labeling. For example, it was relatively easy to detect virus polypeptide (VP) 68 at approximately 48 hr after infection. This viral protein continues to be synthesized at relatively high rates throughout the late phase of infection. At times, even as late as 120 hr after infection, VP68 is synthesized at extremely high relative rates while other viral proteins such as the presumptive major capsid protein, VP155, is synthesized at relatively low rates [29]. The viral protein VP68 constitutes approximately 15% of the protein associated with purified virions and dense bodies. Gibson (personal communication) has proposed that this protein represents a matrix protein necessary for interfacing the nucleocapsid with the outer envelope. There are a few other prominent viral polypeptides such as VP155, VP120 and VP83 that constitute a significant percentage of the virions and dense bodies but the majority of the other proteins are present in relatively low concentrations [29]. These represent a significantly large number of polypeptides since it has been estimated that the HCMV has approximately 35 structural proteins [29].

An estimation of the number of structural polypeptides associated with purified virions is complicated by contamination with dense bodies which are membrane-bound bodies composed of a finely granular, homogeneous, electron-dense material. An analysis of the polypeptide composition of preparations that contain high or low ratios of virions to dense bodies suggests that dense bodies share most of the polypeptides contained in virions [42, 43]. However, dense bodies do not contain the viral DNA genome [42]. It has been proposed that dense bodies represent an aberrant assembly of virion structural proteins [42], while others have proposed that dense bodies represent an aberrant assembly of just the viral envelope and tegument polypeptides [43]. Unfortunately, the nature of these dense bodies and their importance, if any, in the infectious cycle of HCMV remains unclear. What is clear is that virions and dense bodies share antigenic determinants in common as demonstrated by immune electron microscopy [44]. Therefore, dense bodies constitute an immunogen to the human host perhaps as significant as the virions.

The purified virions and dense bodies of HCMV have been analyzed for enzyme activities by Mar et al [45]. The purified particles contain a DNA polymerase activity and a protein kinase activity. The DNA polymerase has the properties of the virus-specified DNA polymerase described above and, therefore, it is not considered a host-cell polymerase. The virus-associated protein kinase activity is preferentially capable of phosphorylating HCMV structural proteins rather than exogenous protein substrates. The biologic roles of these virus-associated enzymes are not known presently.

The membranes of virions and dense bodies were found to be composed of at least eight glycoproteins repeatedly detectable by either denaturing gel electrophoresis or gel filtration [46]. The molecular weights of these viral glycoproteins were 145, 132, 120, 115, 90, 70, 64, 55, and 12×10^3 daltons. Although some of these glycopolypeptides can be differentiated electrophoretically, immunoprecipitation studies using monoclonal antibodies suggested some immunologic relationships between different glycopolypeptides [47]. The location of the glycoprotein genes of HCMV is presently unknown. However, the use of recombinant DNA technology to produce HCMV-specific glycoproteins might offer a new approach towards vaccination. Antibody to the glycoproteins of HCMV can neutralize viral infectivity [46, 47]. Antibody against membrane antigens of CMV-infected cells can be found in the sera of patients with CMV infection [48]. In addition, lymphocytes from CMV-seropositive individuals are stimulated by purified virus or infected cells, whereas lymphocytes from seronegative individuals do not respond [49]. Therefore, an immunologic response to CMV-specified antigens, either on the surface of infected cells or infectious virions, is paramount to controlling this infection in the human host.

CONCLUSION

After entry into a productive or nonproductive cell, the genes of HCMV are sequentially expressed. These genes and their protein products have been placed into three broad categories referred to as IE, early, and late. The IE genes are expressed immediately after infection and reach their highest level of expression within four hr. One of the IE genes is highly expressed relative to the others. It is hypothesized that this viral gene product of approximately 72,000 daltons is a regulatory protein that controls the expression of the other viral genes. Expression of early gene products requires the synthesis of the predominant IE 72,000 dalton protein. A significant number of the early viral genes are expressed in nonproductive cells of human or animal origin. Early viral gene expression is also detectable within four hr after infection. In contrast to other herpesviruses, such as HSV, HCMV has a prolonged phase of early viral gene expression. The same early viral proteins expressed within four to six hr after infection are the predominant viral proteins in the infected cell at 24 hr or later. Late viral gene products are not present in nonproductive cells. Expression of these viral proteins requires viral DNA synthesis. Since newly synthesized viral DNA accumulates in the infected cell slowly, there is also a slow accumulation of late viral proteins that are not easily detectable until 36 to 48 hr after infection. This relatively slow rate of viral DNA synthesis is related directly to the relatively slow accumulation of late viral proteins and infectious virus. Therefore, CMV is a slow replicating virus usually associated with persistent and chronic infections of the human host. There are several stages where control of HCMV infection might be feasible. HCMV presumably requires the predominant IE protein for subsequent viral gene expression. A better understanding of the function(s) of this viral protein may lead to a novel approach to controlling viral infection. HCMV replicates its DNA slowly. Antivirals that would inhibit the synthesis of CMV DNA without affecting the host cell would be valuable for suppressing an acute infection. However, HCMV has the potential to remain latent and, consequently, the virus would likely reappear after termination of antiviral treatment. Therefore, humoral and/or cell-mediated immunity play a very important role in controlling CMV infections. An understanding of the virus-specified glycoprotein genes and the glycoproteins should also contribute important new knowledge toward controlling CMV infections.

REFERENCES

1. Stinski MF, Thomsen DR, Wathen MW: Structure and function of the cytomegalovirus genome. In Nahmias AJ, Dowdle WR, Schinazi RF (eds): "The Human Herpesviruses." New York: Elsevier North Holland, 1981, pp 72–84.
2. Stinski MF: Molecular biology of cytomegaloviruses. In Roizman B (ed): "The Herpesviruses." New York: Plenum Press, 1983, pp 67–113.
3. Stinski MF, Thomsen DR, Stenberg RM, Goldstein LC: Organization and expression of the immediate early genes of human cytomegalovirus. J Virol 46:1–14, 1983.
4. DeMarchi JM: Post-transcriptional control of human cytomegalovirus gene expression. Virology 124:390–402, 1983.
5. Wathen MW, Stinski MF: Temporal patterns of human cytomegalovirus transcription: Mapping the viral RNAs synthesized at immediate early, early, and late times after infection. J Virol 41:462–477, 1982.

6. Stinski MF: Sequence of protein synthesis in cells infected by human cytomegalovirus: Early and late virus-induced polypeptides. J Virol 26:686–701, 1978.

7. Wathen MW, Thomsen DR, Stinski MF: Temporal regulation of human cytomegalovirus transcription at immediate early and early times after infection. J Virol 38:446–459, 1981.

8. Gibson W: Immediate-early proteins of human cytomegalovirus strains AD169, Davis, and Towne differ in electrophoretic mobility. Virology 112:350–354, 1981.

9. Cameron JM, Preston CM: Comparison of the immediate early polypeptides of human cytomegalovirus isolates. J Gen Virol 54:421–424, 1981.

10. Michelson S, Horodniceanu F, Kress M, Tardy-Panit M: Human cytomegalovirus-induced immediate early antigens: Analysis in sodium dodecyl sulfate-polyacrylamide gel electrophoresis after immunoprecipitation. J Virol 32:259–267, 1979.

11. Tanaka S, Otsuka M, Shara S, Malda F, Watanabe Y: Introduction of pre-early nuclear antigen(s) in HEL cells infected with human cytomegalovirus. Microbial Immunol 23:263–271, 1979.

12. Blanton RA, Tevethia MJ: Immunoprecipitation of virus-specific immediate-early and early polypeptides from cells lytically infected with human cytomegalovirus strain AD169. Virology 112:262–273, 1981.

13. Thomsen DR, Stenberg RM, Goins BF, Stinski MF: The promoter-regulatory region of the major immediate early gene of human cytomegalovirus. (Submitted for publication)

14. Payne GS, Bishop JM, Varmus HE: Multiple arrangements of viral DNA and an activated host oncogene in bursal lymphomas. Nature 295:209–214, 1982.

15. Weiker H, König M, Gruss P: Multiple point mutations affecting the simian virus 40 enhancer. Science 219:626–631, 1983.

16. Banerji J, Rosconi S, Schaffner W: Expression of a B-globin gene is enhanced by remote SV_{40} DNA sequences. Cell 27:299–308, 1981.

17. deVilliers J, Schaffner W: A small segment of polyoma virus DNA enhances the expression of a cloned B-globin gene over a distance of 1400 base pairs. Nucleic Acids Res 9:6251–6264, 1981.

18. Michelson-Fiske S, Horodniceanu F, Guillon JC: Immediate early antigens in human cytomegalovirus-infected cells. Nature 270:615–617, 1977.

19. Kamata T, Tanaka S, Watanabe Y: Human cytomegalovirus-induced chromatin factors responsible for changes in template activity and structure of infected cell chromatin. Virology 90:197–208, 1978.

20. DeMarchi JM: Human cytomegalovirus DNA: Restriction enzyme cleavage maps and map locations for immediate early, early, late RNAs. Virology 114:23–38, 1981.

21. McDonough SH, Spector DH: Transcription in human fibroblast permissively infected by human cytomegalovirus strain AD169. Virology 125:31–46, 1983.

22. Stinski MF, Thomsen DR, Rodriguez JE: Synthesis of human cytomegalovirus-specified RNA and protein in interferon-treated cells at early times after infection. J Gen Virol 60:261–270, 1982.

23. St. Jeor S, Hutt R: Cell DNA replication as a function in the synthesis of human cytomegalovirus. J Gen Virol 37:65–73, 1977.

24. Smith JD, DeHarven E: Herpes simplex virus and human cytomegalovirus replication in WI-38 cells. I. Sequence of viral replication. J Virol 12:919–930, 1973.

25. Furukawa T, Fioretti A, Plotkin S: Growth characteristics of cytomegalovirus in human fibroblasts with demonstration of protein synthesis early in viral replication. J Virol 11:991–997, 1973.

26. Furukawa T, Sodatoshi S, Plotkin SA: Human cytomegalovirus infection of WI-38 cells stimulates mitrochondrial DNA synthesis. Nature 262:414–416, 1976.
27. Furukawa T, Tanaka S, Plotkin SA: Stimulation of macromolecular synthesis in guinea pig cells by human CMV. Proc Soc Exp Biol Med 148:211–214, 1975.
28. St. Jeor S, Albrecht TB, Funk FD, Rapp F: Stimulation of cellular DNA synthesis by human cytomegalovirus. J Virol 13:353–362, 1974.
29. Stinski MF: Synthesis of proteins and glycoproteins in cells infected with human cytomegalovirus. J Virol 23:751–767, 1977.
30. Tanaka S, Furukawa T, Plotkin SA: Human cytomegalovirus-stimulated host cell DNA synthesis. J Virol 15:297–304, 1975.
31. Huang ES: Human cytomegalovirus III. Virus-induced DNA polymerase. J Virol 16:298–319, 1975.
32. Miller RL, Rapp F: Distinguishing cytomegalovirus, mycoplasma, and cellular DNA polymerase. J Virol 20:564–569, 1976.
33. Hirai K, Furukawa T, Plotkin SA: Induction of DNA polymerase in WI-38 and guinea pig cells infected with human cytomegalovirus (HCMV). Virology 70:251–255, 1976.
34. Nishiyama Y, Maeno K, Yoshida S: Characterization of human cytomegalovirus-induced DNA polymerase and the associated 3'-to-5' exonuclease. Virology 124:221–231, 1983.
35. Huang ES: Human cytomegalovirus. IV. Specific inhibition of virus-induced DNA polymerase activity and viral DNA replication by phosphonoacetic acid. J Virol 16:1560–1565, 1975.
36. Chién LT, Cannon MJ, Whitley RI, Diethelm AG, Dismukes WE, Scott CW, Buchanan RA, Alford CA: Effect of adenine arabinoside on cytomegalovirus infection. J Infect Dis 130:32–39, 1974.
37. Alford CA, Whitley RT: Treatment of infections due to herpesvirus in humans: A critical review of the state of the art. J Infect Dis 133:101–108, 1976.
38. Kraemer KG, Neiman PE, Reeves WC, Thomas ED: Prophylactic adenine arabinoside following marrow transplantation. Transplant Proc 10:237–240, 1978.
39. Mocarski ES, Stinski MF: Persistence of the cytomegalovirus genome in human cells. J Virol 31:761–775, 1979.
40. Stinski MF, Mocarski ES, Thomsen DR, Urbanowski ML: Membrane glycoproteins and antigens induced by human cytomegalovirus. J Gen Virol 43:119–129, 1979.
41. Tanaka J, Yoshihiko Y, Hatano M: Evidence for early membrane antigens in cytomegalovirus-infected cells. J Gen Virol 53:157–161, 1981.
42. Sarov I, Abady I: The morphogenesis of human cytomegalovirus: Isolation and polypeptide characterization of cytomegalovirus and dense bodies. Virology 66:464–473, 1975.
43. Fiala M, Honess RW, Heiner DC, Heine JW, Murname J, Wallace R, Guze LB: Cytomegalovirus proteins. I. Polypeptides of virions and dense bodies. J Virol 19:243–254, 1976.
44. Craighead JE, Kanich RE, Almeida JD: Nonviral microbodies with viral antigenicity produced in cytomegalovirus-infected cells. J Virol 10:766–775, 1972.
45. Mar EC, Patel PC, Huang ES: Human cytomegalovirus-associated DNA polymerase and protein kinase activities. J Gen Virol 57:149–156, 1981.
46. Stinski MF: Human cytomegalovirus: Glycoproteins associated with virions and dense bodies. J Virol 19:594–609, 1976.
47. Pereira L, Hoffman M, Gallo D, Cremer N: Monoclonal antibodies to human cytomegalovirus: Three surface membrane proteins with unique immunological and electrophoretic properties specify cross-reactive determinants. Infect Immun 36:924–932, 1982.

48. The TH, Largenhuysen MMAC: Antibodies against membrane antigens of cytomegalovirus infected cells in sera of patients with a cytomegalovirus infection. Clin Exp Immunol 11:475–482, 1972.
49. Moller-Larsen A, Andersen HK, Heron I, Sarov I: In vitro stimulation of human lymphocytes by purified cytomegalovirus. Intervirology 6:249–257, 1976.

SECTION 2:
NATURAL HISTORY OF CYTOMEGALOVIRUS

Congenital and Perinatal Cytomegalovirus Infections: Clinical Characteristics and Pathogenic Factors*

Sergio Stagno, MD, Robert F. Pass, MD, Meyer E. Dworsky, MD, William J. Britt, MD, and Charles A. Alford, MD

Departments of Pediatrics and Microbiology, The University of Alabama in Birmingham, School of Medicine, Birmingham, AL 35294

CMV is a ubiquitous agent that commonly infects man. Its ability to cause chronic infection of the fetus, newborn, and young infant, leading in some cases to acute disease, and perhaps more important, to late-onset sequelae is an important characteristic of this virus. Weller [1] stated over a decade ago that the social toll attributable to congenital CMV infection alone far exceeds that produced by congenital rubella, and current concepts have proven him correct. The absence of epidemics and the fact that disease occurs only in a small proportion of infected patients contributed to the unawareness of the lay public as to the potential devastating effects of congenital CMV infections. However, the situation is rapidly changing, and an increasing number of physicians are beginning to deal with this issue and are being asked to advise or make specific management decisions.

The purpose of this review is to summarize the current knowledge of CMV infection in pregnant women in particular as it relates to clinical expression, virulence, and long-term sequelae of congenital and perinatal CMV infections. These observations are based in part on previously published data [2,3].

*Supported by grants from the National Institutes of Child Health and Human Development (#HD10699), General Clinical Research Center (5 M01 RR32) and from the March of Dimes Birth Defects Foundation (#6-372).

Birth Defects: Original Article Series, Volume 20, Number 1, pages 65–85

CONGENITAL INFECTION

CMV is the most frequent known cause of congenital viral infections in man [2]. It is endemic throughout the world, occurring in approximately 1% of all newborn infants. However, as illustrated in Table 1, the incidence of congenital CMV infection ranges widely among the different populations. Contrary to what may have been expected, there is a direct rather than inverse relationship between incidence of congenital CMV and the rate of preexisting maternal immunity. This phenomenon results from the fact that maternal immunity does not prevent CMV from reactivating during pregnancy and, more importantly, cannot reliably prevent transmission to the fetus [4–6]. Therefore, there is a higher incidence of congenital infections in lower socioeconomic sectors of developed countries and in developing nations of the world.

Symptomatic Infection

Only about 5% of the infants with congenital CMV infection have typical cytomegalic inclusion disease (CID), another 5% have atypical involvement, and 90% have no clinical manifestations at birth [7]. Early studies focused on symptomatic infections, and congenital CMV was considered a rare and often fatal disease [8–11]. Many of the patients included in the early reports were not diagnosed until late in infancy, and it is conceivable that some represent postnatally acquired infections. More troublesome from the clinical point of view, many patients were referred to the investigators because of

TABLE 1. Incidence of Congenital CMV Infection According to Rate of Maternal Immunity*

Location	No. Infants Studied	% Congenital CMV Infection	Rate Maternal Immunity
Manchester, England, 1978	6,051	0.24	25%
Aarhus-Voborg, Denmark, 1979	3,060	0.40	52%
Hamilton, Canada, 1980	15,212	0.42	44%
Halifax, Canada, 1975	542	0.55	37%
Birmingham, AL (upper socioec.), 1981	2,698	0.60	60%
Houston, TX (upper socioec.), 1980	461	0.60	50%
London, England, 1973	720	0.69	58%
Houston, TX (low socioec.), 1980	493	1.20	83%
Abidjam, Ivory Coast, 1978	2,032	1.38	100%
Sendai, Japan, 1970	132	1.40	83%
Santiago, Chile, 1982	118	1.70	98%
Helsinki, Finland, 1977	200	2.0	85%
Birmingham, AL (upper socioec.), 1980	1,412	2.20	85%

*From Stagno S et al: Clin Obstet Gynecol 25:563, 1982, [3], with permission.

developmental problems which may have automatically selected a group of patients at a higher risk for persistent abnormalities and neurologic damage. More sensitive and specific methods of diagnosis, particularly viral isolation, have allowed prospective longitudinal study of both symptomatic and initially asymptomatic patients. This has resulted in increased awareness of the infection and its clinical spectrum. Clinically apparent infections are characterized by involvement of multiple organs, in particular reticuloendothelial and central nervous systems. Weller and Hanshaw [8] defined the abnormalities found most frequently in infants with CID as hepatomegaly, splenomegaly, microcephaly, jaundice and petechiae. As illustrated in Table 2, a combination of petechiae, hepatosplenomegaly, and jaundice are the most frequently noted presenting signs. In addition, the magnitude of the prenatal insult is noted by the occurrence of microcephaly with or without cerebral calcification, intrauterine growth retardation, and prematurity. Inguinal hernia in males and chorioretinitis with or without optic atrophy are less common. Pneumonitis, a common clinical manifestation of CMV infection following bone marrow and renal transplants in adults, is not usually a part of the clinical presentation of congenital CMV infection in newborn infants. In our experience, diffuse interstitial pneumonitis occurs in < 1% of congenitally infected infants, even when the most severely affected cases are considered [12]. As will be discussed in greater detail later, CMV-associated

TABLE 2. Newborn Clinical Findings in 34 Patients with Congenital CMV Infection all of Whom Were Symptomatic by 2 wk of Age

Abnormality	Positive/Total Examined (%)	
Petechiae	27/34	(79)
Hepatosplenomegaly	25/34	(74)
Jaundice	20/32	(63)
Microcephaly*	17/34	(50)
Small for gestation age[†]	14/34	(41)
Prematurity[‡]	11/32	(34)
Inguinal hernia	5/19[§]	(26)
Chorioretinitis	4/34	(12)

(From Pass RF et al: Outcome of symptomatic congenital cytomegalovirus infection: Results of long-term longitudinal follow-up. Pediatrics 66:758–762, 1980, with permission.)

*Less than tenth percentile based upon Colorado Intrauterine Growth Charts, for premature newborns, Lubechenco et al., or more than 2 SD below mean for term babies based upon Nelhaus.

[†]Weight less than tenth percentile for gestational age.

[‡]Gestational age less than 38 wk.

[§]Males.

pneumonitis is more likely to develop in infants with perinatal CMV infections.

There are reports suggesting an association between CMV and congenital anomalies involving various organs. Most of the studies are retrospective or in the form of single case reports. To date, with the exception of inguinal hernias occurring in males, anomalies of the 1st branchial arch, structural defects of the CNS, and a defect of tooth enamel which becomes apparent when teeth erupt, there is little evidence that CMV can be considered a teratogen [13].

Laboratory findings in patients with symptomatic infection indicate frequent involvement of hepatobiliary, immunologic, hematologic, and central nervous systems [7]. The following are found decreasing in order of frequency: increased cord IgM ($>$ 20 mg/dl), atypical lymphocytosis ($\geqslant$ 5%), elevated SGOT ($>$ 80 μU/ml), thrombocytopenia ($<$ 100,000 platelets/ mm^3), conjugated hyperbilirubinemia (direct serum bilirubin $>$ 2 mg/dl) and increased CSF protein ($>$ 120 mg/dl).

Among the most severely affected infants mortality may be as high as 30%. It may occur in the neonatal period or months later [7]. More importantly, the likelihood of survival with normal intellect and hearing sensitivities following symptomatic congenital CMV infection is small. Of the original group of 17 patients described by Weller and Hanshaw [8], only two were normal at 14 and 20 months of age. One infant had subnormal vision due to chorioretinitis and optic atrophy. The remaining 14 had various degrees of mental retardation with or without other sequelae like seizures, blindness, paraparesis or diplegia. Subsequent reports also demonstrated a high rate of CNS damage in infants with CID [10,11]. In addition, they described disorders of hearing, language, and learning. Combining these reports with our prospective study of 52 patients with CID, nearly 100 cases can be tabulated. As illustrated in Table 3, microcephaly, usually combined with mental retardation or a significant delay in psychomotor development, has occurred in nearly 70% of the cases. In addition, sensorineural hearing loss (bilateral or unilateral, severe to profound) and ocular abnormalities have occurred in 50% and 14% of cases, respectively. As the children have aged it is evident that hearing loss is of a progressive nature in some. Williamson et al [14] recently reported on their longitudinal study of 17 patients with symptomatic congenital CMV. In addition to the abnormalities described by previous investigators, they found that 14 children had expressive language delays. In 11, this could be related to hearing loss or cognitive deficits, but three other children had delayed expressive language skills with normal or disproportionately high language skills with normal or disproportionately high language

TABLE 3. Outcome of Infants and Children Presenting With Symptomatic and Asymptomatic Congenital CMV Infection

Complications	Symptomatic %	Asymptomatic %
Fatal	20	0
Psychomotor retardation or neuromuscular disorder	70	2–7
Hearing loss	50	10
bilateral	25	5
unilateral	25	5
Chorioretinitis or optic atrophy	14	1
Learning disability	20	4
Dental defects	33	3
Total with one or more complications	90–95	5–15

comprehension that could not be directly attributed to auditory or mental impairment. Also, learning disabilities and visual motor dysfunction were exhibited by four school-age children with normal intelligence and hearing loss.

Asymptomatic Infection

As indicated in the previous section, most infants with congenital CMV infections have no early clinical manifestations and their long-term outcome is much better. Nevertheless, there is now solid evidence derived from controlled prospective studies that at least 5%, and perhaps as many as 15%, are at risk for developing a multitude of developmental abnormalities, such as sensorineural hearing loss, microcephaly, motor defects such as spastic diplegia or quadriplegia, mental retardation, chorioretinitis, and dental defects. These abnormalities usually become apparent within the first two years of life. Table 3 illustrates results based upon four prospective longitudinal studies of nearly 250 patients with asymptomatic congenital infection and followed by using serial clinical, psychometric, and audiometric, and visual assessments [2,15–18]. The great majority of these patients and their controls were from low socioeconomic background. Consequently, we should be careful not to extrapolate these findings to the population at large, at least until more extensive studies are carried out in other groups. The single most important late-appearing abnormality in children born with subclinical congenital CMV is sensorineural hearing loss. The impairment is bilateral in nearly half the cases and of significant magnitude (50–100 dB) to produce serious difficulties with verbal communication and learning. Another alarming observation is that in at least 25% of these patients, hearing impairments have either developed or become severe after the first year of life, the same as happened with the symptomatic group. This progressive deterioration raises the possibility that the overall incidence, as well as the magnitude of the auditory defects in those already less severely involved, may increase with time. From an audiologic viewpoint, this phenomenon implies that an assessment of hearing sensitivity done within the first year of life does not rule out the possibility of hearing impairments in the future. Consequently, children at risk, whether symptomatic or not, should have careful, serial audiometric examinations.

These prospective studies of children with subclinical congenital CMV infection have also revealed a wide but significant spectrum of neurologic complications. It has been estimated that within the first two years of life an additional 2% to 7% of the infants in this group develop microcephaly with various degrees of mental retardation and neuromuscular defects. How often milder forms of brain damage, such as learning or behavioral difficulties, will occur as these patients grow older is presently unknown. Asymptomatic congenital CMV infections have a low risk of being complicated by chorioretinitis. Current estimate is that it occurs in 1% of these children and, like the hearing loss, may not be present at the outset.

Recently, we have observed a striking dental defect in association with congenital CMV infection [13]. Clinically, the defect of tooth structure is more common in children with the symptomatic form of the infection than in those born with asymptomatic infections. It is also more severe since when it occurs in patients of the former group, all or nearly all, of the teeth are affected. The defect is characterized by generalized yellowish discoloration. The enamel is opaque and apparently hypocalcified. In many cases, the enamel is simply absent, and affected teeth tend to wear down rapidly or to fracture. Rampant dental caries is also frequently seen in both groups of affected children. The group of patients is too young for clinical determination of whether enamel defects will occur in permanent teeth.

The definition of how many children born with asymptomatic congenital infection develop these complications required carefully conducted longitudinal studies. We have found that an important variable in this respect is the screening method used to identify patients. In our original communication on this subject [18] we reported that 25% of 16 patients with asymptomatic congenital infection had developed sensorineural hearing loss. These patients had been selected for viral cultures because they had elevated cord blood IgM levels. In a later phase of the study, when more patients had been identified by screening for viruria within the first week of life, sensorineural hearing loss was found in 15% of 51 patients [19]. Now that the majority of our patients have been identified by screening for CMV excretion as opposed to other screening methods the proportion of patients with hearing loss has decreased to 7%. It appears that asymptomatic newborns with increased levels of IgM or positive IgM-CMV antibodies in cord blood have a more severe form of congenital CMV infection. In this regard, these markers for intrauterine infection may reflect increased antigenic stimulation and viral load, and thus select a subgroup of patients at higher risk [4].

In summary, these observations underscore the need for longitudinal follow-up of patients with congenital CMV infection regardless of its clinical presentation at the outset. Careful assessments of perceptual functions, psychomotor development, and learning abilities must be carefully evaluated in order to recognize the full impact of CMV. With early identification of a problem corrective measures can be instituted to reduce school and psychosocial problems.

PERINATAL INFECTIONS

Perinatal infections refer to those naturally acquired during the course of delivery (natal) from exposure to infected maternal genital secretions [20], or during the postnatal period from ingestion of breast milk that contains CMV [21–23], or iatrogenically acquired as a result of blood transfusions [24,25]. Perinatal CMV infection occurs in approximately 40% to 60% of infants of seropositive mothers who are breast-fed for over one month [21, 23], and in 25% to 50% of those exposed to CMV in the birth canal [20]. Given current rates of seropositivity of the mothers, prevalence of CMV excretion in the genital tract at delivery, and the prevalence of breast-feeding, in the United States approximately 10% to 15% of infants begin to shed virus into urine by six months of age. The incubation period of perinatal CMV infection ranges between four and 12 weeks. Although the quantity of virus excreted by infants with perinatal infection is less than that seen with intrauterine acquisition, the infection is also of a chronic nature, with viral shedding persisting for years [2]. The vast majority of infants with naturally acquired perinatal CMV infections remain asymptomatic. However, recent reports indicate that this infection may be temporally associated with protracted interstitial pneumonitis. In recent years, we have observed that, of 45 prospectively studied infected infants, four developed pneumonitis. Three of these patients had evidence of coinfection with *Chlamydia trachomatis*; in the fourth infant, only CMV could be found. In a study that was subsequently undertaken to define the possible association of CMV and other potential respiratory pathogens with pneumonia in hospitalized infants less than three months of age, 20% (21 of 104) of the patients with pneumonitis were excreting CMV [12]. In 12 of these cases, CMV was the only identifiable infectious agent, while in nine patients we documented coinfection with *C trachomatis* (four), *P carinii* (two), *U urealyticum* (two), and enterovirus (one). In these and other studies, CMV had no adverse effect on growth, perceptual functions, or on motor or psychosocial development.

In premature infants who require prolonged and intensive medical care, blood transfusions are an important iatrogenic cause of CMV infection. In Dr. Yeager's experience [24], 13.5% of 74 infants of seronegative mothers who were exposed to one or more seropositive blood donors acquired CMV infection. The risk of infection increased to 24% for those patients who received more than 50 ml of packed red blood cells, and who were exposed to at least one seropositive donor. Among infants of seropositive mothers exposed to seropositive blood donors, the rate of infection was 15%.

In contrast, none of the infants of seronegative mothers exposed to blood from seronegative donors became infected. What is remarkable is that fatal or serious illness occurred in 50% of the seronegative infants who became infected, and in none of the infected infants of seropositive mothers. This observation indicates that passive antibody cannot always prevent the infection but can ameliorate its clinical expression. In infected infants CMV excretion usually begins 30 and 150 days postexposure, with a mean of approximately 50 days. Symptoms associated with this iatrogenic infection are characterized by rapid deterioration, septic appearance, hepatosplenomegaly, pneumonitis or exacerbation of pulmonary problems, atypical lymphocytosis, thrombocytopenia, and hemolytic anemia [24, 25]. Death may occur in as many as 10% of these patients. From this data it follows that CMV must be considered in the differential diagnosis of any preterm infant who, after progressing satisfactorily, suddenly begins to deteriorate.

PATHOGENESIS OF CONGENITAL AND PERINATAL INFECTIONS

Why some infants are severely affected whereas others remain symptom-free is not fully understood. Continuous viral replication, vasculitis and/or immunologic mediated injury are some of the possibilities that may operate in utero or during postnatal life. Because of the low-grade virulence of this infection, it is conceivable that some of the late-appearing complications are simply delayed manifestations of damage incurred during gestation. In this regard, other possible factors which are now under scrutiny include, either singly or in combination, the type of maternal infection during pregnancy (primary or recurrent), fetal age at the time of transmission in utero, host genetic factors that control immune responses, and difference in the virulence of viral strains.

Chronic Viral Replication

The hallmark of congenital and perinatal CMV infection is chronicity characterized by years of continuous viral shedding followed by a state of latency that may be disturbed by periodic exacerbations [2]. Certainly, continuous low-grade viral replication in critical organs leading to significant damage over time is the most evident mechanism but not necessarily the most important. As illustrated in Table 4, comparative virologic studies have demonstrated the striking chronicity of both congenital and perinatal CMV infections. In infants with congenital infection, irrespective of clinical status, and with perinatally acquired infections, viruria persists for years. Likely, viral replication also persists in other sites that are less accessible to routine virologic examination.

The duration of viral excretion is little influenced by the time or mode the infection was acquired. However, the quantity of virus excreted in the urine does reflect the time of acquisition and the resultant disease state. Infants with symptomatic congenital infection excrete significantly higher quantity of CMV at birth and during the early months of life [2]. After six months of age all three groups of patients excrete essentially similar amounts of virus.

Pharyngeal shedding is also universal at birth in the congenitally infected and appears, like viruria, after a mean incubation period of six weeks in the perinatally infected. In contrast to urinary excretion, continuous pharyngeal shedding is not as prolonged.

TABLE 4. Frequency of Viruria According to Age and Patient Category

| Age (mo) | Congenital Infection | | Perinatal Infection (%) |
	Symptomatic (%)	Asymptomatic (%)	
Birth	18/18 (100)	65/65 (100)	0/25 (0)
3	18/18 (100)	75/75 (100)	24/25 (96)
6	14/14 (100)	58/60 (97)	24/24 (100)
12	15/15 (100)	35/37 (95)	15/15 (100)
24	12/12 (100)	22/24 (92)	18/18 (100)
36	16/17 (94)	35/41 (85)	22/23 (96)
48	7/8 (88)	24/37 (65)	15/15 (100)
60	5/7 (71)	14/27 (52)	10/16 (63)
72	3/5 (60)	9/16 (56)	5/10 (50)

(From Stagno et al: Congenital and perinatal cytomegalovirus infections. Semin Perinatol 7:31–42, 1983, with permission.)

Immune Response

Serial assessment of infants with congenital and perinatal infections has shown that the humoral immune system is grossly intact and responding, albeit overstimulated in patients with congenital CMV infections. Serial quantifications of immunoglobulins in this group of patients has demonstrated that the postnatal development of IgG and IgM is accelerated, as compared to uninfected controls [20]. In keeping with their increased viral load in early life, sick, congenitally infected infants have an even more accelerated development of IgG and IgM. IgA development appears to be similar to that of the control group. Though Ig development only grossly gauges antigenic load, it provides an indirect means for estimating the magnitude of the immune response and perhaps of the persistent antigenic stimulation.

The specific humoral immune response, as assessed with a variety of serologic assays, is substantial and prolonged whether the infection is productive or latent. To further characterize the humoral antibody response at the molecular level, we studied the ability of sera obtained from patients with congenital (symptomatic and asymptomatic) and perinatal CMV infections to precipitate polypeptides extracted from CMV-infected cells [26]. As illustrated in Figure 1, sera obtained from patients with symptomatic congenital infections immune precipitated larger quantities of at least 11 polypeptides ranging in molecular weight (MW) from 20,000 to 150,000. Polypeptides with apparent MWs of 140,000, 66,000 and 47,000 comigrate with glycoproteins, and those with MWs of 140,000 and 66,000 contain the neutralizing sites. Sera from patients with either asymptomatic congenital or perinatal CMV infections not only precipitate smaller amounts of polypeptides, but polypeptides with apparent MWs of 74,000, 49,000 34,000, and 25,000 are not detected or are present in trace amounts. These differences are more striking if we consider that the sera from all patients were obtained between 12 and 15 months of age, all patients were shedding CMV at the time sera were obtained, and their antibody titers measured by anticomplement immunofluorescence (ACIF) were very similar. When sequential sera from these three groups of patients were studied, the differences became even more pronounced. In patients with symptomatic congenital infection, the appearance of precipitating antibodies was delayed up to 12 months of age. However, once these antibodies developed they precipitated viral polypeptides in greater number, in larger quantities, and for longer periods of time. These observations could lead to the development of serologic assays that could identify patients at risk of developing sequelae later in life, something that present techniques are not able to do.

Patients with both congenital and perinatally acquired CMV infections have also been noted to have diminished or absent in vitro lymphocyte

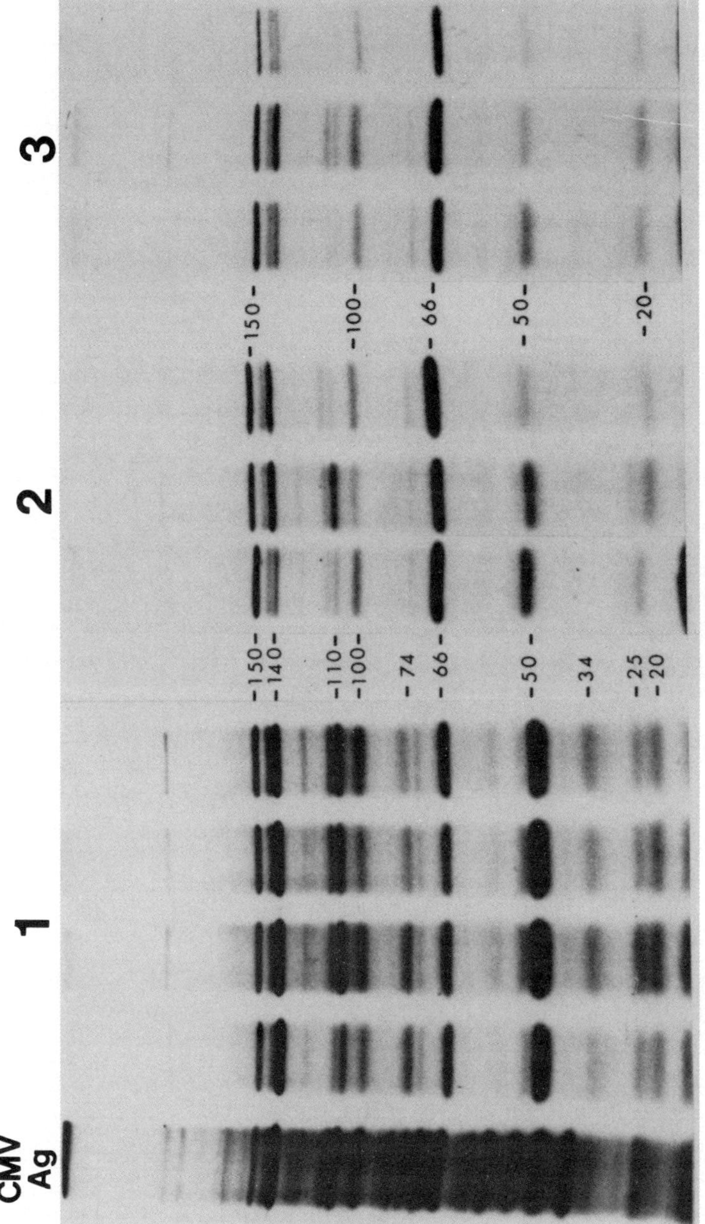

Fig. 1. Electrophoretically separated polypeptides immunoprecipitated from [^{35}S] methionine-labeled CMV-infected cell extracts. Sera are from children with congenital symptomatic (Col. 1), congenital asymptomatic (Col. 2), and perinatal (Col. 3) CMV infections. Numbers give apparent molecular weights (10^3).

transformation responses to CMV antigens [27–30]. This defect is not the consequence of a global immune deficiency, since CMV-specific antibody levels are elevated, and these patients have a normal ability to recognize other bacterial and viral antigens like HSV. In this regard, the impairment of CMI is highly specific for CMV. Moreover, clinical and laboratory evidence indicates normal T-lymphocyte function in most of these patients, and normal distribution between helper and suppressor subpopulations. This defect in blastogenic response occurs irrespective of clinical presentation, but it appears to be more intense and long lasting in patients with symptomatic congenital infection. Typically, in both groups of CMV congenitally infected patients there is no proliferative response in infancy. In this regard, the defect appears to be directly related to viral excretion. Infants and young children who generally excrete the largest amount of virus have a significantly higher prevalence of negative responses than do older children who have ceased to excrete CMV.

The continued replication of virus in the face of a sustained and broad humoral immune response, which in certain aspects is overstimulated, is an excellent milieu for immune complex formation. There is now evidence that during the first year of life immune complexes circulate in a significant proportion of infants with congenital and perinatal CMV infections [31]. Immune complexes appear to be of heavier MW in sick infants, as opposed to asymptomatically infected infants in whom intermediate size complexes (12-16 S) are found. Moreover, in a few symptomatic infants who died of CMV infection, deposition of immune complexes was demonstrated in renal glomeruli. Conceivably, this immunologically mediated mechanism could contribute to progressive organ disease by interfering with host defense mechanisms or by direct tissue damage in concert with continued viral replication.

Virulence of CMV Strains

Intrauterine transmission in the face of maternal immunity has been attributed to reactivation of endogenous virus, but the possibility of reinfection by an exogenous strain of virus cannot be excluded. The analyses of genetic homology of strains of CMV isolated from unrelated persons are almost always genetically different [32,33]. In contrast, the viruses recovered from related individuals like mother–baby pairs, or repeatedly from the same individual, are most often identical [34]. In some cases this homology remains after intervals of up to six years. Of particular interest is our observation that the viruses isolated from each of four pairs of congenitally or perinatally infected sibs were genetically identical. In two of the three pairs of infected sibs the first-born baby was severely affected, while the second-born sib was subclinically infected. In addition, in a study of Huang and colleagues (personal communication), the virulence of congenital infections was not strain-dependent. Reactivation of latent virus appears as the dominant mechanism responsible for intrauterine transmission in immune women. However, until a much larger number of strains is analyzed, it would be inappropriate to conclude that reinfections play an insignificant role.

Type of Maternal Infection

Recent studies have clearly demonstrated that preexisting maternal immunity does not prevent CMV from reactivating during pregnancy and, more importantly, cannot reliably prevent intrauterine transmission [6]. Despite this imperfection, we have shown that congenital infections resulting from a recurrence of CMV during pregnancy are less likely to be clinically apparent than those resulting from primary maternal infection [6]. On a worldwide basis, the vast majority of congenitally infected infants who are symptomatic at birth and/or develop sequelae at a later time are believed to be the result of primary maternal CMV infections. As illustrated in Table 5, at our institution we have identified 84 infants with congenital CMV infections that resulted from well-documented primary or presumed primary infections in 52, and from proven recurrent or presumed recurrent infections in 32. Twenty-nine of the mothers with primary infections and all those with recurrent infections were prospectively and longitudinally studied during pregnancy. The remaining 23 mothers with primary infection had donated blood either before conception or early in gestation, and also at the time of delivery. Thus, following delivery it was possible to classify their infection

TABLE 5. Severity of Congenital CMV Infection According to Type of Maternal Infection During Pregnancy

Type of Maternal Infection	Symptomatic at Birth	Sequelae
Primary[1]	4/40 (10%)	4/30 (13%)
Presumed primary[2]	3/12 (25%)	4/12 (33%)
Total	7/52 (13%)	8/42 (19%)
Recurrent[3]	0/15 (0%)	0/15 (0%)
Presumed recurrent[4]	0/17 (0%)	2/17 (11%)
Total	0/32 (0%)	2/32 (6.2%)

[1]Seroconversion during pregnancy.
[2]Seropositive patient with positive IgM antibody test in early gestation.
[3]Patient known to be seropositive before conception.
[4]Seropositive before 12 weeks of gestation with negative IgM antibody tests at time of enrollment.

as primary, but documentation of infection in the neonate was the initial step in identifying these women. Because of this retrospective component of our studies, it would be inappropriate to accept as accurate the figures shown for neonatal disease and complications at a later time for the entire group of women with primary infection. Nevertheless, it is striking that the few infants with clinically apparent disease at birth were born only to women with primary infections. There is also a significant difference for the risk of later sequelae associated with primary maternal infection. Notably, the two infants with sequelae (one with unilateral chorioretinitis and the other with hearing loss) in the recurrent infection group were born to mothers with presumed rather than proven recurrent infections, based on the absence of IgM antibody in the mother at 12 weeks of gestation. As previously shown, the reliability of the RIA method used in these cases to detect maternal IgM antibodies at this stage of pregnancy has an accuracy of 91% [35]. Considering only those women who were seropositive before conception (15), or who were lacking IgM antibody in sera collected no later than eight weeks of gestation (nine), all their infants have remained disease-free. Additional evidence for the protective, albeit imperfect, role of maternal seroimmunity to CMV was provided by a retrospective comparative analysis of death attributed to CMV [36]. Briefly, in Chile, in a population which was highly immune to CMV (98% seropositive), congenital infection occurred in 1.7% of infants examined, but no death could be attributed to CID among 407 autopsy records examined. Moreover, in recent years this diagnosis has not been confirmed by means of viral isolation in several newborn infants who presented with a clinical syndrome compatible with congenital infection. Most of them turned out to be congenital toxoplasmosis, syphilis, or Chagas disease. In contrast, in Birmingham, Alabama, CMV infection was found in nearly 1% of the 938 neonatal deaths examined. Moreover, these infants were born of women in the middle-to-high income bracket who are known to be more susceptible to CMV. However, because of the small numbers involved we cannot exclude the possibility that recurrent maternal infection can cause a lesser degree of fetal damage, particularly regarding subtle or late-onset sequelae. In fact, one such circumstance has already been described [37].

To better define the role of primary infection as cause of fetal damage, we summarize here the current data from our ongoing studies and compare them to four other similar investigations. For this analysis we have only included those studies which clearly indicate the number of women followed throughout pregnancy, particularly those that were serosusceptible, and the number of newborn infants adequately examined for the presence and outcome of congenital CMV infection (P.D. Griffiths, personal communication and [6,

38–41]). Case reports and data collected in a retrospective manner were not included. For this reason, the information summarized here is of greater relevance and can be safely utilized in patient management and to establish the need for prophylactic measures. Of these five large-scale prospective, longitudinal studies, three were done in Britain (P.D. Griffiths, personal communication, and [38–40]), one in Sweden [41], and one in the United States [6]; the latter included two populations of different racial and socioeconomic compositions. As illustrated in Table 6, these studies included more than 31,000 women. Obviously the women who were examined differ significantly in several of their demographic characteristics, socioeconomic background, and mean gestational age at the time of first prenatal visit. The serologic methods used to define CMV immune status in these studies were of comparable sensitivity and specificity.

The results of these five investigations warrant several important comments. The rate of susceptible women ranged from a low 18.5% for the predominantly black American population of low socioeconomic status to 45.5% for one of the British cohorts. Nearly 10,000 of the susceptible women enrolled completed the study (84.5%). As noted in Table 6, the rates of seroconversion during the period of observation (range 5 to 7.5 months) varied from 0.7% to 4.1%, both occurring in British cohorts. The 1.9% average rate of seroconversion calculated from these studies extrapolates to an average of 2.6% for the full nine months of gestation, or to 3.5% per year. At least in our study, the 2.5% rate of seroconversion per year obtained for the cohort of middle-class background is similar to the attack rates for physicians in training (2.7%) and nurses working in a newborn nursery (3.3%), but lower than the rate (5.5%) observed in nonpregnant women of

TABLE 6. Primary CMV Infection During Pregnancy and Risk of Intrauterine Transmission

| | | | No. | Seroconversions | |
| | No. Women | % of | Seronegatives | No. of | Fetal |
Study	Enrolled	Seronegatives	Followed (%)	Patients (%)	Infection (%)
Stern et al	1,040	33.4	270 (78)	11 (4.1)	5/11 (45)
Griffiths et al	10,847	41.9	3,481 (90)	29 (0.8)	9/26 (35)
Grant et al	4,446	45.5	1,841 (91)	13 (0.7)	5/13 (38)
Ahlfors et al	4,382	28.0	1,175 (96)	14 (1.2)	6/14 (43)
Stagno et al A[1]	8,555	44.0	2,870 (76)	39 (1.4)	17/39 (44)
B[2]	2,515	18.5	353 (76)	11 (3.0)	3/9 (33)
Total	31,785	35.2	9,990 (84.5)	117 (1.9)	45/112 (40)

[1]Middle-upper socioeconomic background.
[2]Low socioeconomic background.

similar socioeconomic background who had at least one child living at home [42]. Taken as a whole, these observations support the contention that pregnancy per se does not increase the risk of acquiring CMV infection. Among the highly immune, low-income group, the rate of seroconversion during pregnancy was more than twice the attack rate of the middle-class cohort, a reflection of their sustained higher degree of exposure to CMV at all times. The differences encountered among the groups may simply reflect factors which account for degree of exposure to CMV such as race, socio-economic factors, age, prevalence of infection in the community, exposure to infants and toddlers, and sexual practices, among others.

In CMV infection, as in other infections during pregnancy, there appears to be an innate barrier against vertical transmission. In the five studies summarized in Table 6, primary maternal CMV infection resulted in demonstrable fetal involvement in only 45 of the 112 cases (40%, range 33% to 45%). In other congenital infections, namely rubella, toxoplasmosis, and syphilis, the rate of transmission and virulence of infection are profoundly influenced by gestational age. Although the information on CMV is still limited, it appears that gestational age exerts no influence on the rate of intrauterine infection following primary infection.

Four of these five prospective longitudinal studies reported on the fate of the infants who were congenitally infected as a result of primary maternal infection. Only six of the 51 infants (11.7%) had clinical manifestations of CMV infection at birth, but only three of them had organ involvement characteristic of CID. More significantly, five of these 51 (10%) congenitally infected infants have developed sequelae clearly linked to CMV infection: hearing loss (1), mental retardation (4), neurologic complications (2), or dental defects (1) singly or in combinations. Because the period of follow-up is too short, this figure must be viewed as preliminary. Likewise, due to the small number of women studied, the effect of gestational age on fetal disease cannot be ascertained with accuracy. Suffice it to say that symptomatic infections at birth have occurred after primary infections acquired both early and late in gestation.

PRACTICAL CONSIDERATIONS

Although preexisting maternal immunity does not prevent the virus from reactivating and leading to intrauterine infection, it affords some protection against overwhelming systemic infection of the fetus [6]. For all practical purposes, there are no simple virologic or immunologic markers to identify women who may transmit CMV to their newborn infants when reactivation occurs. Thus, women known to be seropositive before conception do not need to be assessed by either virologic or serologic means, nor do they need to be unduly worried. In the United States, at least 50% to 60% of patients of middle-class background and 70% to 85% of those from the low socioeconomic sector have CMV antibodies.

In contrast, approximately 45% and 18% of women of middle-class and low socioeconomic background, respectively, are susceptible to CMV. Diagnosis of primary infection can be confirmed reliably by serologic tests. However, in order to decide if serologic screening for CMV as part of routine prenatal care for all pregnant women is justified, it is necessary to define the impact of this infection in the fetus and developing infant. As previously discussed, among susceptible women of different socioeconomic backgrounds primary CMV infection occurs at a rate of 1.8% to 4.5% for the nine months of gestation. Therefore, approximately 81 primary infections can be anticipated to occur in a group of 10,000 unselected women studied throughout pregnancy. Because under these circumstances in utero transmission occurs in only 40% of primary infections, we can expect 32 congenital infections. Fortunately, the clinical impact for the fetus and developing infant is low (approximately 10%). Thus, frank cytomegalic inclusion disease can be anticipated in only three to four our of 10,000 infants born to unselected women. Considering that 90% of those with overt disease at birth, and that approximately 10% to 15% of those with asymptomatic congenital infection develop complications and sequelae at a later time, then five to seven out of every 10,000 infants are at risk for developmental abnormalities caused by primary maternal CMV infection.

These findings indicate that the cost-effectiveness of serologic screening for CMV as part of routine prenatal care of all pregnant women is still questionable, particularly in the absence of safe, effective therapeutic or preventive measures. More importantly, how would one determine whether the virus would be transmitted in utero and which infants would be damaged in a single pregnancy complicated by primary CMV infection? Besides, the fear of delivering a damaged baby—even though the chances were slim— would likely lead to an inordinate number of unnecessary therapeutic abortions.

In order to diagnose asymptomatic primary infections, at least two antibody determinations are required, one as soon as possible after conception, the other preferably at delivery. Without evidence that gestational age at the time of infection has any effect on intrauterine transmission and fetal morbidity, serial antibody determinations would only increase the cost of a screening program. How to manage a seropositive patient at her first prenatal visit is even more confounding. The use of specific and sensitive serologic assays to detect IgM antibodies to designate primary maternal infection is still limited to research laboratories [35]. The diagnosis of a primary maternal CMV infection should always be suspected in women with a heterophile negative mononucleosis-like syndrome. The diagnosis can be confirmed reliably by serologic tests. However, this syndrome is rarely recognized, and it is unclear whether this form of primary infection leads to an increased risk of intrauterine transmission and/or fetal damage. Careful studies are needed to define the effect of gestational age, the value of amniocentesis, and the use of noninvasive procedures to estimate degree of fetal morbidity. Without an answer to these problems it is difficult to forsee the success of a screening program to detect CMV infection in pregnant women.

Undoubtedly, knowing that the fetus has been potentially exposed in utero is important for the pediatrician who will care for the infant. The diagnosis of congenital CMV infection is easy to confirm by virus isolation [1]. Knowing that the infant is infected would encourage the pediatrician to more carefully assess for subtle acute and chronic damage. Serial examinations for late-onset perceptual and psychomotor difficulty is especially important so that corrective measures can be instituted to overcome future school and psychosocial problems.

The information summarized here also emphasizes the problems associated with developing preventive measures for the control of congenital CMV infection, particularly in regard to the use of live vaccines [13]. Beside the usual problems of assessing immunogenicity, reactogenicity, compliance, and cost-effectiveness, a candidate vaccine must be capable of preventing primary maternal infection without persisting in host tissues; vaccine virus should not be shed nor be able to spread to the fetus even at a later time through reactivations. Vaccine-induced immunity must be capable of preventing reinfections with wild strains [14, 15]. For some of these reasons, and because to reduce the impact of congenital infection vaccine-induced immunity would be required only for the childbearing years, perhaps it would be more useful to consider developing new vaccines using modern technologies ie, potent specific viral protein vaccines, or a live CMV vaccine genetically engineered for immunogenicity, but lacking oncogenicity, and with a reduced ability for latency or reactivation.

REFERENCES

1. Weller TH: The cytomegaloviruses: Ubiquitous agents with protean clinical manifestations. N Engl J Med 285:203–241, 1971.

2. Stagno S, Pass RF, Dworsky ME, Alford CA: Congenital and perinatal cytomegalovirus infections. Semin Perinatol 7:31–42, 1983.
3. Stagno S, Pass RF, Dworsky ME, Alford CA: Maternal cytomegalovirus infection and perinatal transmission. Clin Obstet Gynecol 25:563–576, 1982.
4. Stagno S, Reynolds DW, Huang E-S, Thames SD, Smith RJ, Alford CA Jr: Congenital cytomegalovirus infection: Occurrence in an immune population. N Engl J Med 296:1254–1258, 1977.
5. Schopfer K, Lauber E, Krech U: Congenital cytomegalovirus infection in newborn infants of mothers infected before pregnancy. Arch Dis Child 53:536–539, 1978.
6. Stagno S, Pass RF, Dworsky ME, Henderson RE, Moore EG, Walton PD, Alford CA: Congenital cytomegalovirus infection: The relative importance of primary and recurrent maternal infection. N Engl J Med 306:945–949, 1982.
7. Pass RF, Stagno S, Myers GJ, Alford CA: Outcome of symptomatic congenital cytomegalovirus infection: Results of long-term longitudinal follow-up. Pediatrics 66:758–762, 1980.
8. Weller TH, Hanshaw JB: Virological and clinical observations on cytomegalic inclusion disease. N Engl J Med 266:1233, 1964.
9. Medearis TN: Observations concerning human cytomegalovirus infection and disease. Bull Johns Hopk Hosp 114:181, 1964.
10. McCracken GH, Shinefeld HR, Cobb K, Rausen AR, Dische MR, Eichenwald F: Congenital cytomegalic inclusion disease: A longitudinal study of 20 patients. Am J Dis Child 117:522–539, 1969.
11. Berenberg W, Nankervis G: Long-term follow-up of cytomegalic inclusion disease of infancy. Pediatrics 37:403, 1970.
12. Stagno S, Brasfield DM, Brown MB, Cassell GH, Pifer LL, Whitley RJ, Tiller RE: Infant pneumonitis associated with cytomegalovirus, *Chlamydia*, pneumocystis, and *Ureaplasma* - A prospective study. Pediatrics 68:322–329, 1981.
13. Stagno S, Pass RF, Thomas JP, Navia JM, Dworsky ME: Defects of tooth structure in congenital cytomegalovirus infection. Pediatrics 69:646–648, 1982.
14. Williamson WD, Desmond MM, LaFevers N, Taber LH, Catlin FI, Weaver TG: Symptomatic congenital cytomegalovirus: Disorders of language, learning and hearing. Am J Dis Child 136:902–905, 1982.
15. Kumar ML, Nankervis GA, Gold E: Inapparent congenital cytomegalovirus infection, a follow-up study. N Engl J Med 288:1370,1973.
16. Melish ME, Hanshaw JB: Congenital cytomegalovirus infection: Developmental progress of infants detected by routine screening. Am J Dis Child 126:190, 1973.
17. Saigal S, Luynk O, Larke B, Chernesky MA: The outcome in children with congenital cytomegalovirus infection: A longitudinal follow-up study. Am J Dis Child 136:896–901, 1982.
18. Reynolds DW, Stagno S, Stubbs KG, Dahle AJ, Livingston MM, Saxon SA, Alford CA: Inapparent congenital cytomegalovirus infection with elevated cord IgM levels: Causal relationship with auditory and mental deficiency. N Engl J Med 290:291–296, 1974.
19. Stagno S, Reynolds DW, Amos CA, Dahle AJ, McCollister FP, Mohindra I, Ermocilla R, Alford CA: Auditory and visual defects resulting from symptomatic and subclinical congenital cytomegaloviral and toxoplasma infections. Pediatrics 59:669–678, 1977.
20. Reynolds DW, Stagno S, Hosty TS, Tiller M, Alford CA: Maternal cytomegalovirus excretion and perinatal infection. N Engl J Med 289:1–5, 1973.
21. Stagno S, Reynolds DW, Pass RF, Alford CA: Breast milk and the risk of cytomegalovirus infection. N Engl J Med 302:1073–1076, 1980.

22. Hayes K, Danks DM, Gibas J, Jack I: Cytomegalovirus in human milk. N Engl J Med 287:177, 1972.
23. Dworsky ME, Yow M, Stagno S, Pass RF, Alford CA: Cytomegalovirus infection of breast milk and transmission in infancy. Pediatrics (In press).
24. Yeager AS, Grumet FC, Hafleigh EB, Arvin AM, Bradley JS, Prober CG: Prevention of transfusion-acquired cytomegalovirus infections in newborn infants. J Pediatr 98:281–287, 1981.
25. Ballard RA, Drew WL, Hufnagle KG, Riedel PA: Acquired cytomegalovirus infection in preterm infants. Am J Dis Child 133:482–485, 1979.
26. Pereira L, Stagno S, Hoffman M, Volanakis JE: Cytomegalovirus infected cell polypeptides immune precipitated by sera from children with congenital and perinatal infections. Infect Immun 39:100–108, 1983.
27. Reynolds DW, Dean PH, Pass RF, Alford CA: Specific cell-mediated immunity in children with congenital and neonatal cytomegalovirus infection and their mothers. J Infect Dis 140:493–499, 1979.
28. Starr SE, Tolpin MD, Friedman HM, Paucker K, Plotkin SA: Impaired cellular immunity to cytomegalovirus in congenitally infected children and their mothers. J Infect Dis 140:500–505, 1979.
29. Gehrz RC, Knorr SO, Marker SC, Kalis JM, Balfour HH Jr: Specific cell-mediated immune defect in active cytomegalovirus infection of young children and their mothers. Lancet 2:844–847, 1977.
30. Pass RF, Dworsky ME, Whitley RJ, August AM, Stagno S, Alford CA Jr: Specific lymphocyte blastogenic responses in children with cytomegalovirus and herpes simplex virus infections acquired early in infancy. Infect Immun 34:166–170, 1981.
31. Stagno S, Volanakis JE, Reynolds DW, Stroud R, Alford CA: Immune complexes in congenital and natal CMV infections of man. J Clin Invest 60:838–845, 1977.
32. Huang E-S, Kilpatrick BA, Huang YT, Pagano JS: Detection of human cytomegalovirus and analysis of strain variation. Yale J Biol Med 49:29–43, 1976.
33. Kilpatrick BA, Huang E-S, Pagano JS: Analysis of cytomegalovirus genomes with restriction endonucleases HinD III and EcoR-I. J Virol 18:1095–1105, 1976.
34. Huang E-S, Alford CA, Reynolds DW, Stagno S, Pass RF: Molecular epidemiology of cytomegalovirus infections in women and their infants. N Engl J Med 303:958–962, 1980.
35. Griffiths PD, Stagno S, Pass RF, Smith RJ, Alford CA: Infection with cytomegalovirus during pregnancy: Specific IgM antibodies as a marker of recent primary infection. J Infect Dis 145:647–653, 1982.
36. Stagno S, Torres J, Dworsky ME, Mesa T, Hirsh T: Prevalence and importance of congenital cytomegalovirus infection in three different populations. J Pediatr 101:897–900, 1982.
37. Ahlfors K, Harris S, Ivarsson S, Svanberg L: Secondary maternal cytomegalovirus infection causing symptomatic congenital infection. N Engl J Med 305:284, 1981.
38. Stern H, Tucker SM: Prospective study of cytomegalovirus infection in pregnancy. Br Med J 2:268–270, 1973.
39. Grant S, Edmond E, Syme J: A prospective study of cytomegalovirus infection in pregnancy. I. Laboratory evidence of congenital infection following maternal primary and reactivated infection. J Infect Dis 3:24–31, 1981.
40. Griffiths PD, Campbell-Benzie A, Heath RB: A prospective study of primary cytomegalovirus infection in pregnant women. Br J Obstet Gynaecol 87:308–314, 1980.

41. Ahlfors K: Epidemiological studies of congenital cytomegalovirus infection. Thesis, Department of Medical Microbiology, University of Lund, Malmo General Hospital, Malmo, Sweden, 1982.
42. Dworsky M, Welch K, Stagno S, Cassady G: Occupational risk of seroconversion to cytomegalovirus (CMV). (Abstract #1090). Pediatric Res 17:268A, 1982.

The Relationship of Epidemiology and Treatment Factors to Infection and Allograft Survival in Renal Transplantation*

Robert F. Betts, MD

Infectious Diseases Unit, Department of Medicine, University of Rochester School of Medicine, Rochester, NY 14642

CMV has been a part of the renal transplant program almost since its inception. Morphologic evidence [1] soon confirmed by virus isolation [2] was documented within two or three years of the program initiation. The number of patients who shed HSV after renal transplantation approaches in frequency the number who shed CMV, yet almost all of the attention has been focused on CMV. The reasons are severalfold, and these will be discussed. Furthermore, the factors that lead to CMV infection and the complications that CMV seems to produce are complex and interdependent. This manuscript will address and discuss these complex interactions as well.

TYPES OF INFECTION POSTTRANSPLANT

Reactivation of latent infection from the recipient or from the donated allograft accounts for most infection [3–5]. Shedding posttransplant in an individual who was seropositive prior to transplant will be referred to as nonprimary infection and shedding and seroconversion will be referred to as primary infection. Nonprimary is much more common than primary infection [3,5]. In most instances, primary infection is derived from the donated

*Supported in part by a grant from the George Link, Jr. Foundation.

Birth Defects: Original Article Series, Volume 20, Number 1, pages 87–99
© **1984 March of Dimes Birth Defects Foundation**

allograft [3–5]. When an allograft donor is seropositive and a recipient is seronegative, primary infection will develop in 65% to 75% of such pairings (Table 1). The age of the seropositive donor which presumably reflects duration of latent infection in the donor does not seem to affect frequency of reactivation, although living related donor virus may be less frequently reactivated than virus from cadaver donor. In some instances, blood transfusions administered around the time of the transplantation are the probable source of virus. If the donor and recipient are both seronegative and no blood or only frozen blood [6,7] is used, primary infection, for all practical purposes, does not occur.

The actual site of latency in the allograft is not known. Attempts at virus rescue from explants of renal parenchyma have been unsuccessful [8,9]. The only report suggesting that CMV was demonstrable in renal tissue also concluded that HSV was detectable by similar methods [10]. The complete lack of evidence that HSV does transmit with the allograft raises the question of a technical problem with the assays used by those investigators. Occasionally, allografts are removed for technical reasons during the first two weeks posttransplant from individuals where the risk of CMV transmission is present. Primary CMV infection and the syndrome still have occurred, raising the question of whether circulating cells trapped in the kidney, which then escape after transplant, are the source of virus.

Whatever the source of virus, it is clear that the serology of the donor is important in predicting primary infection. One question this raises is whether the CMV serologic status of the donor might also be important to CMV seropositive recipients [11,12]. There is some indirect evidence of "superinfection" in these pairings based on the higher frequency of IgM antibody development in those seropositives who receive seropositive kidneys compared to those who receive seronegative kidneys (Table 2) [11,12]. No studies analyzing DNA fingerprinting of viruses in different sites of excretion from these individuals have been conducted. Clearly, though, dialysis patients who

TABLE 1. Risk of CMV Infection Defined as Seroconversion or Virus Shedding Posttransplant

Donor	Recipient	Nonfrozen Blood	Number Infected/Total
−	−	no	1/46 [6]
−	−	yes	25/40[*]
+	−	no	21/30 [6]
?	+	?	62/70 [4, 6, 13, 20]

[*]Data from Dr. Robert Rubin, Massachusetts General Hospital.

TABLE 2. Frequency of Development of Cytolytic Anti-CMV Antibody* to CMV-Infected Cells in Patients Grouped by Donor Status and Posttransplant Virus Shedding

Donor	Recipient	Virus Posttransplant	#+/# Tested
−	−	−	0/41
−	+	+	1/14
+	−	−	0/ 9
+	−	+	20/22
+	+	+	12/23[†]

*IgM and not IgG mediates this reaction.
[†]Data from Rochester and Massachusetts General Hospital.

receive CMV Towne strain vaccine and subsequently receive kidneys from seropositive donors do become "superinfected" with the transplanted virus.

SHEDDING OF CMV AFTER TRANSPLANT

The frequency with which shedding in nonprimary infection is detected depends both on the immunosuppressant regimen after transplant and the vigor with which attempts at virus isolation are conducted. If specimens of saliva, urine, and blood are obtained from patients weekly, if the tissue culture is cared for diligently and kept for 4 wk, if the specimens are blind passed and observed for an additional 4 wk, then 80% to 100% of seropositive recipients will shed virus at least once from at least one site [3]. In roughly 50% to 60% of nonprimary infection, shedding is more easily detected and persists for longer periods. In those 50% to 60%, virus is detected even if only looked for casually. It is not known whether there are differences in virus shedding in seropositives who receive seropositive kidneys versus those who receive kidneys from seronegative donors.

In primary infection, shedding is more prolonged and more often associated with viremia than in nonprimary infection [3]. In fact, we, as well as others, have observed CMV shedding 5 to 10 years after transplantation. A corollary of the prolonged and frequent shedding of CMV is the fact that when practically anything happens in a transplant recipient, CMV can be isolated and, therefore, is likely to be blamed for the process at hand. This prolonged shedding also explains why CMV has gained so much more attention than HSV.

EPIDEMIOLOGY OF CMV INFECTION IN NORMALS

Because shedding in nonprimary infection is dependent on the epidemiology of CMV in the recipient and development of primary infection is dependent on the epidemiology of CMV in both the donor and recipient, these issues of epidemiology will be addressed.

In the United States, geographic location of the transplant program is not nearly as important as the race or the socioeconomic status of the individuals in the program (Fig. 1). Frequency of past CMV infection in middle-class white renal transplant recipients is lower than in blacks in whom it is quite high. By contrast, potential susceptibility to primary infection would be quite the opposite. These differences become less pronounced among older transplant candidates because of progressive increase in antibody frequency with age. Thus, one could predict likelihood of primary or nonprimary CMV infection after transplant in a given group. For example, cadaver recipients, as a group, tend to be older because for the most part, those individuals with

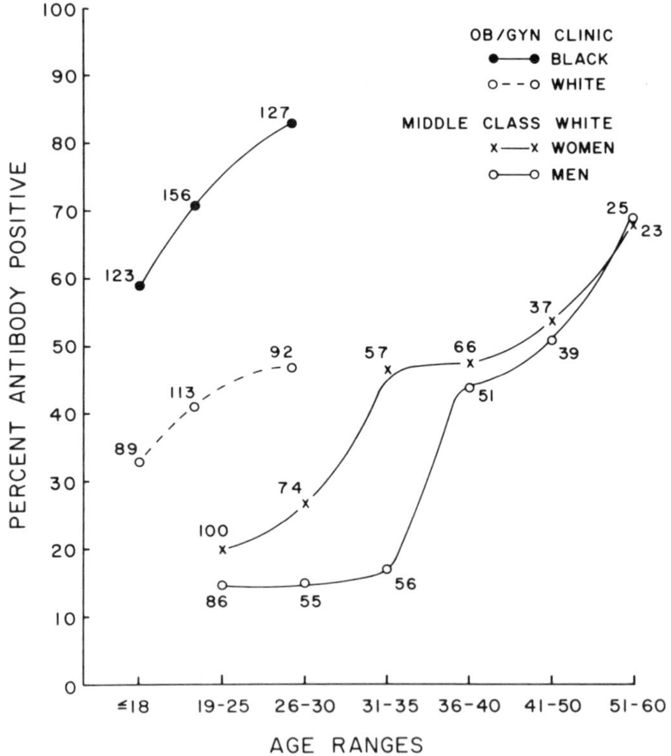

Fig. 1. Relationship of age, sex, and socioeconomic status to frequency of antibody to CMV.

no suitable young parent or sib resort to cadaver donations. Hence, nonprimary infection is common. By contrast, young white recipients have a very low frequency of latent CMV; therefore, the donor epidemiology becomes very important. Cadaver donors are very often young accident victims. Their youth is an important factor in their being considered for donation, and also means that they infrequently (20%) have latent CMV [3]. This combination of factors is responsible for the low incidence of primary infection in cadaver recipients. It is also relatively uncommon for a seropositive cadaver recipient to receive a graft from a seropositive donor. By contrast, in blacks, nonprimary infection is quite common, especially in individuals over age 25.

While nonprimary infection or no infection are the two most likely possibilities in cadaver recipients, primary infection is more common when parent child pairings are carried out [6]. This is true because the parent, being older, has a high incidence and the child a low incidence of latent infection. Therefore, primary infection occurs most commonly in a group that has an otherwise good prognosis. Considering these epidemiologic factors, it is important not to compare a group with a high incidence to a group with low incidence of primary infection when trying to determine outcomes.

VIRAL-ASSOCIATED ILLNESS AFTER TRANSPLANT

Illness is closely related to the onset and duration of viremia and, hence, is quite common in primary infection (Table 3) [6,13]. Whether or not the infection is primary, other factors govern the extent of infection as well. The immunosuppressive regimen plays an important role. When antithymocyte globulin (ATG) is used with azathioprine and corticosteroids in seropositive recipients, frequency of viremia as well as duration of shedding are greater than when ATG is not used [13,14]. Although less frequent, disease can be equally severe in nonprimary infection when ATG is administered.

The most prominent symptom in CMV infection is fever followed in frequency and time by a number of symptoms, signs, and/or laboratory

TABLE 3. Illness 30 to 90 Days Posttransplant in Patients Grouped by Different Criteria [6, 13]

Antibody Status Pretransplant	Posttransplant Virus Shedding	ATG Used	Percent Ill
−	no	yes or no	12
−	yes	no	87
+	yes	no	18
+	yes	yes	34

features (Table 4). Arthralgia and sometimes frank arthritis, chills, and severe lassitude are common [6,15]. Although it is rare for severe hepatitis to develop, mild elevation in serum glutamic oxalic transaminase is common and develops almost simultaneous to the appearance of new antibody in primary infection [6]. Mild-to-moderate leukopenia, sometimes associated with pneumonia, either focal or diffuse, may occur [6,16]. When complications do not develop, the febrile clinical illness can be of short duration or can persist for two to four weeks. In most instances, the mononucleosis-like illness is self-limited with no other superimposed features. In very unusual circumstances, disseminated CMV infection develops which can be fatal [17]. There has been some indication that individuals with severe disseminated infection do not form antibody to CMV, but well-documented death from disseminated CMV can occur in those with brisk antibody response.

Although disseminated CMV accounts for some of the mortality after transplant, more commonly the leukopenia which occurs with the CMV syndrome then predisposes the individual to secondary bacterial or fungal infection [16,18] (Table 4). It is this secondary bacterial or fungal infection that contributes in a greater way to mortality. As with the CMV mononucleosis syndrome, individuals with primary infection are at greater risk to develop

TABLE 4. Clinical and Laboratory Abnormalities in CMV Illness Posttransplant

Abnormality	Approximate Percentage of Subjects With Abnormalities
Symptoms	
Fever	100[*]
Chills	80
Sore throat	10
Joint discomfort	20
Cough	35
Signs	
Lymphadenopathy	0
Pharyngitis	0
Splenomegaly	30†
Hepatomegaly	20
Rales	10
Laboratory	
Leukopenia	30
Lymphocytosis	40
SGOT rise	55
Abnormal chest xray	15

[*]Required to be included.
†Of those without splenectomy.

this complication than are those with reactivation infection [16,18], although the latter are certainly not free of this complication.

ASSOCIATION OF VIRUS INFECTION WITH REJECTION

The clinical illnesses listed above first drew attention to CMV, but it is the proposed association of virus infection with allograft failure that has sustained this interest. Debate has occurred on whether it is the treatment of acute rejection that leads to virus infection or vice versa [6,19,20]. Gradually, this question is being resolved, but even now the most consistent thread is that CMV infection interacts with other factors that play a role in transplant success. Quite clearly, previous studies have shown that the effect of CMV on allograft outcome cannot be judged in isolation. In fact, a recent cooperative serologic study supervised by Dr. Robert H. Rubin of the Massachusetts General Hospital (personal communication) in which 50 hospitals are participating, once again suggests that a complex interaction of factors occurs.

To address this question, it is first important to consider non-CMV factors that are associated with allograft outcome (Table 5). Administration of multiple blood transfusions before transplantation is of benefit. In this regard, whole blood appears to be better than frozen blood [21–25]. Two separate studies [26,27] have demonstrated that if blood transfusion and CMV factors are considered together in patients grouped by these phenomena, the group that receives blood transfusion and is free of CMV antibody before transplant has the greatest success; those who have CMV antibody and have received transfusion are intermediate; and those who do not receive transfusion have the poorest outcome whether or not they remain free of antibody. The type of infection does not seem to be important. In one of these two studies [26], 90% of the cadaver recipients with infection had nonprimary infection and

TABLE 5. Factors in Allograft Success

Beneficial
  Living related donor kidney [6]
  Pretransplant transfusion [21–27]
  ATG [14, 28]
  MLC negativity [29]
  Splenectomy [31]
Adverse
  Primary CMV plus ATG[*]
  Viremia [32]
  Glomerulopathy and decreased function [33]

[*]Data provided by Dr. Robert Rubin.

most had no clinical illness. In that study, almost none of the subjects received ATG.

A second maneuver that appears beneficial is the administration of ATG to recipients [14,28]. However, when this was examined by Cheeseman and co-workers [14], ATG had its greatest benefit in individuals with no CMV infection. A larger cooperative study among several centers, including the above center, showed that poorest outcome occurred in individuals with primary CMV infection who received ATG (Dr. Robert H. Rubin, personal communication). All other combinations of ATG and nonprimary or no infection had similar outcomes. Other factors that have been evaluated for their contribution to success in transplantation such as MLC negativity [29], method of preservation of cadaver kidneys [30], or splenectomy [31] have not been evaluated in CMV-positive and CMV-negative groups.

MECHANISMS IN CMV-ASSOCIATED ILLNESS AND ALLOGRAFT FAILURE

Insights into the interaction of the above mechanisms remain to be elucidated; however, the mechanisms by which illness and allograft failure occur have been investigated (Table 5). The development of viremia is an event common to those with primary infection and those with nonprimary infection who receive ATG. However, illness does not always develop in the presence of viremia and viremia can persist as illness wanes. Another phenomenon common to primary infection patients is the development of IgM cytolytic anti-CMV antibody which by destroying cells may contribute to some of the symptoms observed [11]. Some individuals with primary infections do not develop cytolytic antibody and some with cytolytic antibody do not become ill [11]. There must be additional factors that account for these discrepancies that are as yet not recognized.

Studies bearing on this point have been conducted by Richardson and co-workers [32], who described a posttransplant glomerulopathy in which deposits of Ig along the basement membranes of glomeruli and in the mesangial regions of the allograft occur. Both IgM and, to a lesser degree, IgG have been detected. IgG remains detectable but in decreased quantity for several months. Similar findings have been reported by Baldwin et al [33] in patients with primary CMV infection. Although the initial observations by Richardson indicated that CMV viremia was an associated feature, subsequent studies [34] have not confirmed that point. The apparent association between CMV infection and loss of allograft function correlates with the mere presence of CMV infection, a finding that May and colleagues [20], and Andrus and colleagues [26] had reported previously. In the study reported by Schooley and colleagues [34], inversion of T-cell subset ratio to < 1, an inversion produced by the combination of OKT4 (helper/inducer) decrease and OKT8 (cytotoxic/suppressor) increase was closely correlated with the structural changes in the glomerulus. In this study, the sequence of events began with ATG-induced reactivation of herpesvirus, especially CMV but also HSV and EBV. This reactivation was followed by inversion of the T-cell subset ratio. This usually preceded the identification of glomerulopathy. By contrast, if glomerular changes were not detected in kidney tissue obtained by biopsy, T-cell subset ratios were usually > 1. Thus, ATG-induced T-cell subset changes may be due to ATG-induced reactivation of virus. Furthermore, association of CMV infection, leukopenia, and opportunistic infection may, in fact, be due to the reversed T-cell subset ratio which provides the setting for development of opportunistic infection. The interesting observation that CMV can be isolated from T cells of actively infected renal transplant patients [35] provides a potential mechanism by which T-cell subset changes could be produced. CMV syndrome may either precede or follow the development of these abnormalities noted on biopsy, and when these abnormalities occur, if renal dysfunction develops, nearly three fourths of these individuals will lose their allograft [34]. The number of patients in this series is small and further work will be needed to corroborate these observations. However, the potential to use a laboratory test to help outline a therapeutic strategy in the event renal dysfunction develops is provided. Although it is not yet known how the reversal of the T-cell subset ratios leads to the glomerular changes nor is the nature of the IgM (and IgG for that matter) in the kidney biopsies understood, it would appear that the materials are in hand for evaluation of these questions.

PREVENTION AND TREATMENT OF CMV INFECTION

A variety of measures have been offered as a means to control CMV infection: donor selection, vaccine, hyperimmune globulin/plasma, IFN, and other antivirals. Donor selection [3–5,20,30,36] is the easiest and most straightforward of these but is only clearly relevant to prevention of primary CMV and to a degree possibly primary EBV. Unfortunately, there is a somewhat limited population to which this applies and, as outlined previously, for many of those it could mean elimination of kidneys from a living related donor. However, when more than one living related donor is equally matched, CMV serology could be the tie breaker. For the potential recipient of a cadaver kidney who is seronegative, donor selection has potential relevance. The CMV-negative individual could expect little delay if transplantation is postponed until a seronegative donor is found, because the pool of seronegative donors is relatively large. Furthermore, there are screening antibody tests now available [36] that can provide a result as quickly as the results from a cross match.

Another potential intervention is hyperimmune serum or plasma [37]. The apparent value of transplacental antibody in babies [38] and the preliminary data in bone marrow recipients, suggesting value of hyperimmune plasma [37], raises this measure as a possibility. However, until the nature of the mechanism producing the glomerular changes reported by Richardson et al [32] and by Schooley et al [34] is defined, therapy will be kept on hold.

Still another consideration is vaccine. CMV vaccine has attracted much interest [39], but several factors need to be considered. First, the data from Schooley et al [34], May et al [20], and Andrus et al [26] suggest that natural immunity does not prevent the allograft loss associated with CMV. Second, CMV vaccine does not prevent allograft-derived infection. Third, the vaccine might not be useful since the immunosuppressive regimen decreases cell-mediated natural or vaccine-induced immunity just when it is needed most [40]. In addition, the long-term effects of a live attenuated vaccine in a group receiving immunosuppressive therapy is not known. Many questions remain to be answered.

The above methods are aimed at prevention of CMV. Methods which have been suggested as treatment include IFN [14]. Data pertaining to IFN therapy has suggested a decreased incidence of viremia and a postponement of onset of CMV shedding in nonprimary infection among recipients of IFN [14]. Schooley and colleagues [34] commented on a lower incidence of symptomatic viral infection in IFN recipients but made no mention of the effect of IFN on glomerulopathy. Other possible uses of IFN would be the prevention of primary CMV infection.

Besides the use of IFN, other antivirals have been suggested as having some benefit [41–43]. However, to date, the effect of anti-CMV antivirals has been limited. When and if either IFN or another antiviral is found to be effective, it will be important to define the transplant population at risk of developing problems with viral infection and who might benefit from antiviral IFN treatment.

Assuming that the data analyzing T-cell subsets are confirmed as reported by Schooley and colleagues [34], the selection of potential patients for possible antiviral chemotherapy could be made based on those T-cell subset ratios, long before other techniques to identify those at risk were available. Both confirmation and effective antiviral agents are eagerly awaited.

UNANSWERED QUESTIONS

Much of the work in renal transplantation has focused on CMV. Certainly, with respect to viruses, CMV is the major player on this stage with HSV and EBV as supporting viruses. Clearly the variety of other interventions also play an important part. When studies are conducted concerning the value (or the risk) of any alteration in the transplant program, critics must keep their diagnostic/analytic eye on all of the important performers.

The major unanswered questions include the following: In what way do viruses and various processes, such as transfusion, interact; how do they relate to exert their combined effect? How does the use of ATG lead to reactivation of CMV? What is the nature of IgM in the kidney with glomerulopathy [33,34]? Is it reacting with an antigen? Is it a cause of the glomerulopathy? If the glomerulopathy in renal transplantation is due to antibody and CMV antigen, why does glomerulopathy not occur in bone marrow recipients? Is an inactivated vaccine a worthwhile consideration? Can latent virus in the donated allograft be eliminated by removing all circulating cells from the interstices?

A final question which is of major importance: Are kidneys from seropositive donors really satisfactory for use in seropositive recipients or does superinfection from these grafts cause problems [11,12,36]? There is much work yet to be done to answer these questions. The final act of this play should be fascinating.

REFERENCES

1. Rifkind D, Starzl TE, Marchino TL, Waddell WR, Rowlands DT Jr, Hill RB Jr: Transplantation pneumonia. JAMA 189:808–812, 1964.
2. Hedley-Whyte ET, Craighead JE: Generalized cytomegalovirus inclusion disease after renal homotransplantation. N Engl J Med 272:473–475, 1965.
3. Betts FR, Freeman RB, Douglas RG Jr, Talley TE, Rundell B: Transmission of cytomegalovirus infection with allograft. Kidney Int 8:387–394, 1975.
4. Ho M, Suwansirikul S, Dowling JN, Youngblood LA, Armstrong JA: The transplanted kidney as a source of cytomegalovirus infection. N Engl J Med 293:1109–1112, 1975.
5. Pass RF, Long WK, Whitley RJ, Soong SJ, Diethelm AG, Reynolds DW, Alford CA Jr: Productive infection with cytomegalovirus and herpes simplex virus in renal transplant recipients: Role of source of kidney. J Infect Dis 137:556–563, 1978.
6. Betts RF, Freeman RB, Douglas RG Jr, Talley TE: Clinical manifestations of renal allograft derived primary cytomegalovirus infection. Am J Dis Child 131:759–763, 1977.
7. Thomas F, Lee HM, Wolf JS, Mendez-Picon G, Thomas J: Monitoring and modulation of immune reactivity in human transplant recipients. Surgery 79:408–413, 1976.
8. Schultz J, Bernik MB, Earle DP, Jennings RB: Absence of virus in renal biopsy specimens of patients. Nephrologie 5:329–338, 1968.

9. Naraqui S, Jacdson GG, Jonasson O, Rubenis M: Search for latent cytomegalovirus in renal allografts. Infect Immun 19:669–702, 1978.
10. Orsi EV, Howard JL, Batway N, Ende N, Ribot S, Eslami H: High incidence of virus isolation from donor and recipient tissues associated with renal transplantation. Nature 272:372–373, 1978.
11. Betts RF, Schmidt SD: Evaluation of cytolytic antibody to cytomegalovirus infected cells in patients undergoing renal transplantation. In "Transplantation and Clinical Immunology." Amsterdam: Excerpta Medica, 1980, vol xii, p 55.
12. Betts RF, George SD: Cytolytic IgM anticytomegalovirus antibody in primary cytomegalovirus infection in man. J Infect Dis 143:821–826, 1981.
13. Pass RF, Whitley RJ, Diethelm AG, Whelchel JD, Reynolds DW, Alford CA: Cytomegalovirus infection in patients with renal transplants: Potentiation by antithymocyte globulin and an incompatible graft. J Infect Dis 142:9–17, 1980.
14. Cheeseman SH, Rubin RH, Stewart JA, Tolkoff-Rubin NE, Cosimi AB, Cantell K, Gilbert J, Winkle S, Herrin JT, Black PH, Russell PS, Hirsch MS: Controlled clinical trial of prophylactic human-leukocyte interferon in renal transplantation. N Engl J Med 300:1345–1349, 1979.
15. Fiala M, Payne JE, Berne TV, Moore TC, Henle W, Montgomerie JZ, Chatterjee SN, Guze LB: Epidemiology of cytomegalovirus infection after transplantation and immunosuppression. J Infect Dis 132:421–433, 1975.
16. Rubin RH, Cosimi AB, Tolkoff-Rubin NE, Russell PS, Hirsch MS: Infectious disease syndromes attributable to cytomegalovirus and their significance among renal transplant recipients. Transplantation 24:458–464, 1977.
17. Simmons RL, Matas AJ, Rattazzi LC, Balfour HH Jr, Howard RJ, Najarian JS: Clinical characteristics of the lethal cytomegalovirus infection following renal transplantation. Surgery 82:537–546, 1977.
18. Chatterjee SN, Fiala M, Weiner J, Stewart JA, Stacey B, Warner N: Primary cytomegalovirus and opportunistic infections. JAMA 240:2446–2449, 1978.
19. Lopez C, Simmons RL, Mauer SM, Najarian JS, Good RA, Gentry S: Association of renal allograft rejection with virus infections. Am J Med 56:280–288, 1974.
20. May AG, Betts RF, Freeman RB, Andrus CH: An analysis of cytomegalovirus infection and HLA antigen matching on the outcome of renal transplantation. Ann Surg 187:110–117, 1978.
21. Briggs JD, Canavan JSF, Dick HM, Hamilton DNH, Kyle KF, Macpherson SG, Paton AM, Titterington DM: Influence of HLA matching and blood transfusion on renal allograft survival. Transplantation 25:80–85, 1978.
22. Fuller TC, Delmonico FL, Cosimi AB, Huggins CE, King M, Russell PS: Impact of blood transfusion on renal transplantation. Ann Surg 187:211–218, 1978.
23. Opelz G, Terasaki PI: Prolongation effect of blood transfusions on kidney graft survival. Transplantation 22:380–383, 1976.
24. Speers EK, Vaughn WK, Williams GM, Filo RS, McDonald JC, Mendez-Pilon G, Niblack G: Effect of blood transfusion on cadaver renal transplantation. Transplantation 30:455–463, 1980.
25. Van Es AA, Balner H: Effect of pretransplant transfusion on kidney allograft survival. Transplant Proc 11:127–137, 1979.
26. Andrus CH, Betts RF, May AG, Freeman RB: Cytomegalovirus infection blocks the beneficial effect of pretransplant blood transfusion on renal allograft survival. Transplantation 28:451–456, 1979.

27. Flechner SM, Novick AC, Steinmuller D: Improved cadaver allograft survival in transfused recipients who remain serologically negative for cytomegalovirus. J Urol 127:644–647, 1982.
28. Cosimi AB, Wortis HH, Delmonico FL, Russell PS: Randomized clinical trial of antithymocyte globulin in cadaver renal allograft recipients: Importance of T-cell monitoring. Surgery 80:155–163, 1976.
29. Vincenti F, Duca RM, Amend W, Perkins HA, Cochrum KC, Feduska NJ, Salvatierra O Jr: Immunological factors determining survival of cadaver-kidney transplants. N Engl J Med 299:793–798, 1978.
30. Burleson RL, Jones DB, Yenkikimshian AM, Cornwall C, DeVoe C, DiRito J: Clinical renal preservation by cryoperfusion with an albumin perfusate. Arch Surg 113:688–692, 1976.
31. Fryd DS, Sutherland DER, Simmons RL, Fergusson RM, Kjellstrand CM, Najarian JS: Results of a prospective randomized study on the effect of splenectomy versus no splenectomy in renal transplant patients. Transplant Proc 13:48–56, 1981.
32. Richardson WP, Colvin RB, Cheeseman SH, Tolkoff-Rubin NE, Herrin JT, Cosimi AB, Collins AB, Hirsch MS, McCluskey RT, Russell PS, Rubin RH: Glomerulopathy associated with cytomegalovirus viremia in renal allografts. N Engl J Med 305:57–63, 1981.
33. Baldwin WM, Van Es A, Valentijn RM, Van Gamert GW, Daha MR, Van Es LA: Increased IgM and IgM immune complex-like material in the circulation of renal transplant recipients with primary cytomegalovirus infections. Clin Exp Immunol 50:515–524, 1982.
34. Schooley RT, Hirsch MS, Colvin RB, Cosimi AB, Tolkoff-Rubin NE, McCluskey RT, Burton RC, Russell PS, Herrin JT, Delmonico FL, Giorgi JV, Henle W, Rubin RH: Association of herpesvirus infections with T-lymphocyte-subset alterations, glomerulopathy, and opportunistic infections after renal transplantation. N Engl J Med 308:307–313, 1983.
35. Garnett HM: Isolation of human cytomegalovirus from peripheral blood T cells of renal transplant patients. J Lab Clin Med 99:92–97, 1982.
36. Burleson RL, Lamberson HV, Hubbel C, Burleson A: Prevention of primary CMV infection in renal transplant patients by antibody screening of donors and recipients. (Abstract). This volume.
37. Winston DJ, Pollard RB, Ho WG, Gallagher JG, Rasmussen LE, Huang SN, Lin CH, Gissett TG, Merigan TC, Gale RP: Cytomegalovirus immune plasma in bone marrow transplantation. Ann Intern Med 97:11–18, 1982.
38. Yeager AS, Grumet FC, Hafleigh EB, Arvin AM, Bradley JS, Prober CG: Prevention of Tx-acquired cytomegalovirus infections in newborn infants. J Pediatr 98:281–287, 1981.
39. Glazer JP, Friedman HM, Grossman RA, Starr SE, Barker CF, Perloff LJ, Huang ES, Plotkin SA: Live cytomegalovirus vaccination of renal transplant candidates. Ann Intern Med 91:676–683, 1979.
40. Linnemann CC Jr, Kauffman CA, First MR, Schiff GM, Phair JP: Cellular immune response to cytomegalovirus infection after renal transplantation. Infect Immun 22:176–180, 1978.
41. Pollard RB, Egbert PR, Gallagher JG, Merigan TC: Cytomegalovirus retinitis in immunosuppressed hosts. Ann Intern Med 93:655–670, 1980.
42. Balfour HH Jr, Bean B, Mitchell CD, Sacko GW, Boen JR, Edelman CK: Acyclovir in immunocompromised patients with cytomegalovirus disease: A controlled trial in one institution. Am J Med 73(1A):241–248, 1982.
43. Spector SA, Tyndall M, Kelley E: Effects of acyclovir combined with other antiviral agents on human cytomegalovirus. Am J Med 73 (1A):36–39, 1982.

Cytomegalovirus Infection Following Marrow Transplantation: Risk, Treatment, and Prevention*

Joel D. Meyers, MD

Fred Hutchinson Cancer Research Center and the University of Washington School of Medicine, Seattle, WA 98104

CMV infection of the compromised host has commanded increasing attention, either because the wider availability of methods for specific virologic diagnosis has increased recognition of CMV infection, or because the importance of CMV as a pathogen has indeed increased due to the use of more potent immunosuppressive regimens and to the widespread application of organ allografting. CMV infection is associated with syndromes of fever and leukopenia, hepatitis, arthritis and arthralgias, and a predisposition to bacterial, fungal, and protozoan superinfections among patients receiving renal or cardiac transplants [1–6]. Among patients receiving kidney allografts, CMV infection has been associated with a higher risk of graft loss [1,2,7], apparently due in part to circulating antigen-antibody complexes which may contain CMV [8]. Neonatal CMV infection is associated with fever, hepatitis, prolongation of hospitalization, and, occasionally, death due to disseminated infection with pneumonia [9]. Most recently, CMV has been recognized as one of a number of pathogens affecting patients with AIDS [10]. In these patients it may be the most common pathogen and has been considered for an initiating role in this syndrome, though proof of causality is lacking at this

*Supported by grants CA 18029, CA 30924, and CA 26966 awarded by the National Cancer Institute, DHHS. Dr. Meyers is the recipient of Young Investigator Award AI 15689 from the National Institute of Allergy and Infectious Diseases.

Birth Defects: Original Article Series, Volume 20, Number 1, pages 101–117
© 1984 March of Dimes Birth Defects Foundation

time. CMV is also the most common infectious agent identified after allogeneic (non-twin) marrow transplantation, and has been associated with more deaths than any other single agent.

EPIDEMIOLOGY OF CMV INFECTION

The occurrence of CMV *infection* is determined by epidemiologic factors which are shared by several groups of immunosuppressed patients, while the occurrence of severe CMV *disease* is determined by immunologic factors which may be peculiar to the marrow transplant patient and which are discussed below. The average incidence of CMV infection, defined as recovery or identification of virus in patient specimens or as a significant rise in antibody titer to CMV, is approximately 50% after marrow transplant [11–13]. The incidence is similar among patients transplanted for leukemia or aplastic anemia [13], and although the data are less complete, patients receiving syngeneic (twin) transplants for leukemia appear to have a similarly high risk of infection [14]. The median time of first virus recovery is 8 wk after transplant (Fig. 1), whereas seroconversion occurs at a median of 9 wk (Fig. 2). The median time of CMV pneumonia, the most serious manifestation of CMV disease, is also 8–9 wk after transplant (see below).

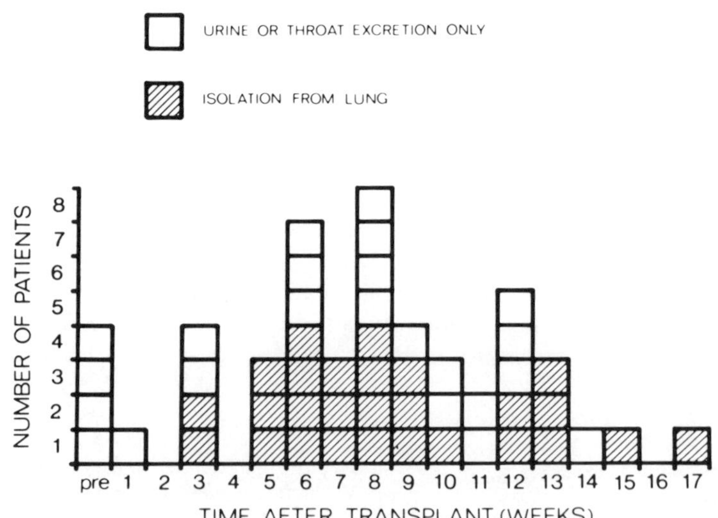

Fig. 1. Time of first isolation of CMV by week before or after marrow transplant. (From Meyers JD et al: Cytomegalovirus infection and specific cell-mediated immunity after marrow transplant. J Infect Dis 142:816–824, 1980, with permission.)

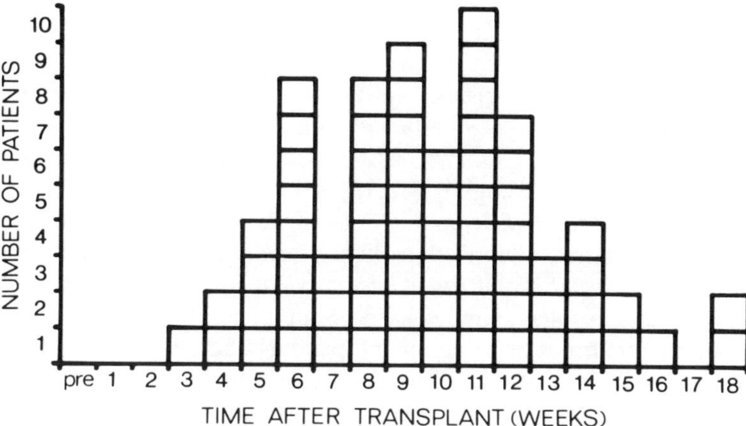

Fig. 2. Time of seroconversion to CMV by week after marrow transplant.

The incidence of infection is lowest among patients who do not have detectable antibody before transplant and who presumably do not harbor latent CMV. Although some seronegative patients may be shown to have antibody if more sensitive serologic techniques are used, the incidence of CMV infection in the first 3 months after transplant among those who are seronegative by complement-fixation assay is 33%, while among seropositive patients the incidence is significantly higher at 62% [15]. Because other sources of CMV infection (eg, sexual transmission) are unlikely immediately following transplant, the presumed source of virus in the seronegative patients is leukocyte-containing blood products. Seropositive patients are also subject to reactivation of latent virus, thereby explaining their higher risk of infection. Seronegative patients who develop CMV infection have been shown to have received a somewhat larger quantity of transfusions than seronegative patients who remain uninfected [16]. These transfusions usually include more than 100 units of platelets taken from random donors. The restriction endonuclease pattern of CMV isolates from ten different patients in one study [17] and from five in another (J.K. McDougall, unpublished data) were all shown to be different, confirming that nosocomial transmission is not occurring.

The risk of infection among seronegative patients who receive prophylactic granulocyte transfusions taken from seropositive donors increases significantly to 75%, whereas the use of granulocytes from seropositive donors for seropositive patients does not affect the incidence of infection [15]. A similar relationship can be shown with the use of *therapeutic* granulocyte transfusions (Table 1). These patients were given granulocytes taken from single donors. These data confirm the association between granulocyte transfusions and CMV infection observed when multiple random donors are used [18], and clearly show that the risk of infection is due to virus acquired from antibody-positive donors. A significantly increased risk of infection due to marrow from seropositive donors has not been found, though the incidence of infection does increase slightly [13,15].

CMV may be recovered from a variety of sites including urine, throat or other upper respiratory sites, conjunctiva, sinus aspirates, rectal swabs, and blood, as well as a variety of tissue specimens including lung, liver, spleen, kidney, adrenals, esophagus, bowel, and brain. The likelihood of recovering virus from either throat or urine among patients excreting CMV is approximately equal at 75%. The frequent recovery of virus from the oropharynx or other upper respiratory sites in marrow transplant patients compared with renal allograft recipients parallels the higher risk of CMV pneumonia observed after marrow transplant. Though most patients excrete CMV only transiently, some become chronic excretors and shed CMV for 1–2 years, or even longer, after transplant.

MANIFESTATIONS OF CMV

As in other immunocompromised hosts, recovery of virus from sites other than tissue does not prove that CMV is the cause of a particular clinical syndrome [19]. Even the recovery of CMV from sites, such as the conjunctiva among patients with conjunctivitis or from sinus aspirates from patients with sinusitis, may not prove that it is the responsible pathogen, since there

TABLE 1. Incidence of CMV Infection Among Seronegative Marrow Transplant Recipients*

		CMV Antibody Titer of Granulocyte Donor	
Patient Group	No. Granulocytes	Negative	Positive
Control group	37/113 (.33)[†]		
Prophylactic granulocytes		16/46 (.35)[‡]	21/28 (.75)[‡]
Therapeutic granulocytes		2/11 (.18)[§]	3/3 (1.00)[§]

*Data adapted from Hersman et al [15].
[†]Number infected/total number in group (proportion infection).
[‡]P = 0.005.
[§]Exact P = 0.027.

are multiple causes of these syndromes after marrow transplant. One such cause is GVHD, which may itself increase the occurrence or severity of CMV disease. It is clear that many patients have truly asymptomatic excretion of CMV from urine or throat.

Patients who acquire primary infection appear to have a higher incidence of clinical symptomatology than patients who excrete CMV in the presence of preexisting antibody. However, the concept of primary infection is complex in the marrow transplant patient, since the responding immune system is that of the marrow donor. Thus, it may be more appropriate to define primary infection based on the serologic status of the marrow *donor* rather than of the patient, even though the virus may be reactivated from latent sites within the patient, and even though the patient's plasma cells may persist and make antibody for some time after transplantation. Conversely, because it appears that the new immune system must repeat its ontogeny [20] after transplant, it may be appropriate to consider *all* CMV infections after marrow transplant as primary infections regardless of the pretransplant serology of patient *or* donor. Despite these *caveats,* it appears that clinical symptoms are more common among seronegative patients who exhibit new antibody production in response to CMV infection after transplant.

In an occasional patient, symptoms are limited to transient myalgias or arthralgias, although we have observed two patients with monoarticular joint effusions. More commonly, patients develop a syndrome consisting of fever, abnormal liver function tests, and transient leukopenia. These symptoms and signs are often attributed to other causes such as acute GVHD, viral hepatitis, or drug (cotrimoxazole or methotrexate) toxicity, until seroconversion becomes apparent. More significant marrow suppression, as well as marrow graft rejection, may also be temporally associated with CMV infection. Among 22 patients transplanted in 1977–1978 who required either additional marrow infusions to "boost" initial engraftment or a second transplant, 14 (64%) had associated CMV infection compared with only 18 of 44 (41%) temporally matched control patients. When these two groups are analyzed together, 16 of 27 patients (59%) with either seroconversion or tissue infection with CMV had a significant fall in neutrophil or platelet count, compared with only 14 of 39 patients (36%) without such CMV infections. These data cannot distinguish between marrow suppression which is due to CMV infection, and CMV infection which is reactivated or exacerbated by graft rejection. However, they do suggest an association of CMV infection with graft suppression or rejection following marrow transplant, similar to graft rejection observed following kidney transplant.

CMV infection has been increasingly recognized as a cause of GI infection after marrow transplant. Ulcerative disease of the esophagus, stomach [21], small intestine, and colon have been observed. Mixed infections of the esophagus, stomach, or bowel with HSV, adenovirus, or *Candida* also occur. Patients with CMV esophagitis may have persistent, debilitating infections even without more widespread virus dissemination. Approximately one third of patients with CMV esophagitis develop subsequent CMV pneumonia, an incidence of dissemination similar to other forms of CMV infection (see below). A small number of patients have developed diffuse bowel involvement with CMV and have died of massive GI bleeding. As noted above, patients with an antibody response to CMV often develop abnormal liver function tests, though clear implication of CMV compared with other causes of hepatic disease, such as acute GVHD, is difficult. We have never recovered CMV from needle biopsies of the liver, although postmortem specimens may yield virus; thus, the diagnosis of CMV hepatitis is usually presumptive in infected patients.

Finally, between one quarter and one third of patients with CMV infection have detectable viremia. Some of these patients have asymptomatic infection despite viremia, and only about one third of viremic patients progress to CMV pneumonia. However, more than one half of patients with pneumonia have viremia, and the mortality rate among patients with pneumonia and viremia appears to be higher than among those without detectable viremia [22].

CMV PNEUMONIA

The most important manifestation of CMV infection after allogeneic marrow transplant is CMV pneumonia. In a review of 952 allogeneic marrow transplant recipients, CMV pneumonia occurred in 147 (15%) and made up 44% of all nonbacterial causes of pneumonia [23]. Approximately one third of all infected patients develop CMV pneumonia. Risk is highest between 5 and 13 wk after transplant, with the peak risk at 8 wk (Fig. 3). Multiple risk factors have been associated with the CMV pneumonia. Among allogeneic graft recipients, the risk is significantly higher among patients transplanted for leukemia than among patients transplanted for aplastic anemia. This difference is attributed primarily to the use of total body irradiation for conditioning among leukemics. Furthermore, the addition of *either* total body irradiation or antithymocyte globulin (ATG) and procarbazine to the conditioning regimen, in addition to the standard use of high-dose cyclophosphamide, significantly increases the risk of CMV pneumonia among patients transplanted for aplastic anemia (Fig. 4). Conversely, there have been no cases of CMV pneumonia among twins transplanted for leukemia even

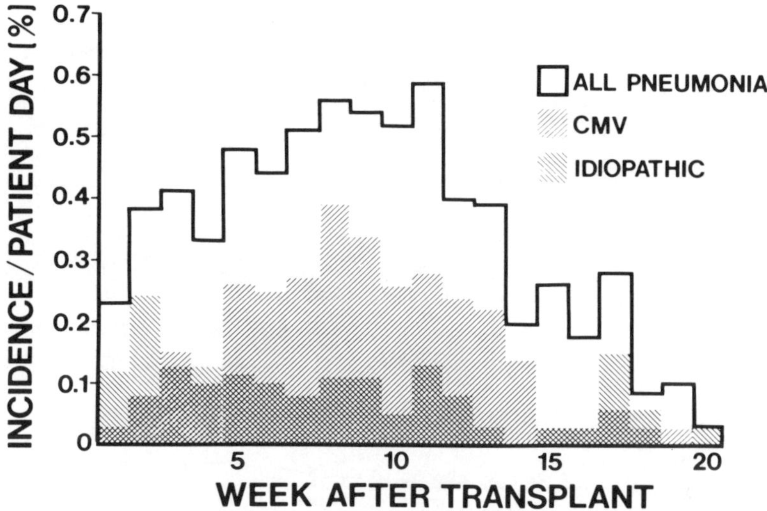

Fig. 3.   Incidence of CMV, idiopathic, and all nonbacterial pneumonias among 952 allogeneic graft recipients expressed as percentage per patient day for each week after marrow transplant. (Figs. 3, 5, and 6 from Meyers JD et al: Biology of interstitial pneumonia after marrow transplantation. In Gale RP (ed): "Recent Advances in Bone Marrow Transplantation." New York: Alan R Liss, 1983, p 405, with permission.)

though they also receive total body irradiation and have a similar overall incidence of CMV infection [14].

The occurrence of more severe acute GVHD also increases the risk of CMV pneumonia (Fig. 5), and treatment with ATG increases this risk even further. Additional risk factors include: older age, seropositivity before transplant, and use of cytotoxic agents in addition to cyclophosphamide for conditioning of patients with leukemia. The risk associated with seropositivity is presumably due to the higher infection rate in that group. The risk associated with age is not explained but is *not* due to an increasing proportion of seropositives among older patient groups [23]. The presumed explanation for many of these observations is the presence or absence of a specific immune response to CMV after transplant (see below).

Most patients with CMV pneumonia develop diffuse reticular-nodular or interstitial infiltrates, hypoxia, and fever. However, localized segmental, alveolar, and nodular infiltrates have all been observed. Open-lung biopsy must be performed to provide the specific diagnosis of CMV pneumonia and to rule out other causes of diffuse pulmonary infiltrates. Although cells bearing characteristic CMV inclusions or with CMV antigen detected by immunofluorescence [24] have been obtained by endotracheal aspiration or

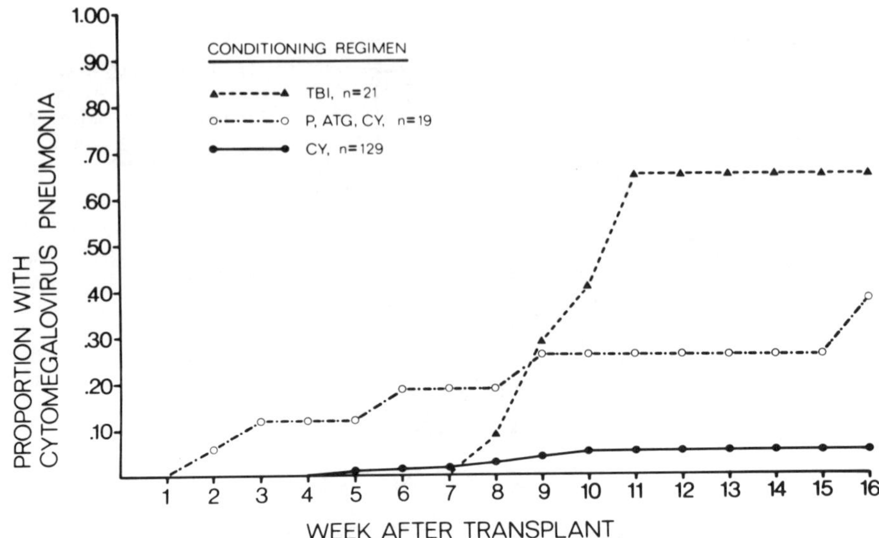

Fig. 4. Kaplan-Meyer product limit estimate of the risk of developing CMV pneumonia after allogeneic marrow transplant for aplastic anemia, by conditioning regimen. (From Meyers JD, Flournoy N, Thomas ED: Nonbacterial pneumonia after allogeneic marrow transplantation: A review of ten years' experience. Rev Infect Dis 4:1119–1132, 1982, with permission.)

bronchopulmonary lavage in patients with CMV pneumonia, the sensitivity and specificity of these tests for the diagnosis of CMV pneumonia are not yet known. In particular, bronchoscopic biopsies have not been reliable [25]. The median survival of patients with CMV pneumonia is three weeks or less from onset, and the case fatality rate is 88%.

Although defective immune responses appear to be the primary reason for the high incidence of CMV pneumonia after marrow transplant, there is also evidence that CMV has a predilection for the lung. Drew et al [26] have shown that CMV replicates better than HSV in pulmonary macrophages in vitro. Studies using in situ hybridization for detection of CMV-specific RNA in tissue showed a higher density of CMV RNA in lung tissue compared with other organs such as liver or spleen, even among patients with disseminated infection [23,27]. The higher incidence of CMV pneumonia among marrow allograft recipients compared with recipients of renal or cardiac transplants is probably due to a multitude of factors, possibly including an increased propensity for CMV to replicate in the lungs of patients who have received total body irradiation.

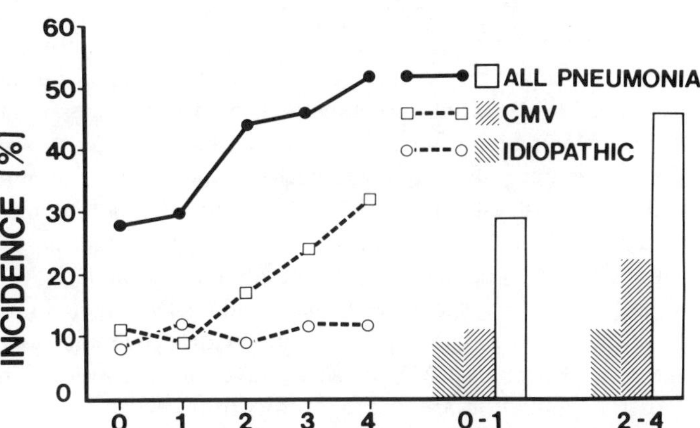

Fig. 5. Incidence of CMV, idiopathic, and all nonbacterial pneumonias by grade of acute GVHD. The incidence of CMV and of all pneumonias was significantly higher (P = 0.00005) among patients with grades 2 to 4 GVHD compared to those with grades 0 to 1.

IMMUNE RESPONSE TO CMV AFTER MARROW TRANSPLANT

Marrow transplant patients lose both nonspecific and specific immune responsiveness after transplant regardless of type of match (allogeneic *v* syngeneic) or underlying illness (malignancy *v* aplasia) [13,20]. Thereafter, restoration of immunity is dependent on maturation of the transplanted donor marrow and is influenced by many factors, including the occurrence of acute or chronic GVHD and exposure to specific antigens. Many of the risk factors for CMV pneumonia mentioned above, including the occurrence of GVHD and its treatment with ATG, the use of total body irradiation or ATG for conditioning among patients with aplastic anemia, the use of cytotoxic agents in addition to cyclophosphamide for patients with leukemia, and transplantation from syngeneic *v* allogeneic donors, may be mediated through their effects on reconstitution of the immune system.

The immune response, which determines both the severity of, and recovery from CMV disease, has been the subject of several studies. In general, the specific lymphocyte transformation response to CMV does not appear to be the crucial response after allogeneic transplant, although responses are better among patients transplanted for aplastic anemia than among those transplanted for leukemia [13], and survival appears to be correlated with positive transformation responses in recent treatment trials [28,29]. Nonspecific cytotoxic responses to K562 tumor cells (NK activity) have been associated with recovery as determined by Quinnan et al [30,31], though others did not find this relationship [32]. The response of either cytotoxic T cells to CMV-infected and major histocompatibility antigen-matched target cells or of NK cells to CMV-infected target cells has also been associated with recovery from CMV pneumonia [30,31]. It is likely that a combination of these responses are necessary in vivo, perhaps including endogenous IFN production [33]. In contrast, production of antibody has not been associated with either recovery from CMV pneumonia or with prolongation of survival [23], although antibody-dependent cell-mediated cytotoxicity (ADCC) has not been studied with CMV-specific antibody and CMV-infected target cells. Data showing that patients with aplastic anemia or syngeneic donors, who have a lower risk of serious CMV disease, have better cytotoxic responses to CMV after transplantation are lacking at this time.

TREATMENT AND PREVENTION OF CMV INFECTION

A series of trials of antiviral agents for the treatment of biopsy-proven CMV pneumonia are summarized in Table 2. Treatment with these agents has neither changed the ultimate outcome of CMV pneumonia nor prolonged survival (Fig. 6). A consistent decrease in the titer of virus recovered from lung tissue before and after treatment was found only with the treatment regimen of vidarabine and human α (leukocyte) IFN (Table 2), although this regimen was also the most toxic [28]. Whether the surviving patients, or the patients in whom a substantial decrease in virus titer in the lung was found, were infected with strains of CMV unusually sensitive to these agents, remains to be determined. Initial trials with other agents, such as recombinant

TABLE 2. Results of Treatment Trials for CMV Pneumonia After Marrow Transplant*

Treatment Regimen	No. Treated	No. Surviving	Toxicity		Virus Recovered From Lung at	
			Marrow	Neurologic	Biopsy	Autopsy
Vidarabine	9	2	3	1	$3 \times 10^{7\ddagger}$	7×10^6
IFN[†]	8	0	3	0	3×10^4	3×10^3
Vidarabine + IFN[†]	7	1	4	2	5×10^4	1×10^2
Acyclovir	8	1	3	1	1×10^5	2×10^5
Acyclovir + IFN[†]	13	3	5	2	6×10^5	3×10^4

*Adapted from Meyers et al [23].
[†]Cantell α (leukocyte) IFN.
[‡]Mean tissue culture infectious dose 50%/gm of lung tissue. Figures represent paired lung specimens only.

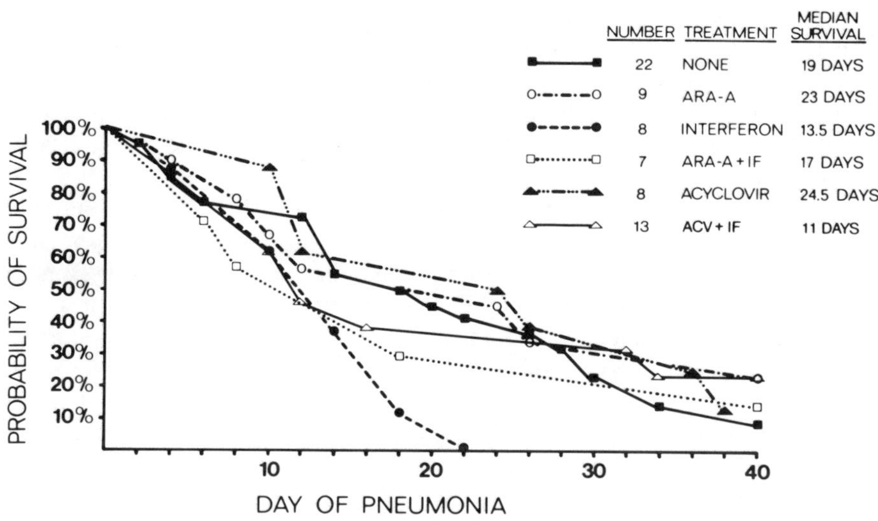

Fig. 6. Probability of survival of pneumonia by day among patients with biopsy-proven CMV pneumonia. Treatment regimen, numbers of patients treated, and median survival are indicated on the figure.

α-IFN or higher doses of purified lymphoblastoid IFN combined with high-dose acyclovir, have been similarly unsuccessful (unpublished data). Although treatment of CMV infection with these agents may prove to be successful in less immunosuppressed patients, neither agent appears to be beneficial in profoundly immunosuppressed marrow transplant recipients with established severe CMV infection.

Prophylaxis with these antiviral agents has not been extensively studied. A trial of the intermittent use of vidarabine given at doses of 5 mg/kg/d for periods of up to ten days did not substantially decrease the incidence of serious CMV infection [34]. Although acyclovir used for the treatment or prophylaxis of HSV infection has not affected the occurrence of subsequent CMV infection after marrow transplant [35–37], the use of higher doses of acyclovir given for a prolonged period after marrow transplant has not yet been studied.

Human leukocyte IFN given prophylactically has been successful in reducing the incidence and severity of CMV infection after renal transplant [38] and remains a candidate for the prophylaxis of CMV infection after marrow transplant. However, preliminary analysis of an ongoing trial of α (Cantell) IFN given beginning 2–3 wk *after* allogeneic transplant for acute lymphocytic leukemia has not demonstrated a reduction in overall incidence or severity of

CMV infection, though a slight delay in time to excretion or seroconversion was found [39]. It is possible that IFN or other antiviral agents started *before* transplant may be effective for the prophylaxis of CMV infection. This would be especially important among seropositive patients in whom infections may be due to reactivation of latent CMV occurring at the time of total body irradiation.

As discussed above, patients without antibody to CMV before transplantation acquire infection through exposure to exogenous virus, presumably through the large number of leukocyte-containing blood products used after transplant. Although it is not possible to identify donors or specific blood units which contain latent CMV, it is possible to avoid the use of blood taken from antibody-positive donors. Among neonates born to seronegative mothers, use of whole blood taken solely from seronegative donors was effective in eliminating CMV infection [9]. The use of leukocyte-depleted blood or frozen, deglycerolyzed blood has also been shown to reduce CMV infection rates [40,41]. Though the number of transfusions, especially platelets, given after transplant is very large, it should be possible to reduce or eliminate infection due to exogenous CMV among seronegative patients through the sole use of seronegative blood products.

A parallel approach is passive immunization of seronegative patients before exposure to these blood products. Two such studies have been reported. Human plasma with a high antibody titer to CMV was shown to decrease the occurrence of CMV pneumonia among seronegative recipients, though the incidence of all CMV infections was unchanged [42]. A specific immunoglobulin with high antibody titers to CMV has been found to reduce infection rates significantly after marrow transplant in a randomized trial [16]. In this study, globulin was given IM three times before transplantation and then weekly after transplant through week 11. Among patients who received no granulocyte transfusions, globulin recipients developed significantly fewer CMV infections compared with control patients (Table 3 and Fig. 7). No protection was seen among patients who received granulocytes from seropositive donors, while the number of patients receiving granulocytes from seronegative donors was insufficient to draw any firm conclusions. Even among patients who received no granulocytes, the effect was seen only among those who received marrow from seronegative, but not seropositive, marrow donors. This last observation, as well as the lack of effect among recipients of granulocytes from seropositive donors, may suggest a dose-response effect. These studies are continuing, with both commercially available "nonimmune" globulins [43] and high-titer immunoglobulins given IV [44]. Though not expected to be effective among seropositive

TABLE 3. Incidence of CMV Infection Among Seronegative Globulin Recipients and Control Patients by Use of Prophylactic Granulocyte Transfusions*

Granulocyte Use	Globulin Recipients	Control Patients
Seropositive granulocytes[†]	7/8[‡]	6/7
Seronegative granulocytes[†]	1/5	0/6
No granulocytes	2/17 (12%)[§]	8/19 (42%)[§]

*From Meyers JD et al: Successful prevention of cytomegalovirus infection after marrow transplant with cytomegalovirus immune globulin. Ann Intern Med 98:442–446, 1983, with permission.

†Seropositive and seronegative granulocytes refer to the serologic status of the granulocyte donor.

‡Number infected/total number in group.

§Difference significant at P = 0.05 by Fisher's exact test and P = 0.03 by Mantel-Cox test (see Fig. 7).

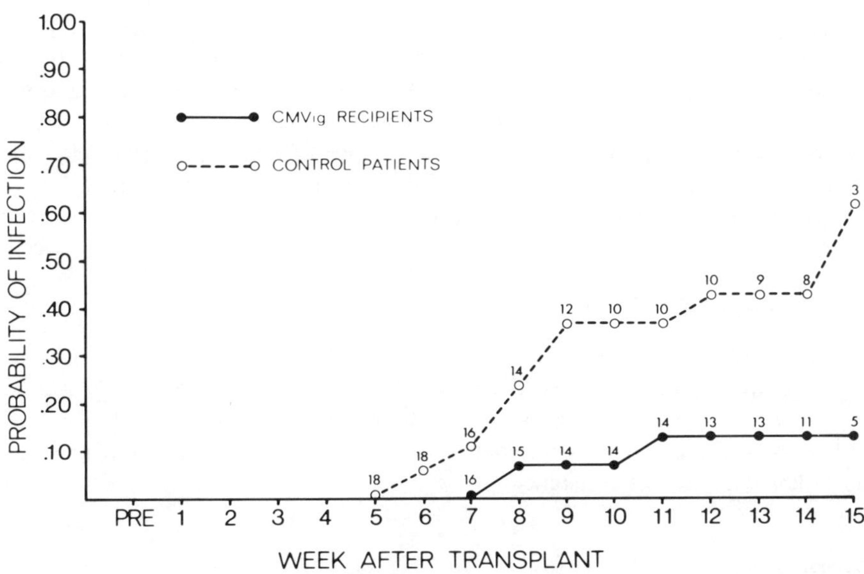

Fig. 7. Probability of acquiring CMV infection by week after transplant among globulin recipients (closed circles) and control patients (open circles) who did not receive prophylactic granulocyte transfusions. The numbers indicate the number of patients still at risk of infection at the beginning of each interval. The risk is different at P = 0.03 by Mantel-Cox test. (From Meyers JD et al: Successful prevention of cytomegalovirus infection after marrow transplant with cytomegalovirus immune globulin. Ann Intern Med 98:442–446, 1983, with permission.)

marrow transplant patients who have reactivation of latent virus in the presence of endogenous antibody, this approach should be effective in reducing infection rates among patients who are seronegative before transplantation.

CONCLUSIONS

CMV infection is a common and often serious infection after marrow transplantation, producing a variety of clinical manifestations from fever and leukopenia to possible graft rejection or fatal pneumonia. The occurrence of serious CMV disease requires both exposure to (or reactivation of) CMV and a host sufficiently immunosuppressed to allow dissemination of infection. It appears that cytotoxic immune responses are important in recovery from CMV infection after marrow transplant, although patients with a lower incidence of serious CMV infection, such as twins or patients transplanted for aplastic anemia, must be studied further to confirm these early suggestions. Use of presently available antiviral agents, including IFN, has not been effective in treating manifest CMV infection, though extensive prophylactic trials have not yet been performed. Reduction in the significance of CMV infection following marrow transplant will depend on better understanding of the immunologic correlates of severe infection and recovery, better treatment (or prevention) of complications of marrow transplant such as acute GVHD, development of antiviral agents that are more effective against CMV, and reduction of exposure to exogenous virus through screening of blood products or the prophylactic use of immune globulins.

ACKNOWLEDGMENTS

We gratefully acknowledge the assistance of Kimberly B. Porter, Lila M. Day, Judith Anderson, Sreelekha Devarayalu, Barbara Newton, R.N., James C. Wade, M.D., and the nurses and physicians of the Seattle Marrow Transplant Team in the performance of these studies. Lisa Eldred provided excellent manuscript assistance.

REFERENCES

1. Rubin RH, Cosimi AB, Tolkoff-Rubin NE, Russell PS, Hirsch MS: Infectious disease syndromes attributable to cytomegalovirus and their significance among renal transplant recipients. Transplantation 24:458–464, 1977.
2. Betts RF, Freeman RB, Douglas RG Jr, Talley TE: Clinical manifestations of renal allograft derived primary cytomegalovirus infection. Am J Dis Child 131:759–763, 1977.

3. Fiala M, Payne JE, Berne TV, Moore TC, Henle W, Montgomerie JZ, Chatterjee SN, Guze LB: Epidemiology of cytomegalovirus infection after transplantation and immunosuppression. J Infect Dis 132:421–433, 1975.

4. Peterson PK, Balfour HH Jr, Marker SC, Fryd DS, Howard RJ, Simmons RL: Cytomegalovirus disease in renal allograft recipients: A prospective study of the clinical features, risk factors and impact on renal transplantation. Medicine 59:283–300, 1980.

5. Rand KH, Pollard RB, Merigan TC: Increased pulmonary superinfections in cardiac-transplant patients undergoing primary cytomegalovirus infection. N Engl J Med 298:951–953, 1978.

6. Chatterjee SN, Fiala M, Weiner J, Stewart JA, Stacey B, Warner N: Primary cytomegalovirus and opportunistic infections. Incidence in renal transplant recipients. JAMA 240:2446–2449, 1978.

7. Fryd DS, Peterson PK, Ferguson RM, Simmons RL, Balfour HH Jr, Najarian JS: Cytomegalovirus as a risk factor in renal transplantation. Transplantation 30:436–439, 1980.

8. Richardson WP, Colvin RB, Cheeseman SH, Tolkoff-Rubin NE, Herrin JT, Cosimi AB, Collins AB, Hirsch MS, McCluskey RT, Russell PS, Rubin RH: Glomerulopathy associated with cytomegalovirus viremia in renal allografts. N Engl J Med 305:57–63, 1981.

9. Yeager AS, Grumet FC, Hafleigh EB, Arvin AM, Bradley JS, Prober CG: Prevention of transfusion-acquired cytomegalovirus infections in newborn infants. J Pediatr 98:281–287, 1981.

10. Durack DT: Opportunistic infections and Kaposi's sarcoma in homosexual men. N Engl J Med 305:1465–1467, 1981.

11. Neiman PE, Reeves W, Ray G, Flournoy N, Lerner KG, Sale GE, Thomas ED: A prospective analysis of interstitial pneumonia and opportunistic viral infection among recipients of allogeneic bone marrow grafts. J Infect Dis 136:754–767, 1977.

12. Winston DJ, Gale RP, Meyer DV, Young LS, and the UCLA Bone Marrow Transplantation Group: Infectious complications of human bone marrow transplantation. Medicine 58:1–31, 1979.

13. Meyers JD, Flournoy N, Thomas ED: Cytomegalovirus infection and specific cell-mediated immunity after marrow transplant. J Infect Dis 142:816–824, 1980.

14. Appelbaum FR, Meyers JD, Fefer A, Flournoy N, Cheever MA, Greenberg PD, Hackman R, Thomas ED: Nonbacterial nonfungal pneumonia following marrow transplantation in 100 identical twins. Transplantation 33:265–268, 1982.

15. Hersman J, Meyers JD, Thomas ED, Buckner CD, Clift R: The effect of granulocyte transfusions upon the incidence of cytomegalovirus infection after allogeneic marrow transplantation. Ann Intern Med 96:149–152, 1982.

16. Meyers JD, Leszczynski J, Zaia JA, Flournoy N, Newton B, Snydman DR, Wright GG, Levin MJ, Thomas ED: Successful prevention of cytomegalovirus infection after marrow transplant with cytomegalovirus immune globulin. Ann Intern Med 98:442–446, 1983.

17. Huang ES, Winston DJ, Miller MJ, Ho WG, Gale RP: Molecular analysis of cytomegalovirus isolates from bone marrow transplant recipients. (Abstract #817) Programs and Abstracts of the 21st Interscience Conference on Antimicrobial Agents and Chemotherapy. Chicago, IL, November 4–6, 1981.

18. Winston DJ, Ho WG, Howell CL, Miller MJ, Mickey R, Martin WJ, Lin C-H, Gale RP: Cytomegalovirus infections associated with leukocyte transfusions. Ann Intern Med 93:671–675, 1980.

19. Friedman HM: Cytomegalovirus: Subclinical infection or disease? Am J Med 70:215–217, 1981.

20. Noel DR, Witherspoon RP, Storb R, Atkinson K, Doney K, Mickelson EM, Ochs HD, Warren RP, Weiden PL, Thomas ED: Does graft-versus-host disease influence the tempo of immunologic recovery after allogeneic human marrow transplantation? An observation on 56 long-term survivors. Blood 51:1087–1105, 1978.

21. Strayer DS, Phillips GB, Barker KH, Winokur T, DeSchryver-Kecskemeti K: Gastric cytomegalovirus infection in bone marrow transplant patients: An indication of generalized disease. Cancer 48:1478–1483, 1981.

22. Meyers JD, Wade JC, McGuffin RW, Springmeyer SC, Thomas ED: The use of acyclovir for cytomegalovirus infections in the compromised host. J Antimicrob Chemother (In press).

23. Meyers JD, Flournoy N, Wade JC, Hackman RC, McDougall JK, Neiman PE, Thomas ED: Biology of interstitial pneumonia after marrow transplantation. In Gale RP (ed): "Recent Advances in Bone Marrow Transplantation." New York: Alan R Liss, 1983, p 405.

24. Goldstein LC, McDougall J, Hackman R, Meyers JD, Thomas ED, Nowinski RC: Monoclonal antibodies to cytomegalovirus: Rapid identification of clinical isolates and preliminary use in diagnosis of cytomegalovirus pneumonia. Infect Immun 38:273–281, 1982.

25. Springmeyer SC, Silvestri RC, Sale GE, Peterson DL, Weems CE, Huseby JS, Hudson LD, Thomas ED: The role of transbronchial biopsy for the diagnosis of diffuse pneumonias in immunocompromised marrow transplant recipients. Am Rev Respir Dis 126:763–765, 1982.

26. Drew WL, Mintz L, Hoo R, Finley TN: Growth of herpes simplex and cytomegalovirus in cultured human alveolar macrophages. Am Rev Respir Dis 119:287–291, 1979.

27. Medeiros ER, Neiman PE, McDougall JK, Thomas ED: Detection of cytomegalovirus RNA in lung tissue from patients with interstitial pneumonia following bone marrow transplantation. (Abstract) International Conference on Human Herpesviruses. Atlanta, GA, March 17–21, 1980.

28. Meyers JD, McGuffin RW, Bryson YJ, Cantell K, Thomas ED: Treatment of cytomegalovirus pneumonia after marrow transplant with combined vidarabine and human leukocyte interferon. J Infect Dis 146:80–84, 1982.

29. Wade JC, Hintz M, McGuffin RW, Springmeyer SC, Connor JD, Meyers JD: Treatment of cytomegalovirus pneumonia with high-dose acyclovir. Am J Med 73(1A):249–256, 1982.

30. Quinnan GV Jr, Kirmani N, Esber E, Saral R, Manischewitz JF, Rogers JL, Rook AH, Santos GW, Burns WH: HLA-restricted cytotoxic T lymphocyte and nonthymic cytotoxic lymphocyte responses to cytomegalovirus infection of bone marrow transplant recipients. J Immunol 126:2036–2041, 1981.

31. Quinnan GV Jr, Kirmani N, Rook AH, Manischewitz JF, Jackson L, Moreschi G, Santos GW, Saral R, Burns WH: HLA-restricted T-lymphocyte and non-T-lymphocyte cytotoxic responses correlate with recovery from cytomegalovirus infection in bone-marrow-transplant recipients. N Engl J Med 307:6–13, 1982.

32. Livnat S, Seigneuret M, Storb R, Prentice RL: Analysis of cytotoxic effector cell function in patients with leukemia or aplastic anemia before and after marrow transplantation. J Immunol 124:481–490, 1980.

33. Levin MJ, Parkman R, Oxman MN, Rappeport JM, Simpson M, Leary PL: Proliferative and interferon responses by peripheral blood mononuclear cells after bone marrow transplantation in humans. Infect Immun 20:678–684, 1978.

34. Kraemer KG, Neiman PE, Reeves WC, Thomas ED: Prophylactic adenine arabinoside following marrow transplantation. Transplant Proc 10:237–240, 1978.
35. Saral R, Burns WH, Laskin OL, Santos GW, Lietman PS: Acyclovir prophylaxis of herpes-simplex-virus infections. A randomized, double-blind, controlled trial in bone-marrow-transplant recipients. N Engl J Med 305:63–67, 1981.
36. Wade JC, Newton B, McLaren C, Flournoy N, Keeney RE, Meyers JD: Intravenous acyclovir to treat mucocutaneous herpes simplex virus infection after marrow transplantation: A double-blind trial. Ann Intern Med 96:265–269, 1982.
37. Wade JC, Newton B, Flournoy N, Meyers JD: Oral acyclovir prophylaxis of herpes simplex virus infections after marrow transplant. 22nd Interscience Conference on Antimicrobial Agents and Chemotherapy. Miami, FL, October, 1982.
38. Cheeseman SH, Rubin RH, Stewart JA, Tolkoff-Rubin NE, Cosimi AB, Cantell K, Gilbert J, Winkle S, Herrin JT, Black PH, Russell PS, Hirsch MS: Controlled clinical trial of prophylactic human-leukocyte interferon in renal transplantation. Effects on cytomegalovirus and herpes simplex infections. N Engl J Med 300:1345–1349, 1979.
39. Meyers JD, McGuffin RW, Thomas ED: Prophylactic human leukocyte interferon (HLI) after allogeneic marrow transplant: Immunologic and virologic effects. 22nd Interscience Conference on Antimicrobial Agents and Chemotherapy. Miami, FL, October 1982.
40. Lang DJ, Ebert PA, Rodgers BM, Boggess HP, Rixls RS: Reduction of post-perfusion cytomegalovirus-infections following the use of leukocyte depleted blood. Transfusion 17:391–395, 1977.
41. Tolkoff-Rubin NE, Rubin RH, Keller EE, Baker BP, Stewart JA, Hirsch MS: Cytomegalovirus infection in dialysis patients and personnel. Ann Intern Med 89:625–628, 1978.
42. Winston DJ, Pollard RB, Ho WG, Gallagher JG, Rasmussen LE, Huang SN-Y, Lin C-H, Gossett TG, Merigan TC, Gale RP: Cytomegalovirus immune plasma in bone marrow transplant recipients. Ann Intern Med 97:11–18, 1982.
43. Winston DJ, Ho WG, Rasmussen LE, Lin C-H, Chu CL, Merigan TC, Gale RP: Use of intravenous immune globulin in patients receiving bone marrow transplants. J Clin Immunol 2 (April suppl):42S–46S, 1982.
44. Snydman DR, McIver J, Leszczynski J, Grady GF, Berardi VP, Wright GG, Cho S, Logerfo F: Pharmacokinetics and safety of an intravenous cytomegalovirus immune globulin (CMVIG-IV) in renal transplant recipients. (Abstract #332) 22nd Interscience Conference on Antimicrobial Agents and Chemotherapy. Miami, FL, October 1982.

SECTION 3:
PATHOGENESIS OF CYTOMEGALOVIRUS

Sexual Transmission of CMV and Its Relationship to Kaposi Sarcoma in Homosexual Men

W. Lawrence Drew, MD, PhD

Clinical Laboratory and Infectious Diseases, Mount Zion Hospital and Medical Center, San Francisco, CA 94120

In populations of low socioeconomic status or in underdeveloped countries, postneonatal infection with CMV is common, apparently as a result of overcrowded living conditions and/or exposure to CMV-positive breast milk [1]. In the United States these sources of infection are less important; if a child escapes congenital and perinatal infection with CMV, he may avoid infection by this virus for many years. In general, only 10%–15% of American adolescents are seroimmune. However, during young adulthood the rate of infection rapidly increases, so that, by age 35, approximately 50% show serologic evidence of past infection [2]. There is increasing evidence that many of these infections are sexually transmitted. This evidence may be summarized as follows:

1) The virus does not spread readily among adults by ordinary, nonsexual, person-to-person contact [3], even during prolonged exposure to individuals known to be excreting the virus [3,4]. Wenzel et al [3] reported only 1% seroconversion among a group of military recruits during a 14-week training program. In similar settings, agents such as *Mycoplasma pneumoniae* and adenovirus spread readily. In two dialysis units where hospital personnel were regularly exposed to CMV-infected patients, transmission to seronegative individuals did not occur [4,5]. In a study of pediatric nurses exposed to CMV-infected infants and children, there was a trend toward a higher rate of seroconversion among the nurses compared to nonpatient-care personnel, but the differences were not statistically significant, despite the fact that no seroconversion occurred in the latter group over an average of 29 months of

Birth Defects: Original Article Series, Volume 20, Number 1, pages 121–129
© **1984 March of Dimes Birth Defects Foundation**

follow-up [6]! This finding was rather remarkable, since several studies have documented an approximately 2% rate of seroconversion per year among women aged 15 to 35 years.

2) Rates of seroconversion are highest among those attending clinics for sexually transmitted diseases. The rate of seroconversion for women attending a venereal disease clinic was 28% per year [7] *v* a rate of approximately 2% for women attending nonvenereal disease clinics. Among heterosexual men, we have shown a higher prevalence of seropositivity in those attending a venereal disease clinic (54%) *v* random blood donors of similar age (43%) (Table 1) [8].

3) There is a high rate of CMV isolation from the cervix of women attending clinics for suspected venereal disease. CMV has been cultured from the cervix of 13% to 25% of women undergoing gynecologic examination for suspected sexually transmitted disease [7,9,10], and recovery of CMV from the cervix was significantly more likely in women with documented past or active gonococcal infection. In contrast, none of 76 women undergoing routine or required gynecologic examination was CMV-positive [9].

4) Sexual contacts of women whose cervix cultures are CMV-positive are more likely to have the virus in their semen. In a study at a venereal disease clinic, Handsfield et al [7] determined that 4 of 21 (19%) male sexual contacts of women whose cervix was CMV-positive had the virus in their semen or urine. In contrast, CMV culture was negative in all but one of 48 male sexual partners of women whose cervix was culture-negative (P = 0.027). Restriction enzyme mapping from two partner pairs revealed definite similarity of isolates from sexual contacts which were, in turn, distinct from epidemiologically unrelated strains [7]. Chretien et al [11] reported CMV mononucleosis in two men after sexual contact with a woman whose cervix and urine were CMV-positive. Evidence of recent CMV infection was also found in

TABLE 1. Prevalence of Antibody to CMV Among Homosexual and Heterosexual Men Attending a Venereal Disease Clinic and Volunteer Male Blood Donors

Age (yr)	No. Positive/No. Tested (%)		
	Heterosexual	Homosexual	Blood Donors
18–29	18/38 (47.4)	70/75 (93.3)	10/28 (35.7)
≥30	20/32 (62.5)	60/64 (93.8)	34/75 (45.9)
Total	38/70 (54.3)	130/139 (93.5)	44/103 (42.7)

NOTE: Differences between homosexual men and both heterosexual men and volunteer male blood donors are statistically significant (P < 0.005) for each age group and for totals. Blood donors were unselected as to sexual orientation.

another female sexual contact of one of the two male patients, whereas two roommates of these patients, who were not their sexual contacts, had negative CMV CF antibody titers.

5) CMV infection is highly prevalent among homosexual men. Because sexually transmitted diseases may occur with an especially high frequency in homosexual men, we prospectively studied the prevalence of cytomegaloviruria in homosexual men. The initial documentation of high rates of CMV infection in gay men resulted from prevalence studies performed by us at the San Francisco Venereal Disease Clinic in 1979 [8]. We observed urinary excretion of CMV in 14 of 90 (7.4%) homosexual men, but in none of 101 heterosexual men attending the same clinic (P < 0.005). Similarly, antibody to CMV was detected in 130 of 139 (93.5%) homosexual, but in only 38 of 70 (54.3%) heterosexual men (P < 0.005). Subsequently, we have studied prospectively 237 homosexual men [12].

On initial testing, 206 of the 237 men (86.9%) had CMV antibody. Of the 31 initially seronegative men, 22 had seroconverted by the ninth month of the study for an attack rate of 71% during this time period. During a mean follow-up period of 14.3 months (range = 2–20), 66 of the 206 initially seropositive men (32%) excreted CMV in their urine on one or more occasions. In a separate study, simultaneous urine and semen specimens were obtained from 52 homosexual men. CMV was recovered from 18 of the semen specimens, but from only four of the corresponding urine samples (Table 2). Specimens from a single individual grew CMV from the urine, but not from the semen. Semen would therefore appear to be approximately five times as sensitive as urine in detecting the presence of CMV. Clearly, the widespread occurrence of CMV viruria and virus in semen in this population makes exposure to the virus all but inevitable, and accounts for the extraordinarily high attack rate of CMV infections among seronegative homosexual men.

CMV IgM antibody was detected on one or more occasions in the sera of over 90% of the study subjects. In contrast, IgM antibody to CMV was

TABLE 2. Recovery of CMV From Simultaneously Collected Urine and Semen Specimens From 52 Homosexual Men

Urine Culture	Semen Culture	
	Positive	Negative
Positive (4)	3	1
Negative (48)	15	33

P = 0.001 (McNemar's test)

detected in only 3.8% of 103 sera randomly collected from volunteer male blood donors. In the homosexual men, IgM antibody tended to appear, disappear, then reappear again over the course of time. There was no temporal correlation between the presence of CMV viruria and serum IgM antibody titers. The high prevalence of CMV IgM antibody in longstanding seropositive men suggests that homosexuals are continually being reexposed to (and possibly reinfected with) exogenous strains of the virus.

Questionnaires concerning demographic data, clinical histories, and sexual practices were completed by 78 subjects (54 initially seropositive; 24 initially seronegative, including 17 of the 22 seroconverters and 7 of the 9 who remained persistently seronegative).

None of 17 CMV seroconverters reported clinical illness during a three-month period encompassing the time of their seroconversion. We can therefore surmise that primary infection with CMV produces symptomatic illness in less than 6% of cases.

Information was obtained regarding the frequency of participation in the following sex practices: Kissing; oral-anal contact (oral role); oral-anal contact (anal role); fellatio (oral role); fellatio (genital role); anal intercourse (active role); and anal intercourse (passive role) (Table 3). Only passive anal intercourse correlated with the initial presence of anti-CMV antibody or with seroconversion to this virus during the course of the study. CMV antibody was present in 96.6% of 59 men who engaged in passive anal intercourse, but in only 73.7% of men who did not (P < 0.01). The latter figure does not differ significantly from the prevalence of CMV antibody among heterosexual men attending a venereal disease clinic (Table 2). These data suggest that exposure of the anorectal mucosa to CMV-infected semen constitutes the major route of acquisition of CMV infection by homosexual men.

These accumulated results provide a background against which to evaluate the reports documenting CMV infection in homosexual men with AIDS and Kaposi sarcoma (KS) [13,14].

Over 300 cases of malignant KS have been reported since the beginning of the AIDS epidemic. The identity of the putative transmissible agent causing immune deficiency in AIDS patients is altogether unknown, although CMV is a candidate. Whether or not this virus is the etiologic agent of immune deficiency, there is increasing evidence that in a suitably predisposed (ie, immunocompromised) host, CMV is capable of causing oncogenic transformation of endothelial cells leading to KS. This conclusion is based on three lines of evidence:

a) *The oncogenic potential of CMV.* CMV has been considered a possible oncogenic virus by virtue of its ability to stimulate synthesis of DNA and

TABLE 3. Prevalence of CMV IgG Antibody Among 78 Homosexual Men According to Sexual Practice

Sexual Practice	No. of Men	No. Antibody-Positive*	
Kissing			
Yes	77	70 (91)	NS
No	1	1 (100)	
Oral-genital contact (active)			
Yes	78	71 (91)	NS
No	0	—	
Oral-genital contact (passive: with ejaculation)			
Yes	71	64 (90)	NS
No	7	7 (100)	
Oral-genital contact (passive: no ejaculation)			
Yes	75	68 (91)	NS
No	3	3 (100)	
Anal-genital contact (active)			
Yes	74	67 (91)	NS
No	4	4 (100)	
Anal-genital contact (passive: with ejaculation)			
Yes	59	57 (97)	$P = 0.008$[†]
No	19	14 (74)	
Anal-genital contact (passive: no ejaculation)			
Yes	57	54 (95)	NS
No	21	17 (81)	
Oral-anal contact (active)			
Yes	47	44 (94)	NS
No	31	27 (87)	
Oral-anal contact (passive)			
Yes	66	61 (92)	NS
No	12	10 (83)	

*Numbers in parentheses denote percentage.
[†]Fisher's exact test.
NS = not significant.

RNA in host cells [15], and its ability to transform human embryo fibroblasts, which then grow as sarcomatous tumors when transplanted to immunosuppressed mice [16]. Recently, Nelson et al [17] have refined the latter observation by identifying the transforming segment of the CMV genome.

b) *Epidemiologic evidence associating CMV with KS.* The epidemiologic evidence for CMV involvement in KS derives from the heightened prevalence of this tumor in two groups of individuals, renal transplant patients and homosexual men, who share the twin features of immunosuppression and extremely high rates of active CMV infection. There have been at least 36 reports of KS in renal transplant patients [18–21]; it is estimated that KS accounts for more than 3% of all malignancies occurring in organ transplant recipients [19]. Although CMV studies have not been specifically reported in these patients, renal transplant recipients as a group are subject to extremely high rates of primary or reactivated CMV infection [22], and all these patients are, of course, immunosuppressed during the posttransplant period. KS appears an average of 16 to 36 months after transplantation, suggesting an approximate incubation period for the development of the tumor in immunocompromised patients.

High rates of CMV infection are well documented in homosexual men [8, 13]. To date, we have studied 57 homosexual men with KS for CMV antibody, and all are positive. Of 39 who have had appropriate secretion cultures, 24 (62%) have been positive. Zur Hausen [23] has stated "it is likely that the epigenetic burden of persisting viral DNA increases with the number of infections and is therefore correlated with *age* and *exposure.*" In light of this, it is striking that the average age of homosexual men with KS is 36 years, and that they have been homosexual for an average of 17 years [24]. A quantitative estimate of the extent of CMV exposure among gay men can be inferred from the finding that, even on a single sample, the semen of 25% of homosexual men is CMV culture-positive [12]. The high geometric mean titer of CMV antibody seen in homosexual men *v* heterosexual controls, and the frequent finding of CMV IgM antibody in sera from homosexual men, also support the concept of frequent reexposure.

A further epidemiologic clue linking CMV to KS is the marked discrepancy in the incidence of KS cases among homosexual *v* heterosexual AIDS patients. In New York City, KS accounts for 45% of the AIDS cases in homosexual men, but only 8% of AIDS in heterosexual men [24]. This striking discrepancy suggests that a cofactor may be present in homosexual men that is not present in heterosexuals. This cofactor may be CMV infection since, in contrast to homosexual men, IV drug users, most of whom are heterosexual, do not have high rates of CMV infection. Of 81 IV drug users we have tested, 58 (72%) were seropositive, a rate similar to that observed in heterosexual men in a clinic for sexually transmitted diseases. Other factors, including genetic (HLA-DR5 haplotype, Italian ancestry), may contribute to the disproportionate number of KS cases among homosexual men, but do not provide a total explanation.

The last bit of circumstantial evidence linking CMV to KS stems from work previously reported by Giraldo et al [25]. A significantly higher prevalence of CMV antibody was detected in 46 elderly European and American patients with KS than in two age-matched control groups without KS.

c) *Direct evidence of CMV gene products in KS biopsies.* The best evidence for an association of CMV with KS derives from the demonstration of CMV nucleic acids and antigens in KS tumor biopsies. Boldogh et al [26] detected CMV DNA in six of 12, and RNA in three of nine KS biopsies from African patients. EBV and HSV type 2 sequences were not detected. We reported the presence of CMV RNA by in situ hybridization in two of three KS biopsies from homosexual men whose tumor cultures were negative for replicating CVM [13]. Fenoglio et al [27] confirmed our results by detection of CMV RNA in a KS biopsy from a single homosexual man. Boldogh et al [26] also reported the presence of CMV nuclear antigen by anticomplement immunofluorescence (ACIF) in 14 of 16 KS biopsies from African patients. We have reported detection of CMV antigen by a similar procedure in six of nine biopsy specimens from homosexual men [13], and more recently have found this antigen in an additional nine of 18 cases examined. It is important to note that all of these biopsies were negative for CMV by culture, indicating that CMV genome is present in a nonreplicative—and hence more likely oncogenic—state. Moreover, biopsies of normal skin from all but one of 22 of these patients were negative for CMV antigen, suggesting that the positive biopsies were not simply the result of disseminated CMV infection or a tropism of the virus for skin tissue.

None of the data presented here proves a causal relationship between CMV and KS. Indeed, the presence of the virus or its gene products may only reflect reactivation of latent CMV in tumor tissue, or an affinity of CMV for neoplastic tissue, or carriage of the virus as a passenger within tumor cells. However, detection of CMV RNA and antigen, as in the KS tissues reported here, suggests that the virus is not merely a dormant passenger but is actually directing the synthesis of viral protein(s). Definitive proof of an etiologic role for CMV in the genesis of KS would require the demonstration of protection by a vaccine.

If the hypothesis that CMV is the cofactor which produces KS in homosexual men is correct, then measures for the prevention of CMV infection in this group should be considered. We have shown that at least 25% of homosexual men have CMV in their semen and that the highest risk factor for CMV transmission among homosexual men is anal receptive intercourse, presumably as a result of the introduction of virus-containing semen onto traumatized rectal mucosa. If this sexual practice were avoided, the cycle of CMV transmission might be interrupted. The use of condoms to block CMV transmission has not been studied but might provide an alternative means to avoid exposure of orifices (oral, anal) to semen. Most importantly, reducing the number of sex partners would reduce the chances of contacting the virus-positive semen. Finally, CMV vaccine might be used to prevent acquisition of "wild" CMV infection. Indeed, homosexual men, with their extremely high rate of CMV infection, would be an ideal group in which to test the protective efficacy of a vaccine. Even a killed or subunit vaccine might be useful, since these recipients would subsequently experience multiple live virus challenges.

It may be many years before the putative AIDS agent is identified. In the meantime, homosexual men should initiate protective measures which might at least retard the transmission of a likely cofactor in the genesis of Kaposi sarcoma.

REFERENCES

1. Stagno S, Reynolds DW, Pass RF, Alford CA: Breast milk and the risk of cytomegalovirus infection. N Engl J Med 302:1073–1076, 1980.
2. Wentworth BB, Alexander ER: Seroepidemiology of infections due to members of the herpesvirus group. Am J Epidemiol 94:496–507, 1971.
3. Wenzel RP, McCormick DP, Davies JA, Berling C, Beam WE: Cytomegalovirus infection: A seroepidemiologic study of a recruit population. Am J Epidemiol 97:410–414, 1973.
4. Tolkoff-Rubin NE, Rubin RH, Keller EE, Baker GP, Stewart JA, Hirsch MS: Cytomegalovirus infection in dialysis patients and personnel. Ann Intern Med 89:625–628, 1978.
5. Betts RF, Cestero RVM, Freeman RB, Douglas RG: Epidemiology of cytomegalovirus infection in end stage renal disease. J Med Virol 4:89–96, 1979.
6. Yeager AS: Longitudinal, serological study of cytomegalovirus infections in nurses and in personnel without patient contact. J Clin Microbiol 2:448–451, 1975.
7. Handsfield HH, Chandler CC, Caine VA, McDougall J: Cytomegalovirus infection in sexual partners. Submitted for publication.
8. Drew WL, Mintz L, Miner RC, Sands M, Ketterer B: Prevalence of cytomegalovirus infection in homosexual men. J Infect Dis 143:188–192, 1981.
9. Jordan MC, Rousseau WE, Noble GR, Stewart JA, Chin TDY: Association of cervical cytomegalovirus with venereal disease. N Engl J Med 288:932–934, 1973.
10. Wentworth BB, Bonin P, Holmes KK, Gutman L, Wiesner P, Alexander ER: Isolation of viruses, bacteria and other organisms from venereal disease clinic patients: Methodology and problems associated with multiple isolations. Health Lab Sci 10:75–81, 1973.

11. Chretien JH, McGinniss CG, Muller A: Venereal causes of cytomegalovirus mononucleosis. JAMA 238:1644–1645, 1977.

12. Mintz L, Drew WL, Miner RC, Braff E: Epidemiology of cytomegalovirus infection in homosexual men. Ann Intern Med 99(3):326–329, 1983.

13. Drew WL, Miner RC, Ziegler JL, Gullett JH, Abrams DI et al: Cytomegalovirus and Kaposi's sarcoma in young homosexual men. Lancet 2:125–127, 1982.

14. Ziegler JL, Drew WL, Miner RC, Mintz L, Rosenbaum E et al: Outbreak of Burkitt's-like lymphoma in homosexual men. Lancet 2:631–633, 1982.

15. St. Jean SC, Albrecht TB, Frank FD, Rapp R: Stimulation of cellular DNA synthesis with human cytomegalovirus. J Virol 13:353–362, 1974.

16. Geder L, Lausch R, O'Neill F, Rapp F: Oncogenic transformation of human embryo lung cells by human cytomegalovirus. Science 192:1134–1137, 1976.

17. Nelson J, Fleckenstein B, Galloway DA, McDougall JK: Transformation of NIH3T3 cells with cloned fragments of human cytomegalovirus AD-169. J Virol 43:83, 1982.

18. Myers BD, Kessler E, Levi J, Pick A, Rosenfeld JB, Tikvah P: Kaposi sarcoma in kidney transplant recipients. Arch Intern Med 133:307–311, 1974.

19. Penn I: Kaposi's sarcoma in organ transplant recipients. Transplantation 27:8–11, 1979.

20. Gange RW, Jones EW: Kaposi's sarcoma and immunosuppressive therapy: An appraisal. Clin Exp Dermatol 3:135–146, 1978.

21. Harwood AR, Osoba D, Hofstader SL et al: Kaposi's sarcoma in recipients of renal transplants. Am J Med 67:759–765, 1979.

22. Fiala M, Payne JE, Berne TV et al: Epidemiology of cytomegalovirus infection after transplantation and immunosuppression. J Infect Dis 132:421–432, 1975.

23. Zur Hausen H: The role of viruses in human tumors. Adv Cancer Res 33:77–107, 1980.

24. Marmor M, Friedman-Kien AE, Laubenstein L, Byrum RD, William DC et al: Risk factors for Kaposi's sarcoma in homosexual men. Lancet 1:1083–1086, 1982.

25. Giraldo G, Beth E, Henle W et al: Antibody patterns to herpesviruses in Kaposi's sarcoma. II. Serological association of American Kaposi's sarcoma with cytomegalovirus. Int J Cancer 22:126–131, 1978.

26. Boldogh I, Beth E, Huang E-S, Kyalwazi SK, Giraldo G: Kaposi's sarcoma. IV. Detection of CMV DNA, CMV RNA, and CMNA in tumour biopsies. Int J Cancer 28:469–474, 1981.

27. Fenoglio CM, Oster MW, Lo Gerfo P, Reynolds T, Edelson R et al: Kaposi's sarcoma following chemotherapy for testicular cancer in a homosexual man: Demonstration of cytomegalovirus RNA in sarcoma cells. Hum Pathol 13:955–959, 1982.

Immunology of Cytomegalovirus: Immunosuppressive Effects During Infections

Monto Ho, MD

Departments of Infectious Diseases and Microbiology, Graduate School of Public Health and Division of Infectious Diseases, Department of Medicine, School of Medicine, University of Pittsburgh, Pittsburgh, PA 15261

It is neither possible nor desirable to cover comprehensively all immunologic aspects of CMV in this paper. The subject has been reviewed recently [1], and this volume will cover recent aspects of CMV.

A great deal has been learned recently about the immune responses to CMV. As the structure of the virus becomes better understood, more will be learned about immune responses to specific subunits. Monoclonal antibodies against these have been developed [2]. Regarding humoral immunity, I will only review briefly the clinical significance of some serologic tests.

Most of this paper will concern the cellular immune responses against CMV, a large number of which, depending on different functions of subsets of lymphocytes and macrophages, have been described. Rather than considering each one, I will review the immunosuppressive responses of CMV infection in animals, normal subjects, pregnant women, infants, and in transplant recipients. Some of our data on CMV infection and its immunologic correlates in transplant patients on the new immunosuppressive drug, cyclosporine, will be presented.

ANTIBODY PATTERN IN DIFFERENT TYPES OF INFECTIONS

IgG antibody has been measured by a large number of tests, such as complement-fixation (CF) tests, the immunofluorescence assay (IFA) against early and late antigens, the indirect hemagglutination assay (IHA), and neutralization tests. These antibodies almost always show a conversion or a

Birth Defects: Original Article Series, Volume 20, Number 1, pages 131–147
© **1984 March of Dimes Birth Defects Foundation**

rise depending on the previous serologic state of the patient (Table 1 and [1]).

Besides so-called "summary late antigens," a number of other antigens have been described which elicit specific antibody. For example, membrane antigen (MA) elicits an IgM antibody response which appears one to 13 days after illness in most patients with CMV infections [4]. Others, described below, purport to indicate specific states of infection. There are still a great number of questions about their significance. Betts et al [5] described a complement-dependent cytolytic IgM antibody against unknown late antigens which correlates with symptomatic disease.

Early Antigen

Early antigen (EA) can be demonstrated in infected cells early in infection in the absence of DNA synthesis. The et al [6] thought that its presence indicated current primary infection, but Ten Napel and The [7] showed that it could remain elevated as long as 250 days after a proven CMV mononucleosis in a normal patient.

Stagno et al [8] followed the antibody titers of infected neonates by the IFA-LA, IFA-EA, neutralization IHA, and CF tests. If the mother were seropositive, titers in the neonate were measurable, but normally decreased after birth. In the perinatally infected baby, titers against IFA-EA would rise diagnostically after an initial fall. This rise was more reliable and more rapid

TABLE 1. Antibody Responses Indicating Different States of HCMV Infections

Association	Early Antigens		Late Antigens					
	EA	IEA(PENA)	CF	IFA(ACIF)	IHA	IgM	IgA	IgM Cytolytic
Rise after infection	+	+	+	+	+	+	+	±
Particularly useful after perinatal and congenital infection	+					+		
Associated with persistent viral proliferation	+	+						
May be diminished or absent in severe infection			+	+		+		
Indicates recent infection or reactivation						+	+	
Indicates symptomatic infection								+

than rises in antibody detected by other tests. This pattern was distinguished from that shown by the congenitally infected baby, whose IFA-EA antibody titer did not decrease after birth but remained elevated.

Immediate Early Antigen and Pre-Early Nuclear Antigen

Pre-early antigens are also called immediate early antigens (IEA), one of which is prenuclear early antigen (PENA) determined by the anticomplement immune fluorescence (ACIF) test [9]. These antigens develop in cells 20 minutes to one hour after infection, even earlier than EA. IEA was identified by the indirect immunofluorescence test [10] or by the immunoperoxidase test [11]. PENA may resemble Epstein-Barr virus nuclear antigen (EBNA), but the exact significance of antibodies to IEA or PENA is still unclear.

Some authors [11] believe that the presence of antibody against EA is closely associated with active viral proliferation in patients who may be chronically secreting virus. Others do not believe that antibodies to EA, IEA, or PENA are that specific [12,13]. They were detected in some asymptomatic volunteers in vaccine trials. It would be very useful to have an antibody test indicating active infection, but it is uncertain whether there is a valid one.

CMI RESPONSES

Like the humoral immune response, different measures of specific CMI are increased after infection. In the mouse, the specific lymphocyte proliferative effect [14], and the specific cytotoxic T-cell response [15] may be detected a few days to a week after infection. Specific cytotoxic T lymphocytes (CTL) obtained from infected mice and passively transferred to syngeneic mice will protect against infection [16]. These are T-lymphocyte responses. Other responses are mediated by non-B, non-T cells. Murine CMV infection will enhance the NK and ADCC responses and induce IFN [17].

I would like to concentrate on the immunosuppressive reactions of CMV infection in man and in animals. Almost all of these may be regarded as immunologic responses because they are specific results of infection. Many may turn out to be the result of changes of lymphocyte subsets or their functions. Since we do not know much about these mechanisms, I will discuss immunosuppression primarily from the pathogenic point of view.

Immunosuppression by Infection in Animals (Table 2)

In the mouse, acute CMV infection will depress antibody formation, suppress IFN induction by a heterologous virus, and suppress the lymphocyte

TABLE 2. Immunosuppressive Effects of Acute CMV Infection in Animals

Phenomenon	Observation	References
Antibody formation to SRBC	decreased antibody plaque formation	Osborn and Medearis [18]
Skin graft across H-Y or H-2 barrier	decreased rejection	Howard et al [19]
Lymphocyte response to PHA, PWM, Con A	decreased ^{3}H-thymidine uptake	Howard et al [19] Booss and Wheelock [20]
IFN induced by NDV	decreased 2–12 days	Osborn and Medearis [18]
Clearance of *Pseudomonas aeruginosa*, *E coli*	decreased	Hamilton et al [21] Bale et al [22]
Survival after infection with *P aeruginosa*, *S aureus*, *Candida albicans*, *E coli* (i.n.)	decreased	Hamilton et al [21] Bale et al [22]
Number of leukocytes in peritoneal infection with *E coli*	decreased	Bale et al [22]
Development of cytotoxic T cells against ectromelia or EL4 tumor	decreased	Ho [16] Hamilton [23]
Effect of MCMV infection of macrophage on phago-cytosis of *Staphylococci*	decreased	Shanley and Pesanti [24]
NK enhancement by IFN	decreased	Ho [1, 3]
Phagocytosis and H_2O_2 re-lease from PMNs of guinea pigs*	decreased	Yourtee et al [25]

*Only observation not made in mice using MCMV as infecting agent. MCMV = murine cytomegalovirus.

response to nonspecific mitogens such as PHA, PWM, and Con A. Skin grafts are better tolerated.

A series of studies from Lowell Glasgow's laboratory by Hamilton, Bale and colleagues [21–23] show that during acute infection, the mouse is less able to clear a number of pathogenic microbial agents from the blood stream, such as *Pseudomonas*, *Candida*, and *Escherichia*. This is accompanied by decreased survival after infection by these agents. The mechanism for this decreased clearance is unknown, although studies both in mice and guinea pigs suggest that phagocytic mobilization and function may be directly affected by infection. Neutrophils from infected mice are less able to phago-cytize *Staphylococci* and to generate H_2O_2 [25]. Macrophages from guinea pigs directly infected with their virus also lose phagocytic function [24]. It is notable that most of these effects are only present during acute infection, usually lasting not more than two weeks. Other functions, such as generation of cytotoxic T cells against heterologous viruses or against histoantigens, are also lost [16,23].

We recently have been interested in the resistance of NK cells to IFN as a response to virus infection. Figure 1 shows the spleen NK-cell activity directed against YAC-1 (mouse lymphoma) cells at various times following MCMV infection. The solid dot indicates a rise in such activity two to three days following virus infection, an observation originally made for lymphocytic choriomeningitis virus by Welsh [26], and for MCMV by Quinnan et al [15]. We found, however, that these NK cells lose their enhancement response to IFN five days after infection, and that this refractoriness remains

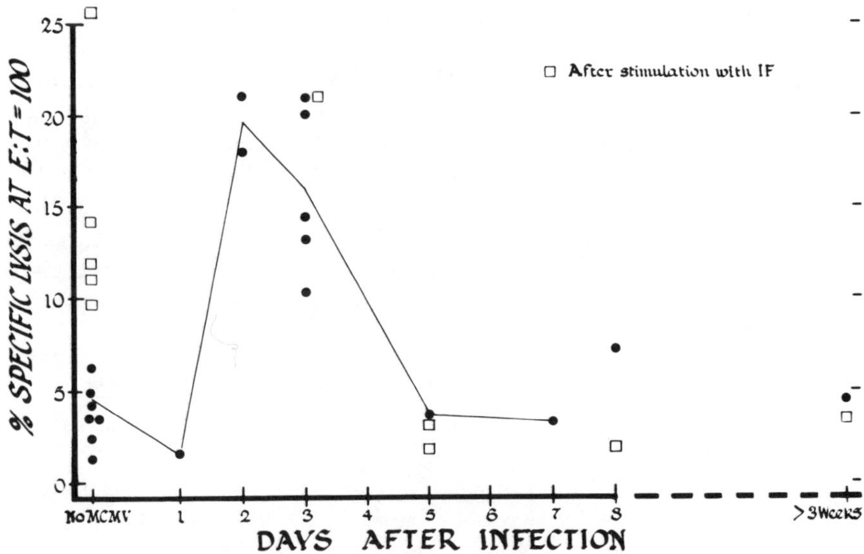

Fig. 1. Effect of MCMV infection on mouse NK cells (Reprinted from Ho [3]). NK cells were assayed at an effector:target ratio of 100:1. Effector cells were obtained from spleens of BALB/c mice. ^{51}Cr-labeled YAC-1 cells were the target cells for lysis. IFN stimulation: 10^7 spleen cells were incubated with 10^3 units of mouse IFN in 1 ml at 37°C for 3 hr. This figure illustrates a number of points about NK cells and their relationship to IFN. The closed dots represent spleen lymphocyte NK levels; the open squares represent NK levels after in vitro stimulation with IFN. 1) Lymphocytes from normal uninfected mice have a low base-line NK activity which could be stimulated by IFN. 2) NK activity rose 2 to 3 days after mice were infected with 10^4 PFU of CMV intraperitoneally. This rise fell rapidly to low-normal levels by day 5. IFN did not stimulate this activity any more. 3) A state of resistance to stimulation by IFN developed after virus infection. The reason for this is unclear.

for some time [3]. Similar responses have been found for Newcastle disease virus (NDV) in mice [27]. These cells also do not produce IFN upon exposure to various IFN inducers, a "hyporeactivity" which is a well-known phenomenon [28].

Immunosuppression by Infection in Normal Subjects (Table 3)

There is now an impressive body of evidence which indicates that while there are specific humoral and cellular immune responses following CMV infection in normal subjects, they may develop slowly and later than other virus infections, and a number of nonspecific parameters are suppressed acutely.

In the early stages of infection in normal subjects, the lymphocyte proliferative responses to heterologous antigens such as HSV, VZV, and nonspecific mitogens, such as PHA, Con A, and PWM are decreased compared with uninfected subjects [29,30]. For about two months after infection, the proliferative response to specific CMV antigens remains below that of the uninfected seropositive individual. In the peripheral blood, there may be a decrease in the absolute number of T lymphocytes, and the skin reactivity to mumps and other common antigens may be lost [31]. The production of IFN induced by CMV or nonspecific mitogens is reduced [30]. Analysis of PBL subsets indicates that there is a decrease in T-helper cells with reversal of the T-helper/suppressor cell ratio [33]. This interesting finding is also present in patients with AIDS [35]. Active CMV infection is frequently present in

TABLE 3. Immunosuppressive Effects of Acute CMV Infections in Normal Subjects

Phenomenon	Observation	References
Proliferative response to CMV	decreased compared to seropositive normals	Levin et al [30] Rinaldo et al [29]
Proliferative response to HSV, VZV	decreased for about 2 months	Rinaldo et al [29]
Proliferative response to PWA, Con A	decreased compared to normals	Rinaldo et al [29]
Absolute number of T cells	decreased to 7%	Oill et al [31]
Skin reactivity to mumps	lost	Oill et al [31]
IFN response to CMV, PHA, PWM, Con A	decreased	Levin et al [30] Rinaldo et al [32]
T-lymphocyte helper/ suppressor ratio	decreased with lower number of helpers, may last 10 months	Carney et al [33]
Leukocyte migration inhibition	decreased with viruria in children	Fiorilli et al [34]

patients with AIDS, although it has not been proven that AIDS is caused by CMV infection.

Immunosuppressive Effects of CMV Infection in Pregnancy and During Infancy (Table 4)

One important pathogenic property of CMV is that it is able to cross the placenta to infect the unusually susceptible fetus. A possible explanation is that acute infection, particularly of the primary type, depresses immunity to the point where the placental barrier is compromised. While there are many indications of important immunologic changes during pregnancy, Gehrz et al [41] found that the CMV-specific lymphocyte proliferation response is decreased in normal uninfected seropositive mothers during the 2nd and 3rd trimesters, while responses to other antigens remained normal. This may indicate a peculiar inability of pregnant women to mount cellular immune responses to CMV at certain times during pregnancy. How this might promote susceptibility to intrauterine infection is as yet unknown. It is interesting that Chong and Mims [42] report that delayed hypersensitivity to MCMV in pregnant or lactating mice is greatly depressed.

In view of what we know about the specific proliferative response in infected normal subjects, it is not surprising that it is also depressed in infected pregnant women, as well as in congenitally infected babies [40]. Seropositive children up to about five years of age do not appear to respond

TABLE 4. Immunosuppressive Effect of CMV in Infancy and in Pregnancy

Phenomenon	Observation	References
CMV-specific lymphocyte transformation in seropositive subjects	decreased at < 1 year and 1–5 years	Tamura et al [36] Pass et al [37]
This response in con- genitally viruric children	decreased to absent response	Gehrz et al [38] Reynolds et al [39]
IFN response in congenitally infected and their mothers	decreased response especially in symptom- atic children	Starr et al [40]
Response to PHA, Con A, PWM in viruric children and mothers	normal	Gehrz et al [38]
CMV-specific response in seropositive mothers	decreased even in non- viruric at 2nd and 3rd trimesters	Gehrz et al [41]
CMV-specific response in mothers of infected babies	decreased	Gehrz et al [38] Starr et al [40]

as well as normal [36]. By and large, the degree of immunosuppression is more severe in younger infants and in the symptomatically infected.

Immunosuppressive Effects of CMV Infection After Transplantation (Table 5)

These immunosuppressive effects are complicated by the presence of immunosuppressants universally used in patients after transplantation. It is often impossible to be sure whether any particular response is due to infection, immunosuppressants, or both. Nevertheless, in view of what we know about the infection in normal subjects and uninfected transplant recipients, it seems quite clear that seropositive subjects may lose their proliferative response to CMV, as well as to heterologous antigens and mitogens.

Severe primary infections are particularly prone to produce profound immune depression. Patients may fail to respond with specific IgG or IgM synthesis. Quinnan et al [48] have correlated severe infections with decreased NK, ADCC, as well as with decreased specific T-cell cytotoxic response in

TABLE 5. Immunosuppressive Effects of CMV After Transplantation

Phenomenon	Observation	References
Proliferative response to CMV, HSV, PHA, PWM, Con A	lost or depressed after transplantation,	Linnemann et al [43] Haahr et al [44]
IFN production induced by CMV, HSV and mitogens	further depressed with CMV infection, may remain so for months to 1–2 years	Pass et al [45] Levin et al [46] Meyers et al [47]
Specific T-cytotoxic response in marrow and	decreased in severe infections	Quinnan et al [48]
renal transplants	decreased in patients on cyclosporine	Breinig et al, unpublished
NK-cell response	decreased in severe infections	Quinnan et al [48]
ADCC response	decreased in severe infections	Quinnan et al [48]
Skin sensitivity to PPD, mumps, strepto- kinase	decreased to lost	Rytel et al [49]
Antibody response to CMV	decreased to lost in severe or fatal infection	Craighead et al [50] Neiman et al [51]
Severe bacterial infections	increased in cardiac transplants with primary CMV	Rand et al [52]
Severe fungal infections	increased in renal transplant patients	Chatterjee et al [53]

BMT recipients. Patients who recovered from their infections had normally enhanced responses following infection. We found, however, that the specific cytotoxic T-cell response may be depressed in renal transplant patients on cyclosporine who may be asymptomatically infected (Breinig, Camp, Dummer, and Ho, abstract, this volume).

In transplant patients there is evidence that the immunosuppressive effect of CMV infection, particularly primary CMV infection, is clinically significant. Severe bacterial and fungal infections are increased in cardiac and renal transplant patients when they have CMV infection, particularly when it is of the de novo primary type [52,53].

EFFECT OF CYCLOSPORINE ON CMV INFECTION

It is well known that both primary and reactivated CMV infections occur frequently after organ transplantation. In a review of various series totalling 1,145 renal transplant recipients, 53% of 505 who were initially seronegative acquired primary infection. Of the remainder who were seropositive (640), 85% acquired reactivated infection [1]. The degree of morbidity from this almost universal infection after transplantation varies a great deal.

I would like to report our experience at the Presbyterian-University Hospital of Pittsburgh with patients put on cyclosporine (cyA), which is a unique new immunosuppressant that has supplanted azathioprine at our institution. Unlike azathioprine, this drug is not marrow suppressive, and selectively inhibits certain T-cell functions, such as the production or action of IL [54,55].

In a study of 122 renal, liver, and cardiac transplant recipients done at our institution in 1981–1982, we still found a significant number of all types of infections [56]. In a direct comparison of renal transplant patients randomized to either azathioprine or cyA, those on cyA had fewer grampositive, particularly *Staphylococcal*, infections. Liver transplant patients had a great deal of fungal infections.

In terms of CMV infections, the renal transplant patients who received cyA had 44% primary and 80% reactivated CMV infections. For all patients on cyA, which included 60 renal, 13 cardiac, and 18 liver transplant recipients, there were 58% primary and 82% reactivated infections. Forty percent of all cyA patients were viremic for CMV, and 35% were symptomatic. In our experience, we see no difference in frequency and severity of CMV infections in patients on cyA. Symptomatic infections included febrile illness, pneumonitis, and at least one cardiac patient whose death was attributable to CMV. It is interesting that as a group, the cardiac transplant patients had more infection, more viremia and more symptomatic disease.

EFFECT OF CYCLOSPORINE AND CMV ON NK-CELL ACTIVITY

The NK activities of peripheral leukocytes of normal controls, previously normal subjects with CMV mononucleosis, renal transplant patients on azathioprine, and renal transplant patients on cyA are summarized in Table 6. To be noted is the relatively high NK activity as well as its further enhancement by IFN in normal controls and normal subjects with CMV mononucleosis. Others have already shown that NK activity in renal transplant patients on azathioprine may be depressed for years after transplantation [57,58]. We found similar depression of NK activity in patients on cyA. To be noted, however, is the more severe impairment of NK cells enhanced by IFN.

The NK activity and the effect of IFN is shown in Figure 2. There is a wide range of NK activities. During the first six weeks after transplantation, when 992 mg/day of cyA was used, there was no enhancement. Between 7–18 weeks, 725 mg/day was given. However, after 18 wk, when a mean of 429 mg/day was given, or less than half of the initial dose, enhancement was much improved, although the level of NK activity was not appreciably higher. We feel that the abnormality of the NK system in the many types of patients we have studied, but in particular those on cyA, is more appreciable by measuring IFN enhancement. In a separate study in mice, we have shown that NK enhancement by IFN can be inhibited in vitro by IFN (Breinig, Camp, Dummer, and Ho, abstract, this volume).

How much of the abnormality in the NK system is due to CMV infection? As noted, most patients have either primary or reactivated infection. In this particular series (Fig. 3), 12 of 14 patients were infected at some time by one

TABLE 6. Mean NK-Cell Responses in Normal and Immunosuppressed Subjects

Group	Subject	Immuno-suppression	No. subjects	No. samples	NK Activity in % S.R. (25:1)	NK Activity After IFN	Enhancement in % S.R. by IFN
1	Normal	none	11	16	44.5 ± 4.4	58.0 ± 4.4	13.5 ± 1.8
2	CMV mono.	none	7	8	40.7 ± 5.5	57.0 ± 4.3	16.3 ± 2.9
3	Transplant	azathioprine	18	23	16.9 ± 3.9	24.8 ± 4.9	7.9 ± 2.1
4	Transplant	cyA	19	59	24.6 ± 1.9	27.4 ± 1.9	2.8 ± 1.02

The NK activities represent means from all the tests and their standard error. For NK activity: Group 1 was significantly different from Groups 3 or 4 (P < 0.01). Groups 3 and 4 were not significantly different. For enhancement: Group 1 was significantly different from Groups 3 or 4 (P < 0.05). Groups 3 and 4 were also significantly different (P < 0.05).
S.R. = specific release.

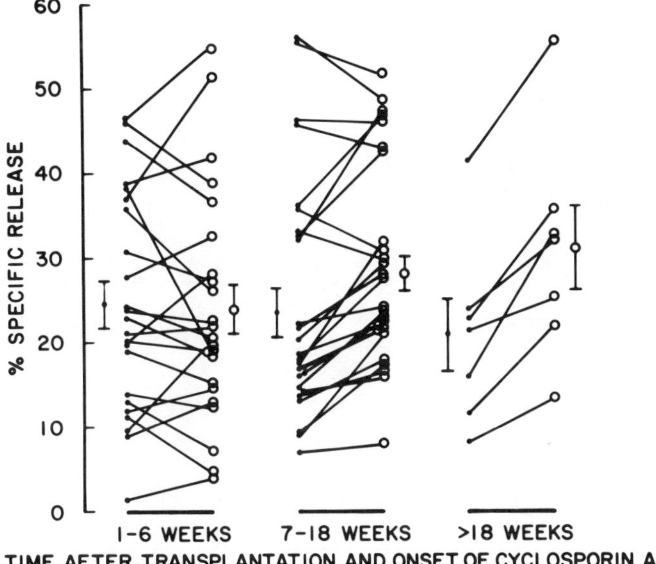

Fig. 2. NK activity and IFN enhancement of NK activity of renal transplant patients on cyA. The solid dots represent circulating NK activity of PBML, and the open circles represent NK activity after in vitro incubation with IFN. Lines connect tests on individual samples. The mean and standard error of NK activity and enhancement values are given for samples collected for the three time periods indicated.

criterion or another. We analyzed our samples depending on whether they were obtained before or after infection, as determined by viremia. Figure 3 shows that after cessation of viremia, the enhancement levels were closer to normal, while no enhancement occurred during viremia. Viremia may thus depress enhancement, although the depression may have been contributed to by cyA. Thus, before viremia, which chronically corresponds to times when higher doses of cyA were given, we saw no enhancement. We do not feel infection alone is a sufficient explanation, since, in addition, normal patients with CMV mononucleosis and most patients on azathioprine can enhance their NK activity with IFN (see above).

EFFECT OF CYCLOSPORINE AND CMV INFECTION ON IFN INDUCTION

We have been following the ability of leukocytes from cardiac transplant patients on cyA to produce IFN after induction in vitro with NDV. It is well known that after organ transplantation in patients on azathioprine, IFN induction is inhibited (Table 5). From Figure 4, we see that in 20 cardiac

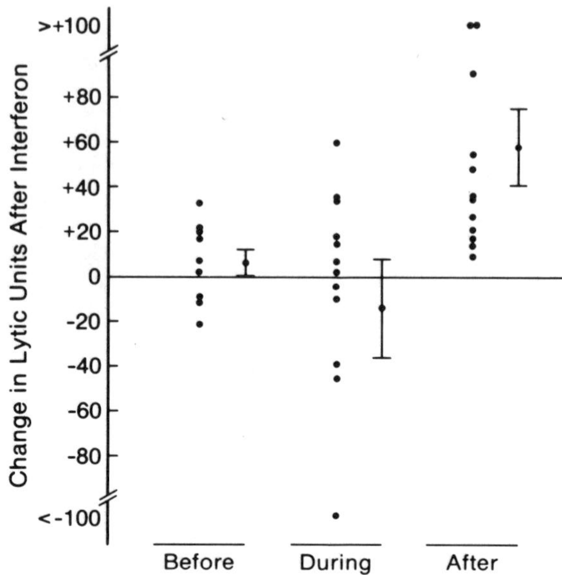

Fig. 3. Effect of the presence of CMV viremia in renal transplant patients on cyA on the change of NK activity after incubation with IFN. Each dot represents a sample collected from 10 patients before, during, and after viremia. The NK activity was measured against K-562 cells in a 16-hr assay. Lytic titers were expressed in 30% lytic units in 10^7 effector cells graphically obtained. For each sample, NK titers with and without incubation with 1,000 units of α-IFN were obtained, and the differences plotted. Positive values represent enhancement, 0 represents no change, and negative values represent depression.

transplant recipients on cyA, the response to NDV is essentially eliminated. The group includes not only patients who have CMV infection, but also patients early after transplantation who were not infected. Hence, the deficit is due to cyA or their basic disease. Only four samples out of 33 show any IFN production. It is interesting that of the four responders, three were 10 to 13 months after transplantation when they were no longer excreting virus. Figure 4 shows that production of γ-IFN in response to enterotoxin A is also inhibited.

Suppression of IFN induction may be even more sensitive to cyA and/or infection than enhancement of NK activity by IFN. We are now working on the hypothesis that these two phenomena, hyporeactivity to IFN inducers and hyporesponsiveness of NK activity to enhancement by IFN, may be related.

SUMMARY

Acute CMV infection in the mouse results in depressed antibody production, IFN induction, lymphocyte proliferation responses to mitogens, alloge-

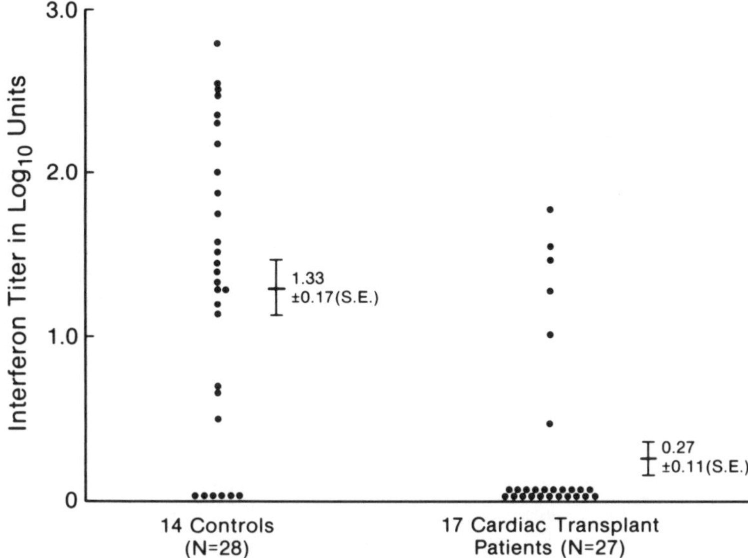

Fig. 4.   Induction of IFN in peripheral leukocytes by enterotoxin A. Each sample represents IFN produced by 10^5 cells induced by 0.1 μg/ml enterotoxin A.

neic skin graft rejection, and clearance of certain bacteria and fungi from the blood stream. CMV mononucleosis in humans is associated with decreased lymphocyte proliferation responses to mitogens and herpesvirus antigens, decreased IFN production, and reversal of the T-helper to suppressor cell ratio. In recent studies, we have shown that NK activity is depressed after renal transplantation and the use of cyA, and is poorly enhanced by the addition of IFN to in vitro assays. In vitro induction of α-IFN as well as γ-IFN by NDV and enterotoxin-A is also inhibited. These deficits may contribute to the severity of CMV infections in this patient population.

ACKNOWLEDGMENTS

Results cited from our laboratory represent the work of Xi-en Gui, J. Steve Dummer, Ann Hardy, Mary Kay Breinig, Charles R. Rinaldo, Jr., Linda White, and John A. Armstrong, in addition to that of the writer.

REFERENCES

1. Ho M: "Cytomegalovirus: Biology and Infections." New York: Plenum Press, 1982, 309 pp.

2. Pereira L, Hoffman M, Gallo D, Cremer N: Monoclonal antibodies to human cytomegalovirus: Three surface membrane proteins with unique immunological and electrophoretic properties specify cross-reactive determinants. Infect Immun 36:924–932, 1982.
3. Ho M: Recent advances in the study of interferon. Proc Symposium on Recent Advances in Biological and Medical Sciences, 15–23, Academica Sinica, Taipei, Taiwan, 1982.
4. The TH, Langenhuysen MMAC: Antibodies against memrane antigens of cytomegalovirus infected cells in sera of patients with a cytomegalovirus infection. Clin Exp Immunol 11:475–482, 1972.
5. Betts RF, Schmidt SG: Cytolytic IgM antibody to cytomegalovirus in primary cytomegalovirus infection in humans. J Infect Dis 143:821–826, 1981.
6. The TH, Klein G, Langenhuysen MMAC: Antibody reactions to virus-specific early antigens (EA) in patients with cytomegalovirus (CMV) infection. Clin Exp Immunol 16:1–12, 1974.
7. Ten Napel CHH, The TH: Acute cytomegalovirus infection and the host immune response. I. Development and maintenance of cytomegalovirus induced in vitro lymphocyte reactivity and its relationship to production of cytomegalovirus antibodies. Clin Exp Immunol 39:263–271, 1980.
8. Stagno S, Reynolds DW, Tsiantos A, Fuccillo DA, Long W, Alford CA: Comparative serial virologic and serologic studies of symptomatic and subclinical congenitally and natally acquired cytomegalovirus infections. J Infect Dis 132:568–577, 1975.
9. Chiba S, Motokawa T, Tamura T, Hanazono H, Kamada M, Chiba Y, Nakao T: Seroconversion to virus-specific pre-early nuclear antigens in infants with primary CMV infection. Infect Immun 30:135–139, 1980.
10. Michelson-Fiske S, Horodniceanu F, Guillon JC: "Immediate early" antigens in human cytomegalovirus infected cells. Nature 270:615–617, 1977.
11. Gerna G, Cereda PM, Cattaneo E, Achilli G, Revello MG: Immunoglobulin G to virus-specific early antigens in congenital, primary and reactivated human CMV infections. Infect Immun 22:833–841, 1978.
12. Friedman AD, Furukawa T, Plotkin SA: Detection of antibody to cytomegalovirus early antigen in vaccinated, normal volunteers and renal transplant candidates. J Infect Dis 146:255–259, 1982.
13. Friedman AD, Michelson S, Plotkin SA: Detection of antibodies to pre-early nuclear antigen and immediate-early antigens in patients immunized with cytomegalovirus vaccine. Infect Immun 38:1068–1072, 1982.
14. Kelsey DK, Overall JC Jr, Glasgow LA: Correlation of the suppression of mitogen responsiveness and the mixed lymphocyte reaction with the proliferative response to viral antigens of splenic lymphocytes from cytomegalovirus-infected mice. J Immunol 121:464–470, 1978.
15. Quinnan GV, Manischewitz JE, Ennis FA: Cytotoxic T lymphocyte response to murine cytomegalovirus infection. Nature 273:541–543, 1978.
16. Ho M: Role of specific cytotoxic lymphocytes in cellular immunity against murine cytomegalovirus. Infect Immun 27:767–776, 1980.
17. Quinnan GV, Manischewitz JE: The role of natural killer cells and antibody-dependent cell-mediated cytotoxicity during murine cytomegalovirus infection. J Exp Med 150:1549–1554, 1979.
18. Osborn JE, Medearis DN Jr: Suppression of interferon and antibody and multiplication of Newcastle disease virus in cytomegalovirus infected mice. Proc Soc Exp Biol Med 124:347–353, 1967.

19. Howard RJ, Miller JJ, Najarian JS: Cytomegalovirus-induced immune suppression. II. Cell-mediated immunity. Clin Exp Immunol 18:119–126, 1974.
20. Booss J, Wheelock EF: Progressive inhibition of T-cell function preceding clinical signs of cytomegalovirus infection in mice. J Infect Dis 135:478–481, 1977.
21. Hamilton JR, Overall JC Jr, Glasgow LA: Synergistic effect on mortality in mice with murine cytomegalovirus and *Pseudomonas aeruginosa, Staphylococcus aureus* or *Candida albicans* in mice. Infect Immun 14:982–989, 1976.
22. Bale JF Jr, Kern ER, Overall JC Jr, Glasgow LA: Enhanced susceptibility of mice infected with murine cytomegalovirus to intranasal challenge with *Escherichia coli;* Pathogenesis and altered inflammatory response. J Infect Dis 145:525–531, 1982.
23. Hamilton JD, Fitzwilliam JF, Cheung KS, Shelburne J, Lang DJ, Amos DB: Viral infection-homograft interactions in a murine model. J Clin Invest 62:1303–1312, 1978.
24. Shanley JD, Pesanti EL: Replication of murine cytomegalovirus in lung macrophages: Effect of phagocytosis of bacteria. Infect Immun 29:1152–1159, 1980.
25. Yourtee EL, Bia FJ, Griffith BP, Root RK: Neutrophil response and function during acute cytomegalovirus infection in guinea pigs. Infect Immun 36:11–16, 1982.
26. Welsh RM: Cytotoxic cells induced during lymphocytic choriomeningitis virus infection of mice. I. Characterization of natural killer cell induction. J Exp Med 148:163–181, 1978.
27. Melder RJ, Ho M: Modulation of natural killer cell activity in mice after interferon induction: Depression of in vitro enhancement by interferon. Infect Immun 36:990–995, 1982.
28. Ho M, Kono Y, Breinig MK: Tolerance to the induction of interferons by endotoxin and virus: Role of a humoral factor. Proc Soc Exp Biol Med 119:1227–1232, 1965.
29. Rinaldo CR Jr, Black PH, Hirsch MS: Interactions of virus with mononucleosis due to cytomegalovirus. J Infect Dis 136:667–678, 1977.
30. Levin MJ, Rinaldo CR Jr, Leary PL, Zaia JA, Hirsch MS: Immune response to herpesvirus antigens in adults with acute cytomegaloviral mononucleosis. J Infect Dis 140:851–857, 1979.
31. Oill PA, Fiala M, Schofferman J, Byfield PA, Guze LB: Cytomegalovirus mononucleosis in a healthy adult. Association with hepatitis, secondary Epstein-Barr virus antibody response and immunosuppression. Am J Med 62:413–417, 1977.
32. Rinaldo CR Jr, Carney WP, Richter BS, Black PH, Hirsch MS: Mechanisms of immunosuppression in cytomegaloviral mononucleosis. J Infect Dis 141:488–495, 1980.
33. Carney WP, Rubin RH, Hoffman RA, Hansen WP, Healey K, Hirsch MS: Analysis of T lymphocyte subsets in cytomegalovirus mononucleosis. J Immunol 126:2114–2116, 1981.
34. Fiorilli M, Sirianni MC, Iannetti P, Pana A, Divizia M, Aiuti F: Cell-mediated immunity in human cytomegalovirus infection. Infect Immun 35:1162–1164, 1982.
35. Gottlieb MS, Schroff R, Schanker HM et al: *Pneumocystis carinii* pneumonia and mucosal candiasis in previously healthy homosexual men. N Engl J Med 305:1425–1431, 1981.
36. Tamura T, Chiba S, Abo W, Chiba Y, Nakao T: Cytomegalovirus-specific lymphocyte transformations in subjects of different ages with primary immunodeficiency. Infect Immun 28:49–53, 1980.
37. Pass RF, Dworsky ME, Whitley RJ, August AM, Stagno S, Alford CA: Specific lymphocyte blastogenic responses in children with cytomegalovirus and herpes simplex virus infections acquired early in infancy. Infect Immun 34:166–170, 1981.
38. Gehrz RC, Marker SC, Knorr SO, Kalis JM, Balfour HH Jr: Specific cell-mediated immune defect in active cytomegalovirus infection of young children and their mothers. Lancet 2:844–847, 1977.

39. Reynolds DW, Dean PH, Pass RF, Alford CA: Specific cell-mediated immunity in children with congenital and neonatal cytomegalovirus infection and their mothers. J Infect Dis 140:493–499, 1979.

40. Starr SE, Tolpin MD, Friedman HM, Paucker K, Plotkin SA: Impaired cellular immunity to cytomegalovirus in congenitally infected children and their mothers. J Infect Dis 140:500–505, 1979.

41. Gehrz RC, Christianson WR, Linner KM, Conroy MM, McCue SA, Balfour HH Jr: Cytomegalovirus-specific humoral and cellular immune responses in human pregnancy. J Infect Dis 143:391–395, 1981.

42. Chong KT, Mims CA: Delayed hypersensitivity to murine cytomegalovirus and its depression during pregnancy. Infect Immun 37:54–59, 1982.

43. Linnemann CC Jr, Kaufmann CA, First MR, Schiff GM, Phair JP: Cellular immune response to cytomegalovirus infection after renal transplantation. Infect Immun 22:176–180, 1978.

44. Haahr S, Møller-Larsen A, Anderson HK, Spencer ES: Cell-mediated and humoral immune responses to herpes simplex virus and cytomegalovirus in renal transplant patients. J Clin Microbiol 10:267–274, 1979.

45. Pass RF, Reynolds DW, Whelchel JD, Diethelm AG, Alford CA: Impaired lymphocyte transformation response to cytomegalovirus and phytohemagglutinin in recipients of renal transplants: Association with antithymocyte globulin. J Infect Dis 143:259–265, 1981.

46. Levin MJ, Parkman R, Oxman MN, Rappeport JM, Simpson M, Leary PL: Proliferative and interferon response by peripheral blood mononuclear cells after bone marrow transplantation in humans. Infect Immun 20:678–684, 1978.

47. Meyers JD, McGuffin RW, Neiman PE, Singer JW, Thomas ED: Toxicity and efficacy of human leucocyte interferon for treatment of cytomegalovirus pneumonia after marrow transplantation. J Infect Dis 141:555–562, 1980.

48. Quinnan GV, Kirmani N, Esber E, Saral RR, Manischewitz JE, Rogers JL, Rook AH, Santos GW, Burns WH: HLA-restricted cytotoxic T lymphocyte and non-thymic cytotoxic lymphocyte responses to cytomegalovirus infections of bone marrow transplant recipients. J Immunol 126:2036–2041, 1981.

49. Rytel MW, Aguilar-Torres FG, Balay J, Heim LR: Assessment of the status of cell-mediated immunity in cytomegalovirus-infected renal allograft recipients. Cell Immunol 37:31–40, 1978.

50. Craighead JE: Pulmonary cytomegalovirus infection in the adult. Am J Pathol 63:487–504, 1971.

51. Neiman PE, Reeves W, Ray G, Flournoy N, Lerner KG, Sale GE, Thomas ED: A prospective analysis of interstitial pneumonia and opportunistic viral infection among recipients of allogeneic bone marrow grafts. J Infect Dis 136:754–767, 1977.

52. Rand KH, Pollard RB, Merigan TC: Increased pulmonary superinfections in cardiac transplant patients undergoing primary cytomegalovirus infection. N Engl J Med 298:951–953, 1978.

53. Chatterjee SN, Fiala M, Weiner J, Stewart JA, Stacey B, Warner N: Primary cytomegalovirus and opportunistic infections. Incidence in renal transplant recipients. JAMA 240:2446–2449, 1978.

54. Borel JF, Feurer C, Gubler HU, Stahelin H: Biological effects of cyclosporin A: A new antilymphocyte agent. Agents Action 6:468–475, 1976.

55. Bunjes D, Hardt C, Rollinghoff M, Wagner H: Cyclosporin A mediates immunosuppression of primary cytotoxic T cell responses by impairing the release of interleukin 1 and interleukin 2. Eur J Immunol 11:657–661, 1981.

56. Dummer JS, Hardy A, Poorsattar A, Ho M: Early infection in kidney, heart and liver transplant recipients on cyclosporine. Transplantation (In press).
57. Lipinski M, Tursz T, Kreis H, Finale Y, Amiel JL: Dissociation of natural killer cell activity and antibody-dependent cell-mediated cytotoxicity in kidney allograft recipients receiving high-dose immunosuppressive therapy. Transplantation 29:214–218, 1980.
58. Guillau PJ, Hegarty J, Ramsden C, Davison AM, Will EJ, Giles GR: Changes in human natural killer activity early and late after renal transplantation using conventional immunosuppression. Transplantation 33:414–421, 1982.

Immune Balance in the Cytomegalovirus-Infected Host: In Vitro Studies of Virus-Lymphocyte Interactions and the Effects on Specific Lymphocyte Function*

Paolo Casali[†], MD, George P.A. Rice[‡], MD, and Michael B.A. Oldstone, MD

Department of Immunology, Scripps Clinic and Research Foundation, La Jolla, CA 92037

BACKGROUND AND INTRODUCTION OF THE PROBLEM

An interesting aspect of CMV as a human pathogen lies in its propensity for producing disease in persons with impaired or immature immunity. When immune defense in a human host loses the upper hand, as during pregnancy, the congenital, neonatal, or perinatal periods, or at times of renal, bone marrow or other allograft transplantation, the balance frequently tips to favor CMV infection. More than half of all individuals given bone marrow trans-

*This is Publication Number 2997-IMM from the Department of Immunology, Scripps Clinic and Research Foundation, La Jolla, California 92037. This research was supported by GCRC grant no. MO1 RR-00833, and USPHS grants AI-07007 and NS-12428.

†P.C. is the recipient of a Clinical Investigator Award from the Medical Group of Scripps Clinic and Research Foundation, and is supported by funds from the Weingart Foundation.

‡G.P.A.R. is a recipient of a Centennial Fellowship from the Medical Research Council of Canada.

Birth Defects: Original Article Series, Volume 20, Number 1, pages 149–159

plants (BMT) acquire CMV infection, which is often fatal. In humans and experimental animals, both the specific immune response and nonspecific natural mechanisms of defense act to limit viral infection and thereby tip the immune balance to favor the infected host's survival. The specific immune response may limit viral growth by various effector mechanisms: virus inactivation by antibodies, complement-mediated lysis of enveloped viral particles or virus-infected cells coated with appropriate antibody, lysis of infected cells by antibody-dependent cell-mediated cytotoxicity (ADCC) and specific cytotoxic T-lymphocytes (CTLs) [1]. Cytotoxic lymphocytes may lyse infected cells early in the virus's replicative cycle before infection reaches surrounding fluids and may abort cell-to-cell spread of virus. Both mechanisms serve as highly effective ways of limiting infection. Such CTLs are specific for glycoproteins of the virus that generated them and for the major histocompatibility complex (MHC) antigens. Generation of CTLs requires activation of T cells by a specific viral antigen presented on accessory cells, such as macrophages. A lag period, usually of seven to ten days, is required before T cells develop peak reactivity, which thereafter rapidly abates. ADCC, as well as complement-mediated lysis of infected cells, require the presence of antibodies specific for structures expressed at the surfaces of infected cells. Because of the requirement for antibody (against viral glycoproteins expressed on the cell surface), ADCC effector mechanisms and complement-dependent lysis take place only after a delay, comparable to that for generation of specific CTLs.

In addition to these virus-specific responses, nonspecific host mechanisms of defense may play a role against viral infections when specific immunologic memory is absent (primary infection) and/or in early phases of infection when the immune response is not yet fully expressed. Natural resistance can be mediated by soluble factors such as molecules of the complement system (eg, the binding of C3 to infected cells promotes their opsonization), IFNs and other lymphokines, and by cellular effectors such as macrophages, polymorphonuclear leukocytes (PMNLs), and NK cells. Among such nonspecific mechanisms of defense, NK cells figure importantly [2]. NK cells do not show restricted specificity for viral glycoproteins and MHC antigens. They constitute an early line of defense against microorganisms during primary infection preceding the generation of a specific immune response or on reexposure to microbial agents before the secondary immune response develops. Cell populations mediating NK mechanisms are heterogeneous and overlap with cells involved in ADCC.

In general, an antibody response that is specific for CMV develops in individuals after asymptomatic, primary, or secondary CMV infection [3,4].

Frequently, high titers of antibodies to CMV occur in patients with AIDS, in those who excrete CMV in body fluids, and even in transplant patients who die from CMV infection [4,5]. However, the quality of the response with respect to binding of various CMV glycoprotein epitopes is unknown. Transfer of antibody to CMV in patients undergoing transplantation or into experimental animals [6,7] indicates that such antibody may limit CMV infection.

In addition to antibody, cytotoxic lymphocytes appear to be important in recovery from CMV infection. CTLs, NK cells, and cells involved in ADCC function less actively in patients who die from CMV infection after BMT [5] than in those who survive. Further, lymphocyte function is altered during CMV infection. For example, during acute CMV-mononucleosis infection, lymphocyte proliferative responses to CMV antigens and mitogens are depressed [8], and the T-suppressor-cytotoxic lymphocyte subset (OKT8$^+$) expands, compared with the T-helper lymphocyte subset (OKT4$^+$) [9,10].

Questions emanating from such observations were whether CMV is directly responsible for suppressing the immune system, or whether the preexisting suppression of immune responses favors primary CMV infection or reactivation of latent virus. To address this issue, we have initiated studies of CMV-lymphocyte interactions. In this chapter, we will present our results concerning CMV, influenza virus, and measles virus infection on such selected lymphocyte functions as cytotoxicity, proliferation and antibody production in vitro. We also report here a new, practical, and sensitive assay for measuring antibodies to CMV.

EXPERIMENTAL OBSERVATIONS
Effects of CMV, Influenza Virus and Measles Virus on Lymphocyte Functions in Vitro

To evaluate cytotoxicity, proliferation, and Ig synthesis by infected lymphocytes, we used PBMC from human volunteers, removed adherent cells, and incubated these lymphocytes with either CMV, influenza virus, or measles virus at a multiplicity of infection (MOI) of two to three. The infected cells were then cultured for 24, 48, or 72 hr in RPMI medium containing 10% FBS and washed in warm medium. We first analyzed functional alterations by using K-562 cells and human fibroblasts to measure NK activity, and P-815 cells coated with IgG antibody to P-815 cell surfaces to measure ADCC. Table 1 shows that CMV induced NK activity and IFN release by human PBLs in vitro. In addition, NK activity increased in these cultures for as long as 72 hr. Like NK activity, ADCC occurred during CMV exposure throughout the 72-hr observation period. In contrast to CMV, measles virus

TABLE 1. Cytotoxicity Activity of Lymphocytes Cultured With HCMV*

PBL Cultured in Medium Containing:	% Specific ^{51}Cr Release From:									
			Human Fibroblasts				P-815 Cells			
	K-562 Cells		+ Medium		+ IFN†		+ PBS		+ Ab	
(48 hr)										
Nil	69 ± 6‡	38 ± 1§	12 ± 4	2 ± 1	47 ± 7	29 ± 2	4 ± 1	3 ± 1	78 ± 5	63 ± 4
Virion	81 ± 2	57 ± 4	46 ± 14	27 ± 3	44 ± 4	32 ± 2	5 ± 1	4 ± 1	75 ± 4	71 ± 5
(72 hr)										
Nil	58 ± 5	40 ± 7	8 ± 2	‖	60 ± 9	71 ± 3	27 ± 6	‖	69 ± 3	67 ± 4
Virion	66 ± 3	46 ± 6	30 ± 5	‖	66 ± 2	70 ± 3	48 ± 6	‖	65 ± 5	100 ± 9

*Results observed with PBL from one donor. Similar results were found with four different donors studied.

†100 IU/ml of human α-leukocyte IFN present throughout the assay

‡Mean value ± 1 SE. Effector to target cell ratio, 50:1.

§Effector to target cell ratio, 15:1

‖Not done

TABLE 2. Inhibition of Cell-Mediated Cytotoxicity by Measles Virus

PBL Cultured in Medium Containing:	K-562 Cells		% Specific ^{51}Cr Release From: Human Fibroblasts + Medium		+ IFN*		P-815 Cells + PBS		+ Ab	
(24 hr)										
Nil	73.4†	29.7‡	1.5	0.9	28.7	9.0	2.7	1.4	76.7	64.9
Virion	61.2	17.9	6.7	2.0	8.1	0.9	2.5	1.9	77.7	56.8
(48 hr)										
Nil	76.7	36.9	3.9	0.2	51.4	16.8	0.4	0.2	65.0	51.4
Virion	21.8	5.6	2.8	0.1	9.0	1.7	2.0	1.3	64.5	60.8
(72 hr)										
Nil	78.2	39.1	2.8	0.1	35.6	1.2	0.4	0.7	63.7	61.9
Virion	2.8	1.3	0.0	0.4	0.0	0.7	0.6	2.2	64.0	60.5

*100 IU of human α-IFN present throughout the cytotoxicity assay.
†Effector to target cell ratio, 50:1
‡Effector to target cell ratio, 10:1

completely inhibited the NK activity of PBL over the 72-hr period (Table 2). PBL incubated with influenza virus behaved similarly to those cultured with CMV, in that cytotoxic lymphocyte (NK, ADCC) activity was fully preserved (Fig. 1). In all these experiments, the viability of PBL incubated with the three different viruses for 72 hr was > 90%. In other experiments [11], the abrogation of lymphocyte cytotoxicity by measles virus was attributed to the direct effect of virus on effector cells.

The second function of PBL we investigated was mitogen-driven proliferation. One $\times$ 10^6 PBL were cultured with purified PHA and one each of the three viruses, and then the cultures were pulsed with ^{3}H-thymidine. After 96 hr in culture, the lymphocyte viability was approximately 90%, equivalent to that of lymphocytes cultured with mitogen in the absence of added virus. Mitogen-driven proliferation of these PBL was markedly inhibited by both measles virus and influenza virus, but was not affected by CMV (Table 3). These results with CMV in vitro contrast to studies performed in vivo on lymphocytes harvested from patients with acute CMV infection with unresponsiveness to mitogens [8].

The third lymphocyte function analyzed was synthesis of Ig in vitro by T-cell-dependent B lymphocytes. The test involved culturing purified syngeneic B and T lymphocytes at a 1:3 ratio in the presence of PWM for six days. The different viruses were added at a MOI of one. The amount of Ig synthesized (IgM and IgG antibody released into culture fluid) was then analyzed by an ELISA system. As one sees in Table 4, CMV did not decrease Ig synthesis, but in several experiments (data not shown) appeared to slightly

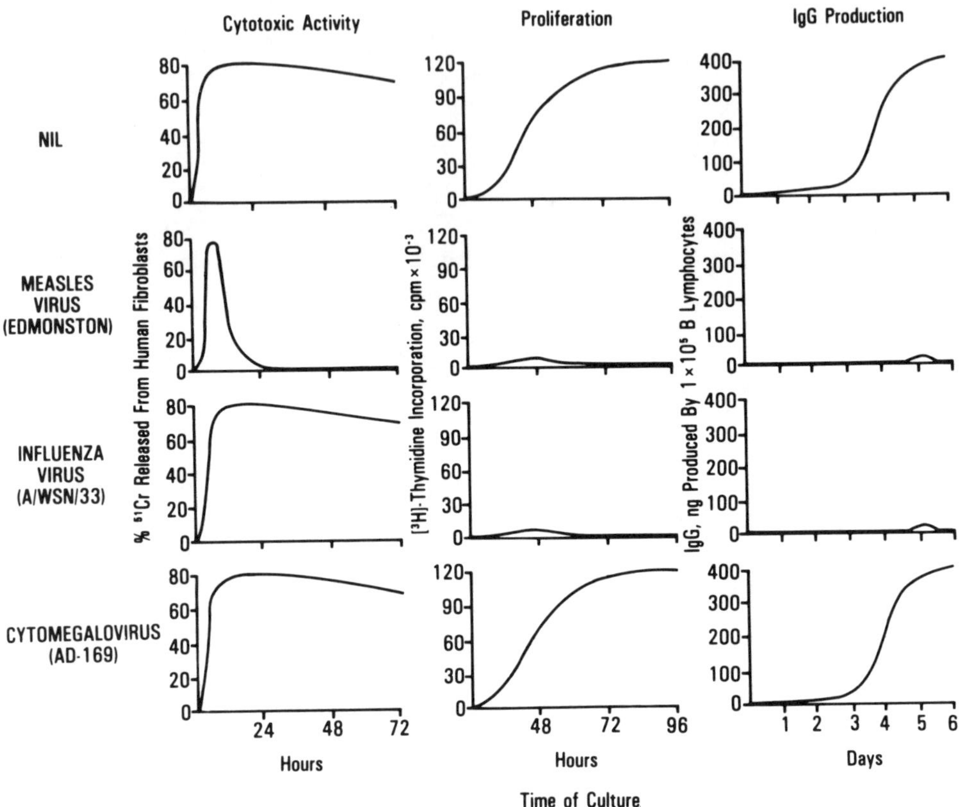

Fig. 1. In vitro alteration of human lymphocyte function by virus.

augment the synthesis of IgG. In contrast, both influenza virus and measles virus significantly lowered Ig synthesis by B cells (Table 4, Fig. 1).

CMV (AD169) clearly does not affect several in vitro lymphocyte functions that are markedly impaired by either measles virus or influenza virus. Primary or secondary (following activation of latent virus) CMV infection is frequently associated with immunosuppression [12–14]. However, our data suggest, in part, that CMV may not directly depress immunity, but rather that immunosuppression from other sources may provide the milieu for CMV activation. Our results were formulated with laboratory-adapted CMV. An

TABLE 3. Mitogen-Driven Proliferation of Human Lymphocytes* Cultured With:

	Measles Virus		Influenza Virus		CMV	
	PBS	PHA	PBS	PHA	PBS	PHA
Nil	2,850† ± 235	112,500 ± 5,671	1,317 ± 118	97,340 ± 4,824	3,616 ± 1,335	86,226 ± 5,259
Virion	10,632 ± 3,536	6,250 ± 1,310	1,694 ± 155	1,410 ± 73	11,134 ± 3,882	79,925 ± 5,855

*PBL, 3×10^5/well. PHA, 1 μg/ml. Similar results were obtained with PBL from 15 donors in three different experiments.
†^{3}H-thymidine incorporation, mean value ± 1 SE.

TABLE 4. T-Cell-Dependent Ig Production by Human Lymphocytes Cultured With Virus

PBL From Donor	No Virus	Measles Virus	Influenza Virus	CMV
1	140*	6	4	120
2	303	6	4	367
3	167	12	15	†

*ng of Ig produced by 1×10^5 B lymphocytes after six days of culture.
†Not done

alternative explanation is that AD169 is a selected variant that may not reflect CMV-lymphoid effects in vivo with wild-type virus. If this is so, then the sequence differences between AD169 or other laboratory-used CMV strains and wild-type virus may be of value in understanding basic mechanisms of lymphocyte reactivity.

Measles virus significantly altered several lymphocyte functions, including the generation of cytotoxic lymphocytes and antibody (Ig) synthesis. This occurred without evidence of expression of measles virus gene products, production of infectious virions, or change in lymphocyte viability. Thus, measles virus altered the differentiated functions of lymphocytes without altering their vital function. These observations aid in understanding the von Pirquet phenomenon of measles virus-associated inhibition of the tuberculin reaction [15]. Similarly, influenza virus abrogated Ig synthesis by lymphocytes, although failing to alter their cytotoxic activity. These results are summarized in Figure 1.

A New, Practical, and Sensitive Assay for Measuring Antibodies to CMV

Antibodies to CMV are usually detected either by immunofluorescence or CF techniques. Recently, we have developed an ELISA [16] that provides greater sensitivity and ease of handling than its predecessors. This ELISA accurately measures total specific antibodies as well as defining the amount of each class and subclass of such antibodies. In this system, uninfected or infected fibroblasts harvested at the time of maximum cytopathology are placed in 96-well microtiter plates with phosphate-buffered saline and allowed to dry. Appropriate dilutions of the sera to be tested are applied for two hr. After several washes, the Ig bound specifically to the solid-phase antigen is detected by adding an enzyme-linked probe. After addition of the appropriate substrate [16], the amount of enzyme-labeled probe bound is measured by colorimetric analysis. The process of antigen dessication does not impair the binding of specific antibodies to the solid-phase antigen. Indeed, some experiments suggest that dessication may improve the quality of antigen presentation. An unusual, practical, and significant benefit of this assay is that dried plates can be stored at least three to six months at room temperature.

Test serum is subjected to the assay at three different dilutions on both CMV-infected and mock-infected fibroblasts. The value of specific optical density (ie, O.D. of sample on infected cells - O.D. of same on uninfected cells) for each dilution is plotted (y-axis) *v* the log of its dilution factor (x-axis). By linear regression, the reciprocal value defined by the intercept on the x-axis is considered the serum titer. In addition to providing highly reproducible results, this method allows characterization of the antibody's reactivity. By altering antigen concentration, one can estimate the avidity of CMV-specific antibodies in test serum, which may be useful in evaluating antibody in sera from patients with CMV, especially in learning why transplant patients have died with CMV infection despite normal or high titers of the antibodies. Results from the ELISA procedure described above correlate with CMV-antibody titers observed by conventional immunofluorescence assay (Table 5) (Spearman R = 0.9), although titers from the former are usually higher.

The specific proliferative response of lymphocytes to CMV antigens indicates prior immune exposure and occurs in individuals who have preexisting antibodies to the virus [17,18]. We have observed a positive correlation between the antibody titer in this ELISA assay and the extent of T-cell proliferation from a given patient in response to CMV antigens. For investigation, we cultured patients' PBMCs in 96-well plates with free virions as a source of CMV antigen, or with fluids from mock-infected cultures, and assessed specific proliferative responses. As seen in Table 6, after four days a quantitative correlation was evident between the proliferation index and the antibody titer in serum from individual donors.

TABLE 5. Correlation of Antibody Titers to CMV Determined by ELISA and Immunofluorescence Techniques*

Titer by Immunofluorescence	Titer by ELISA
< 16†	< 20
< 16	< 20
< 16	< 20
< 16	< 20
< 16	< 20
< 16	< 20
< 16	< 20
< 16	< 20
< 16	< 20
32	3,000
64	300
64	760
128	840
128	1,400
128	2,000
128	2,520
256	3,300
256	4,300
512	1,400
512	2,560
512	5,600
2,048	1,700
8,192	19,000
16,384	6,000
16,384	20,000

*Immunofluorescence assays were determined with the Electronucleonics CMV Antibody# kit. In this assay, antigen from infected fibroblasts is dried on a glass slide. The amount of IgG bound is measurable with a fluorescein-conjugated antibody to human IgG. The ELISA was performed as described in the text [16].

†Reciprocal of dilution. Each line represents an individual patient sample. We tested and compared 25 individual samples.

CONCLUSIONS

Dissection of CMV-specific immune responses is needed to better understand the ability of the host to control or fail in its control of CMV infection. The rapid advance in immunologic technology using clonal analysis of antibody and cytotoxic lymphocytes should provide new insight in the future.

TABLE 6. Correlation of Antibody Titers Determined by ELISA Technique With in Vitro Proliferation Response to CMV*

Titer by ELISA	Stimulation Index
< 20	1.2
< 20	1.0
< 20	1.4
< 20	1.23
< 20	0.5
< 20	1.6
< 20	0.8
< 20	0.4
300	1.8
1,900	2.2
1,900	1.9
2,560	4.0
2,560	4.2
6,000	3.3
9,000	6.3

*3×10^5 PBMCs from each donor were incubated for four days in RPMI supplemented with 5% FBS, with CMV antigen, or control antigen. Tritiated thymidine incorporation was measured in the last 24 hr of culture. The index is determined by dividing the counts per min of lymphocytes cultured in the presence of CMV by the counts per min of lymphocytes cultured in the absence of CMV. ELISA was performed as outlined in the text. Each line represents an individual patient sample.

Further, a comparison of virus-lymphocyte interactions between the conventional laboratory strains of CMV and fresh CMV isolates from patients is clearly needed.

REFERENCES

1. Notkins AL, Oldstone MBA (eds): "Concepts in Viral Pathogenesis." New York: Springer-Verlag (In press).
2. Casali P, Trincheri G: Natural killer cells in viral infection. In Notkins AL, Oldstone MBA (eds): "Concepts in Viral Pathogenesis." New York: Springer-Verlag (In press).
3. Levin MJ, Rinaldo CR, Leary PL, Zaia JA, Hirsch MS: Immune response to herpesvirus antigens in adults with acute cytomegalovirus mononucleosis. J Infect Dis 140: 811–857, 1979.
4. Rasmussen L, Kelsall D, Nelson R, Carney W, Hirsch M, Winston D, Preiksaitis J, Merigan TC: Virus-specific IgG and IgM antibodies in normal and immunocompromised subjects infected with cytomegalovirus. J Infect Dis 145:191–199, 1982.

5. Quinnan GV Jr, Kirmani N, Rook AH, Manischewitz JF, Jackson L, Moresch G, Santos GW, Saral R, Burns WH: Cytotoxic T cells in cytomegalovirus infection. HLA-restricted T-lymphocyte and non-T-lymphocyte cytotoxic responses correlate with recovery from cytomegalovirus infection in bone-marrow-transplant recipients. N Engl J Med 307:6–13, 1980.
6. Meyers J, Leszcznski J, Zaia J, Levin J, Smydam D, Wright G, Thomas ED: Successful immunoprophylaxis of cytomegalovirus infection after marrow transplant with CMV immune globulin. Clin Res 30:374A, 1981.
7. Shanley J, Jordan C, Stevens J: Modification by adaptive humoral immunity of murine cytomegalovirus infection. J Infect Dis 143:231–237, 1981.
8. Pass RF, Dworsky ME, Whitley RJ, August AM, Stagno S, Alford CA Jr: Specific lymphocyte blastogenic responses in children with cytomegalovirus and herpes simplex virus infections acquired early in infancy. Infect Immun 34:166–170, 1981.
9. Carney WP, Rubin RH, Hoffman RA, Hansen WP, Healey K, Hirsch MS: Analysis of T lymphocyte subsets in cytomegalovirus mononucleosis. J Immunol 126:2114–2116, 1981.
10. Carney WP, Iacoviello V, Hirsch MS: Functional properties of T lymphocytes and their subsets in cytomegalovirus mononucleosis. J Immunol 130:390–393, 1981.
11. Casali P, Rice GPA, Oldstone MBA: Alteration of human lymphocyte functions by virus. Differential effect of measles, influenza viruses and cytomegalovirus. Manuscript in preparation.
12. Oill PA, Fiala M, Schofferman J, Byfield PE, Guze LB: Cytomegalovirus mononucleosis in a healthy adult: Association with hepatitis, secondary Epstein-Barr virus antibody response and immune suppression. Am J Med 62:413–417, 1977.
13. Weller TH: The cytomegaloviruses: Ubiquitous agents with protean clinical manifestations. Part I. N Engl J Med 285:203–214, 1971.
14. Weller TH: The cytomegaloviruses: Ubiquitous agents with protean clinical manifestations. Part II. N Engl J Med 285:267–274, 1971.
15. Von Pirquet C: Das Verhalten der kutanen Tuberkulin-reaktion während der Masern. Dtsch Med Wochenschr 34:1297–1300, 1908.
16. Rice GPA, Casali P, Oldstone MBA: A convenient solid phase immunosorbent assay for the detection of antibodies specific to measles virus. J Infect Dis 147:1055–1059, 1983.
17. Wahren B, Robert K-H, Nordlund S: Conditions for cytomegalovirus stimulation of lymphocytes. Scand J Immunol 13:581–586, 1981.
18. Starr SE, Dalton B, Garrabrant T, Paucker K, Plotkin SA: Lymphocyte blastogenesis and interferon production in adult human leukocyte cultures stimulated with cytomegalovirus antigens. Infect Immun 30:17–22, 1980.

Cytomegalovirus–Leukocyte Interactions*

Martin S. Hirsch, MD

Infectious Disease Unit, Department of Medicine, Massachusetts General Hospital, Harvard Medical School, Boston, MA 02114

Cytomegalovirus can interact with human leukocytes in many ways, both to the benefit and detriment of the host. Lymphocytes, monocytes, and granulocytes may all be involved in the control of viral replication, either directly or through the mediation of soluble factors such as antibodies and interferons. The human host response to CMV and CMV-associated antigens will be reviewed by other participants in this volume.

This review will focus on the other aspect, ie, how CMV affects human leukocytes, and how these interactions may influence subsequent host responses. It has been approximately 17 years since CMV transmission was first associated with blood transfusions [1-8] and only six years since CMV's immunosuppressive effects were described [9]. Since those observations were made, a great deal has been learned about how CMV interacts with leukocytes, but fundamental gaps in our knowledge remain. I will focus both on what has been learned and on what questions remain to be answered.

LEUKOCYTE TRANSMISSION

Transmission of CMV by blood transfusion is common, though not often followed by clinical illness. Several studies have evaluated the risk of transfusions [1, 4, 5, 8, 10-15]. Once thought to be related only to extracorporeal

*Supported by NIH grants CA-12464, CA-35020, and contract CP-43222, and by the Mashud A. Mezerhand B. Fund.

Birth Defects: Original Article Series, Volume 20, Number 1, pages 161–173

infusions associated with cardiac surgery, it is now clear that the risks of posttransfusion infection are actually related to the amount of blood transfused, the type of blood product employed, and the serologic status of both the donor and the recipient. Ho [16] has recently compiled 12 studies relating to transfusion-associated CMV infections. Admitting that his figures "must be taken with a grain of salt," he has estimated the likelihood of infections, defined by antibody rises, following moderate-to-large numbers of transfusions (> 3 U per recipient). The overall likelihood of infection was 14% per recipient, 19% for those susceptible to primary infection, and 10% for those susceptible to secondary infection. Symptomatic infection occurred in approximately 4% of recipients, almost exclusively in those without preexisting CMV antibody. Such infections are generally characterized by prolonged fever, malaise, fatigue, splenomegaly, liver function abnormalities, and a heterophile antibody-negative mononucleosis. In addition, 7% of patients in one study developed asymptomatic infection with peripheral blood lymphocytosis and prominent atypical lymphocytes [12]. The risk of infection of recipients of blood from volunteer donors has been estimated by Ho to be approximately 3% per unit transfused [16].

The antibody status of the donor obviously is of importance in determining the likelihood of CMV transmission. Monif et al [14] demonstrated that CMV transmission was tenfold greater when CMV seropositive donors (by CF antibody) were used than when CMV seronegative donors were employed. Yeager et al [17] studied infants receiving blood transfusions, and found that if both mothers and donors were seronegative by IHA, infants did not become infected. However, if either mother or donor were seropositive, the likelihood of infant infection was 13.5%-17.6%. The only symptomatic infections were observed in those infants undergoing primary infection. In the infant population born to seronegative mothers, it would, thus, appear wise to limit donors to those who are also seronegative.

How is CMV transmitted by blood transfusion? In one study, two of 35 healthy donors had CMV isolated from peripheral blood [18]. Several large studies in over 1,500 blood donors have not confirmed these observations [13, 19-23], although in one center cytomegaloviruria was found in 3% of donors [22]. We have observed that CMV viremia can persist two to three months following acute CMV mononucleosis [9], and Cheeseman et al [24] have demonstrated the occurrence of chronic CMV viremia following renal transplantation. Thus, the occasional transfusion of infectious virus in donor blood cannot be excluded. Nevertheless, transmission by latently infected blood would appear far more common.

The association between leukocytes and infectious virus during acute CMV infections is well established. The specific leukocyte types that carry latent CMV in peripheral blood are less clear. During acute CMV mononucleosis and during symptomatic infections in renal transplant recipients, the polymorphonuclear leukocyte (PMNL) is the principal site of virus carriage [9, 25, 26]. Whether this reflects phagocytosis by mature granulocytes or replication in granulocyte precursors is unclear. Peripheral blood monocytes may also harbor infectious virus under these circumstances [27], whereas lymphocytes and other blood elements (erythrocytes, plasma, platelets) appear to be virus-free. In contrast to these studies, Garrett [28] has reported that T-cell-enriched populations from 18 renal transplant recipients harbored CMV, whereas B lymphocytes generally did not; granulocytes and monocytes were not examined in this study.

The situation following latent infection is more obscure. Our attempts to activate CMV from lymphocytes of healthy seropositive subjects have been unsuccessful, despite the use of techniques that induce viruses in other systems, including MLR, mitogen treatment, or use of halogenated pyrimidines [9]. In addition, attempts to infect lymphocytes, or subpopulations thereof, have been unrewarding, in contrast to parallel studies with HSV, where replication in lymphocytes was easily demonstrated [29]. St. Jeor and Weisser [30], however, found low level persistent CMV infections of HPBLs after in vitro exposure, and a CMV-containing B-lymphoblastoid cell line has been established from a congenitally infected child who was also infected with EBV [31]. Moreover, certain B-lymphoblastoid cell lines support CMV replication [32-34], suggesting that the presence of EBV genomes makes B lymphocytes or lymphoblasts more susceptible to infection with CMV. T-lymphoblastoid cell lines appear resistant to CMV infection [29].

No simple conclusions can be drawn from these various studies. It appears that under different circumstances, various PBL populations may carry CMV, and that the source of infection following transfusion may be diverse.

The mechanisms by which CMV becomes activated following transfusion are equally obscure. Early in the 1970s, we demonstrated that murine retroviruses could be immunologically activated during graft-*v*-host and host-*v*-graft reactions [35, 36]. Subsequent studies have suggested that similar mechanisms might be operative in murine CMV infection [37-40], although these conclusions are not universally accepted. Following blood transfusions in humans, allogeneic reactions develop [41], and it is possible that immunologic activation of CMV may occur. However, no evidence to prove this possibility has emerged either in vivo or in vitro.

Since leukocytes are the principal peripheral blood reservoirs for human CMV, two events might appear predictable: 1) leukocyte transfusions would carry a high risk of virus transmission; 2) removal of leukocytes from blood preparations would lower the risk of transmission. Both of these predictions appear valid.

Leukocyte transfusions have been widely employed in neutropenic patients, both as prophylaxis and as therapy against infection. Studies in Los Angeles and Seattle have indicated that this practice is associated with an increased risk of CMV infection. Winston et al [42] showed that 19 of 31 recipients of prophylactic leukocyte transfusions developed CMV infections, compared with 7 of 27 who did not receive leukocytes (P=0.01). Hersman et al [43] found that CMV-seronegative recipients of prophylactic granulocytes from seropositive donors had a much higher incidence of infection (21/28) than seronegative patients who did not receive granulocytes (37/113, P=0.005), or seronegative patients who received granulocytes from seronegative donors (16/46, P=0.05). Thus, leukocyte transfusions carry a high risk for CMV transmission, although many of the subsequent infections may be asymptomatic.

Certain procedures in blood banking can reduce the viability of leukocytes in products for transfusion. We have demonstrated that use of frozen red cells thawed and deglycerolized by a cytoagglomeration technique reduces the risk of CMV seroconversion [15]. In our study none of 21 seronegative dialysis patients who received a total of 157 units of frozen thawed blood developed CMV antibodies, compared with three seronegative recipients of conventional blood, all of whom seroconverted and excreted virus. Lang et al [44] similarly demonstrated a diminished rate of CMV seroconversions in recipients of blood that was partially leukocyte depleted by gravitation and repeated centrifugation techniques.

Several summary points emerge from this review of CMV carriage and transmission:

1. The likelihood of virus infection following blood transfusion is related to the amount of blood administered, the type of blood product employed, and the serologic status of donor and recipient.

2. Leukocyte transfusions are associated with a high risk of CMV transmission, whereas depletion of leukocytes from blood products substantially reduces the risk.

3. Asymptomatic infection following transfusion of CMV-containing blood is far more common than clinical illness.

4. Primary infection is more likely to be symptomatic than secondary infection following blood transfusion.

5. Although infectious CMV may occasionally be transmitted by transfusion, far more common is the transmission and subsequent activation of latent leukocyte-borne virus.

6. During acute CMV infections, the PMNL is the principal reservoir of infectious virus, although certain mononuclear cells (monocytes and possibly T lymphocytes) may occasionally carry virus as well.

7. The site of leukocyte latency in peripheral blood and the mechanisms of subsequent activation remain unclear.

EFFECTS OF CMV ON LEUKOCYTE FUNCTION

CMV infections increase susceptibility to superinfection by other organisms, both in experimental animals and in man. In 1967, Osborn and Medearis [45] first demonstrated that Newcastle disease virus (NDV), ordinarily noninfective for mice in vivo, would replicate to high titers in mice infected with murine CMV. Subsequent studies by Hamilton et al [46, 47] clearly showed that murine CMV infection could markedly increase the lethality of subsequent infection with *Staphylococcus aureus, Pseudomonas aeruginosa,* or *Candida albicans*.

Increased susceptibility to superinfection following HCMV infection has been most clearly demonstrated in transplant recipients [48, 49], but has also been suggested in other populations, including infants with cytomegalic inclusion disease [50], adults with mononucleosis [51], and in patients with AIDS [52]. In renal transplant recipients, a common scenario is a CMV-induced syndrome occurring one to four months following grafting, often characterized by fever and leukopenia, and complicated by a subsequent overwhelming infection with fungi (eg, *Aspergillus, Mucoraceae*), protozoa (eg, *Pneumocystis carinii*), or bacteria. Similar sequences are frequently observed in AIDS patients, although the role of CMV in these patients is less clear. In both transplant and AIDS populations, Kaposi sarcoma (KS) and lymphoid neoplasms also are unusually common [53, 54], and usually follow overt or covert CMV infections. Cytomegalic inclusion disease in infants has also been associated with an enhanced proclivity toward pneumocystis pneumonia [50]. An increased superinfection rate has been reported following CMV mononucleosis [51], but these studies need confirmation.

How does CMV increase susceptibility? Although final answers are not in, studies in patients with CMV mononucleosis have elucidated many of the mechanisms involved. Early studies in our laboratory demonstrated that lymphocyte proliferative responses to the mitogens Con A and PWM are depressed during acute infection and gradually return to normal during convalescence [9]. In collaboration with Dr. Myron Levin, we subsequently found that not only are mitogen responses depressed, but also proliferative and γ-IFN responses to specific antigens of the herpesvirus group (VZ, HS,

CMV) [55]. The development of proliferative responses to CMV in such patients lags well behind the development of CMV-specific antibodies. In convalescence, proliferative and IFN responses return to normal. In contrast to the suppression observed in these lymphocyte responses, PMNL function appears grossly normal, as measured by phagocytosis, reduction of nitroblue tetrazolium, and chemotaxis [56]. Recently, Yourtee et al [57], studying a guinea pig model of CMV mononucleosis, demonstrated more subtle abnormalities of granulocyte function, eg, diminished maximal H_2O_2 release. These studies suggest that a closer look at granulocyte function in HCMV mononucleosis may be indicated.

The ability to generate cytotoxic lymphocytic responses against allogeneic cells has also been studied in CVM mononucleosis [58]. Mononuclear cells from patients or control donors were cultured alone or in the presence of mitomycin C-treated Laz 156 cells (an EBV-transformed B-lymphoblastoid line). On the day of assay, cells were harvested and tested for their capacity to lyse ^{51}Cr labeled Laz 156 cells. During acute CMV mononucleosis, patient cells were significantly less able to lyse target cells, although this capacity returned during convalescence. Whether the defect is in recognition of and sensitization to heterologous antigens, or in lytic capability remains to be determined.

Rinaldo et al [59] have recently studied NK cell cytotoxicity against K562 cells in CMV mononucleosis patients, and found these responses to be intact. Where studied, antibody responses have also been normal [55]. B-lymphocyte responses in vitro have not been extensively examined, although preliminary studies in our laboratory show no marked abnormalities. Thus, the major abnormalities induced by CMV appear to be in T-lymphocyte function involving proliferative and cytotoxic responses, as well as γ-IFN production.

More recently, we have been attempting to study the mechanisms underlying lymphocyte hyporesponsiveness during CMV mononucleosis. Initial efforts were to determine whether suppressor cells or soluble factors help mediate CMV's effects on lymphocyte function. Attempts to define suppressive soluble mediators in patient serum or lymphocyte supernatant fluid by a variety of techniques were unsuccessful. However, preculture of cells from patients with acute CMV mononucleosis for up to seven days before addition of Con A was found to greatly enhance the subsequent blastogenic response to that mitogen, suggesting that a labile suppressor cell may be lost in vitro [26]. Lymphocyte responses were further enhanced by depletion of adherent monocytes after seven days in culture, whereas addition of fresh autologous monocytes to precultured cells could once again depress the Con A responses. Similar suppressive effects were not observed with adherent cells from normal donors in autologous mixing experiments.

Subsequent studies have attempted to show that monocyte-macrophage suppressor activity in vitro could be increased by infection with CMV [27]. Separated monocytes from normal donors were infected in suspension with CMV, and incubated from 5-14 days, after which they were mixed with autologous lymphocytes and assayed for Con A blastogenesis. Although both uninfected and infected monocytes reduced autologous lymphocyte responses to Con A, infected monocytes were generally more suppressive. This was not due to a direct lymphocytotoxic effect of CMV, since culture of lymphocytes with cell-free virus did not suppress proliferative responses. How the infected monocyte interacts with lymphocytes to reduce responsiveness remains a subject for further study.

One of the more important advances in immunologic research in the past five years has been the use of monoclonal antibodies to help define lymphocyte subsets and their functions. We analyzed peripheral blood T lymphocytes from patients in the acute and convalescent stages of CMV mononucleosis using Ortho Pharmaceutical monoclonal antibodies OKT3 (Pan T), OKT4 ("helper-inducer"), OKT8 ("cytotoxic suppressor"), and OKIa ("activation"). Acute CMV infection is associated with a reversal of the normal ratio of T4+ to T8+ cells, reflecting a large absolute increase in T8+ cells, and a smaller decrease in T4+ cells [60]. Ia+ cells were also increased fivefold during acute CMV mononucleosis. During convalescence, Ia+ cells diminish quickly but there is a gradual decline in T8+ cells over several months. Inversions of T4+/T8+ ratios are associated with diminished mitogen responses, though Con A responses return to normal more quickly than the phenotypic alterations.

Recently, in collaboration with Dr. Stanley Plotkin, we have performed similar studies prospectively on healthy recipients of live Towne strain CMV vaccine [61]. Although these subjects develop both humoral and cell-mediated responses to CMV antigens, none of eight vaccine recipients showed significant changes in T-cell subset numbers or blastogenic responses to Con A. Following vaccination, in contrast to CMV mononucleosis, viremia, peripheral excretion, systemic illness, and atypical illness are not observed. Alterations in lymphocyte phenotype and function may thus depend not merely on the presence of CMV infection, but also on the amount of viral burden and the severity of infection.

Studies in renal transplant recipients support this contention [62]. In recipients of kidneys from living related donors, T4+/T8+ ratio inversions were seen only in association with clinically apparent CMV infections. No changes were observed during transient or asymptomatic CMV excretion. In the more heavily immunosuppressed recipients of cadaver kidneys, subset alterations accompanied all primary or reactivated CMV infections. T-cell subset alterations were accompanied by a high likelihood of subsequent opportunistic superinfection or CMV-associated glomerulopathy. Thus, measurement of inverted ratios during CMV infections may suggest the presence of significant immunologic dysfunction. However, all too often T-cell subset phenotype data are considered synonymous with functional characterization. Since not all T4+ cells are helpers, nor all T8+ cells suppressors, functional studies must be performed on individual subsets before such conclusions can be securely drawn.

Among our major current efforts are attempts to better define the functional properties of T-cell subsets in CMV mononucleosis. Are the preponderant T8+ cells functional suppressors, committed cytotoxic cells, or nonfunctional cells? Preliminary studies on populations of cells enriched by complement-mediated lysis for T8+ cells indicate that they are unreactive to Con A whereas T4+-enriched cells are much more reactive [58]. Control lymphocytes showed no such dichotomy in responsiveness. In vitro cultures of PBLS result in a selective loss of T8+, Ia+ cells, so that the remaining T-cell population is composed primarily of Con A responsive T4+ cells. Thus, the previously mentioned return of responsiveness on in vitro culture may be explained by the selective depletion of unresponsive T8+ cells.

Large atypical lymphocytes are characteristic of acute CMV mononucleosis. Their genesis and functional roles are obscure. Recently, we have employed separation techniques to attempt better definition of these cell populations. Preliminary studies suggest that the great majority of atypical lymphocytes belongs to the T8+, Ia+ subpopulation of cells (Carney and Felsenstein, unpublished data).

Considerable efforts have also been directed toward defining immunologic abnormalities during congenital CMV infections. Lymphocytes from infected children appear hyporesponsive in proliferative and IFN responses to CMV antigens, as do lymphocytes from their mothers [63-68]. Responses to mitogens in the infected children and mothers do not appear depressed, in contrast to observations in CMV mononucleosis patients. In some series, the most severe infections were associated with the most suppressed responses [66], whereas others did not find close correlations between symptomatology and immune suppression [68]. Over time, some children developed normal responses despite continued virus excretion, while others remained hyporesponsive for prolonged periods.

Although many gaps remain in our understanding of how CMV infections affect human immune responsiveness, several points have emerged from studies over the past decade:

1. CMV infection often predisposes patients to potentially severe superinfections with other opportunistic pathogens, and possibly to the development of certain neoplasms.

2. CMV's major impact on responsiveness appears to be on T lymphocyte function where it suppresses proliferative and IFN responses to mitogens and antigens, and cytotoxic responses to allogeneic cells.

3. PMNL functions (phagocytosis, nitroblue tetrazolium reduction, chemotaxis) are intact in CMV mononucleosis, as are NK-cell cytotoxicity and antibody production.

4. Suppressor monocyte-macrophages are induced during CMV infections, but soluble suppressor factors have not been detected.

5. T cells with the phenotypic surface markers of activated cytotoxic-suppressor lymphocytes (T8+, Ia+) increase in the peripheral blood of patients with symptomatic CMV infection, while the relative numbers of cells with helper-inducer (T4+)-phenotype decrease. These changes are not observed following immunization with the live Towne strain CMV vaccine.

6. The preponderant T8+, Ia+ lymphocyte present during CMV mononucleosis is virtually unresponsive to mitogen stimulation. The atypical lymphocytes characteristic of this disorder fall largely in this category.

APPROACHES TO REVERSAL OF CMV-INDUCED LYMPHOCYTE DYSFUNCTION

A number of immunomodulatory approaches to CMV infection and its consequences may become feasible once the mechanisms of CMV-induced immunosuppression are more fully clarified. Both in vivo studies and in vitro models of CMV macrophage infection may help unravel how these cells interact with T-lymphocyte subsets to induce hyporesponsiveness. Are infected monocytes defective in interleukin 1 (IL 1) production? Is IL 2 production by stimulated T4+ lymphocytes impaired? Are aberrant signals produced which stimulate the replication of T8+ cells with atypical morphology and altered function? Are such lymphocytes committed cytotoxic cells for CMV-infected targets, or suppressor cells for T-cell effector functions?

Once answers to these questions are known, a variety of therapeutic or prophylactic avenues might become reasonable, including the exogenous administration of ILs or IFNs, ablative therapy with specific antibodies to individual T-cell or monocyte-macrophage subsets, or the use of prostaglandin inhibitors, immunoadjuvants, or antimetabolites. Many of these same approaches may be useful in other situations such as AIDS where CMV infection may be an important contributing pathogen. Thus, the need for finding answers to the questions raised is pressing, and the impetus for creative studies on CMV-leukocyte interactions persists.

REFERENCES

1. Kaariainen L, Klemola E, Paloheimo J: Rise of cytomegalovirus antibodies in an infectious-mononucleosis-like syndrome after transfusion. Br Med J 2:1270–1272, 1966.
2. Harnden DG, Elsdale TR, Young DE, Ross A: The isolation of cytomegalovirus from peripheral blood. Blood 30:120–125, 1967.
3. Lang DJ, Scolnick EM, Willerson JT: Association of cytomegalovirus infection with the post-perfusion syndrome. N Engl J Med 278:1147–1149, 1968.
4. Paloheimo JA, von Essen R, Klemola E, Kaariainen L, Siltanen P: Subclinical cytomegalovirus infections and cytomegalovirus mononucleosis after open heart surgery. Am J Cardiol 22:624–630, 1968.
5. Embil JA, Folkins DF, Haldane EV, Van Rooyen CE: Cytomegalovirus infection following extra-corporeal circulation in children: A prospective study. Lancet 2:1151–1155, 1968.
6. Foster KM, Jack I: Isolation of cytomegalovirus from the blood leukocytes of a patient with post-transfusion mononucleosis. Aust Ann Med 17:135–140, 1968.
7. Lang DJ, Hanshaw JB: Cytomegalovirus infection and the post-perfusion syndrome. N Engl J Med 280:1145–1149, 1969.
8. Foster KM, Jack I: A prospective study of the role of cytomegalovirus in post-transfusion mononucleosis. N Engl J Med 280:1311–1316, 1969.
9. Rinaldo CR Jr, Black PH, Hirsch MS: Virus-leukocyte interactions in cytomegalovirus mononucleosis. J Infect Dis 136:667–678, 1977.
10. Henle W, Henle G, Scriba M, Joyner CR, Harrison FS, von Essen R, Paloheimo J, Klemola E: Antibody responses to the Epstein-Barr virus and cytomegalovirus after open heart and other surgery. N Engl J Med 282:1068–1074, 1970.
11. Prince AM, Szmuness W, Millian SJ, Davis DS: A serologic study of cytomegalovirus infections associated with blood transfusions. N Engl J Med 284:1125–1131, 1971.
12. Caul EO, Clarke SKR, Mott MG, Perham TGM, Wilson RSE: Cytomegalovirus infections after open heart surgery. Lancet 1:777–780, 1971.
13. Armstrong JA, Tarr GC, Youngblood LA, Dowling JN, Saslow AR, Lucas JP, Ho M: Cytomegalovirus infection in children undergoing open heart surgery. Yale J Biol Med 49:83–91, 1976.
14. Monif GRG, Daicoff GI, Flory LF: Blood as a potential vehicle for the cytomegaloviruses. Am J Obstet Gynecol 126:445–448, 1976.
15. Tolkoff-Rubin N, Rubin RH, Keller EW, Baker GP, Stewart JA, Hirsch MS: Cytomegalovirus infection among dialysis patients and personnel. Ann Intern Med 89:625–628, 1978.
16. Ho M: "Cytomegalovirus—Biology and Infection." New York: Plenum Press, 1982.
17. Yeager AS, Grumet FC, Hafleigh EB, Arvin AM, Bradley JS, Prober CG: Prevention of transfusion-acquired cytomegalovirus infections in newborn infants. J Pediatr 98:281–287, 1981.
18. Diosi P, Moldovan E, Tomescu N: Latent cytomegalovirus infection in blood donors. Br Med J 4:660–662, 1969.

19. Wentworth BB, Alexander ER: Seroepidemiology of infections due to members of the herpes group. Am J Epidemiol 94:496–507, 1971.
20. Perham TGM, Caul EW, Conway PJ, Mott MG: Cytomegalovirus infection in blood donors. A prospective study. Br J Haematol 20:307–320, 1971.
21. Mirkovic R, Werch J, South MA, Benyesh-Melnick M: Incidence of cytomegalovirus in blood bank donors and in infants with congenital cytomegalic inclusion disease. Infect Immun 3:45–50, 1971.
22. Kane RC, Rousseau WE, Noble GR, Tegtmeier GE, Wulff H, Herndon HB, Chin TDY, Bayer WL: Cytomegalovirus infection in a volunteer blood donor population. Infect Immun 11:719–723, 1975.
23. Bayer WL, Tegtmeier GE: The blood donor: Detection and magnitude of cytomegalovirus carrier states and the prevalence of cytomegalovirus antibody. Yale J Biol Med 49:5–12, 1976.
24. Cheeseman SH, Stewart JA, Winkle S, Cosimi AB, Tolkoff-Rubin NE, Russell PS, Baker GP, Herrin J, Rubin RH: Cytomegalovirus excretion 2-14 years after transplantation. Transplant Proc 11:71–74, 1979.
25. Fiala M, Payne JE, Berne TV, Moore TC, Henle W, Montgomerie JZ, Chaterjee SN, Guze LB: Epidemiology of cytomegalovirus infection after transplantation and immunosuppression. J Infect Dis 132:421–433, 1975.
26. Rinaldo CR Jr, Carney WP, Richter BS, Black PH, Hirsch MS: Mechanisms of immunosuppression in cytomegalovirus mononucleosis. J Infect Dis 141:488–495, 1980.
27. Carney WP, Hirsch MS: Mechanisms of immunosuppression in cytomegalovirus mononucleosis II. Virus-monocyte interactions. J Infect Dis 144:47–54, 1981.
28. Garrett HM: Isolation of human cytomegalovirus from peripheral blood T cells of renal transplant patients. J Lab Clin Med 99:92–97, 1982.
29. Rinaldo CR Jr, Richter BS, Black PH, Callery R, Chess L, Hirsch MS: Replication of herpes simplex virus and cytomegalovirus in human leukocytes. J Immunol 120:130–136, 1978.
30. St. Jeor S, Weisser A: Persistence of cytomegalovirus in human lymphoblasts and peripheral leukocyte cultures. Infect Immun 15:402–409, 1977.
31. Joncas JH, Menezes J, Huang E-S: Persistence of CMV genome in lymphoid cells after congenital infection. Nature 258:432–434, 1975.
32. Furukawa T: Persistent infection with human cytomegalovirus in a lymphoblastoid cell line. Virology 94:214–218, 1979.
33. Furukawa T, Yoshimura N, Jean J-H, Plotkin SA: Chronic persistent infection with human cytomegalovirus in human lymphoblasts. J Infect Dis 139:211–214, 1979.
34. Tocci MJ, St. Jeor SC: Susceptibility of lymphoblastoid cells to infection with human cytomegalovirus. Infect Immun 23:418–423, 1979.
35. Hirsch MS, Black PH, Tracy GS, Leibowitz S, Schwartz RS: Leukemia virus activation in chronic allogeneic disease. Proc Natl Acad Sci USA 67:1914–1917, 1970.
36. Hirsch MS, Ellis DA, Kelly AP, Proffitt MR, Black PH, Monaco AP, Wood ML: Activation of C-type viruses during skin graft rejection of the mouse. Int J Cancer 15:493–502, 1975.
37. Wu BC, Dowling JN, Armstrong JA, Ho M: Enhancement of mouse cytomegalovirus infection during host versus graft reaction. Science 190:56–58, 1975.
38. Olding LB, Jensen FC, Oldstone MBA: Pathogenesis of cytomegalovirus infections. I. Activation of virus from bone marrow-derived lymphocytes by in vitro allogeneic reaction. J Exp Med 141:561–572, 1975.

39. Cheung KS, Lang DJ: Transmission and activation of cytomegalovirus with blood transfusion: A mouse model. J Infect Dis 135:841–845, 1977.
40. Dowling N, Wu BC, Armstrong JA, Ho M: Enhancement of murine cytomegalovirus infection during graft versus host reaction. J Infect Dis 135:990–994, 1977.
41. Schechter GP, Soehnlen F, McFarland W: Lymphocyte responses to blood transfusion in man. N Engl J Med 287:1169–1173, 1972.
42. Winston DJ, Ho WG, Howell CL, Miller MJ, Mickey R, Martin WJ, Lin C-H, Gale RP: Cytomegalovirus infections associated with leukocyte transfusions. Ann Intern Med 93:671–675, 1980.
43. Hersman J, Meyers JD, Thomas ED, Buckner CD, Clift R: The effect of granulocyte transfusions on the incidence of cytomegalovirus infection after allogeneic marrow transplantation. Ann Intern Med 96:149–152, 1982.
44. Lang DJ, Ebert PA, Rodgers BM, Boggess HP, Rixse RS: Reductions of post-perfusion cytomegalovirus infections following the use of leucocyte depleted blood. Transfusion 17:391–395, 1977.
45. Osborn JE, Medearis DN Jr: Suppression of interferon and antibody and multiplication of Newcastle disease virus in cytomegalovirus infected mice. Proc Soc Exp Biol Med 124:347–353, 1967.
46. Hamilton JR, Overall JC Jr, Glasgow LA: Synergistic effect on mortality in mice with murine cytomegalovirus and *Pseudomonas aeruginosa, Staphylococcus aureus,* or *Candida albicans* infections. Infect Immun 14:982–989, 1976.
47. Hamilton JR, Overall JC Jr: Synergistic infections with murine CMV and *Pseudomonas aeruginosa* in mice. J Infect Dis 137:775–782, 1978.
48. Braun EW, Nankervis G: Cytomegalovirus viremia and bacteremia in renal allograft recipients. N Engl J Med 299:1318–1319, 1978.
49. Rubin RH, Cosimi AB, Tolkoff-Rubin NE, Russell PS, Hirsch MS: Infectious disease syndromes attributable to cytomegalovirus and their significance among renal transplant recipients. Transplantation 24:458–464, 1977.
50. Seifert G: Weitere Untersuchungen zur Frage der Syntropie von interstitieller Pneumonie und Zytomegalie. Zentralbl Allg Pathol 91:445–450, 1954.
51. Ten Napel CHH, The TH: Acute cytomegalovirus infection and the host immune response. II. Relationship of suppressed in vitro lymphocyte reactivity to bacterial recall antigens and mitogens with the development of cytomegalovirus-induced lymphocyte reactivity. Clin Exp Immunol 39:272–278, 1980.
52. Durack DT: Opportunistic infections and Kaposi's sarcoma in homosexual men. N Engl J Med 305:1465–1467, 1981.
53. Drew WL, Miner RC, Ziegler JL, Gullett JH, Abrams DI, Conant MA, Huang ES, Groundwater JR, Volberding P, Mintz L: Cytomegalovirus and Kaposi's sarcoma in young homosexual men. Lancet 2:125–128, 1982.
54. Penn I: Kaposi's sarcoma in organ transplant recipients: Report of 20 cases. Transplantation 27:8–11, 1979.
55. Levin MJ, Rinaldo CR Jr, Leary PL, Zaia JA, Hirsch MS: Immune response to herpes virus antigens in adults with acute cytomegalovirus mononucleosis. J Infect Dis 140:851–857, 1979.
56. Rinaldo CR Jr, Stossel TP, Black PH, Hirsch MS: Leukocyte function during cytomegalovirus mononucleosis. Clin Immunol Immunopathol 12:331–334, 1979.
57. Yourtee EL, Bia FJ, Griffith BP, Root RK: Neutrophil response and function during acute cytomegalovirus infection in guinea pigs. Infect Immun 36:11–16, 1982.

58. Carney WP, Iacoviello V, Hirsch MS: Functional properties of T lymphocytes and their subsets in cytomegalovirus mononucleosis. J Immunol 130:390–393, 1983.

59. Rinaldo CR Jr, Ho M, Hamoudi WH, Gui X, DeBiasio RL: Lymphocyte subsets and natural killer cell responses during cytomegalovirus mononucleosis. Infect Immun 40:472–477, 1983.

60. Carney WP, Rubin RH, Hoffman RA, Hansen WP, Healey K, Hirsch MS: Analysis of T lymphocyte subsets in cytomegalovirus mononucleosis. J Immunol 126:2114–2116, 1981.

61. Carney WP, Iacoviello VR, Hirsch MS, Starr SE, Fleisher G, Plotkin SA: T lymphocyte subsets and lymphocyte responses following immunization with cytomegalovirus vaccine. J Infect Dis 147:958, 1983.

62. Schooley RT, Hirsch MS, Colvin RB, Cosimi AB, Tolkoff-Rubin NE, McCluskey RT, Burton RC, Russell PS, Herrin JT, Delmonico FA, Giorgi JV, Henle W, Rubin RH: Association of herpesgroup virus infections with T-lymphocyte subset alterations, glomerulopathy, and opportunistic infections following renal transplantation. N Engl J Med 308:307–313, 1983.

63. Gehrz RC, Marker SC, Knorr SO, Kalis JM, Balfour HH Jr: Specific cell-mediated immune defect in active cytomegalovirus infection in young children and their mothers. Lancet 2:844–847, 1977.

64. Reynolds DW, Dean PH, Pass RF, Alford CA: Specific cell-mediated immunity in children with congenital and neonatal cytomegalovirus infection and their mothers. J Infect Dis 140:493–499, 1979.

65. Starr SE, Tolpin MD, Friedman HM, Paucker K, Plotkin SA: Impaired cellular immunity to cytomegalovirus in congenitally infected children and their mothers. J Infect Dis 140:500–505, 1979.

66. Tamura T, Chiba S, Abo W, Chiba Y, Nakao T: Cytomegalovirus-specific lymphocyte transformations in subjects of different ages with primary immunodeficiency. Infect Immun 28:49–53, 1980.

67. Gehrz RC, Christianson WR, Linner KM, Conroy MM, McCue SA, Balfour HH Jr: Cytomegalovirus-specific humoral and cellular immune responses in human pregnancy. J Infect Dis 143:391–395, 1981.

68. Gehrz RC, Linner KM, Christianson WR, Ohm AE, Balfour HH Jr: Cytomegalovirus infection in infancy: Virological and immunological studies. Clin Exp Immunol 47:27–33, 1982.

Cytomegalovirus and Human Cancer*

Fred Rapp, PhD, and Deanna Robbins, PhD

Department of Microbiology and Cancer Research Center, The Pennsylvania State University College of Medicine, Hershey, PA 17033

INTRODUCTION

HCMV belongs to the herpesvirus group of DNA-containing viruses (Table 1), and is known to cause a broad array of human diseases, including classic cytomegalic inclusion disease, intrauterine death, congenital defects, an infectious mononucleosis, postperfusion syndrome and interstitial pneumonia [1,2]. Similar to the other herpesviruses, HCMV is capable of causing persistent and latent infections in man. The organ systems it has been detected in are often targets of malignancy and for many years HCMV has been viewed as a potential human oncogenic virus. There is a strong association between the presence of HCMV and several forms of human neoplasia (Table 2), but as yet, there is no direct evidence of its role in human oncogenesis as has been found for another herpesvirus, EBV, and Burkitt lymphoma [3]. The ubiquitous nature of HCMV infections complicates the issue of its role as a cancer-causing agent. The vast majority of HCMV infections are subclinical and the virus can almost be considered a commensal that is commonly found in people the world over. In this chapter, the evidence that links HCMV with human neoplasia will be presented. The suggestion is made that while a direct etiologic role for HCMV in human oncogenesis has not yet been proven, the complex interactions of this viral agent with its human host merit continued examination.

*Supported by grants CA 18450, CA 27503, and CA 09124.

Birth Defects: Original Article Series, Volume 20, Number 1, pages 175–192

TABLE 1. Cancers Associated with Human Viruses

Malignancy	Virus	Virus Group
Burkitt lymphoma	Epstein-Barr	herpesvirus
Nasopharyngeal carcinoma	Epstein-Barr	herpesvirus
Hepatocellular carcinoma	hepatitis B	hepatitis B
Cervical and vulvar carcinoma	herpes simplex type 2, cytomegalovirus	herpesvirus
Prostatic carcinoma	cytomegalovirus, herpes simplex type 2	herpesvirus
Kaposi sarcoma	cytomegalovirus	herpesvirus
Adenocarcinoma of the colon	cytomegalovirus	herpesvirus
Carcinoma of the lip and oropharynx	herpes simplex type 1	herpesvirus
Squamous cell carcinoma	human papilloma	papovavirus
Laryngeal papilloma	human papilloma	papovavirus
Adult T-cell leukemia	human T-cell leukemia	retrovirus

BIOLOGIC CONSIDERATION

HCMV is an enveloped, double-stranded DNA virus with an icosahedral capsid containing 162 capsomeres. It is species-specific and is strongly cell-associated. These characteristics, and its ability to produce persistent infections place HCMV in the family of herpesviruses—a group of pathogens strongly linked to human cancer (Table 1).

Latent and Persistent Infection by HCMV

Primary infection with HCMV causes serious and sometimes fatal infections in utero and in newborns. Congenital infections with HCMV occur in a significant percentage of pregnant women in the 3rd trimester of pregnancy [4-6]. Infants infected in utero often develop a persistent HCMV infection with a broad spectrum of clinical consequences ranging from "silent," asymptomatic infections to severe, cytomegalic inclusion disease. While the vast majority of these infections are asymptomatic, reactivation of HCMV can produce a more serious disease than the primary infection (excluding cytomegalic inclusion disease which is usually fatal). An example of a disease resulting from reactivation is interstitial pneumonia, which is a serious complication seen in BMT recipients approximately two months after transplantation [7,8].

In vivo studies using a murine model of CMV infection determined that monocytes in the lung contained infectious viral particles that migrated from

TABLE 2. Evidence of HCMV in Humans

Specimen	Evidence of HCMV
Leukocytes	HCMV, HCMV DNA
Lymphoblasts	HCMV
Lymphoblastoid cells	HCMV, HCMV DNA
Skin fibroblasts	HCMV
Colon cancer cells	HCMV DNA
Normal prostate cells	HCMV-specific antigens, HCMV DNA
Malignant prostate cells	HCMV-related antigens
Normal kidney tissue	HCMV DNA
Male and female GU tract	HCMV
Semen	HCMV
Kaposi sarcoma	HCMV, HCMV DNA

capillaries into the alveolar spaces of the lung [9]. An in vitro study has shown that HCMV grows well in human alveolar macrophages [10]. HCMV is also able to persist in circulating PMNLs [11] and, more controversially, in blood lymphocytes [12–14]. The ability of HCMV to infect cells of the immune system has profound implications: CMV is a known immunosuppressant both in the mouse [15] and in man [16], and its effects on CMI are amply noted in the literature. The possible auxiliary role of HCMV in the pathogenesis of human neoplasia will be discussed further in a later section. A versatile virus, HCMV can persist in epithelial cells of salivary glands, in the cervix, and in renal tubules [11], and it also has been detected in nervous tissue [17]. Posttransfusion reactivation of HCMV has been reported by several investigators [18,19], and it is known that a positive correlation exists between the increased risk of HCMV infection and the volume of blood transfused [20]. These clinically significant examples of HCMV reactivation have been corroborated in a number of in vitro studies of HCMV persistence and latency.

The ability of HCMV to establish latent, persistent infections has been studied rather extensively in cultured human cells. In the presence of the antiviral compound, cytosine arabinoside (ara-C), Gönczöl and Váczi [21] detected HCMV in 1% of infected human embryo fibroblasts. By immunofluorescent techniques, about 50% of these cells contained HCMV-specific antigens. Ara-C maintained latent infections indefinitely, and removal of the drug led to the recovery of infectious virus after four or five days [21]. In 1975, Rapp et al [22] established a human cell line (Mj-P) from normal prostatic cells expressing HCMV antigens. Infectious virus could not be "rescued" from these cells. It would appear that the establishment of this cell line is due to either a chronic HCMV infection or to HCMV-induced cell transformation. Hybridization studies detected 10-15 genome equivalents of HCMV DNA per cell. Investigators examining an EBV-positive lymphoblastoid cell line infected with HCMV reported that while there was no detectable expression of HCMV, 8-10 virus genomic equivalents were found per cell [23]. Other lymphoblastoid cell lines and peripheral blood leukocytes have been persistently infected in vitro with HCMV [13,24]. These studies, in addition to many clinical observations, indicate that HCMV induces long-term latent and persistent infections in man. This property along with the ability of HCMV to enhance host cell DNA and RNA synthesis [25,26] suggests that the continuous presence of the virus in human cells can lead to integration of HCMV DNA into the host genome, possibly resulting in malignant transformation.

Oncogenic Characteristics of HCMV

In addition to stimulating host DNA and RNA synthesis, HCMV shares other properties in common with known oncogenic viruses such as: production of many defective particles; persistence in the host for extended periods; ability to transform cells in vitro to malignancy; and induction of tumors in vivo by transformed cells. It was recognized some years ago that HCMV released into the cytoplasm or into the extracellular fluid of cell cultures may contain a high percentage of defective particles [27,28]. The high number of defective particles increases the probability of a nonproductive infection which may allow the virus to remain within cells and cause persistent latent infections.

The oncogenicity of HCMV has been recognized since 1973 when Albrecht and Rapp [29] demonstrated transformation of hamster embryo fibroblasts by ultraviolet-irradiated HCMV. At 20 days postinfection, foci of cells appeared that had lost contact inhibition, a characteristic of malignant cells. Subculture of one of these foci resulted in the establishment of a fibroblastoid cell line, which in later passages showed increasingly aberrant morphology [29]. This finding was corroborated by other investigators using ultraviolet-inactivated HCMV [30].

Later studies showed that noninactivated, infectious HCMV (strain Mj) could also transform human embryo lung cells [31]. Subsequent studies reported that these HCMV-transformed cells were tumorigenic in athymic nude mice. Increased tumorigenicity was noted as the in vitro passage number increased; after passage 20, tumorigenicity ranged from 47% to 100%. Interestingly, the percentage of HCMV-transformed human cells with detectable HCMV antigens gradually decreased to 20% by passage 40 and to 0% by passage 60 [32,33]. When cell lines were derived from tumor tissue, inoculation of low passage cells (1 to 20) back into nude mice resulted in tumors in only 16% of the animals. Passages later than 20 showed a decrease in tumorigenicity that at passage 145 was undetectable. However, in passages higher than 145 oncogenic potential increased, and 66% of the inoculated mice developed tumors. One cell line, in contrast to the parental (original transformed human embryonic lung cells) and other tumor lines, maintained a constant level of HCMV antigen expression until passage 146, when the number of HCMV-positive cells decreased while oncogenicity increased [33]. It appears, therefore, that oncogenicity inversely correlates with HCMV antigen expression and that malignant cells originally transformed by the virus no longer show evidence of HCMV expression at readily detectable levels.

HCMV, its genetic material, or its antigens have been detected in many normal and malignant human cells and in GU secretions (Table 2). However, a direct link between human cancer and HCMV has not yet been established. HCMV has been found in both malignant and nonmalignant tissues of the same individual [34], but there is controversy surrounding the role of HCMV in the development of human cancer. One study has reported that the absence of HCMV in tumor tissue from patients with KS implies that active HCMV infection does not occur in neoplastic cells, but that exposure to HCMV is a primary event leading to oncogenesis [35]. This line of thinking is provocative and is supported by findings of high antibody levels to HCMV in KS patients. However, this hypothesis is purely subjective, as it is based on negative findings. It could be similarly argued that the lack of detectable HCMV particles or antigen expression in malignant human tissue is analogous to the situation observed in nude mice injected with HCMV-derived transformed cell lines; ie, low levels of virus expression (perhaps at undetectable levels) correlate with increased oncogenicity.

The high incidence of HCMV infection in humans, its ability to cause asymptomatic infections and to remain latent for long periods of time before reactivation and subsequent disease, in conjunction with its proven oncogenicity both in vitro and in vivo provide strong indirect evidence that HCMV is a cancer-causing agent in man. However, there are inconsistent as well as negative findings that speak against this supposition. In the following sections, the association of HCMV with certain human cancers will be discussed. An hypothesis is suggested that may be helpful in developing a perspective on the relationship of this oncogenic DNA virus to the development of human cancer.

As listed in Table 1, several human cancers are associated with viruses, many of which are in the herpesvirus group. The presence of virus does not prove direct causation, and in the case of Burkitt lymphoma, EBV has not been isolated successfully from primary explants of tumors. Nevertheless, epidemiologic, biologic, molecular, and immunologic evidence provide a substantial body of observations supporting the hypothesis that viruses play a role in the development of human neoplasms (Table 3).

Genital cancer, including cancer of the prostate and cervical carcinoma, is linked with HCMV by several factors:

Persistent HCMV infections in GU tract;

Sexual transmission;

Seroepidemiologic studies linking HCMV antibodies and genital cancer;

Detection of HCMV particles or HCMV-specific antigens in genital cancer biopsies; and

In vitro transformation studies.

The GU tract is known to support persistent infection by HCMV [36], and the virus has been isolated from the cervix and from semen [5, 37, 38]. It is also known that HCMV persists in the GU tract of the human host in the presence of high titers of anti-HCMV antibody. These and other observations [39] strongly suggest that HCMV can be transmitted sexually.

Prostatic Carcinoma

The incidence of cancer of the prostate has increased more than 20% since the mid-1950s, and statistics from the American Cancer Society show this disease now to be the fourth most prevalent type of cancer in the United States [40]. While there is a strikingly high incidence of prostatic cancer in American blacks, there are as yet no data that definitively link prostatic cancer with race, socioeconomic class, sexual habits, or venereal disease. While HSV has also been isolated from the human male GU tract [41], in

TABLE 3. Evidence for Virus Pathogenesis of Human Cancers

Evidence	Observation
Epidemiologic	association of virus with tumors
Biologic and virologic	tumor cells contain infectious virus
	transformation of cells in vitro
	tumor induction in vivo
Molecular biologic	presence of virus DNA, RNA, and proteins in tumor cells
Immunologic	virus-specific antigens in tumor cells
	anti-virus antibodies in patient serum

contrast to cervical carcinoma, the evidence associating prostatic cancer to HCMV is more abundant. A serologic study of 92 patients firmly established that prostatic cancer patients have significantly higher HCMV antibody titers than control groups, including patients with benign prostatic hyperplasia and nonurogenital cancers [42]. In another in vitro study, it was determined that lymphocytes from patients with prostatic cancer are specifically cytotoxic to cells transformed by HCMV-Mj [43]. As mentioned, this tumorigenic strain of HCMV was isolated from normal prostate tissue subsequently transformed in vitro by the viral isolate [22].

Cervical Carcinoma

The most common cancer of women throughout the world is cervical carcinoma [44]. New cases of in situ carcinoma of the cervix are estimated to reach 45,000 annually, while the estimated number of cases of invasive uterine cancer (invasive cervical cancer and cancer of the uterine endometrium and of the corpus) in 1983 is 55,000 [40]. Epidemiologic studies reported in the 1950s and 1960s established a profile of the female adult most likely to develop this disease [45–47]: the individual is between the ages of 35 and 60, and has had multiple sexual partners beginning at an early age. There is also an association between the disease and low socioeconomic status. Sexual transmission is suggested by the infrequency of cervical carcinoma in celibate women and in Jewish women whose husbands are circumcised.

The evidence linking HCMV and cervical carcinoma is not as strong as that between HSV and this cancer [47–49]. For both viruses, much of the evidence consists of epidemiologic studies and serologic findings. As already described, HCMV has been detected in semen [38] and has also been isolated from the cervix [50]. However, there have been many conflicting reports concerning the association of circulating HCMV antibody levels with cervical cancer [51–54]. The most recent investigation by Hart et al [54] examined sera from 199 patients with abnormal cervical smears and found no correlation between levels of antibody and degree of pathologic findings ranging from several degrees of dysplasia to in situ carcinoma. It was found, however, that increasing age correlated well with percent of seropositivity. The point that is clear from these studies is that antibodies to HCMV are not protective even though they are neutralizing antibodies. The frequent presence of this virus in the GU tract in the absence of cervical carcinoma does not wholly speak against a role for HCMV in the development of the disease, but points out that several unknown factors may exist that possibly initiate or potentiate an early neoplastic event.

Adenocarcinoma of the Colon

Carcinomas of the colon and rectum will account for an estimated 58,000 deaths in 1983. The incidence of these two diseases is second only to lung cancer in the United States [40]. There is epidemiologic evidence suggesting that diet, environmental factors, and genetics play a role in the development of cancer of the colon [55]. Adenomatous polyps are closely associated with this disease in individual patients as well as geographic distribution [56], suggesting that there may be some factor(s) in common with the development of both nonmalignant and malignant tumors. HCMV is known to be present in the GI tract of man [57], and a 1978 study examined colon tissue for HCMV nucleic acid [34]. Using membrane cRNA-DNA hybridization, it was determined that four out of seven tumors contained HCMV DNA, in a range of 1-9 genome equivalents per cell. One of the four patients with colon carcinoma positive for HCMV DNA also had HCMV DNA present in normal colon tissue. In contrast, in patients with Crohn disease, both normal and diseased segments of the colon were negative for HCMV DNA, although two out of three individuals were found to have detectable serum levels of HCMV antibody. Patients with familial polyposis and ulcerative colitis, conditions that predispose to adenocarcinoma of the colon, were also positive for HCMV DNA. While the number of patients in these studies was small, the results indicate an association of HCMV with carcinoma of the colon.

In 1979, Hashiro et al [58] identified HCMV in tumor cell cultures from patients with adenocarcinoma of the colon, strengthening the association of the virus with this type of cancer. Other factors associating HCMV with adenocarcinoma of the colon are:

HCMV persistently infects the GI tract;

HCMV DNA detected in malignant tumors of the colon; and

HCMV DNA found in colon tissues of patients with conditions predisposing for adenocarcinoma of the colon.

The presence of HCMV does not automatically confirm an etiologic role. HCMV, which is known to persistently and latently infect cells, may be reactivated by some, as yet unknown, factor or may be induced by the development of a "neoplastic state" in the host tissues. It is also possible that HCMV may be present in the tumor but have no involvement in the development of the transformed state in vivo. Serologic findings indicate that serum titers to other herpesviruses are also elevated, making difficult the analysis of the association between colon carcinoma and HCMV [59]. It is interesting that these authors found an increased serum titer only to HCMV and not to other herpesviruses when they used complement fixation to detect IgG antibodies. This points out the necessity for care in interpreting serologic findings.

It is also important to note that another study [60] failed to detect HCMV DNA in adenocarcinoma of the colon using, presumably, a more sensitive technique than that used by Huang and Roche [34]. Using a reassociation kinetics assay with a sensitivity of less than one genomic equivalent per cell, Brichácek et al [60] did not detect HCMV DNA in a small number of patients with colon carcinoma. While the authors are careful to point out that their results may be due to the presence of a fragment of the HCMV genome too small to be detected by the method used or to their small patient population, this study further points out the difficulty in assigning an etiologic role to HCMV in the development of this tumor. In a more recent study taking advantage of a battery of modern molecular and biologic techniques, no evidence of HCMV DNA or antigenic expression was found in adenocarcinoma cells [61]. Fourteen tumor specimens from patients with adenocarcinoma of the colon or rectum were studied in parallel with normal tissues from the same patients. Using in situ hybridization of a ^{3}H-labeled HCMV DNA probe to detect HCMV mRNA, immunofluorescence, long-term tumor cell culture, and cocultivation of normal and malignant tissues, these investigators did not detect HCMV. In addition, they fused tumor cells to HCMV-permissive human embryonic lung cells to encourage reactivation of possible latent virus, and treated the fusions with iododeoxyuridine, a known inducer of virus production [62], all with negative results.

It is somewhat difficult to argue a point with essentially negative findings, but this study indicates that the role of HCMV in the development of adenocarcinoma of the colon, if indeed it is more than a bystander, may be highly dependent on the presence or absence of other factors.

Kaposi Sarcoma (KS)

KS (multiple idiopathic pigmented hemangiosarcoma) has been studied as a potential model for virus-associated human malignancy [63]. The disease has a particularly high incidence in equatorial Africa and makes up 3% to 9% of all malignant tumors in Kenya, Tanzania, and Zaire. African cases occur predominantly in children, and are rapidly progressive and fatal, in contrast to European and American cases of KS which are less aggressive. Also, in contrast to African KS, cases of the disease outside the African continent are found predominantly in the 50- to 70-year old age group, particularly in people of Mediterranean descent [64-66]. This malignancy is a disease of males and one study has reported an incidence ratio of males to females as 14:1 [67]. The clustering of the disease strongly suggests that genetic and environmental factors (including an infectious agent) are involved in the etiology of KS. Over 10 years ago, Giraldo et al [68] reported the isolation of HCMV from a KS tissue-derived cell line. Seroepidemiologic studies subsequently have determined that KS patients have HCMV antibodies and do not have antibody patterns characteristic of HSV type 1, HSV type 2, or EBV [66, 69].

More recently, HCMV "nuclear antigens," HCMV RNA, and HCMV DNA sequences have been found in KS tumor biopsies, early passage cells derived from sarcoma tissue, and in DNA extracted from the tumor cells [70, 71]. These studies demonstrated that about 30% of KS biopsy material contains HCMV DNA sequences at a level of 0.7 to 1.0 genomic equivalents per cell. One inherent problem in detecting virus sequences and products in KS tumors and cell lines (as well as in other tumor types) is the lack of a clearly defined population of cells. Tumors often contain a mixture of malignant and nonmalignant cell types, and early passage tumor cell lines can be overgrown with fibroblastic cells. This latter point, combined with the unidentified cell origin of KS, have provoked criticism that HCMV may not be involved in tumorigenesis, and may be a passenger carried by a nonmalignant, latently infected cell. The low levels of HCMV in KS tumor biopsies also may reflect a heterogeneity of cell type that essentially dilutes the level of virus or viral expression detectable. An interesting aspect of the association between HCMV and KS is the fact that patients with this disease have a significantly increased incidence of second, primary tumors, especially of the lymphoreticular system [72]. HCMV can cause immunosuppression in both mice and man [15, 16] and, as will be further discussed below, its interaction with elements of the immune system may also be involved in oncogenesis.

DOES HCMV CAUSE HUMAN CANCER?

The association between HCMV and human cancer is provocative. However, seroepidemiologic studies, reports of virus isolation, and even molecular studies (to be discussed in this section) do not provide conclusive proof for HCMV in the etiology of human malignancy. Three areas of consideration must be included in any evaluation of HCMV as a cause of human cancer. First, HCMV is a ubiquitous virus that many individuals are exposed to early in life—even prenatally. In addition, other DNA viruses commonly infect large numbers of people relatively early in life. Second, many HCMV infections are asymptomatic, but produce low-level persistent infection in many different organ systems studied. Thus, the presence of HCMV in malignant tissue may represent a reactivation of latent virus secondary to the development of neoplasia. Third, there is evidence of geographic and/or socioeconomic clustering in many of the cancers associated with HCMV. Therefore, environmental as well as genetic factors should be considered in any discussion of viral etiology.

Possible Auxiliary Roles for HCMV in Carcinogenesis

Large numbers of agents, including carcinogens, cocarcinogens, and tumor promoters, are found in the environment, sometimes in conjunction with certain occupations [73]. Some investigators have compared high versus low incidences of cancer in specific regions and concluded that a majority of human cancers are due to environmental causes [74,75]. The two-stage model for carcinogenesis proposed by Berenblum in 1941 [76] requires an "initiator" (carcinogen) and a "promoting" substance, both perhaps found in the environment. First described as a model for tumor development in mouse skin, the theory requires that the carcinogen alone does not produce tumors and, similarly, that the promoter itself does not (or rarely) produce malignancy. However, one application of the initiator followed by repeated exposure to a promoter will result in many benign and malignant tumors [77]. Diterpene esters have been described as efficient tumor promoters [76] that enhance transformation of human leukocytes by EBV [78]. In this system, these compounds effectively induce production of virus from persistently infected cells. To date, similar experiments with HCMV and phorbol diesters have not been carried out. This may be due in part to the lack of firm evidence that HCMV can replicate in human leukocytes as can EBV. Nevertheless, interactions of HCMV with chemical carcinogens may be expected to occur as they do for other oncogenic herpesviruses [74,79,80].

There is also evidence suggesting that HCMV-infected cells exhibit selective chromosomal damage [81]. Chromosomes 2, 3, 4, and 21 of HCMV-infected cells show significantly more anomalies than other chromosomes that are not directly proportional to the length of the chromosomes. It is not yet known whether this effect of HCMV infection has direct bearing on the oncogenicity of the virus.

As already mentioned, another role of HCMV in human cancer may involve the immune system. Very recently, a new disorder termed AIDS has been described. This disease has received a great deal of public attention, and has been reported in diverse groups including homosexuals [82–84], Haitian immigrants to the United States [85], hemophiliacs [86], and children of parents who are intravenous drug users [87]. In homosexual patients with AIDS, there is an alarming increase in incidence of KS [82] along with severe acquired cellular immunodeficiency that is hallmarked by a reversal of the helper/suppressor T-cell ratio [83,84,88]. Another characteristic of

AIDS is life-threatening opportunistic infections. HCMV infection is a common denominator in these reports. While other herpesviruses have also been isolated, and in general antibody levels to HSV and EBV are high along with HCMV titers, the association of HCMV and immunosuppression provides a possible role for this virus in human carcinogenesis if indeed a defect in the immune response is involved in early transformational events. While the concept of "immune surveillance" is generally under siege, there is evidence suggesting that alteration of CMI may play a role in the development of neoplasia [reviewed in 89]. Through interaction with leukocytes and/or cells of the monocytic series, HCMV may subtly alter both immunoregulatory and effector functions of cells in the immune system. Little work has been done in this area, and this approach may hopefully provide answers to many of the unknown aspects of the etiology of human cancer.

Current Avenues of Research

As described in this chapter, there is a significant amount of indirect biologic and seroepidemiologic evidence suggesting that HCMV may be involved in human cancer. In addition, molecular biologic techniques have enabled many investigators to identify HCMV DNA and RNA in malignant tumor tissues. However, these studies provide only indirect proof of the involvement of HCMV in cancer pathogenesis. More direct information on the role of several strains of HCMV in cell transformation has been provided by restriction endonuclease mapping, and fragments of the viral genome have been cloned providing a complete gene library [90-94]. These studies are aimed at identification of the viral sequences necessary for cell transformation.

Using cloned fragments of purified DNA to transfect NIH 3T3 cells, a transforming sequence of HCMV strain AD169 has been identified [95]. In this same study, cells transformed by this fragment of viral DNA were tumorigenic in young athymic nude mice. However, when these investigators examined DNA from the transformed cells, they were not able to detect viral sequences homologous to the *Hin*dIII-E fragment used to transform the cells.

In another study, the mechanisms controlling the expression of different HCMV gene products were examined [96]. Earlier work had identified regions of the HCMV genome coding RNAs at various times postinfection, ie, IE, early, and late RNAs [97]. To study HCMV gene regulation at the posttranscriptional level [96], viral transcripts synthesized during the IE, early, and late phases of infection were examined.

Results showed that posttranscriptional controls of viral gene expression in HCMV-infected cells include transcript accumulation, transport to the cytoplasm, preferential association of different RNA transcripts with polysomes, and differences in stability of RNAs. In a recent paper, a major regulatory protein of HCMV transcription has been described [98]. Such molecular approaches to analyze the regulation of the HCMV genome in permissive cells provide valuable methodologies for future examination of the regulation of HCMV activity within persistently and latently infected cells, and ultimately may help clarify the oncogenic characteristics of HCMV and how they relate to human cancer.

CONCLUSIONS

HCMV is an oncogenic DNA virus of the herpesvirus group that causes a broad spectrum of diseases in man. There is a great deal of evidence linking this virus to human cancers—some of this evidence seems stronger for some forms of cancer (KS for example) than for others (such as cervical carcinoma). Recent studies with cloned fragments of HCMV, however, clearly indicate that this virus has the potential to directly transform cells. The mechanism by which HCMV causes transformation is still unknown, and current studies are examining the expression of viral genes within infected human cells. Existing evidence also suggests that HCMV may play different roles in the pathogenesis of various forms of cancer. Rather than being a direct etiologic agent, it may serve as an "initiator," requiring the presence of some as yet unidentified "promoter" or cofactor (perhaps including a genetic variable) to cause neoplasia. There is a possibility (from the number of AIDS victims developing carcinomas) that HCMV may exert an effect on the human immune system that subtly affects the ability of the body to detect and remove transformed, malignant cells.

The difficulty in assessing the relation of HCMV to human cancer stems from its relatively wide distribution as a human pathogen. It has the ability to cause clinically silent but persistent infections that make early detection of primary infection difficult, if not impossible. Its ability to persist in several different organ systems also clouds the issue of its role in oncogenesis and whether it is merely a "passenger" reactivated by some other, early neoplastic event. The low level of detection of its DNA and RNA in malignant tissues has also raised questions as to its etiologic role. Hopefully, improved cell culture techniques that permit cloning of individual transformed cells, as well as more highly purified tumor cell cultures, will provide materials for further studies of the role of HCMV in tumorigenesis. Rapid gains have already been made in understanding how HCMV gene products are expressed in infected cells. Identification of sequences of HCMV DNA with the ability to transform cells in vitro should provide further support for the role of HCMV as a human cancer virus.

REFERENCES

1. Weller TH: The cytomegaloviruses: Ubiquitous agents with protean clinical manifestation. N Engl J Med 285:203–214; 267–274, 1971.
2. Lang DJ: Cytomegalovirus infection in organ transplantation and post-perfusion, An hypothesis. Arch Ges Virusforsch 37:365–377, 1972.
3. Epstein MA, Achong BG, Barr YM: Virus particles in cultured lymphoblasts from Burkitt's lymphoma. Lancet 1:702–703, 1964.
4. Numazaki Y, Yano N, Morizuka T, Taki S, Ishida N: Primary infection with human cytomegalovirus: Virus isolation from healthy infants and pregnant women. Am J Epidemiol 91:410–417, 1970.
5. Montgomery R, Youngblood L, Medearis DN: Recovery of cytomegalovirus from the cervix in pregnancy. Pediatrics 49:524–531, 1972.
6. Reynolds DW, Stagno S, Hosty TS, Tiller M, Alford CA: Maternal cytomegalovirus excretion and perinatal infection. N Engl J Med 289:1–5, 1973.
7. Rubin RH, Russell PS, Levin M, Cohen C: From the National Institutes of Health. Summary of a workshop on cytomegalovirus infections during organ transplantation. J Infect Dis 139:728–734, 1979.
8. Pagano JS: Infections with cytomegalovirus in bone marrow transplantation: Report of a workshop. J Infect Dis 132:114–120, 1975.
9. Murphy GF, Brody AR, Craighead JE: Monocyte migration across pulmonary membranes in mice infected with cytomegalovirus. Exp Mol Pathol 22:35–44, 1975.
10. Drew WL, Mintz L, Hoo R, Finley TN: Growth of herpes simplex and cytomegalovirus in cultured human alveolar macrophages. Annu Rev Respir Dis 119:289–291, 1979.
11. Huang E-S, Pagano JS: Comparative diagnosis of cytomegalovirus. In Kurstak E (ed): "New Approaches in Comparative Diagnosis of Viral Diseases." New York:Academic Press, 1977, pp 241–285.
12. Caul EO, Clarke SKR, Matt MG, Perham TGM, Wilson RSE: Cytomegalovirus infections after open heart surgery. A prospective study. Lancet 1:777–780, 1971.
13. St. Jeor S, Weisser A: Persistence of cytomegalovirus in human lymphoblast and peripheral leukocyte cultures. Infect Immun 15:402–409, 1977.
14. Rinaldo CR, Richter BS, Black PH, Callery R, Chess L, Hirsch MS: Replication of herpes simplex virus and cytomegalovirus in human leukocytes. J Immunol 120:130–136, 1978.
15. Hamilton JR, Overall JC, Glasgow LA: Synergistic effect on mortality in mice with murine cytomegalovirus and *Pseudomonas aeruginosa, Staphylococcus aureus* or *Candida albicans* infections. Infect Immun 14: 982–989, 1976.
16. Carney WP, Rubin RH, Hoffman RA, Hanser WP, Healey K, Hirsch MS: Analysis of T lymphocyte subsets in cytomegalovirus mononucleosis. J Immunol 126:2114–2116, 1981.
17. Duchowny M, Caplan L, Siber G: Cytomegalovirus infection of the adult nervous system. Ann Neurol 5:458–461, 1979.
18. Feinstone SM, Kapikian AZ, Purcell RH, Alter HJ, Holland PV: Transfusion-associated hepatitis not due to viral hepatitis type A or B. N Engl J Med 292:767–770, 1973.
19. Lerner PI, Sampliner JE: Transfusion-associated cytomegalovirus mononucleosis. Ann Surg 185:406–410, 1977.
20. Prince AM, Szmuness W, Millian SJ, David DS: A serologic study of cytomegalovirus infections associated with blood transfusions. N Engl J Med 284:1125–1131, 1971.
21. Gönczöl E, Váczi L: Cytomegalovirus latency in cultured human cells. J Gen Virol 18:143–151, 1973.

22. Rapp F, Geder L, Murasko D, Lausch R, Ladda R, Huang E-S, Webber MJ: Long-term persistence of cytomegalovirus genome in cultured human cells of prostatic origin. J Urol 16:982–990, 1975.

23. Joncas JG, Menezes J, Huang E-S: Persistence of CMV genome in lymphoid cells after congenital infections. Nature 258:432–434, 1975.

24. Tocci MJ, St. Jeor SC: Susceptibility of lymphoblastoid cells to infection with human cytomegalovirus. Infect Immun 15:402–409, 1977.

25. St. Jeor S, Albrecht TB, Funk FD, Rapp F: Stimulation of cell DNA synthesis by human cytomegalovirus. J Virol 13:353–362, 1974.

26. Tanaka S, Furukawa T, Plotkin SA: Human cytomegalovirus stimulates host cell RNA synthesis. J Virol 15:297–304, 1975.

27. Huang AS, Baltimore D: Defective interfering animal viruses. In Fraenkel-Conrat H, Wagner R (eds): "Comprehensive Virology." New York: Plenum Press, 1977, pp 73–116.

28. Stinski MF, Mocarski ES, Thomsen DR: DNA of human cytomegalovirus: Size heterogeneity and defectiveness resulting from serial undiluted passage. J Virol 31:231–239, 1979.

29. Albrecht T, Rapp F: Malignant transformation of hamster embryo fibroblasts following exposure to ultraviolet-irradiated human cytomegalovirus. Virology 55:53–61, 1973.

30. Boldogh I, Gönczöl E, Váczi L: Transformation of hamster embryonic fibroblast cells by UV-irradiated human cytomegalovirus. Acta Microbiol Acad Sci Hung 25:269–275, 1970.

31. Geder L, Lausch R, O'Neill F, Rapp F: Oncogenic transformation of human embryo lung cells by human cytomegalovirus. Science 192:1134–1137, 1976.

32. Geder L, Kreider J, Rapp F: Human cells transformed *in vitro* by human cytomegalovirus: Tumorigenicity in athymic nude mice. J Natl Cancer Inst 58:1003–1009, 1977.

33. Geder L, Laychock A, Gorodecki J, Rapp F: Alterations in biological properties of different lines of cytomegalovirus-transformed human embryo lung cells following *in vitro* cultivation. IARC Sci Publ 24:561–601, 1978.

34. Huang E-S, Roche JK: Cytomegalovirus DNA and adenocarcinoma of the colon: Evidence for latent viral infection. Lancet 1:957–960, 1978.

35. Civantos F, Penneys NS, Haines H: Kaposi's sarcoma: Absence of cytomegalovirus antigens. J Invest Dermatol 79:79–80, 1982.

36. Geder L: Oncogenic properties of human cytomegalovirus. In Rapp F (ed): "Oncogenic Herpesviruses." Boca Raton, FL:CRC Press, 1980, pp 47–60.

37. Amstey MS: Genital herpesvirus infection. Clin Obstet Gynecol 18:89–100, 1975.

38. Lang DJ, Kummer JF: Demonstration of cytomegalovirus in semen. N Engl J Med 287:756–758, 1972.

39. Wilmott FE: Cytomegalovirus in female patients attending a venereal disease clinic. Br J Vener Dis 51:278–280, 1975.

40. Cancer Facts and Figures 1983. American Cancer Society, 1983, p 8.

41. Centifanto YM, Kaufman EH, Zam ZS, Drylie DM, Deardourff SL: Herpesvirus particles in prostatic carcinoma cells. J Virol 12:1608–1611, 1973.

42. Laychock AM, Geder L, Sanford EJ, Rapp F: Immune response of prostatic cancer patients to cytomegalovirus-infected and -transformed cells. Cancer 142:1766–1771, 1978.

43. Dagen JE, Sanford EJ, Rohner TJ, Geder L, Rapp F: Recognition of virally transformed cells by lymphocytes from patients with prostatic cancer. Urology 12:532–536, 1978.

44. Persaud V: Geographical pathology of cancer of the uterine cervix. Trop Geogr Med 29:335–345, 1977.

45. Towne JE: Carcinoma of the cervix in nulliparous and celibate women. Am J Obstet Gynecol 69:606–613, 1955.
46. Martin CE: Epidemiology of cancer of the cervix: II. Marital and coital factors in cervical cancer. Am J. Public Health 57:803–814, 1967.
47. Frenkel N, Roizman B, Cassai E, Nahmias A: A DNA fragment of herpes simplex 2 and its transcription in human cervical cancer tissue. Proc Natl Acad Sci USA 69:3984–3789, 1972.
48. Aurelian L, Schumann B, Marcus RL, Davis HJ: Antibody to HSV-2 induced tumor specific antigens in serum from patients with cervical carcinoma. Science 181:161–164, 1973.
49. Pacsa AS, Kummerländer L, Pejtsik B, Krommer K, Pali K: Herpes simplex virus-specific antigens in exfoliated cervical cells from women with and without cervical anaplasia. Cancer Res 36:2130–2132, 1976.
50. Melnick JL, Lewis R, Wimberly I, Kaufman RH, Adam E: Association of cytomegalovirus (CMV) infection with cervical cancer: Isolation of CMV from cell cultures derived from cervical biopsy. Intervirology 10:115–119, 1978.
51. Fuccillo D, Sever J, Moder F, Chen T-C, Catalano L, Johnson L: Antibodies in patients with carcinoma of the uterine cervix. Obstet Gynecol 38:599–601, 1971.
52. Vestergaard B, Hornsleth A, Dedersen S: Occurrence of herpes and adenovirus antibodies in patients with carcinoma of the cervix uteri. Measurement of antibodies to *Herpesvirus hominis* (types 1 and 2), cytomegalovirus, EB virus and adenovirus. Cancer 30:68–74, 1972.
53. Pasca A, Kummerländer L, Pejtsik B, Pali K: Herpesvirus antibodies and antigens in patients with cervical anaplasia and in controls. J Natl Cancer Inst 55:775–782, 1975.
54. Hart H, Springbett A, Norval M: Lack of association of cytomegalovirus antibody level with carcinoma of the uterine cervix. Gynecol Obstet Invest 14:300–308, 1982.
55. Burkitt DP: Epidemiology of cancer of the colon and rectum. Cancer 28:3–13, 1971.
56. Haenzel WM, Correa P: Cancer of the colon and rectum and adenomatous polyps: A review of epidemiologic findings. Cancer 28:14–24, 1971.
57. Henson D: Cytomegalovirus inclusion bodies in the gastrointestinal tract. Arch Pathol 93:477–482, 1972.
58. Hashiro GM, Horikami S, Loh PC: Cytomegalovirus isolations from cell cultures of human adenocarcinomas of the colon. Intervirology 12:84–88, 1979.
59. Avni A, Haikin H, Feuchtwanger MM, Sacks M, Naggan L, Sarov B, Sarov I: Antibody pattern to human cytomegalovirus in patients with adenocarcinoma of the colon. Intervirology 16:244–249, 1981.
60. Brichácek B, Hirsch I, Závadová H, Procházka M, Faltýn J, Vonka V: Absence of cytomegalovirus DNA from adenocarcinoma of the colon. Intervirology 14:223–227, 1980.
61. Hart H, Neill WA, Norval M: Lack of association of cytomegalovirus with adenocarcinoma of the colon. Gut 23:21–30, 1982.
62. St. Jeor S, Rapp F: Cytomegalovirus replication in cells pretreated with 5-iodo-2′deoxyuridine. J Virol 11:986–990, 1973.
63. Giraldo G, Beth E, Coeur P, Vogel CL, Dhru DS: Kaposi's sarcoma: A new model in the search for viruses associated with human malignancies. J Natl Cancer Inst 49:1495–1507, 1972.
64. Oettle AG: Geographical and racial differences in frequency of Kaposi's sarcoma as evidence of environmental or genetic causes. In Ackerman LV, Murray JF (eds): "Symposium on Kaposi's Sarcoma." New York:Haefner Publishing Company, 1963, pp 330–363.

65. Slavin G, Cameron HM, Singh H: Kaposi's sarcoma in mainland Tanzania: A report of 117 cases. Br J Cancer 23:349–367, 1969.

66. Giraldo G, Beth E, Kourilsky FM, Henle W, Henle G, Miké V, Huraux JM, Anderson HK, Gharbi MR, Kyalwazi SK, Puissant A: Antibody patterns to herpesviruses in Kaposi's sarcoma: Serological Association of European Kaposi's sarcoma with cytomegalovirus. Int J Cancer 15:839–848, 1975.

67. Taylor JF, Smith PG, Bull D, Pike MC: Kaposi's Sarcoma in Uganda: Geographic and ethnic distribution. Br J Cancer 26:483–497, 1972.

68. Giraldo G, Beth E, Haguenau F: Herpes-type virus particles in tissue culture of Kaposi's sarcoma from different geographic regions. J Natl Cancer Inst 49:1509–1526, 1972.

69. Giraldo G, Beth E, Henle W, Henle G, Miké V, Safai B, Huraux JM, McHardy J, de-Thé G: Antibody patterns to herpesviruses in Kaposi's sarcoma. II. Serological association of American Kaposi's sarcoma with cytomegalovirus. Int J Cancer 22:126–131, 1978.

70. Giraldo G, Beth E, Huang E-S: Kaposi's sarcoma and its relationship to cytomegalovirus (CMV). III. CMV DNA and CMV early antigens in Kaposi's sarcoma. Int J Cancer 26:23–29, 1980.

71. Boldogh I, Beth E, Huang E-S, Kyalwazi SK, Giraldo G: Kaposi's sarcoma. IV. Detection of CMV DNA, CMV RNA and CMNA in tumor biopsies. Int J Cancer 28:469–474, 1981.

72. Safai B, Miké V, Giraldo G, Beth E, Good RA: Association of Kaposi's sarcoma with second primary malignancies. Possible etiopathogenic implications. Cancer 45:1472–1479, 1980.

73. Wynder EL, Gori GB: Contribution of the environment to cancer incidence: An epidemiologic exercise. J Natl Cancer Inst 58:825–832, 1977.

74. Higginson J: Present trends in cancer epidemiology. Proc Can Cancer Conf 8:40–75, 1969.

75. Armstrong B, Doll R: Environmental factors and cancer incidence and mortality in different countries with special reference to dietary practices. Int J Cancer 15:617–631, 1975.

76. Berenblum I: The cocarcinogenic action of croton resin. Cancer Res 1:44–48, 1941.

77. Hecker E: Cocarcinogenic principles from the seed oil of *Croton tiglium* and from other Euphorbiaceae. Cancer Res 28:2338–2349, 1968.

78. Yamamoto N, zur Hausen H: Tumour promoter TPA enhances transformation of human leukocytes by Epstein-Barr virus. Nature 280:244–245, 1979.

79. Howett MK, Pegg AE, Rapp F: Enhancement of biochemical transformation of mammalian cells by herpes simplex virus following nitrosomethylurea treatment. Cancer Res 39:1041–1045, 1979.

80. Johnson FB: Chemical interactions with herpes simplex type 2 virus: Enhancement of transformation by selected chemical carcinogens and procarcinogens. Carcinogenesis 3:1235–1240, 1982.

81. Lüleci G, Salízlí M, Günalp A: Selective chromosomal damage caused by human cytomegalovirus. Acta Virol 24:341–345, 1980.

82. Kaposi's sarcoma and *Pneumocystis* pneumonia among homosexual men — New York City and California. Morbid Mortal Weekly Rep 30:305–308, 1981.

83. Gottlieb MS, Schroff R, Schanker HM, Weisman JD, Fan PT, Wolf RA, Saxon A: *Pneumocystis carinii* pneumonia and mucosal candidiasis in previously healthy homosexual men. N Engl J Med 305:1425–1431, 1981.

84. Siegal FP, Lopez C, Hammer GS, Brown AE, Kornfeld SJ, Gold J, Hassett J, Hirschman SZ, Cunningham-Rundles C, Adelsberg BR, Parham DM, Siegal MA, Cunningham-Rundles S, Armstrong D: Severe acquired immunodeficiency in male homosexuals, manifested by chronic perianal ulcerative herpes simplex lesions. N Engl J Med 305:1439–1444, 1981.

85. Opportunistic infections and Kaposi's sarcoma among Haitians in the United States. Morbid Mortal Weekly Rep 31:353–354, 1982.

86. *Pneumocystis carinii* pneumonia among persons with hemophilia A. Morbid Mortal Weekly Rep 31:365–367, 1982.

87. Unexplained immunodeficiency and opportunistic infections infants — New York, New Jersey, California. Morbid Mortal Weekly Rep 31:665–667, 1982.

88. Masur H, Michelis MA, Greene JB, Onorato I, Vande Stouwe RA, Holzman RS, Wormser G, Brettman L, Lange M, Murray HW, Cunningham-Rundles S: An outbreak of community-acquired *Pneumocystis carinii* pneumonia. Initial manifestation of cellular immune dysfunction. N Engl J Med 305:1431–1438, 1981.

89. Herberman RB: Natural killer (NK) cells. In Sell KW, Miller WV (eds): "The Lymphocyte." New York:Alan R Liss, 1981, pp 33–43.

90. Demarchi JM: Human cytomegalovirus DNA: Restriction enzyme cleavage maps and map locations for immediate-early, early and late RNAs. Virology 114:23–38, 1981.

91. Thomsen DR, Stinski MF: Cloning of the human cytomegalovirus genomes as endonuclease XbaI fragments. Gene 16:207–216, 1981.

92. Tamashiro JC, Hock LF, Spector DH: Construction of a cloned library of the *Eco*RI fragments from the human cytomegalovirus genome (strain AD169). J Virol 42:547–557, 1982.

93. Oram JD, Downing RG, Akrig A, Dollery AA, Duggleby CJ, Wilkinson GWG, Greenaway PJ. Use of recombinant plasmids to investigate the structure of the human cytomegalovirus genome. J Gen Virol 59:111–129, 1982.

94. Spector DH, Hock L, Tamashiro JC: Cleavage maps for human cytomegalovirus DNA strain AD169 for restriction endonucleases *Eco*RI, *Bg*lII and *Hin*dIII. J Virol 42:558–582, 1982.

95. Nelson JA, Fleckenstein B, Galloway DA, McDougall JK: Transformation of NIH3T3 cells with cloned fragments of human cytomegalovirus strain AD169. J Virol 43:83–91, 1982.

96. Demarchi JM: Post-transcriptional control of human cytomegalovirus gene expression. Virology 124:390–402, 1982.

97. Demarchi JM, Schmidt CA, Kaplan AS: Patterns of transcription of human cytomegalovirus in permissively infected cells. J Virol 35:277–286, 1980.

98. Stinski MF, Thomsen DR, Stenberg RM, Goldstein LC: Organization and expression of the immediate early genes of human cytomegalovirus. J Virol 46:1–14, 1983.

The Oncogenicity of Human Cytomegalovirus*

Eng-Shang Huang, PhD[†], Eng-Chun Mar, PhD[‡], Istvan Boldogh, PhD[‡], and John Baskar, ScD[‡]

Cancer Research Center[†‡], Department of Medicine[†], Department of Microbiology and Immunology[†], The University of North Carolina at Chapel Hill, Chapel Hill, NC 27514

INTRODUCTION

HCMV has been considered an important pathogen which is associated with a great variety of clinical manifestations ranging from asymptomatic infection to intrauterine death, congenital abnormalities, mental retardation, mononucleosis, and interstitial pneumonia in organ transplant or immuno-compromised patients [1]. As with other herpesviruses, CMV is also capable of establishing latent infection following a primary infection with subsequent recurrence under immunocompromised situations. This virus had never been suspected to have oncogenic potential until Albrecht and Rapp [2] demonstrated its transformation of hamster embryonic fibroblasts with UV-irradiated viruses. Its ubiquitous distribution and often asymptomatic interaction with its host frequently lead scientists to overlook the oncogenic potential of this virus. Recently, there were numerous experimental data and observations reported from various laboratories suggesting that CMV has oncogenic potential comparable to that of other herpesviruses. Therefore, we would like to discuss specifically the oncogenicity of HCMV, and to present possible evidence of its association with human cancer.

*Supported by grants from NCI (CA21773) and NIAID (AI-12712 and AI-00229).

Birth Defects: Original Article Series, Volume 20, Number 1, pages 193–211
© 1984 March of Dimes Birth Defects Foundation

Constrained by Koch postulates, it is extremely difficult to present direct evidence to prove the oncogenicity of HCMV in the human host, especially the causal association between CMV and human cancers. To facilitate the analysis of CMV oncogenicity, we have categorized and interpreted the observations made previously by various investigators from different laboratories, as follows: 1) biochemical interaction of CMV with virus-infected host; 2) oncogenic transformation of mammalian cells by virus and viral DNA fragments in vitro; and 3) molecular epidemiologic analysis of the association of CMV with various human malignancies. We understand that these analyses may not provide definitive conclusions for the causal association of CMV with cancer, but at least they may strengthen the understanding of the role of CMV infection in malignant processes in humans.

BIOCHEMICAL INTERACTION OF CMV WITH VIRUS-INFECTED HOST CELLS

Stimulation of Host-Cell Nucleic Acid Synthesis

It is generally accepted that the ability of a virus to induce host-cell macromolecule synthesis is correlated with its transformation and oncogenic potential. The induction of host-cell DNA synthesis in virus-infected permissive and nonpermissive cells has been demonstrated in oncogenic adenovirus and papovavirus systems. In herpesviruses, the oncogenic HSV type 2 is capable of inducing cellular DNA synthesis under nonpermissive conditions [3, 4] and the cellular DNA synthesis of cultivated well-differentiated peripheral lymphocytes is stimulated by EBV infection [5]. The ability to immortalize a lymphoblastoid cell line by EBV infection was found to correlate with the ability of EBV to induce cellular DNA synthesis in virus-infected cord blood cells [6].

In HCMV, St. Jeor et al [7] first demonstrated that CMV was able to stimulate cellular DNA synthesis in both permissive human embryonic lung (HEL) cells and in nonpermissive monkey kidney cells. Their study indicated that stimulation of cellular DNA was mediated by a semiconservative mechanism and that a viral-coded function expressed after infection was essential for this stimulation [7]. Boldogh et al [8] also demonstrated that the ability of HCMV to stimulate cellular DNA synthesis in permissive and nonpermissive cells was dependent on the expression of very early gene function and was relatively resistant to UV irradiation. Besides the stimulation of cellular DNA synthesis, Tanaka et al [9] also reported that cellular mRNA, tRNA, and ribosomal RNA syntheses were greatly enhanced in CMV-infected permissive WI-38 human fibroblasts and in nonpermissive guinea pig embryonic fibroblasts [10]. They also concluded that virus-specific protein synthesis was required for the stimulation of host-cell macromolecule synthesis. Besides the chromosomal DNA, they found that mitochondrial DNA was also stimulated after CMV infection [11].

In nonpermissive rabbit kidney cell systems, DeMarchi et al [12,13] found that the induction of cellular DNA synthesis occurred only in those cells that synthesized viral-specific antigens. Based on blot hybridization experiments, they further concluded that the viral-specific RNA synthesized in nonpermissive rabbit kidney cells was similar to that found at early stages of virus-infected cells [12,13]. In contrast, in permissive cultures, synthesis of viral antigens and induction cellular DNA synthesis are mutually exclusive; cells productively infected with CMV were not induced to synthesize cellular DNA. The induction of cellular DNA synthesis occurred only in those cells in which viral structural antigen synthesis could not be detected [12,13]. DeMarchi and Kaplan [13] also found that defective virus particles were quite effective in stimulating cellular DNA synthesis.

Based on observations described above, it is obvious that HCMV has the important characteristic of stimulating cellular DNA synthesis both in permissive and nonpermissive hosts. Similarly, host-cell macromolecule synthesis which preceded or followed the cellular DNA synthesis should, therefore, be enhanced.

Stimulation of Host-Cell Enzyme Synthesis

One of the unique biochemical characteristics of HCMV, which differs from HSV, is that HCMV is capable of stimulating numerous cellular proteins and enzyme synthesis in both permissive and nonpermissive CMV-infected cells. Kamata et al [14] discovered that one of the chromatin-associated factors, which are induced in HEL cells at early stages of CMV infection, stimulated template activity of cell chromatin. This factor (factor I) coincided with a major component of "pre-early nuclear antigen" which was detectable within 1 hr after infection by its molecular size, elution properties in various column chromatographies, and reactivity to specific antibody. Whether this novel factor is functionally related to various SV40 T antigens is unclear at the present moment. More defined study is needed.

As a consequence of derepression of host-cell chromatin, numerous cellular enzyme activities have been found markedly enhanced in CMV-infected permissive as well as nonpermissive cells. These include thymidine kinase [15, 16], DNA polymerase [17], DNA-dependent RNA polymerase [18], ornithine decarboxylase [19], plasminogen activator [20], exonuclease, and topoisomerases (our unpublished observations). In CMV-infected fibroblasts, there was a rapid and high level of stimulation of low electrophoretic migration cytosol thymidine kinase (TK). A fast migration mitochondrial TK was also stimulated upon CMV infection, but to a lesser extent. The stimulation of these TK activities was found as early as 12 hr after infection, and reached a plateau at 24 to 48 hr PI. Characteristics of these enzymes with respect to electromobility in polyacrylamide gel, phosphodonor specificity, pH optimal, salt inhibition, and thermostability did not show significant differences from those of normal cellular enzyme [16]. Meanwhile, there was no detectable TK with an electromobility distinguishable from that of host-cell enzymes in CMV-infected cells. These observations suggested that virus-stimulated TK activities in CMV-infected cells were all of cellular origin. In contrast, in the case of HSV type 1 a virus-specific TK with biochemical and biologic characteristics distinguishable from that of host-cell enzymes is induced in virus-infected cells. This HSV-1 specific TK can be separated from host-cell enzymes by various affinity chromatographies, and is able to specifically and preferentially phosphorylate several purine and pyrimidine analogs, such as acyclovir [21,22], 5'-amino-2'-5'-deoxy-5- ioduridine [23], and 5'-allyl-deoxyuridine, [24], which, in turn inhibit HSV-DNA replication. In the case of HCMV, where no virus-specific TK has been detected, the virus DNA replication is relatively resistant to these purine and pyrimidine analogs (our unpublished data).

Infection of WI-38 human fibroblasts with HCMV also led to the stimulation of host-cell α-and β-DNA polymerase synthesis. In addition, a novel virus-specific DNA polymerase was also induced [17,25]. The characteristics of these virus-stimulated α-and β- cellular DNA polymerases did not show significant differences from those of mock-infected cells. In contrast, the virus-specific newly synthesized DNA polymerase exhibits different chromatographic behavior, salt sensitivity, template specificity, and phosphonoacetate (PAA) sensitivity, sufficiently distinctive from that of mock-infected or virus-stimulated α-and β-forms of cellular enzyme. The role of newly stimulated host-cell α-and β-DNA polymerase is still unclear; but it is thought to be associated with the stimulation of host-cell DNA synthesis. Whether these polymerases are also involved in the initiation or elongation of viral DNA synthesis, or act as a core enzyme for the formation of viral-specific DNA polymerase (holoenzyme) in viral DNA synthesis has yet to be investigated.

DNA topoisomerases are a group of enzymes that change the helical structure of circular DNA molecules through the transient breakage and religation of the phosphodiester bond of DNA molecules [26]. These enzymes are believed to be involved in site-specific as well as site-nonspecific recombination, disentanglement of catenated DNA circles, facilitation of

RNA transcription, and knotting and unknotting single-stranded DNA molecules [26]. In the prokaryotic system, type 1 topoisomerases selectively remove negative superhelical turns from supercoiled DNA molecules in the absence of ATP and Mg^{++}. The type 2 enzyme can remove negative superhelical turns and close open circle forms but requires the presence of Mg^{++} and ATP. In the eukaryotic system, topoisomerase type 1 has been found to be associated with chromatin, and is able to use both positive and negative supercoiled DNA as substrate without using ATP and Mg^{++} as cofactors, while eukaryotic type 2 enzyme resembles the prokaryotic type 2 topoisomerase and requires Mg^{++} and ATP as cofactors. In HEL cells, the enzyme levels of both type 1 and type 2 topoisomerases are greatly enhanced after infection with CMV (our unpublished data). These enzymes are frequently copurified with cellular α-form and virus-induced DNA polymerases (authors' unpublished data). The topoisomerase activity associated with virus-induced DNA polymerase did not require Mg^{++} and ATP as cofactors, and was resistant to PAA at concentrations of 50 μg/ml; while virus-specific DNA polymerase was sensitive to PAA at concentrations of 10 μg/ml. The distinction in PAA sensitivity indicates that the active centers for virus-induced DNA polymerase and topoisomerase activity should be different. Whether virus-induced DNA polymerase activity and topoisomerase activity are from a single enzyme or are two copurified enzymes should be further investigated.

Ornithine decarboxylase is an enzyme involved in the first rate-limiting reaction in the biosynthesis of protamine. The activity of the enzyme and the rate of enzyme synthesis are frequently linked to DNA synthesis. The increase of the enzyme activity was found to be associated with and to precede DNA synthesis. The level of this enzyme in normal stationary phase cells usually is relatively low, but increases substantially upon the infection of cells with tumor viruses [19]. In HCMV-infected embryonic fibroblasts, a great degree of stimulation of this enzyme activity was found 12 hr PI [19]. The degree of stimulation was dependent on the MOI and was not inhibited or fed back by the addition of protamine, but was reversibly inhibited by PAA treatment. It was therefore concluded that CMV-induced stimulation of ornithine decarboxylase synthesis was independent of cellular DNA synthesis, and might be related to virus-induced DNA polymerase or viral DNA synthesis [19].

Finally, infection of human and hamster cells with UV-irradiated HCMV also led to the stimulation of plasminogen activator synthesis [20]. The plasminogen activator is an enzyme which is able to convert plasminogen into plasmin, and the plasmin in turn, is able to hydrolyze the fibrin. This enzyme appears to be closely related to malignant transformation. Transformation of cells by DNA and RNA tumor viruses frequently leads to enhancement in the synthesis of plasminogen activator [27,28]. The stimulation of plasminogen activator in HCMV-infected cells does not require virus DNA synthesis. Therefore, it is suggested that the stimulation of the plasminogen activator synthesis is an early gene function of HCMV [20].

In brief, instead of shutting down the host-cell macromolecule synthesis HCMV is able to stimulate the synthesis of numerous enzymes relating to cell proliferation. Enzymes studied include TK, DNA polymerase, DNase, topoisomerase, ornithine decarboxylase, plasminogen activator, etc, as described above. The ability to stimulate the synthesis of these enzymes provides the biochemical criteria for the oncogenic potential of this virus.

MORPHOLOGIC TRANSFORMATION OF MAMMALIAN CELLS IN VITRO BY CMV

Albrecht and Rapp [2] first demonstrated the ability of UV-irradiated HCMV to transform hamster embryonic fibroblasts in vitro. Following the exposure of hamster embryonic cells to UV-irradiated HCMV, foci of lost-contact-inhibited hamster cells were found. Of 16 foci selected by Albrecht and Rapp [2], only one survived for three subsequent subcultures; it was called CX-90-3. On the other hand, cells exposed to untreated CMV showed signs of degeneration and subsequently died. Two distinct cell types were observed in cultures derived from CX-90-3 after 8 passages of in vitro subcultivation. One (CX-90-3A) approached crisis at passage 10 and terminated at passage 13. Another, CX-90-3B, showed lost-contact-inhibition and continued to grow well in vitro [2].

The CX-90-3B transformed cell generated by Albrecht and Rapp [2] was found to be tumorigenic in golden Syrian hamsters. Tumors induced in hamsters were poorly differentiated malignant fibrosarcomas and could be continuously subcultured both in vitro and in vivo. Virus-specific antigens were demonstrated both in the cytoplasm and on the cell membrane of CX-90-3B cells using human convalescent sera [2]. The status of the viral genome in CX-90-3B cells and in induced tumor cell lines is still unclear. After long periods of subcultivation in vitro, the viral genome was undetectable in both CX-90-3B and its induced tumor cell line by DNA-DNA reassociation kinetic analysis with a sensitivity of 0.1 viral genome per cell (our unpublished results, in collaboration with Dr. F. Rapp).

Boldogh et al [8] also demonstrated the transformation of hamster embryonic fibroblast cells using UV-irradiated HCMV. The morphologically transformed cell lines and those derived from the induced tumor did bear CMV-specific cytoplasmic and membrane antigen but no infectious virus or virus-specific nuclear antigens. The genomic status in these transformed cell lines is also unclear.

Spontaneous release of HCMV from cell lines derived from human tissues has been reported on at least two occasions [29,30]. A virus strain called Major (Mj) was spontaneously released from a prostate cell line derived from a child. This prostate cell line grew in vitro to passage level well above the expected life span. Geder et al [31] have speculated that CMV gene function might play a certain role in permitting the life span of this prostate cell line in vitro to be extended beyond the normal level. They have further studied the transforming ability of the Mj-strain CMV by low multiplicity (0.001 PFU/cell) and persistent infection of HEL fibroblasts with this virus. After a crisis period, foci of morphologically transformed cells appeared. From this, at least two transformed cell lines were established, which were designated as CMV-Mj-HEL 1 and 2; both cell lines were tumorigenic in athymic nude mice [31]. CMV-specific membrane antigens could be detected in these transformed cells by immunofluorescent tests with human convalescent serum or by cytotoxicity tests using spleen cells from hamsters bearing isografts of CMV-transformed cells. Perinuclear and paranuclear fluorescences were also observed in most of the transformed cells when anticomplement immunofluorescence (ACIF) techniques were applied. Viral DNA had been found in transformed CMV-Mj-HEL cells at 0.3 genomes equivalent per cell at early passage (p48), but became undetectable after prolonged cultivation in vitro (our unpublished results, in collaboration with Dr. F. Rapp).

MORPHOLOGIC TRANSFORMATION OF MAMMALIAN CELLS BY VIRAL DNA FRAGMENTS

Morphologic transformation of mammalian cells by CMV-DNA fragments has been achieved both in human fibroblasts [32] as well as in NIH 3T3 cells [33]. The efficiency of transformation by DNA fragments is extremely low and is far less than what we expected. In HEL fibroblasts, we were able to obtain transformation foci when total Xba I or HindIII-digested DNA fragments were used for transformation. Unfortunately, thus far we have not been able to transform HEL cells by a single cloned Xba DNA fragment; the study of double or combined fragment transformation is underway.

To prevent the complication of lytic infection, we initially used Xba I digested Towne strain HCMV-DNA fragments for our transformation study;

recently EcoR1 and HindIII-digested DNA fragments were also used. The subconfluent (70-80%) HEL cells were transfected with Xba I CMV-DNA fragments by calcium phosphate precipitation and DMSO shock, as described previously [34,35]. On the fifth day posttransfection, the transfected cells were reseeded in low density in MEM with 3% fetal calf serum with three medium changes a week. Cultures were monitored for morphologically transformed loci for six to seven weeks. Mechanically sonicated CMV-DNA, calf thymus DNA (lately salmon sperm DNA was used) and DMSO treatment [32] were included in our control. A tumor promoter agent, 12-0-tetradeca-noyl-phorbol-13-acetate (TPA), also was used in our study to test whether CMV-initiated transformation requires a cocarcinogen or a promoting factor to facilitate the transformation event [32]. Therefore, some transfected cultures and various controls were treated with TPA at 25 ng/ml for 24 hr on days 18 or 35 after transfection.

In the absence of TPA treatment, the Xba I fragment-transfected culture yielded morphologically transformed foci at a frequency of approximately $1/10^6$ cells when a HEL cell was transfected with 2.5×10^6 μg/cell of Xba I DNA fragments. The TPA-treated culture yielded five to six transforming loci per 10^6 cells. No transforming foci have been found in cells transfected with sonicated CMV-DNA, either in the presence or in the absence of TPA. TPA and DMSO treatment alone did not induce any morphologically transformed foci in HEL cultures [32].

CMV-specific antigen and viral-specific mRNA could be detected in transformed foci by ACIF and by in situ DNA-RNA cytohybridization (Fig. 1d-g). Three continuous transformed cell lines designated as BH19, BH21, and BH47 were established from cultures transfected with Xba I fragments and subsequently treated with TPA. These transformed cell lines were able to grow in soft agar and also able to grow to high densities with short doubling times in medium containing a low serum concentration (2% fetal calf serum). These transformed cell lines are morphologically epithelial, combined with short fibroblasts (Fig. 1b), and are able to induce fibrosarcoma in athymic nude mice. The tumorigenicity of these transformed cells was increased by subsequent passages in nude mice. Metastases consisting of poorly differentiated fibrosarcoma could be found in lung, liver, and spleen of these animals. The cell lines derived from these tumors still bear some virus-specific polypeptides that appeared in the original transformed cells. The karyotype of these tumor cells still retains characteristics similar to those of the original transformed cells.

The TPA treatment seems to be very crucial for CMV-DNA fragments to immortalize the morphologically transformed human cell. Without TPA treat-

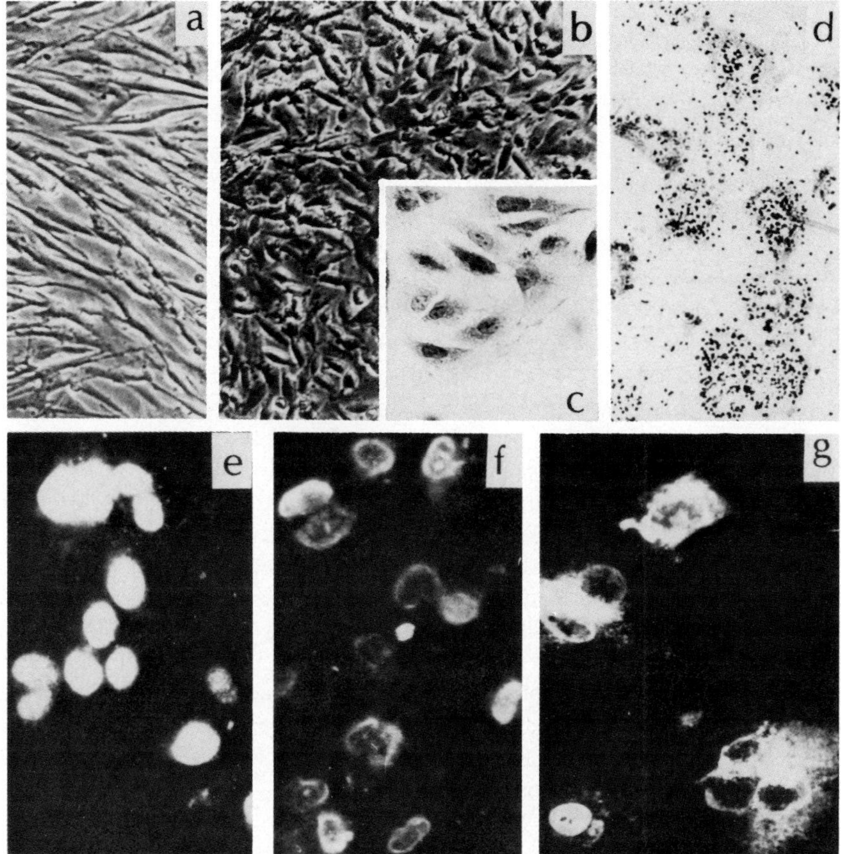

Fig. 1. Photographs of HCMV-DNA fragments (Xba I restricted) transformed cells (Data adapted from ref. [32]); a) mock-transfected normal HEL cells; b) morphologically transformed HEL cells; cell line derived from transformed foci treated with TPA, phase contrast, X96; c) hematoxylin-eosin stained CMV-DNA fragments transformed cell, phase contrast, X125; d) viral-specific RNA as demonstrated by in situ nucleic-acid hybridization and autoradiography, silver grains indicate the specific hybridization; e,f,g) localization of HCMV-specific antigen(s) in morphologically transformed loci by ACIF.

ment, cells from the CMV-transformed foci frequently cease multiplication after a couple of subcultivations. The mechanism of the establishment of CMV-induced transformation, therefore, appears similar to that of other carcinogen-involved multiphase processes [36], ie, that HCMV is capable of initiation of malignant transformation but the maintenance of this malignant state might require the presence of a cocarcinogen, such as a tumor-promoting agent.

In contrast to CMV-DNA fragment transformation of human fibroblasts, we were also able to establish CMV-transformed cell lines without TPA treatment, with a low MOI and extensive subcultivation of HEL cells with infectious viruses of strains BT1757 and Towne CMV. Cell lines derived from BT1757 (2E,4D,5B,6H and 7E) and from Towne (LH1, LH2 and CH5) share a similar biologic nature as those derived from DNA-fragment transformed cells, and are all tumorigenic in athymic nude mice. It appears that the continuous induction of cellular mitotic activity or cellular macromolecule synthesis by frequent subcultivation might function as tumor promoter in assisting CMV in the immortalization of HEL cells.

Nelson et al [33] have recently transfected NIH 3T3 cells with cloned AD169 strain CMV-DNA fragments to identify the transforming region of HCMV [33]. From the mapping and transfection experiments they have found that the transforming region was in the 2.9K subfragment of the HindIII E fragment with map units between 0.123 and 0.14 on the DNA molecule of the AD169 strain CMV. Transformed murine cells selected by 1.2% methylcellulose had high replicating efficiency and were tumorigenic in BALB/c nude mice. However, in their preliminary experiments, Nelson et al [33] were not able to detect viral DNA sequences homologous to the transforming HindIII E fragment with the sensitivity of 0.5 copy HindIII E fragment per cell. Treatment of transfected NIH 3T3 cells with TPA was not necessary in this experiment. It was suggested that the promotion events fulfilled by TPA in HEL cells must reside endogenously in NIH 3T3 cells [33]. This might also explain the high frequency of transformation of NIH 3T3 by numerous tumor viruses.

In Syrian hamster embryo (SHE) cell systems, Rosenthal's group at Georgetown University was also able to morphologically transform SHE cells with cloned Towne strain Xba I E fragment (personal communication, PNAS 80:3826–3830, 1983). This Towne Xba I E fragment was found homologous to Bg1 II transforming fragment N and C of HSV type 2, but lacked homology to the 2.9 kb subfragment of HindIII E as demonstrated by Nelson et al [33]. This Towne strain Xba I E fragment was also able to transform NIH 3T3 cells. The resulting transformed cells were also oncogenic in athymic NIH nude mice (L.J. Rosenthal, personal communication, PNAS 80:3826–3830, 1983).

MOLECULAR EPIDEMIOLOGIC ANALYSIS OF THE ASSOCIATION OF CMV AND VARIOUS HUMAN MALIGNANCIES

Considerable difficulty in the epidemiologic analysis of the association of CMV with various human cancers is the ubiquitous distribution of CMV, together with a high prevalence of CMV antibodies in an asymptomatic control population. It is almost impossible to conclude whether CMV has causal association with a particular human cancer, as analyzed by biostatistical approaches. Therefore, the data presented here from our studies and that of others may only reflect the epidemiologic association rather than etiology or causal association.

To date, HCMV has been implied to be associated with Kaposi sarcoma [37–42], prostatic adenocarcinoma [43,44], adenocarcinoma of the colon [45–47], and cervical cancer [32,48]. Seroimmunology and nucleic acid hybridization were the technologies most employed for studying the association.

Kaposi Sarcoma (KS)

Kaposi sarcoma is a multifocal idiopathic pigmented hemorrhagic sarcoma with an extremely obscure nature [49,50]. This tumor is characterized by the appearance of multicentric, violaceous tumor masses over the skin and sometimes in the internal viscera of adult males. Extensive involvement of the peripheral lymph nodes with or without cutaneous lesion is often found in children [51]. The detailed histopathology and clinical manifestation of KS are described elsewhere [49–53].

In general, the incidence of classic KS is extremely high in blacks in some equatorial countries of Africa. It is one of the most common solid malignant tumors in Kenya and constitutes close to 2.5% of all malignant tumors [53]. The prevalence rate is also higher among Italian or Jewish descendants compared to other races in Europe and America [49,51]. In Africa, KS attacks both young as well as old people with relatively aggressive symptoms; while in the United States it appears to attack older people with less aggressive clinical symptoms. Besides the classic endemic KS, there are two more groups of KS that have been discussed recently. One group arises as the result of aggressive immunosuppressive therapy in organ transplantation, or as the result of disorders of the immune system with a broad spectrum of age and sex ratio distribution. Another group of KS occurs predominantly in homosexual or bisexual men with no known immunosuppressive disease or therapy. The KS in this group is frequently accompanied with another rare disease, Pneumocystis carinii pneumonitis, and is fatal. HCMV has been consistently found to be the most frequent infectious agent associated with these two rare diseases [54].

In searching for viral agents associated with KS, Dr. Giraldo and his colleagues [37,38] demonstrated the herpesvirus particle, and subsequently isolated HCMV (strain K9V) from tissue culture cell lines derived from classic African KS. Through an extensive seroepidemiologic study, Giraldo and his colleagues [39,40] have subsequently showed a significant association between CMV infection and KS in European and American KS patients. No significant association between KS and other herpesvirus infections could be demonstrated statistically [39,40]. In collaboration with Giraldo, we examined classic KS tumors biopsied for CMV-specific nucleic acid sequences and viral-specific macromolecules by nucleic acid hybridization and ACIF. At the onset of the study, viral DNA and/or viral RNA could be detected in five out of ten tumor biopsies, and viral-specific antigens located in the nuclei could be demonstrated in 80% of the specimens [42]. In contrast, no HSV type 2 and EBV-DNA sequences or virus-specific macromolecules could be detected in these specimens [42]. To date, we have examined 17 classic type KS specimens; among them six biopsied tumors carried CMV genomes at a level of 0.25 to one genome equivalent per cell.

In the recent study of homosexual men with KS, Drew and his colleagues [54] found that CMV could be isolated from body secretion, semen or blood of seven out of nine patients. Viral cultures of KS biopsied specimens were negative, but CMV-specific antigens and viral RNA could be demonstrated by immunofluorescence and by in situ nucleic acid hybridization tests in six out of nine and two out of three tested, respectively. Normal tissue specimens from three KS patients were negative for CMV-specific antigens [54].

In an independent observation, Fenoglio and her colleagues [55] also demonstrated the existence of CMV-RNA in KS cells derived from a biopsy specimen of one of the skin lesions of a 35-year-old white Jewish homosexual man who had undergone surgery and chemotherapy for an embryonic carcinoma of the testis and who subsequently developed Kaposi sarcoma.

Prostatic Adenocarcinoma and Benign Hypertrophy of the Prostate

Adenocarcinoma and benign hypertrophy of the prostate are the most common illnesses of the American male. The etiology of these diseases is still unknown. Some studies suggest that these diseases may be related to an endocrine imbalance, but, to date, no conclusions have been made [56]. Some preliminary observations imply that HSV and HCMV might play some roles in the induction of prostatic adenocarcinoma. Lymphocytes from patients with prostatic adenocarcinoma were cytotoxic to CMV-infected and CMV-transformed cells which bore CMV-specific membrane antigens [43]. The peripheral lymphocytes from 84% of patients with prostatic carcinoma were able to kill CMV-transformed cells. In addition, sera from prostatic carcinoma patients were able to block the specific cytotoxicity generated by their lymphocytes [43]. These cellular immunologic data strongly suggest the possible association of CMV with the process of adenocarcinoma of the prostate. Besides, a long-term persistence of an oncogenic CMV strain (Major) in a cell line derived from prostatic tissue [29] makes this speculation more attractive. To obtain more conclusive information, we have performed a molecular epidemiologic study to investigate the existence of viral DNA and viral-specific macromolecules in normal, benign hypertrophy and adenocarcinoma of the prostate.

Surgically removed specimens from 13 normal, nine benign hypertrophy of the prostate (BHP) and ten prostatic adenocarcinoma (ACP) were analyzed for the presence of CMV and MSV type 2 DNA and viral-specific RNA, and antigens by DNA-DNA reassociation kinetics analysis in situ nucleic-acid hybridization, and ACIF, respectively [44]. Experimental results showed three out of nine (33%) BHP and four out of ten (40%) ACP carried CMV-DNA and/or CMV-specific macromolecules, while only two out of 13 (15.4%) in normal prostates. HSV-2 specific products were also found in two out of ten (20%) prostatic tumors, and one out of 13 normal prostates (8%). It is worth noting that 60% of the prostatic tumors show the existence of herpes group viral macromolecules (CMV or HSV-2).

Cervical Cancer

Considerable seroepidemiologic and biologic data suggest a strong causal association between HSV-2 and cervical cancer [57,58]. HSV-2 DNA, mRNA, and protein markers have been found in human cervical cancer, in exfoliated tumor cells, and in cells undergoing neoplastic change [59–61]. On the other hand, the seroepidemiologic data from some geographic areas did not always support the close association of HSV-2 with cervical cancer [48]. Therefore, the multifactorial etiology of cervical cancer was suggested [48,62]. HCMV frequently has been found in cervices and vaginal discharge, especially in Asia where the association of HSV-2 and cervical cancer is not very obvious. Virus was isolated from cervical tumor biopsies (our unpublished data) and from cell cultures derived from tumor biopsies [48]. In view of the oncogenic potential of CMV as demonstrated in vitro, we have performed a molecular epidemiologic survey of CMV-DNA in cervical cancer and in normal cervices from various geographic regions by nucleic-acid hybridization.

In collaboration with Dr. E. Russell Alexander, we examined eight cervical cancers and six normal cervix specimens from Taiwan. CMV-DNA was found in seven out of eight (88%) cancer specimens at a level between 0.4 and 6.6 genome equivalent per cell, while three out of six (50%) normal cervices showed positive at 0.2 to one genome per cell. Infectious CMV was isolated from one tumor specimen which carried CMV-DNA at 6.6 genome per cell. No HSV-2-DNA sequence could be detected in either cervical cancers or normal cervices from Taiwan (Table 1) [32].

As for specimens from Africa (in collaboration with Dr. G. de-Thé), we found CMV-DNA sequence in nine out of 19 cervical cancers, and five out of ten normal cervices at 0.1 to 1, and 0.5 to 1 genome equivalent per cell, respectively. HSV-2-DNA was found in one out of 12 cervical cancers, and in one out of four normal cervices (Table 1). In specimens from Finland and the United States, HCMV-DNA was detected in one out of 11, and two out of 13 cervical cancers, respectively. No HSV-2-DNA was detected in either normal or cervical specimens from Finland and the United States. The CMV-DNA positive rate is significantly lower in specimens from Finland and the United States in comparison with that from Taiwan and Africa. This might reflect the socioeconomic status of each population. Nevertheless, the frequency of the positive CMV rate in cervical cancer was higher than that of HSV-2, and the rate of CMV-positive specimens in cervical cancers from Taiwan was also higher than those from normal cervices. However, the number of specimen studies was limited. It is essential to examine more specimens in order to come up with conclusive data. Again, with the ubiquitous nature of CMV, it is extremely difficult to presume any causal association, especially with cervical cancer; nevertheless, we cannot overlook the possibility. Based on the extremely high frequency of positive CMV-DNA in both cervices and the cervical cancers, we can at least conclude that the human cervix might be a site for latent CMV infection.

TABLE 1. HCMV and HSV Type 2 DNA in Normal Cervices and Cervical Cancers from Various Geographic Regions

Sources of Specimens		CMV-DNA Positive/Total (Genome/Cell)	HSV-2-DNA
Asia	cervical cancer	7/8 (0.4–6.6/cell)	0/8
(Taiwan)	normal	3/6 (0.2–1/cell)	0/6
Africa/ Middle East	cervical cancer	9/19 (0.1–1/cell)	1/12 (1/cell)
Uganda, Iran, Tunisia	normal	5/10 (0.5–1/cell)	1/4 (1/cell)
Finland	cervical cancer	1/11 (0.7/cell)	0/11
	normal	0/8	0/8
United States	cervical cancer	2/13 (0.3–1/cell)	0/13
	normal	NA	NA

Data adapted from ref [32].

Carcinoma of the Colon

Through extensive epidemiologic analysis, it was suggested that enivronmental, as well as genetic, factors might play important roles in the initiation of colon cancer [63–65]. However, the precise nature of the factors or genes involved is still undetermined. By cytologic observation and virus isolation, CMV has been detected in the intestinal wall of patients with ulcerative colitis [65,66], a disease suspected of being associated with colon cancer [67]. By nucleic-acid hybridization techniques, in collaboration with Dr. J.K. Roche of Duke University [45–47], we have shown the presence of viral DNA sequence in the diseased bowel of patients with ulcerative colitis, familial polyposis, and carcinoma of the colon. In contrast, results were negative for the CMV genome in the bowel of Crohn disease patients [45,46]; such patients have little or no increase in cancer risk. Although CMV was detected in the majority of patients with colon cancers, we have found that it frequently existed in some histologically normal and nonneoplastic diseased tissues of colon cancer patients [47]. These observations make the interpretation of the association of CMV with colon cancer extremely difficult. It is more likely that the detected CMV was probably latent or harbored in the intestinal tissues of the majority of the patients. The fact that this virus is widely distributed also does not rule out the possible oncogenic role since close association of virus with host cells may give the virus an excellent opportunity to induce neoplastic transformation of its host during its long-term persistence.

CONCLUSION

The oncogenic potential of HCMV is strongly suggested by its ability to stimulate the synthesis of various host-cell macromolecules; such as cellular DNA, RNA, and the enzymes associated with cell proliferation, and by its ability to transform human as well as other mammalian cells in vitro. All of the CMV-transformed human as well as other mammalian cells were found tumorigenic in athymic nude mice. Although CMV-DNA, RNA, and virus-specific antigens were found frequently in KS, prostatic adenocarcinoma, cervical, and colon cancers, its causal and etiologic roles with these cancers are still unclear. The possibility of the preferential replication of CMV in these neoplastic tissues and reactivation of latent virus in patients with malignancy still exists. Due to the widespread CMV infections, it is also very difficult to study the causal association of CMV with human malignancies by sero- or molecular-epidemiologic approaches. Nevertheless, the connection between CMV and some human malignancies is impossible to dismiss.

The obvious complication of CMV infection in several cancer patients definitely requires more attention.

ACKNOWLEDGMENTS

We thank Drs. E. Russell Alexander, G. de-Thé, J. Roche, G. Giraldo, and T.I. Malinin for their collaboration, and for providing valuable tumor specimens; and Shu-Mei Huong and Barbara Leonard for technical assistance and manuscript preparation.

REFERENCES

1. Weller T H: The cytomegaloviruses: Ubiquitous agents with protean clinical manifestations. N Engl J Med 285:203-214, 1971.
2. Albrecht T, Rapp F: Malignant transformation of hamster embryo fibroblasts following exposure to ultraviolet-irradiated human cytomegalovirus. Virology 55:53–61, 1973.
3. Yamanishi K, Ogino T, Takahashi M: Induction of cellular DNA synthesis by a temperature-sensitive mutant of herpes-simplex virus type 2. Virology 67:450–462, 1975.
4. Melvin P, Kucera L S: Induction of human cell DNA synthesis by herpes simplex virus type 2. J Virol 15:534–539, 1975.
5. Gerber P, Hoyer B H: Induction of cellular DNA synthesis in human leukocytes by Epstein-Barr virus. Nature 231:46–47, 1971.
6. Miller G, Robinson J, Heston L, Lipman M: Differences between laboratory strains of Epstein-Barr virus based on immortalization, abortive infection and interference. Proc Natl Acad Sci USA 71:4006–4010, 1974.
7. St. Jeor S, Albrecht T B, Funk F D, Rapp F: Stimulation of cellular DNA synthesis by human cytomegalovirus. J. Virol 13:353–362, 1974.
8. Boldogh I, Gonczol E, Vaczi L: Transformation of hamster embryonic fibroblast cell by UV-irradiated human cytomegalovirus. Acta Microbiol Acad Sci Hung 25:269–275, 1978.
9. Tanaka S, Furukawa T, Plotkin S A: Human cytomegalovirus stimulates host cell RNA synthesis. J Virol 15:297–304, 1975.
10. Furukawa T, Tanaka S, Plotkin S: Stimulation of macromolecular synthesis in guinea pig cells by human CMV. Proc Soc Expo Biol Med 148:211–214, 1975.
11. Furukawa T, Sakuma S, Plotkin SA: Human cytomegalovirus infection of WI-38 cells stimulates mitochondrial DNA synthesis. Nature 262:414–416, 1976.
12. DeMarchi JM, Ben-Porat T, Kaplan AS: Expression of the genome of noninfectious particles in stocks of standard and defective interfering pseudorabies virus. Virology 97:457–463, 1979.
13. DeMarchi JM, Kaplan AS: The role of defective cytomegalovirus particles in the induction of host cell DNA synthesis. Virology 82:93–99, 1977.
14. Kamata T, Tanaka S, Watanabe Y: Human cytomegalovirus-induced chromatin factors responsible for changes in template activity and structure of infected cell chromatin. Virology 90:197–208, 1978.
15. Zavada V, Erban V, Rezacova D, Vonka V: Thymidine kinase in cytomegalovirus infected cells. Arch Virol 52:333–339, 1976.

16. Estes JE, Huang E-S: Stimulation of cellular thymidine kinases by human cytomegalovirus. J Virol 24:13–21, 1977.
17. Huang E-S: Human cytomegalovirus. III. Virus-induced DNA polymerase. J Virol 16:298–310, 1975.
18. Tanaka S, Ihara S, Watanabe Y: Human cytomegalovirus induces DNA-dependent RNA polymerases in human diploid cells. Virology 89:179–185, 1978.
19. Isom H J: Stimulation of ornithine decarboxylase by human cytomegalovirus. J Gen Virol 42:265-278, 1979.
20. Yamanishi K, Rapp F: Production of plasminogen activator by human and hamster cells infected with human cytomegalovirus. J Virol 31:415–419, 1979.
21. Elion GB, Furman P, Fyfe JA, deMiranda P, Beauchamp L, Schaeffer JJ: Selectivity of action of an antiherpetic agent, 9-(2-hydroxy-ethoxymethyl) guanine. Proc Natl Acad Sci USA 74:5716–5720, 1977.
22. Fyfe JA, Keller PM, Furman PA, Miller RL, Elion GB: Thymidine kinase from herpes simplex virus phosphoxylates the new anti-viral compound 9-(2-hydroxyethoxymethyl)–guanine. J Biol Chem 253:8721–8727, 1978.
23. Cheng YC, Goz B, Neenan JP, Ward DC, Prusoff WH: Selective inhibition of herpes simplex virus by 5′-amino-2′-5′-deoxy-5-iodouridine. J Virol 15:1284–1286, 1975.
24. Cheng YC, Domin BA, Sharma RA, Bobek M: Studies on the antiviral action and cellular toxicity of four thymidine analogs: 5-ethyl, 5-vinyl, 5-propyl and 5-allyl-deoxyuridine. Antimicrob Agents Chemother 10:119–122, 1976.
25. Hirai K, Furukawa T, Plotkin SA: Induction of DNA polymerase in WI-38 and guinea pig cells infected with human cytomegalovirus (HCMV). Virology 70:251–255, 1976.
26. Pulleyblank DE, Ellison MJ: Purification and properties of type 1 topoisomerase from chicken erythrocytes: Mechanism of eukaryotic topoisomerase action. Biochemistry 21:1155–1161, 1982.
27. Unkeless JC, Tobia A, Ossowski L, Quigley JP, Rifkin PB, Reich E: An enzymatic function association with transformation of fibroblasts by oncogenic viruses. I. Chick embryo fibroblast cultures transformed by avian RNA tumor viruses. J Exp Med 137:85–111, 1973.
28. Ossowski L, Quigley JP, Reich E: Fibrinolysis associated with oncogenic transformation: Morphological correlates. J Biol Chem 249:4312–4320, 1974.
29. Rapp F, Geder L, Murasko D, Lausch R, Ladda R, Huang E-S, Webber MM: Long-term persistence of cytomegalovirus genome in cultured human cells of prostatic origin. J Virol 16:982–990, 1975.
30. Williams LL, Blakeslee JR, Huang E-S: Isolation of a new strain of cytomegalovirus from explanted normal skin. J Gen Virol 47:519–523, 1980.
31. Geder L, Lausch R, O'Neill F, Rapp F: Oncogenic transformation of human embryo lung cells by human cytomegalovirus. Science 192:1134–1137, 1976.
32. Huang E-S, Boldogh I, Mar E-C: Human cytomegaloviruses: Evidence for possible association with human cancer. In Philips LA (ed): "Viruses Associated With Human Cancer." New York: Marcel Dekker, 1983, pp 161–193.
33. Nelson JA, Fleckenstein B, Galloway DA, McDougall JK: Transformation of NIH 3T3 cells with cloned fragments of human cytomegalovirus strain AD169. J Virol 43:83–91, 1982.
34. Graham FL, Veldhuisen G, Wilkie NM: Infectious herpes DNA. Nature 245:265–266, 1973.
35. Stow ND, Wilkie NM: An improved technique for obtaining enhanced infectivity with herpes simplex virus type 1 DNA. J Gen Virol 33:447–458, 1976.

36. Bereblum I: Established principles and unresolved problems in carcinogenesis. J Natl Cancer Inst 60:723–726, 1978.

37. Giraldo G, Beth E, Coeur P, Vogel CL, Dhru DS: Kaposi's sarcoma: A new model in the search for viruses associated with human malignancies. J Natl Cancer Inst 49:1495–1507, 1972.

38. Giraldo G, Beth E, Haguenau F: Herpes-type virus particles in tissue culture of Kaposi's sarcoma from different geographic regions. J Natl Cancer Inst 49:1509–1513, 1972.

39. Giraldo G, Beth E, Kourilsky FM, Henle W, Henle G, Mike V et al: Antibody patterns to herpesvirus in Kaposi's sarcoma: Serological association of European Kaposi's sarcoma with cytomegalovirus. Int J Cancer 15:839–848, 1975.

40. Giraldo G, Beth E, Henle W, Henle G, Mike V, Safai B, Huraux JM, McHardy J, de-Thé G: Antibody patterns to herpesviruses in Kaposi's sarcoma. II. Serological association of American Kaposi's sarcoma with cytomegalovirus. Int J Cancer 22:126–131, 1978.

41. Giraldo G, Beth E, Huang E-S: Kaposi's sarcoma and its relationship to cytomegalovirus (CMV). III. CMV DNA and CMV early antigens in Kaposi's sarcoma. Int J Cancer 26:23–29, 1980.

42. Boldogh I, Beth E, Huang E-S, Kyalwazi KS, Giraldo G: Kaposi's sarcoma. IV. Detection of CMV DNA, CMV RNA and CMNA in tumor biopsies. Int J Cancer 28:469–474, 1981.

43. Sanford EJ, Dagen JE, Geder L, Rohner JT, Rapp E: Lymphocyte reactivity against virally transformed cells in patients with urologic cancer. J Urol 118:809–810, 1977.

44. Boldogh I, Baskar JF, Mar E-C, Huang E-S: Human cytomegalovirus and herpes simplex type 2 virus in normal and adenocarcinomatous prostate glands. J Natl Cancer Inst 70:819–825, 1983.

45. Roche JK, Huang E-S: Viral DNA in inflammatory bowel disease: CMV-bearing cells as a target in immune-mediated enterocytolysis. Gastroenterology 72:228–233, 1977.

46. Huang E-S, Roche JK: Cytomegalovirus DNA and adenocarcinoma of the colon: Evidence for latent viral infection. Lancet 1:957–960, 1978.

47. Roche JK, Cheng KS, Huang E-S, Lang DL: Cytomegalovirus: Detection in human colonic and circulating mononuclear cells in association with gastrointestinal disease. Int J Cancer 27:659–667, 1981.

48. Melnick JL, Lewis R, Wimberly I, Kaufman RH, Adams E: Association of cytomegalovirus (CMV) infection with cervical cancer: Isolation of CMV from cell cultures derived from cervical biopsy. Int Virol 10:115–119, 1978.

49. Safai B, Good R: Kaposi's sarcoma: A review and recent development. CA 31:2–12, 1981.

50. Kaposi M: Idiopathisches multiple pigment Sarkom der Haut. Arch Derm Syph (Berl) 4:265–273, 1872.

51. Haverkos HW, Curran JW: The current outbreak of Kaposi's sarcoma and opportunistic infections. CA 32:330–339, 1982.

52. Taylor JF, Templeton AC, Vogel CL et al: Kaposi's sarcoma in Uganda: A clinical pathological study. Int J Cancer 8:122–135, 1971.

53. Kungu A, Gates DG: Kaposi's sarcoma in Kenya: A retrospective clinicopathological study. Antibiot Chemother 29:38–55, 1981.

54. Drew WL, Conant MA, Miner RC, Huang E-S, Ziegler JL, Groundwater JR, Gullett JH et al: Cytomegalovirus and Kaposi's sarcoma in young homosexual men. Lancet 2:125–127, 1982.

55. Fenoglio CM, Oster MW, Gerfo PL, Reynolds T, Edelson R, Patterson JAK et al: Kaposi's sarcoma following chemotherapy for testicular cancer in a homosexual man: Demonstration of cytomegalovirus RNA in sarcoma cells. Hum Pathol 15:955–959, 1982.
56. Rubin P: Cancer of urogenital tract: Prostatic cancer: Current concepts in cancer. JAMA 210:320–1072, 1969.
57. Rawls WE, Adam E, Melnick JL: An analysis of seroepidemiological studies of herpesvirus type 2 and carcinoma of cervix. Cancer Res 33:1477–1482, 1973.
58. Nahmias AJ, Naib ZM, Josey WE: Epidemiological studies relating genital herpetic infection to cervical cancer. Cancer Res 34:1111–1117, 1974.
59. Frenkel N, Roizman B, Cassai E, Nahmias A: A DNA fragment of herpes simplex 2 and its transcription in human cervical cancer tissue. Proc Natl Acad Sci USA 69:3784–3789, 1972.
60. McDougall JK, Galloway DA, Fenoglio CM: Cervical carcinoma: Detection of herpes simplex virus RNA in cells undergoing neoplastic change. Int J Cancer 25:1–8, 1980.
61. Dressman GR, Burek J, Adam E, Kaufman RH, Melnick JL, Powell KL, Purifoy DJM: Expression of herpesvirus-induced antigens in human cervical cancer. Nature 283:591–593, 1980.
62. Alexander ER: Possible etiologies of cancer of the cervix other than herpesvirus. Cancer Res 33:1486–1496, 1973.
63. Hanszel W, Correa P: Cancer of the colon and rectum and adenomatous polyps: A review of epidemiologic finding. Cancer 28:14–24, 1971.
64. Burdette WJ: Identification of antecedents to colorectal cancer. Cancer 28:51–59, 1971.
65. Powell RD, Warner NE, Levine RS, Kirsner JB: Cytomegalic inclusion disease and ulcerative colitis. Am J Med 30:334–340, 1961.
66. Levine RS, Wanner NF, Johnson CF: Cytomegalic inclusion disease in the gastrointestinal tract of adults. Ann Surg 159:35–48, 1964.
67. Farmer GW, Vincent MM, Fuccillo DA: Viral investigations in ulcerative colitis and regional enteritis. Gastroenterology 65:8–18, 1973.

Equine Cytomegalovirus: Genomic Structure, Protein Composition and Role in Oncogenic Transformation and Persistent Infection*

John Staczek, PhD, Gretchen B. Caughman, PhD, and Dennis J. O'Callaghan, PhD

University of Mississippi Medical Center, Department of Microbiology, Jackson, MS 39216

BIOLOGIC PROPERTIES OF ECMV

Equine herpesvirus type 2 (equine cytomegalovirus, ECMV), which is worldwide in distribution [1], is an infectious agent of horses, but the role of ECMV in the production of clinical disease remains uncertain. The virus can be isolated from the respiratory tract of foals, yearlings, and adult horses exhibiting naturally occurring respiratory diseases [2] or experimentally induced ECMV respiratory tract infections [3, 4] and from the conjunctival sac of horses with conjunctivitis [5]. ECMV has also been isolated from the leukocytes (buffy coat) of apparently healthy horses [6]; from routine cell culture preparations derived from equine kidney [7–9], spleen and testicular [5] tissue; and from nasal and genital swabs of healthy and clinically ill horses [see 1, 5, 13]. The observation that ECMV could be isolated from the leukocytes of 71 out of 80 (89%) apparently healthy horses [6] and that 507 of 523 (97%) horses had ECMV complement-fixing antibodies [10] supports

*Research in our laboratory was supported by research grants AI 02032, S-507-RR05386 and AI 19415 from the NIH and a grant from the Grayson Foundation. G.B.C. is supported by a Postdoctoral Fellowship (1 F32 CA 07210-01) from the National Cancer Institute.

Birth Defects: Original Article Series, Volume 20, Number 1, pages 213–231

the concept that most, if not all, horses become infected with ECMV during their lifetime [5]. The pathogenesis of ECMV infection remains to be elucidated, but it is believed that ECMV is acquired horizontally via inhalation and that the virus infects the respiratory epithelium and disseminates throughout the body. The horse then becomes persistently infected or latently infected as evidenced by reports that ECMV has been recovered from washings of leukocytes or isolated from kidney cell cultures only after prolonged maintenance in vitro.

The virus isolated from spontaneously degenerating equine kidney cultures [7–9] or from the washings of equine leukocytes [6] was initially characterized as a novel and unique herpesvirus based on several criteria. The cytopathology produced by this virus was typical of a herpes infection since rounded, highly refractile cells containing Cowdry Type-A intranuclear inclusion bodies and marginated cellular chromatin were readily observed [5–7, 9]. The virus was ether sensitive [6, 9], heat labile [6] and contained DNA [5, 9], and electron micrographs of primary isolates depicted a virus particle with typical herpes-like structure [5–7]. However, this virus was not neutralized by antibodies to equine rhinopneumonitis virus (ERV, tentatively classified EHV-4), and antibodies to this novel virus failed to neutralize other EHV types [6, 11]. Consequently, the new virus isolate was classified as a herpesvirus and was designated equine herpesvirus type 2 (EHV-2) in recognition of its serologic distinctness.

The replication of EHV-2 in tissue culture monolayers demonstrated many of the general characteristics commonly associated with in vitro CMV replication and, therefore, the virus has become known as ECMV [12, 13]. As is typical for CMVs, the in vitro host range for ECMV replication was found to be restricted. ECMV replicated in primary and secondary equine cells (Kentucky equine dermis, equine testes, equine dermis, and equine kidney) as well as in continuous equine (equine transitional cell carcinoma) and rabbit kidney (LLC-RK$_1$) cell lines. ECMV failed to replicate in mouse L-M cells, baby hamster kidney (BHK) cells, or cells of human origin (WI-38) [5, 12]. CMVs also have been associated with a prolonged replication cycle. Primary isolates of ECMV from leukocytes required 14 to 28 days postinoculation to demonstrate cytopathic effects on indicator cells [6] and the spontaneous degeneration of primary equine kidney cells associated with the release of ECMV occurred 60 to 80 days after the cells were introduced into tissue culture [8]. Once adapted to cell culture, ECMV exhibited a replication cycle of three to seven days in duration [12], which is significantly longer than that of the more cytocidal EHVs [13, 14].

In ECMV-infected equine cell cultures, viral cytopathology was first observed at approximately 48 hr PI and was characterized by spreading foci of cytomegalic cells. Plaques on equine cells were uniform in size, although irregular in shape, and had cytomegalic cells at the periphery of the plaque. When examined by electron microscopy, infected cells were found to exhibit margination of cellular chromatin and to contain several large basophilic inclusions. Three morphologic types of nucleocapsids were observed in the nuclei of infected cells: 1) empty capsids, 2) capsids with an electron-lucent, cross-shaped core, and 3) capsids with an electron dense core. The capsids which contain an electron dense core were usually found in apposition with the inner lamina of the nuclear membrane. Apparently these morphologically mature nucleocapsids can become enveloped by either of two processes: 1) the nucleocapsids either bud out through the nuclear membrane to obtain an envelope or 2) convolutions of the nuclear membrane invaginate into the nucleoplasm and react with the nucleocapsid. Both of these processes appeared to function independently of each other as both were observed within the same infected cell [12]. ECMV replication in equine cells had an eclipse period of 48 hr, and maximum titers (10.7 PFU/cell) of infectious virus were reached 96 hr PI. Approximately 50% of the infectious virus remained cell associated.

STRUCTURAL PROTEINS OF ECMV

Studies have been initiated to catalog and characterize the structural proteins of ECMV. Since ECMV replicates to only low titers and has some tendency to remain cell associated, it was necessary to develop procedures suitable for large scale purifications of virions and nucleocapsids. ECMV virions were purified using the method of Perdue et al [15] with some modifications. Briefly, medium which contained virions released from ECMV-infected RK cell monolayers was collected, clarified by low-speed centrifugation, and adjusted to 8% polyethylene glycol-6000 and 2.3% NaCl (W/V, final concentration). The resulting virus-containing precipitate was collected and resuspended via dialysis against low ionic strength buffer (0.001 M sodium phosphate, pH 7.4), and the virions were subjected to one or more cycles of rate velocity centrifugation in 5%–30% dextran-10 gradients. The dextran-banded virus preparation was further purified by isopyknic centrifugation in 28%–40% potassium tartrate gradients. In order to verify the efficiency of this protocol, ^{35}S-methionine-radiolabeled RK cellular proteins were added to crude virus preparations, and the removal of the cellular proteins was monitored throughout the purification. As shown in Table 1, each step resulted in successive reduction in radioactive cellular contamination, and the final virion preparation was 99.99% free of cellular proteins.

TABLE 1. Efficiency of Purification Procedures for Virions and Nucleocapsids of ECMV

Purification Step	^{35}S-Methionine-Labeled Cellular Protein*	
	Total CPM (^{35}S)	% CPM Remaining
I. Virions		
Sonicated suspension of ^{35}S-labeled RK cells	1.1×10^9	
Combined infected and labeled PEG-6000 precipitate	1.2×10^8	100.00
Dextran-10 rate velocity centrifugation	1.3×10^6	1.10
Potassium tartrate isopyknic banding	1.4×10^4	0.01
II. Nucleocapsids		
Infected cell pellet	8.3×10^7	100.00
Nuclear fraction	1.3×10^7	15.70
Solubilization, clarification	1.2×10^7	14.40
Centrifugation through 35% sucrose	1.2×10^6	1.40
1st Renografin gradient	7.5×10^4	0.09
2nd Renografin gradient	2.6×10^4	0.03

*RK cells grown for 96 hr in methionine-deficient EMEM supplemented with ^{35}S-methionine (20 μCi/ml, 1194 Ci/mM) were scraped and washed with EMEM. One half of the cells was added to the infected cell pellet for nucleocapsid purification. The other half was sonicated 2 min, returned to the labeling medium, and added to the infected cell medium for extracellular virus purification.

The procedure for purification of ECMV nucleocapsids was adapted from that of Atherton et al [16]. ECMV-infected RK cells were disrupted by sonication and the nuclei were pelleted by centrifugation. This nuclear fraction was solubilized (0.5 M urea, 0.5% W/V sodium deoxycholate), clarified, and centrifuged through 35% sucrose cushions. The nucleocapsid pellet was resuspended and subjected to one or two cycles of isopyknic banding in 45%–70% (W/V) Renografin-76 density gradients. Again, cellular contamination was monitored throughout the procedure by mixing ^{35}S-methionine-radiolabeled cellular proteins with the infected cell-starting material; as shown in Table 1, 99.96% of the contaminating radiolabel was removed.

Purified preparations of ECMV virions and nucleocapsids were solubilized in SDS-sample buffer containing 2-mercaptoethanol [17] at 100°C for 3 min and the viral polypeptides were subjected to discontinuous polyacrylamide gel electrophoresis (PAGE) [17]. Samples were run on 6%, 9%, and 10% gels as well as 6%–12% linear gradient gels in order to obtain accurate MWs over the entire range of proteins. Typical polypeptide profiles and migration patterns of virion and nucleocapsid proteins in 9% PAGE are shown in Figure 1. In the nucleocapsid preparation, nine capsid proteins were easily discernable, ranging in MW from 18,000 to 148,000. To determine the relative amount of each protein present, nucleocapsids were prepared from RK cells infected with ECMV in the presence of a mixture of ^{3}H-amino acids, and samples of the radiolabeled preparation were electrophoresed into 9% gels. Total radioactivity of the proteins was analyzed by preparing the gels for fluorography and subjecting the resulting fluorograms to densitometric analysis as well as by determining the radioactivity of solubilized 1-mm gel slices. Based on these analyses, five (average MWs = 148K, 46K, 38.5K, 27K, and 18K) of the nine nucleocapsid proteins have been categorized as major proteins, and together these five proteins comprised > 75% of total nucleocapsid protein (Table 2). Of particular interest was the 148K protein which constituted 47.3% of the total nucleocapsid protein and therefore appeared similar in MW to the major capsid proteins reported for other herpesviruses [see 13]. Four capsid proteins (52K, 49.5K, 43.5K, and 20K) were present in minor amounts and together made up 13.4% of the nucleocapsid protein. The remaining 11% of total protein consisted of nine proteins present in trace amounts. Since these trace proteins corresponded in MW to virion proteins, they may represent the presence of small amounts of maturing virions in the nucleocapsid preparations.

ECMV particles (virions) were composed of at least 35 proteins ranging in MW from 14,000 to 251,000 (Table 3). Initial studies using ^{3}H-glucosamine-labeled virions indicated that 11 of these 35 proteins were glycosylated (Table 3). The three most heavily glycosylated polypeptides (83K, 78K, 73.5K) comigrated with a nonglycosylated 71K protein in N,N'-methylenebisacrylamide (MBA) crosslinked gels, but they could be separated by electrophoresis in gels crosslinked with N,N'-diallyltartardiamide (DATD).

PHYSICAL PROPERTIES OF ECMV DNA

ECMV DNA has been purified from infected cells by the Hirt fractionation procedure [18], by extraction from isolated nucleocapsids and, less frequently, from released virions purified by one cycle of differential centrifugation and isopyknic banding in potassium tartrate gradients [12]. As determined by CsCl analytic ultracentrifugation, viral DNA obtained from these sources has a buoyant density of 1.7165 g/cm^3, which agrees with the value of 1.717 g/cm^3 previously reported by Plummer et al [19, 20]. This buoyant density corresponds to a guanosine + cytosine content of 57.7%.

The MW of the ECMV genome has been measured by several methods, including sedimentation analysis in neutral sucrose gradients, restriction

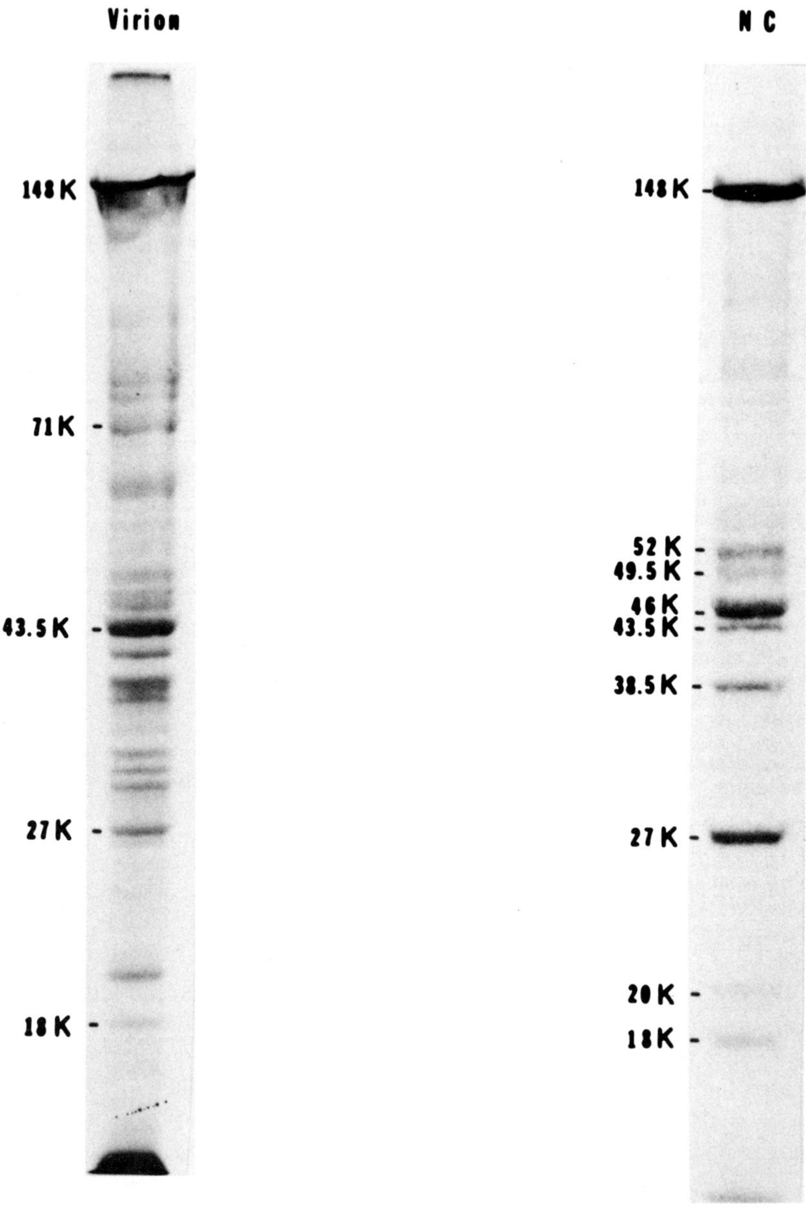

Fig. 1. Structural polypeptides of ECMV virions and nucleocapsids. ^{3}H-amino acid-labeled ECMV virions and nucleocapsids were purified and solubilized as described in the text, and the resultant polypeptides were separated by electrophoresis in a 9% SDS-polyacrylamide slab gel. The approximately 32 virion proteins (MW range = 15.5K to 251K), stained with Coomassie brilliant blue, are shown on the left. A fluorogram depicting the five major (148K, 46K, 38.5K, 27K, 18K) and four minor (52K, 49.5K, 43.5K, 20K) proteins of the nucleocapsid is shown on the right.

TABLE 2. Protein Composition of ECMV Nucleocapsids

Molecular Weight $\times~10^{-3}$	Average % Composition[a]	Molar Ratio[b]	Relative Molar Ratio[c]
A. Major proteins			
148.0	47.3	0.3196	1.99
46.0	7.4	0.1609	1.00
38.5	6.9	0.1792	1.11
27.0	10.2	0.3778	2.35
18.0	3.8	0.2111	1.31
	75.6[d]		
B. Minor proteins			
52.0	4.8	0.0923	0.57
49.5	2.5	0.0505	0.31
43.5	3.4	0.0782	0.49
20.0	2.7	0.1350	0.84
	13.4[d]		

[a]Based on the amount of radioactivity in peaks on electropherograms of ^{3}H-amino acid-labeled nucleocapsid proteins.
[b]Obtained by dividing the average percent composition by the MW; values were multiplied by 1,000.
[c]Obtained by setting the molar ratio of the 46K protein at 1.0.
[d]The remaining 11% of total protein consists of nine proteins present in trace amounts (average relative molar ratio = 0.10). Since these proteins correspond in MW to virion proteins, they may indicate the presence of small amounts of maturing virions in the nucleocapsid preparations.

enzyme analysis, and electron microscopic examination. For these analyses, ECMV DNA was purified by CsCl isopyknic centrifugation, and unit length viral DNA was obtained by subjecting the DNA to rate velocity centrifugation in linear glycerol gradients. ECMV DNA purified in this manner cosedimented with T4 DNA in neutral sucrose gradients and, consequently, was assigned a sedimentation coefficient (S) of approximately 61.8 [12]. Using several formulations that correlate the sedimentation coefficient to MW [21–25], the MW of ECMV DNA was calculated to be as large as 129 megadaltons (md).

Restriction endonuclease digestion of ECMV DNA has also been used to measure the MW of ECMV DNA and to further characterize the physical structure of the ECMV genome. Digestion of ECMV DNA with the restriction endonucleases *Bam*HI, *Eco*RI, *Hin*dIII, or *Sal*I resulted in the production of 21, 18, 14, and 5 fragments, respectively, ranging in size from 0.8 to 44 md. Although most of the restricted DNA fragments were present at a molar ratio of 1, several fragments were present at a molar ratio of 2 and several

TABLE 3. Structural Proteins in ECMV

Average MW $\times 10^{-3}$	Glycoprotein	Presence in Nucleocapsids
251.0		
239.0		
220.0		
203.0	+[a]	
152.0		
148.0		+ (major)
111.0	+ +	
92.5		
83.0*	+ + +	
79.5		
78.0*	+ + +	
73.5*	+ + +	
71.0		
68.0	+ +	
66.0		
61.0	+ +	
58.0		
56.5		
52.0		+ (minor)
49.5	+ +	+ (minor)
47.5		
46.0		+ (major)
43.5	+	+ (minor)
41.0	+ +	
38.5		+ (major)
37.5		
34.5		
32.5		
31.5		
30.0		
27.0		+ (major)
26.0		
23.0		
20.0		+ (minor)
18.0	+	+ (major)
14.0		

[a]Indicates the relative intensities of fluorographic bands developed after SDS-PAGE analysis of purified ^{3}H-glucosamine labeled virions.

*Indicates glycoproteins which comigrated with the 71K protein in MBA-crosslinked gels, but which were separated by electrophoresis in gels crosslinked with DATD.

fragments were present at submolar ratios. The MWs of individual restriction enzyme-digested fragments summed to 126 md for the entire ECMV genome.

Measurements of intact ECMV DNA molecules in the electron microscope using SV40 and EHV-1 DNAs as MW markers yielded unit length measurements that equated to a MW of 123 to 126 md. This value was in good agreement with results of restriction enzyme digestion analyses and indicated that ECMV has a genome that is approximately 30%–35% greater in size than those of EHV-1 (equine abortion virus) and EHV-3 (equine herpesvirus type 3; equine coital exanthema virus).

The presence of submolar fragments in restriction endonuclease digests of ECMV DNA suggested that the genome may undergo isomerization. This possibility was supported by electron microscopic studies which indicated the presence of inverted repeat sequences located around one region of the viral DNA. When single-stranded viral DNA was permitted to self-anneal under conditions which enhance intramolecular reannealing, a 3-md double-stranded region encompassing a single-stranded loop region of approximately 6 md was observed in electron micrographs (Ruyechan, unpublished observations). The presence of inverted repeat regions (the double-stranded regions in the electron micrographs) has been associated with the ability of a DNA molecule to undergo isomerization. Whether these inverted repeat sequences are associated with the submolar restriction endonuclease-generated fragments and whether the ECMV DNA molecule can undergo isomerization remain to be determined. Although tentative restriction enzyme maps of genomic ECMV DNA have been constructed (Staczek et al in preparation), these maps are being verified by using the Hutchison cross blotting technique as modified by Pero et al [26] and by hybridization of isolated radiolabeled restriction enzyme generated fragments to Southern blots [27] of restricted genomic ECMV DNA and to dot blots of isolated restricted ECMV DNA fragments.

GENETIC RELATEDNESS OF ECMV DNA AND DNAs OF EHV-1 AND EHV-3

In a recent study [28], reassociation kinetic analyses and thermal dissociation measurements revealed that ECMV DNA has sequence homology to the genomes of EHV-1 and EHV-3. These experiments indicated that ECMV is homologous to 2.0% (1.8 md) of the EHV-1 genome and 2.0% (1.9 md) of the EHV-3 genome. Conversely, EHV-1 was determined to hybridize to 2.9% (3.7 md) of the ECMV genome and EHV-3 was found to hybridize to 1.0% (1.3 md) of the ECMV genome. Therefore, ECMV and EHV-1 share 1.8 md to 3.7 md of DNA, and ECMV and EHV-3 share 1.3 md to 1.9 md of DNA. When the ECMV × EHV-1 and ECMV × EHV-3 heteroduplexes were isolated and subjected to thermal denaturation analysis to determine the extent of homology within the heteroduplexes, the thermal denaturation profiles of the heteroduplexes closely paralleled those of ECMV × ECMV, EHV-1 × EHV-1, or EHV-3 × EHV-3 homoduplexes. These data indicated that all three EHV genomes have limited regions of very high homology. The observation that the EHVs are genetically related is very interesting in light of recent reports that all three viruses have oncogenic potential [29–33], and it will be of great interest to ascertain whether the type shared sequences are those associated with transforming potential.

COESTABLISHMENT OF ONCOGENIC TRANSFORMATION AND PERSISTENT INFECTION BY ECMV

Under standard conditions of infection at input multiplicities of 20 PFU/cell or less, primary LSH hamster embryo cells are not permissive for ECMV replication [12] and infection does not result in transformation. However, infection of hamster embryo cells with ECMV preparations that have been UV-irradiated under conditions in which only 0.05% of total virus remained infectious resulted in the development of dense foci of rapidly growing cells [33]. Three cell lines, designated EC-1, EC-2, and EC-3 (EC: equine cell), independently established from foci were selected for detailed study. Several biologic properties of these UV-irradiated ECMV-infected hamster embryo cell lines have been examined and compared to the biologic properties of secondary hamster embryo cell cultures (Table 4). The UV-irradiated ECMV-infected cells displayed many of the biologic characteristics associated with the transformed state, such as immortalization, growth to high saturation densities, decreased generation time, decreased dependency on serum for rapid growth, formation of colonies in semisolid medium, and resistance to superinfection by homologous or heterologous virus. More specifically, the EC-1, EC-2, and EC-3 cell lines were immortalized, and all cell lines have been in continuous culture for a minimum of two years and passaged more than 70 times (approximately 350 cell divisions). These transformed cells have saturation densities that are 60%–70% greater than the saturation density obtained by normal hamster embryo cells, and the UV-irradiated ECMV infected cells have generation times that are approximately one half that of the control hamster embryo cells. The EC-1, EC-2, and EC-3 cell lines were capable of growing rapidly in either low (0.5%) or high (5.0%) serum concentrations, which was in contrast to the failure of secondary hamster embryo cells to grow in 1% serum. Furthermore, the EC-1, EC-2, and EC-

3 cell lines were capable of forming colonies at very high plating efficiencies in agarose, whereas primary or secondary hamster embryo cells could not (Table 4). Also, the EC-1, EC-2, and EC-3 cell lines were resistant to superinfection with ECMV and EHV-1 [33]. The fact that these cell lines were resistant to superinfection with ECMV was not very surprising considering the observations that, during routine conditions of infection, ECMV does not normally replicate in hamster cells and that the establishment of these EC cell lines was the result of ECMV infection of primary hamster embryo cells using extraordinary conditions of infection (1200 UV-irradiated ECMV particles per cell). However, the observation that the EC-1, EC-2, and EC-3 cell lines were also resistant to superinfection with the heterologous virus, EHV-1, was quite unexpected as EHV-1 has very limited homology with ECMV (see above) and replicates to high titers in hamsters [14] and LSH hamster embryo cells [29]. The resistance of EC-1, EC-2, and EC-3 cells to superinfection with ECMV or EHV-1 does not reflect a general resistance to all herpesviruses, since HSV-1 replicates to high titers in these cells [33]. Therefore, by all of the criteria mentioned thus far, the EC-1, EC-2, and EC-3 cell lines were transformed.

The EC-1, EC-2, and EC-3 transformed cell lines were tested for the spontaneous release of infectious virus by inoculating culture supernatants from transformed cells or extracts of disrupted EC cells onto RK or equine dermis cells (both of which are permissive for ECMV replication) and monitoring for the development of cytopathology. In the case of the EC-1 cell line, no cytopathic effects were observed, even after two weeks of monitoring the permissive cells. This failure to detect spontaneously released infectious virus was reproducible at either low-cell passages (< 10) or high-cell passages (> 60). Also, attempts to detect infectious virus in the EC-1 cell line by infectious center assay and to detect viral particles by repeated electron microscopic examination of these cells were unsuccessful. However, this failure to detect virus in the EC-1 cell cultures was in contrast to the detection of spontaneously released infectious ECMV from the supernatants of EC-2 and EC-3 cultures. Both the EC-2 and EC-3 culture supernatants contained infectious virus in titers as great as 1×10^4 PFU/ml. Several observations confirmed that the released virus was ECMV: 1) the released virus grew in RK cells but not baby hamster kidney cells; 2) the morphology of the plaques produced by the virus released from the persistently infected EC-2 and EC-3 cells was identical to that of ECMV; 3) electron microscopic examination of EC-2 and EC-3 cells revealed the presence of nucleocapsid species that had a typical herpesvirus structure; and 4) restriction endonuclease profiles of DNA extracted from virus released by the EC-3 cell line

TABLE 4. Biologic Properties of ECMV-Transformed and Tumor Cell Lines

Property	Cell Line						
	HE	EC-1	EC-2	EC-3	EC-1T	EC-2T	EC-3T
Morphology	Normal fibroblast	Fibroblast	Fibroblast	Fibroblast	Mixed	Mixed	Fibroblast
Immortality[a]	12	>70	>70	>70	>40	>40	>40
Saturation density[b]	1.8	3.3	3.2	3.0	NT	NT	NT
Generation time [c] (hours)	21	11	12	12	NT	NT	NT
Serum dependence[d] (growth index)	yes (1.0)	no (3.0)	no (3.2)	no (4.0)	no	no	no
Colony formation in soft agar[e] (% efficiency)	no (0.2%)	yes (50%)	yes (50%)	yes (50%)	NT	NT	NT
Immunofluorescence[f]	no	yes	yes	yes	yes	yes	yes
Superinfection with[g]							
ECMV	no (1)	no (4)	no (20)	no (25)	no (1)	no (1.3)	no (6.6)
EHV-1	yes (10^4)	no (16)	(NT)	no (5)	no (30)	no (5)	no (3.3)
HSV-1	yes ($>10^4$)	yes ($>18^4$)	yes (10^5)	yes (10^4)	yes (10^4)	yes (10^4)	yes ($>10^4$)
Virus production[h]							
PFU/ml	none	none	1×10^4	1×10^4	none	none	none
infectious center assay	0%	0%	2%	5%	NT	NT	NT
electron microscopic examination	0%	0%	0.5%	0.8%	0%	0%	0%
Tumor production[i]	no	yes (12/12)	yes (6/6)	yes (6/6)	yes (8/8)	yes (3/4)	yes (8/8)
ECMV plaque reduction assay[j] (% reduction)	0%	50%	30%	30%	30%	70%	60%
Viral sequences[k] (genome equivalents/cell)	no	yes (<0.05)	yes (0.16)	yes (15)	yes (<0.05)	yes (<0.05)	yes (0.05)

[a]Current number of passages in culture.

[b]Cultures of cells were grown at 37°C in Eagle minimal essential medium-10% fetal bovine serum (EMEM-10) for the HE cells and EMEM-5 for the transformed cells to maximum confluency. The cells were harvested with trypsin (0.25%), washed $1\times$ and counted. The saturation density is expressed as the number of cells $\times 10^6$ per 25-cm^2 flask.

[c]Cells were seeded at 2.0×10^5 per 25-cm^2 plastic culture flasks and allowed to grow at 37°C. Cells were harvested every 12 hr over a 4-day interval. The generation time is expressed as the hours required for the cell population to increase twofold.

[d]Transformed cells were grown in EMEM-0.5 or EMEM-5, monitored for cell growth and counted daily. The cell growth index is expressed as follows: No. of cells at 48 hr/No. of cells at 12 hr.

[e]Assays for the formation of colonies in soft agar were conducted as described by Staczek et al [33]. The efficiency of colony formation was expressed as follows: (No. of colonies formed in 25-cm^2 flasks/No. of cells seeded into 25-cm^2 flasks) $\times$ 100%.

[f]ECMV-transformed cells and control cells grown on coverslips were reacted with complement inactivated hamster anti-ECMV-infected RK cell extracts for 30 min at 37°C in a humidified atmosphere. The coverslips were washed in PBS and the cells were reacted with fluorescein-conjugated rabbit anti-hamster Ig for 30 min at 37°C in a humidified atmosphere. The coverslips were washed in PBS, mounted in 50% glycerol and examined with a Leitz Ortholux II fluorescent microscope.

[g]ECMV-transformed cells were seeded in triplicate at a density of 2.5×10^5 cells/2.5-cm^2 well. Confluent monolayers were decanted and infected with 5-20 PFU/cell of EHV-1, ECMV, or HSV-1. After 1 hr adsorption at 37°C, the monolayers were washed three times with medium, overlaid with fresh medium, and incubated for 6 days at 37°C. Pooled aliquots of 0.1 ml from each of the triplicate monolayers were removed at 2 hr PI and at 24-hr intervals thereafter and stored at -70°C until assayed for PFUs on permissive RK cells. The viral growth index is expressed as PFU recovered at 96 hr/PFU recovered at 2 hr.

[h]The assays for infectious virus in the medium of cultured cells are as follows: Triplicate 0.1 ml aliquots of medium (5 ml/25 cm^2 flasks) were taken daily and plaque assayed as described by Staczek et al [33]. Infectious center assays and electron microscopic examinations were performed as described by Staczek et al [33].

[i]The cells were tested for their tumorigenicity by the injection of 5×10^5 to 5×10^6 cells/animal. The animals were monitored daily for palpable tumors.

[j]Tumor-bearer sera from LSH hamsters inoculated with 10^5-10^6 cells/animal were obtained by cardiac puncture. Complement inactivated sera (56°C, 30 min) were incubated with 2,400 PFU of ECMV at 36°C for 30 min. The residual infectivity of the sample was determined by plaque assay on RK cells. The ability for the tumor bearer sera to neutralize ECMV is expressed as the percent reduction in ECMV titer.

[k]Reassociation kinetic and Southern blot hybridization analyses were used to detect and quantitate ECMV sequences in ECMV-transformed cells [33].

were very similar to those of the ECMV genome. However, some of the restriction fragments generated from the DNA of released EC-3 virus were present in greater molar ratios than those found in standard ECMV DNA digests. The possibility that both standard ECMV and defective interfering particles of ECMV are being released by these persistently infected cells remains to be tested. In this regard, it should be noted that hamster embryo cells persistently infected with EHV-1 have been shown to release EHV-1 defective interfering (DI) particles which seem to play a role in maintaining the persistent infection [31].

Both infectious center assays and electron microscopic studies have confirmed the production of ECMV in the EC-2 and EC-3 transformed cell lines and have permitted the quantitation of virus-producing cells in the ECMV persistently infected cultures (Table 4). The results of these two assays were in agreement and indicated that 0.5%–2% of the EC-2 cells contained virus particles or infectious virus and that 0.8%–5% of the EC-3 cells contained virus particles or infectious virus. The observation that only a small percentage of the EC-2 or EC-3 cells contained and released virus was supported by our observation that none of the 50 clones tested to date which were derived from single cell isolates of EC-2 or EC-3 cell lines released detectable levels of infectious virus. Thus, the minor population of virus-producer cells within the EC-2 and EC-3 transformed cell lines maintained the state of ECMV persistent infection. These two cell lines have continued to release ECMV during extensive passage (> 60).

The transformed EC-1, EC-2, and EC-3 cells were found to be highly oncogenic when inoculated into syngeneic, immunocompetent LSH hamsters (Table 4), and palpable tumors were detected at the inoculation sites in less than three weeks. Histopathologic examinations of the tumor tissue and major organs of tumor-bearing animals revealed that the tumors were fibrosarcomas which were capable of metastasizing to several major organs, especially the lung. Tumors were excised from selected animals and were used to establish tumor cell lines, designated EC-1T, EC-2T, and EC-3T. When tumor cells were inoculated into LSH hamsters, palpable tumors developed within three days, indicating that all tumor cell lines are highly oncogenic. The ability of the transformed EC cells to produce tumors was independent of the cell's phenotypic classification as either a virus nonproducer (EC-1) or a virus producer (EC-2 and EC-3). However, when each of the tumor cell lines was assayed for the presence of released infectious ECMV on permissive RK cells, no viral cytopathology could be detected after several weeks of monitoring (Table 4). Furthermore, failure to detect virus by cocultivation assays or by examination of the EC-1T, EC-2T and EC-3T cells by electron microscopy supported the finding that all tumor cell lines were virus nonproducers. In addition, when the tumor cell lines were challenged with ECMV or EHV-1 at multiplicities of infection of 10-20 PFU/cell, all tumor cell lines, like the parental transformed cells, failed to exhibit cytopathic effects and to support virus replication (Table 4). These findings indicated that the persistently infected phenotype of the EC-2 and EC-3 cell lines was lost upon passage in an animal (tumorigenesis). This was in contrast to the findings that the transformed EC-2 and EC-3 cells continued to release virus at passage levels as high as 60 and after freezing and storage at −70°C.

Immunofluorescence tests and plaque reduction assays of tumor-bearer sera were used to determine whether ECMV-specific antigens were expressed in EC-transformed and tumor cells (Table 4). Indirect immunofluorescence assays using antiserum to ECMV-infected RK cell extracts demonstrated that at least 75%–80% of the EC-transformed cells expressed ECMV antigen(s). Interestingly, approximately 1% of the EC-2 and EC-3 immunofluorescent-positive cells had a rounded morphology and stained very intensely, suggesting that these rounded cells were the producer cells. Immunofluorescent-positive rounded cells were not observed in the virus-nonproducer cell line, EC-1. Although the staining of the EC tumor cells was not as intense as the staining of the EC-transformed cells, the tumor cells were judged to be immunofluorescent-positive when compared to the background staining of control hamster or RK cells. Approximately 60% of the cells within each of the EC tumor cell lines were immunofluorescent positive.

To determine whether the transformed and tumor cells were expressing ECMV antigens during passage in vivo (tumorigenesis), sera from tumor-bearing animals were used in an ECMV plaque reduction assay. Aliquots of complement-inactivated sera from tumor-bearing hamsters were incubated with 2,400 PFU of ECMV prior to titration on RK cells, and as can be seen in Table 4, all tumor-bearer sera neutralized ECMV. The percent reductions in ECMV titer ranged from 30% to 70%; these reductions were substantial when one considers the large amount of virus (2,400 PFU) used for the plaque reduction assay. These data supported the concept that ECMV antigens were expressed during tumorigenesis.

In order to verify the presence of ECMV sequences in EC-transformed and tumor cells, nucleic acid hybridization methodologies were employed (Table 4). Reassociation kinetic analysis of the virus nonproducer EC-1 transformed cell line (passages 50 to 60) indicated that viral sequences were present but in amounts < 0.05 ECMV genome equivalents per cell. Experiments are in progress to identify the organization of these viral sequences. Preliminary findings using radiolabeled ECMV DNA probes in Southern blot hybridization analyses have indicated that a small fraction of the ECMV genome is present in low passage (< 10) EC-1 cells. The finding that EC-1 cells contained only subgenomic ECMV sequences would explain the failure to detect or induce virus in these cells.

Reassociation kinetic analyses of the persistently infected cell lines EC-2 and EC-3 indicated that the EC-2 cells averaged 0.16 genome equivalents per cell and that the EC-3 cells contained as much as 15 ECMV genome equivalents per cell. The virus released from the virus-producing population has been characterized as ECMV (see above). However, reassociation kinetic analysis cannot discriminate between those cells that are producing infectious virus and those cells that may be latently infected. Since only a minor population (< 5%) of cells within the persistently infected cell lines were producing infectious virus, it may be possible that the virus-nonproducer cell population contains subgenomic ECMV sequences. Clones derived from single cell isolates of EC-2 and EC-3 cell lines were tumorigenic and were classified as virus nonproducers. These clones are currently being examined for the presence of ECMV DNA and for the expression of ECMV antigens. Analysis of these clones should provide information about the nature of the viral sequences present within the virus-nonproducing population of the EC-2 and EC-3 persistently infected cell lines.

Reassociation kinetic analyses using cellular DNA extracted from high level passage (40 to 50) EC tumor cells have indicated that the tumor cell lines contained < 0.05 ECMV genome equivalents per cell [33]. Preliminary findings suggest that ECMV sequences are detectable by Southern blot analyses using highly labeled ECMV DNA probes and cellular DNAs of low passage (15 to 18) tumor cells. Both of these findings supported the concept that ECMV DNA was present within tumor cells and that ECMV sequences were retained during tumorigenesis. In the case of the transformed EC-1 cell line and the progeny EC-1T tumor cell line, the ECMV DNA sequences have been retained through ten passages in EC-1 transformed cells, one passage in the hamster (tumorigenesis), and 17 passages in the EC-1T cells. Although these ECMV sequences appear to be retained during tumorigenesis, it is apparent that other viral sequences had been lost during tumorigenesis since the viral DNA present within the tumor cells was genetically less complex than the viral DNA present within the corresponding transformed cell lines.

CONCLUDING REMARKS

We have begun to elucidate the biologic and physiochemical properties of ECMV. Several aspects of the findings obtained to date are particularly interesting and relevant to the varied biologic outcomes resulting from the interaction between a herpesvirus and its host cell. The ability of ECMV to establish oncogenic transformation and/or persistent infection in vitro provides an opportunity to study two different consequences of CMV infection. The development of cell lines that are persistently infected will permit future experimentation designed to obtain more information on the nature of the virus that is released from these cells and on the mediators that function at the molecular level to maintain the persistent infection. The virus-nonproducing transformed cell lines and tumor cell lines are being employed in experiments designed to obtain information on the nature of the viral sequences present in CMV–transformed cell lines and retained during tumorigenesis as well as to characterize viral transcripts and translation products associated with the oncogenic transformation process.

The genetic relatedness of the three EHV is interesting not only with respect to the evolution of these viruses and their distinctly different pathologic sequelae, but also with respect to the observation that all three EHV possess oncogenic potential [29–34]. A most interesting speculation is that these three viruses have arisen from a common ancestor by divergent evolution and thus display diverse pathogenesis in the natural host, but have retained a common set of DNA sequences necessary for the establishment and/or maintenance of oncogenic transformation. Future experiments will be designed to establish the identity and map positions of the shared sequences and the role, if any, that these sequences might have in oncogenesis.

REFERENCES

1. Bagust TJ: The equine bulletin. Vet Bull 41:79–92, 1971.
2. Pálfi V, Belák S, Molnar T: Isolation of equine herpesvirus type 2 from foals showing respiratory symptoms. Zentralbl Veterinarmed [B] 25:165–167, 1978.
3. Blakeslee JR Jr, Olsen RG, McAllister ES, Fassbender J, Dennis R: Evidence of respiratory tract infection induced by equine herpesvirus, type 2, in the horse. Can J Microbiol 21:1940–1946, 1975.
4. Belák S, Pálfi V, Tuboly S, Bartha L: Passive immunization of foals to prevent respiratory disease caused by equine herpesvirus type 2. Zentralbl Veterinarmed [B] 27:826–830, 1980.
5. Studdert MJ: Comparative aspects of equine herpesviruses. Cornell Vet 64:94–122, 1974.
6. Kemeny L, Pearson JE: Isolation of herpesvirus from equine leucocytes: Comparison with equine rhinopneumonitis virus. Can J Comp Med 34:59–65, 1970.
7. Plummer G, Waterson AP: Equine herpes viruses. Virology 19:115–119, 1963.
8. Hsiung GD, Fischman HR, Fong CKY, Green HR: Characterization of a cytomegalovirus-like virus isolated from spontaneously degenerated equine kidney cell culture. Proc Soc Exp Biol Med 130:80–84, 1969.

9. Flammini CF, Allegri G: Herpesvirus from equine kidney tissue culture. Arch Vet Ital 23:93–97, 1972.

10. McGuire TC, Crawford TB, Henson JB: Prevalence of antibodies to herpesvirus types 1 and 2, arteritis and infectious anemia viral antigens in equine serum. Am J Vet Res 35:181–185, 1974.

11. Kemeny LJ: Antigenic relationships of equine herpesvirus strains demonstrated by the plaque reduction and neutralization kinetics tests. Can J Comp Med 35:279–284, 1971.

12. Wharton JH, Henry BE, O'Callaghan DJ: Equine cytomegalovirus: Culture characteristics and properties of viral DNA. Virology 109:106–119, 1981.

13. O'Callaghan DJ, Gentry GA, Randall CC: The equine herpesviruses. In Roizman B (ed): "Herpesviruses," Frenkel-Conrat H, Wagner R (ed): Comprehensive virology. New York: Plenum Press, 1983, pp 215–318.

14. O'Callaghan DJ, Allen GP, Randall CC: Structure and replication of equine herpesviruses. In Bryans JT and Gerber H (eds): "Equine infectious diseases IV." Princeton: Veterinary Publications, 1978, pp 1–32.

15. Perdue ML, Kemp MC, Randall CC, O'Callaghan DJ: Studies of the molecular anatomy of the L-M cell strain of equine herpesvirus type 1: Proteins of the nucleocapsid and intact virions. Virology 59:201–216, 1974.

16. Atherton SS, Sullivan DC, Dauenhauer SA, Ruyechan WT, O'Callaghan DJ: Properties of the genome of equine herpesvirus type 3. Virology 102:18–32, 1982.

17. Laemmeli UK: Cleavage of structural proteins during the assembly of the head of bacteriophage T4. Nature 227:680–685, 1970.

18. Hirt B: Selective extraction of polyoma DNA from infected cell cultures. J Mol Biol 26:365–369, 1967.

19. Plummer G, Bowling CP, Goodheart CR: Comparison of four horse herpesviruses. J Virol 4:738–741, 1969.

20. Plummer G, Goodheart CR, Henson D, Bowling CP: A comparative study of the DNA density and behavior in tissue cultures of fourteen different herpesviruses. Virology 39:134–137, 1969.

21. Rubinstein I, Thomas CA Jr, Hershey AD: The molecular weights of T2 bacteriophage DNA and its first and second breakage products. Proc Natl Acad Sci USA 47:1113–1122, 1961.

22. Doty P, McGill BB, Rice SA: The properties of sonic fragments of deoxyribose nucleic acid. Proc Natl Acad Sci USA 44:432–438, 1958.

23. Eigner J, Doty P: The native, denatured and renatured states of deoxyribonucleic acid. J Mol Biol 12:549–580, 1965.

24. Freifelder D: Molecular weights of coliphages and coliphage DNA. IV. Molecular weights of DNA from bacteriophages T4, T5 and T7 and the general problem of determination of M. J Mol Biol 54:567–577, 1970.

25. Burgi E, Hershey AD: Sedimentation rate as a measure of molecular weight to DNA. Biophys J 3:309–321, 1963.

26. Pero J, Hannett NM, Talkington C: Restriction cleavage map of SP01 DNA: General location of early, middle and late genes. J Virol 31:156–171, 1979.

27. Southern EM: Detection of specific sequences among DNA fragments separated by gel electrophoresis. J Mol Biol 98:503–517, 1975.

28. Staczek J, Atherton SS, O'Callaghan DJ: Genetic relatedness of the genomes of equine herpesvirus types 1, 2 and 3. J Virol 45:855–858, 1983.

29. Robinson RA, Henry BE, Duff RG, 0'Callaghan DJ: Oncogenic transformation by equine herpesviruses (EHV): I. Properties of hamster embryo cells transformed by ultraviolet-irradiated EHV-1. Virology 101:335–362, 1980.

30. Robinson RA, Vance RB, O'Callaghan DJ: Oncogenic transformation by equine herpesviruses: II. Coestablishment of persistent infection and oncogenic transformation of hamster embryo cells by equine herpesvirus type 1 preparations enriched for defective interfering particles. J Virol 36:204–219, 1980.

31. Dauenhauer SA, Robinson RA, O'Callaghan DJ: Chronic production of defective interfering particles by hamster embryo cultures of herpesvirus persistently infected and oncogenically transformed cells. J Gen Virol 60:1–14, 1982.

32. O'Callaghan DJ, Henry BE, Wharton JH, Dauenhauer SA, Vance RB, Staczek J, Atherton SS, Robinson RA: Equine herpesviruses: Biochemical studies on genomic structure, DI particles, oncogenic transformation and persistent infection. In Becker Y (ed): "Developments in Molecular Virology," vol. 1: Herpesvirus DNA. The Hague, The Netherlands: Nijhoff, 1982, pp 387–418.

33. Staczek J, Wharton JH, Dauenhauer SA, O'Callaghan DJ: Co-establishment of persistent infection and oncogenic transformation of hamster embryo cells by equine cytomegalovirus (EHV-2). (Submitted for publication.)

34. Robinson RA, O'Callaghan DJ: A specific viral sequence is stably integrated in herpesvirus oncogenically-transformed cells. Cell 32:569–578, 1983.

The Guinea Pig Cytomegalovirus Model of Congenital Human Cytomegalovirus Infection

Frank J. Bia, MD, MPH, Scott A. Miller, MD, and Kathy H. Davidson

Virology 151/B, West Haven VA Medical Center, West Haven, CT 06516 (F.J.B., K.H.D.); Norfolk Diagnostic Clinic, Norfolk, VA 23502 (S.A.M.)

The purpose of this brief discussion is simply to inform interested clinical and laboratory investigators that a relevant animal model for congenital HCMV infections exists and is well characterized. The guinea pig model for HCMV infections has a scientific history which goes back more than 60 years to some of the earliest work in virology, and it has been the subject of a recent extensive review [1]. Those wishing to consult a more thorough discussion of guinea pig CMV (GP CMV) pathogenesis and the potential applications of this animal model are referred to it [1], and other material which cover the virology of this species [2]. The current paper is specifically concerned with data obtained during recent investigations into the pathogenesis and prevention of congenital CMV infections in the guinea pig model.

GP CMV is certainly not a newcomer to investigative virology. Its earliest descriptions were clearly recorded in 1920 by Leila Jackson [3] in the *Journal of Infectious Diseases,* when it was thought to be a parasitic infection of guinea pig salivary glands. Within a decade, it was shown to be a rather species-specific virus which could be passaged in guinea pigs, and to which they would develop protective immunity [4,5]. However, in 1930 a series of experiments were reported by C.H. Andrewes [6] which gave the first indication that this group of viruses would not be readily controlled by humoral immunity alone. GP CMV, which has been passaged in infected salivary glands, could be neutralized if incubated with immune serum. However, Andrewes [6] found that parenteral administration of the same sera would not prevent generalized spread of experimental GP CMV infection.

Birth Defects: Original Article Series, Volume 20, Number 1, pages 233–241
© **1984 March of Dimes Birth Defects Foundation**

Early investigators learned much about the pathogenesis of GP CMV infection, but the isolation and morphologic characterization of these viruses were to await the development of modern virologic techniques. Most important among these techniques were tissue culture and explant methods for the isolation of infectious virus, and electron microscopy for examination of morphogenesis both within guinea pig tissues and in vitro. Even without these techniques it was evident to some that the virus being so carefully passaged in guinea pigs might have a human counterpart which played an important role in childhood disease. In their studies at Peking Union Medical College, Kuttner and Wang [7] examined several infants who had died with an associated interstitial pneumonia found at autopsy. These investigators were impressed by salivary gland inclusions found in these infants—inclusions which were remarkably similar to those produced by the virus found in guinea pig salivary glands [7]. Subsequent experimental infection of guinea pigs actually demonstrated the production of both interstitial pneumonia and intranuclear inclusions within lungs of an infected animal [8].

Before considering those efforts to elucidate the pathogenesis and prevention of human congenital CMV infections in the guinea pig model, it is helpful to review some initial experimental work on GP CMV pathogenesis. The strain of GP CMV which Hartley isolated in 1957 [9] (No. 22122; American Type Culture Collection, Rockville, MD) has been utilized in published studies since that time. We have arbitrarily designated the virus as GP CMV-SG when passaged in vivo in guinea pig salivary glands, and as GP CMV-TC when passaged in guinea pig embryo (GPE) tissue culture. Hsiung et al [10, 11] made several initial observations regarding the use of GPE cell cocultivation techniques and GP CMV neutralizing antibodies for the isolation and identification of viral isolates. The guinea pig is now known to harbor at least three endogenous herpesviruses which can be distinguished by neutralization testing [2,12].

With these techniques, it was possible to demonstrate both an acute and a chronic persistent phase of GP CMV infection [13]. For purposes of our discussion, the pathogenesis of acute primary GP CMV infection is of greatest interest because its occurrence during pregnancy may result in CMV infection of fetal guinea pigs. Hsiung et al [13] demonstrated that generalized GP CMV infection in nonimmune Hartley guinea pigs resulted in both viremia and generalized CMV infection of these animals. When the acute phase of GP CMV infection was further characterized by Griffith et al [14] it was found to result in an experimental syndrome similar to HCMV-associated mononucleosis, including both granulocytopenia and atypical lymphocytosis (Fig. 1). On fractionation of peripheral blood elements during

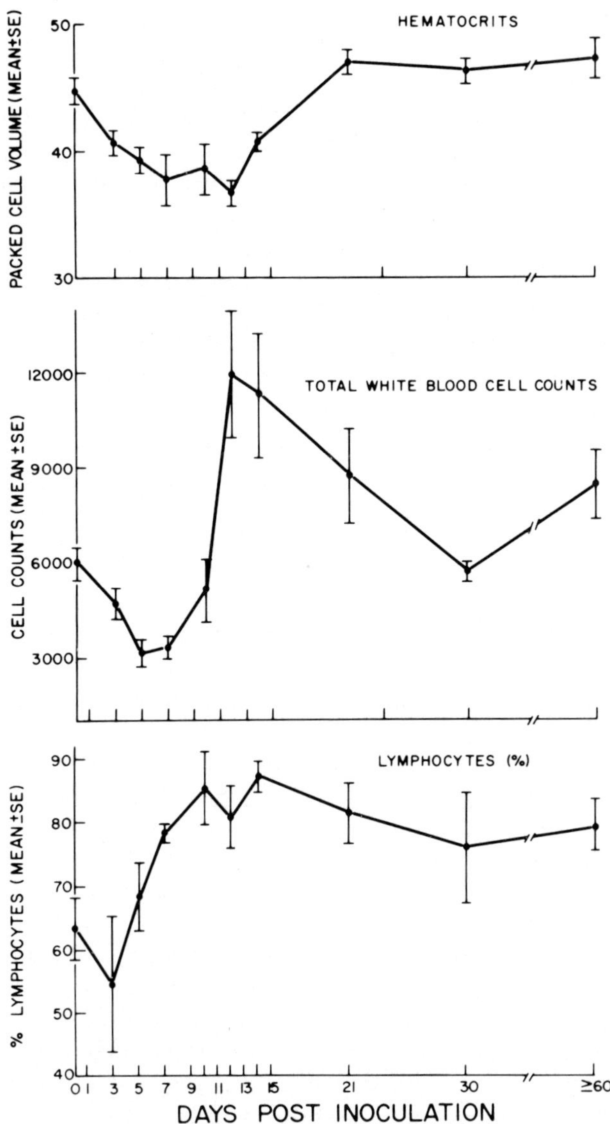

Fig. 1. Peripheral blood counts and hematocrit values in Hartley guinea pigs during acute GP CMV mononucleosis. Anemia and leukopenia are followed by a relative lymphocytosis during the first three weeks after inoculation with GP CMV passaged in salivary gland. Values shown apply to this animal model only. (From Bia FJ et al: Cytomegalovirus infections in the guinea pig: Experimental models for human disease. Rev Infect Dis 5:117–195, 1983, with permission of the publisher and copyright holder, The University of Chicago Press.)

acute GP CMV infection, the virus could be isolated from both PMNLs and mononuclear cells. In fact, this model for acute CMV infection proved useful for studies of PMNL response and function [15], and more recently for delineating the effects of experimental CMV infection on the function of pulmonary alveolar macrophages [16].

However, for our purposes these studies were of considerable interest, because they demonstrated the potential for using this CMV model to investigate the pathogenesis of congenital CMV infection. The possible connection between a salivary gland virus and human fetal infection had been made in the 1930s by Markham and Hudson [17,18] who produced generalized fetal infection in guinea pigs by intraplacental inoculations of GP CMV. Later, it was appreciated that the guinea pig placenta was similar to that of humans [19]. Experimental transplacental transmission of GP CMV was attempted in this animal, which has a relatively long gestation period of approximately 65 to 70 days. Transplacental GP CMV transmission was accomplished, and reported by three groups of independent investigators. In each case it appeared that the production of experimental maternal infection during pregnancy resulted in documentable fetal CMV infection [20–22]. In Choi and Hsiung's study [20], GP CMV recovery from fetuses was accomplished only when maternal CMV infection was initiated during pregnancy. However, transplacental virus transmission could be reliably induced by primary infection throughout pregnancy (days 26 to 60). Kumar and Nankervis [21] experimentally infected mothers during the latter half of pregnancy and showed CMV infection was present in 40% of their litters. Johnson and Connor [22] were also able to infect guinea pig mothers with GP CMV and document fetal infection in guinea pig fetuses which were close to term.

For more detailed experimentation into both the pathogenesis and prevention of CMV infection during pregnancy it was necessary to determine the optimum time following initiation of maternal infection to detect CMV in the developing fetus [23]. Maternal CMV infection can be shown to be viremic during the first two weeks following experimental virus inoculation. With adequate sampling of buffy coat blood obtained during these first two weeks, viremia can be demonstrated in nearly all nonimmune mothers. The generalized infection which ensues includes placental infection. In tissues obtained from animals between days 7 and 15 following experimental virus inoculation 39/79 (49%) placentas had CMV isolated and 34/87 (39%) fetuses or newborns had virus isolated from their tissues. In contrast, only 4/30 (13%) placentas obtained from mothers infected 16 to 30 days previously showed CMV infection, and 7/35 (20%) fetuses or newborns had virus present when tested using cocultivation techniques ([23,24] and Table 1).

TABLE 1. Time Course of Transplacental Transmission of GP CMV

No. of Days After Maternal Inoculation With CMV	No. of Mothers With CMV in Indicated Tissue/No. Tested		No. of Placentas With Virus/No. Tested	No. of Fetuses or Newborns With Virus/No. Tested
	Blood	Other*		
7–10	6/11	11/11	21/44	11/49
11–15	3/9	9/9	18/35	23/38[†]
16–30	0/11	11/11	4/30	7/35

*Other tissues tested were spleen, thymus, liver, lung, kidney, pancreas, brain, and salivary glands.
[†]Ten animals had virus in the brain.
(Tables 1 and 2 from Bia FJ et al: Cytomegalovirus infections in the guinea pig: Experimental models for human disease. Rev Infect Dis 5:177–195, 1983, with permission of the publisher and copyright holder, The University of Chicago Press.)

The trimester during which maternal infection was initiated was associated with a varying incidence of stillbirths. The rate of stillbirths (no. of stillbirths/ total no. of progeny) increased from 1/43 (2%) in mothers inoculated during their 1st trimester to 19/32 (59%) in mothers inoculated during their 3rd trimester [23,24]. In contrast, if both virus recovery from newborn animals and evidence of fetal histopathology were used as indices of CMV infection, the percentages of newborns with evidence of infection were 54%, 50%, and 55% during the 1st, 2nd, and 3rd trimesters, respectively. This indicates an average percent offspring with documentable congenital CMV infection of 54% [24]. With the GP CMV model thus characterized it not only became possible to study pathogenesis but also to attempt various means for prevention of transplacental CMV transmission. The results of those studies may prove pertinent to the future use of a live attenuated HCMV vaccine for the prevention of primary maternal CMV infection during pregnancy.

During vaccination studies, female guinea pigs were immunized prior to pregnancy and subsequently challenged with virulent GP CMV-SG during pregnancy [25]. In nonimmune pregnant animals which were challenged with GP CMV-SG during pregnancy 39/94 (41%) maternal tissues showed CMV infection and 7/26 (27%) fetuses were infected with GP CMV. In contrast, for animals who had previously been vaccinated with a low passage GP CMV-TC vaccine (passage 11 in GPE cells), and subsequently challenged during pregnancy with virulent virus, the degree of generalized CMV infection was less. Only 12% of maternal tissues showed CMV infection, and 1/25 (4%) fetuses tested had GP CMV infection. Although animals who had been vaccinated with a nonliving envelope antigen vaccine or had been given passive immunization with GP CMV antiserum fared better than controls, live vaccine appeared to be most effective at reducing the degree of generalized maternal CMV infection ([25] and Table 2).

There were additional important aspects of vaccination against primary CMV infection during pregnancy, which could be evaluated in this animal model. The CMVs are DNA-containing viruses with the potential for producing both chronic persistent and latent infection; hence, vaccination against these viruses is of even greater concern when issues surrounding pregnancy are involved. Recent work in our laboratories indicates that GP CMV-SG can be isolated from saliva of guinea pigs many months following the initiation of experimental infection [26]. In addition, pregnant Hartley guinea pigs were found at sacrifice to have higher titers of GP CMV in their salivary glands when compared to nonpregnant controls. If tissue culture-passaged HCMV behaved in a similar fashion in humans, it could jeopardize the usage of CMV vaccine. Several experiments have been directed at these issues, using the guinea pig model. The passaged GP CMV-TC vaccine which was used in our previous studies with demonstrable efficacy for the prevention of transplacental CMV transmission was not entirely analogous to human vaccines in current use. The latter have a longer passage history in tissue culture

TABLE 2. Maternal Viremia, Distribution of GP CMV, Titer of Neutralizing Antibody, and Evidence of Fetal Infection After Challenge of Immune, Pregnant Hartley Strain GP CMV-SG

Immunizing Material (No. of Animals Immunized)	After GP CMV-SG Challenge*			
	No. of Animals With Viremia/ No. Challenged	No. of CMV-Infected Tissues/ No. Studied (%)[†]	Average Antibody Titer Before/After Challenge[‡]	No. of Fetuses With CMV Infection/No. Tested (%)
None (controls) (20)	9/10	39/94 (41)	<5/<5	7/26 (27)
Live GP CMV-SG (27)	1/14[§]	19/139 (14)	86/107	0/48
Live GP CMV-TC (22)[‖]	2/9	13/110 (12)	78/269	1/25 (4)
Noninfectious, envelope antigen vaccine (13)	9/10	29/115 (25)	10/73	0/16
Passive immunization with guinea pig antiserum to GP CMV (9)	5/9	17/79 (22)	6/5	0/25

*All animals were tested four to 14 days after challenge with GP CMV-SG.
[†]Includes urine, kidneys, lymph nodes, thymus, spleen, liver, lungs, pancreas, salivary glands, cervix, mammary glands, and placentas.
[‡]Reciprocal of arithmetic mean titers of neutralizing antibody for each group of immunized mothers.
[§]Isolate was identified as guinea pig herpes-like virus, not GP CMV.
[‖]Tissue culture-passaged GP CMV.

and have been administered in lower doses than those given to guinea pigs. With this in mind, we passaged GP CMV-TC more than 30 times in tissue culture to ultimately develop an analogous experimental vaccine.

Clinical immunity could then be assessed using the same system as that to demonstrate efficacy during pregnancy for a low-passage vaccine. The actual test of successful clinical immunity was based on these challenge experiments during pregnancy. Results of these studies have thus far been encouraging. Control mothers developed generalized CMV infections, in which 33% of tissues were positive for CMV when tested using cocultivation techniques. One-third of their progeny were adversely affected by acute maternal CMV infection as evidenced by stillbirths, intrauterine abortions, and/or CMV infections of the fetus [24]. In contrast, vaccinated animals did not develop generalized CMV infection, and CMV was isolated from only 2% of tissues tested. In addition, virus was not isolated from any of the 42 fetuses tested, although six were stillborn. Virus isolation attempts on placentas obtained from these animals showed that GP CMV was isolated from 7/32 (22%) in the unvaccinated control group, and 0/36 in the vaccinated group. Histopathologic examination of these placentas further supported a protective role for this vaccine in that tissue necrosis and cellular infiltrates were widespread in placentas obtained from nonimmune guinea pigs, but not in those obtained from immune mothers. Also, low-passage GP CMV-TC vaccine appeared to reactivate during pregnancy, whereas the higher passage vaccine, administered in dosages similar to those given to humans, did not reactivate.

The guinea pig model for HCMV infection has proven to be a useful one for the investigation of CMV pathogenesis. Congenital infection has been of particular interest to those working with the model because the transplacental transmission of the virus is so readily demonstrated in controlled experiments. This, in turn, has resulted in vaccine trials which appear to indicate that under experimental circumstances it is possible to produce effective CMV vaccines which do not cause chronic persistent CMV infection in animal models or reactivate during pregnancy. Whether the same proves true for human vaccine development remains to be seen.

REFERENCES

1. Bia FJ, Griffith BP, Fong CKY, Hsiung GD: Cytomegalovirus infections in the guinea pig: Experimental models for human disease. Rev Infect Dis 5:177–195, 1983.
2. Hsiung GD, Bia FJ, Fong CKY: Viruses of guinea pigs: Considerations for biomedical research. Microbiol Rev 44:468-490, 1980.
3. Jackson L: An intracellular protozoan parasite of the ducts of the salivary glands of the guinea pig. J Infect Dis 26:347-350, 1920.

4. Cole R, Kuttner AG: A filterable virus present in the submaxillary glands of guinea pigs. J Exp Med 44:855–873, 1926.

5. Kuttner AG: Further studies concerning the filterable virus present in the submaxillary glands of guinea pigs. J Exp Med 46:935–956, 1927.

6. Andrewes CH: Immunity to the salivary virus of guinea pigs studied in the living animal and in tissue culture. Br J Exp Pathol 11:23–34, 1930.

7. Kuttner AG, Wang SH: The problem of the significance of the inclusion bodies found in the salivary glands of infants, and the occurrence of inclusion bodies in the submaxillary glands of hamsters, white mice, and wild rats (Peiping). J Exp Med 60:773–791, 1934.

8. Kuttner AG, T'ung T: Further studies on the submaxillary gland viruses of rats and guinea pigs. J Exp Med 62:805–822, 1935.

9. Hartley JW, Rowe WP, Huebner RJ: Serial propagation of guinea pig salivary gland virus in tissue culture. Proc Soc Exp Biol Med 96:281–285, 1957.

10. Hsiung GD, Tenser RB, Fong CKY: Comparison of guinea pig cytomegalovirus and guinea pig herpes-like virus: Growth characteristics and antigenic relationship. Infect Immun 13:926:933, 1976.

11. Tenser RB, Hsiung GD: Comparison of guinea pig cytomegalovirus and guinea pig herpes-like virus: Pathogenesis and persistence in experimentally infected animals. Infect Immun 13:934–940, 1976.

12. Bia FJ, Summers WC, Fong CKY, Hsiung GD: A new endogenous herpesvirus of guinea pigs: Biological and molecular characterization. J Virol 36:245–253, 1980.

13. Hsiung GD, Choi YC, Bia FJ: Cytomegalovirus infection in guinea pigs. I. Viremia during acute primary and chronic persistent infection. J Infect Dis 138:191–196, 1978.

14. Griffith BP, Lucia HL, Bia FJ, Hsiung GD: Cytomegalovirus induced mononucleosis in guinea pigs. Infect Immun 32:857–863, 1981.

15. Yourtee EL, Bia FJ, Griffith BP, Root RK: Neutrophil response and function during acute cytomegalovirus infection in guinea pigs. Infect Immun 36:11-16, 1982.

16. Miller S, Coleman D, Metcalf J, Root RK, Bia FJ: Pulmonary macrophage function during CMV interstitial pneumonia in guinea pigs. Abstract #44, 22nd ICAAC, 4-6 October 1982, Miami Beach, FL.

17. Markham FS, Hudson NP: Susceptibility of the guinea pig fetus to the submaxillary gland virus of guinea pigs. Am J Pathol 12:175–181, 1936.

18. Markham FS: A study of the submaxillary gland virus of the guinea pig. Am J Pathol 14:311–321, 1938,

19. Enders AC: A comparative study of the fine structure of the trophoblast in several hemochorial placentas. Am J Anat 116:29–67, 1965.

20. Choi YC, Hsiung GD: Cytomegalovirus infection in guinea pigs. II. Transplacental and horizontal transmission. J Infect Dis 138:197–202, 1978.

21. Kumar ML, Nankervis GA: Experimental congenital infection with cytomegalovirus: A guinea pig model. J Infect Dis 138:650-654, 1978.

22. Johnson KP, Connor WS: Guinea pig cytomegalovirus: Transplacental transmission. Brief report. Arch Virol 59:263–267, 1979.

23. Griffith BP, Hsiung GD: Cytomegalovirus infection in guinea pigs. IV. Maternal infection at different stages of gestation. J Infect Dis 141:787–793, 1980.

24. Bia FJ, Miller SA, Lucia HL, Tarsio M, Hsiung GD: Vaccination against transplacental CMV transmission: Vaccine reactivation and efficacy in guinea pigs. J Infect Dis (Submitted for publication)

25. Bia FJ, Griffith BP, Tarsio M, Hsiung GD: Vaccination for prevention of maternal-fetal infection with guinea pig cytomegalovirus. J Infect Dis 142:732–738, 1980.
26. Griffith BP, Lucia HL, Tillbrook JL, Hsiung GD: Enhancement of cytomegalovirus infection during pregnancy in guinea pigs. J Infect Dist 147:990–998, 1983.

SECTION 4:
VACCINATION AGAINST CYTOMEGALOVIRUS

The Importance of Cytotoxic Cellular Immunity in the Protection From Cytomegalovirus Infection

Gerald V. Quinnan, Jr., MD, and Alain H. Rook, MD

The Division of Virology, Office of Biologics, National Center for Drugs and Biologics, Food and Drug Administration, Bethesda, MD 20205

During the past several years, we have performed studies to define the nature of CMI in CMV infections and to define the role of specific immune functions in determining recovery from these infections. In these studies we have confirmed the widely held clinical impression that CMI is much more important than humoral immunity in determining the outcome of infection. In anticipation of this finding, we have designed our studies to determine which defects in effector cells correlate with a poor outcome of infection, and then to study the specific defects responsible for ineffective immune responses. The principal immune functions that have emerged as important correlates with outcome of infection are various types of HLA-restricted CTLs and nonrestricted non-T lymphocytes with characteristics of NK cells or antibody-dependent killer cells [1]. This review will summarize the general characteristics of these responses, the evidence that they are important in determining the outcome of CMV infection, and the immune processes required for their development. In regard to the latter aspect, we will review the approach used to define the reasons for defective cytotoxic responses when they occur.

The approach we have used has been to study several groups of high-risk and healthy individuals prospectively throughout the course of CMV infections. By performing a variety of immunologic studies at repeated intervals, we have been able to define the frequencies with which different responses occur and their relationship to each other, as well as to define which responses correlate most strongly with recovery from infection. The one assay

Birth Defects: Original Article Series, Volume 20, Number 1, pages 245–261

procedure which was newly developed is that for measurement of HLA-restricted CMV-specific cytotoxic T cells [2]. The methods used for that assay are summarized in Figure 1. The procedure is actually quite routine and similar to most chromium release microcytotoxicity assays. As in any such test, the essential components are effector cells and target cells. The effector cells consist of suspensions of PBL or of fractions of these cells prepared by rosetting with sheep erythrocytes, passage through nylon wool columns, treatment with monoclonal antibodies, or other common procedures. In this way, characteristics of the cells mediating any killing found in the assay can be defined. The target cells in this case are human diploid fibroblasts prepared from skin biopsies from HLA-typed donors. Different roller bottles of cells derived from a given skin biopsy are either infected with CMV and frozen in aliquots or harvested while uninfected and frozen. At the time of the assay, these cells are thawed, labeled with chromium, washed, and aliquoted to wells in the assay plate. In each case, several pairs of infected and uninfected cells are used to enable demonstration of whether or not killing is HLA-restricted.

The principle of HLA-restriction is demonstrated in Figure 2. Classically, cytotoxic T cells are antigen-specific in that they only kill target cells with the appropriate surface antigens. In 1974, Doherty and Zinkernagel [3], using a murine system, demonstrated that this cytotoxic effect was not only antigen-specific, but was restricted to killing of syngeneic or semiallogeneic target cells, and that these murine lymphocytes had to be matched to the target cells for one or more H2-D- or K-locus antigens. These loci are analogous to the HLA-A and B loci, and restriction of human CTL by these antigens has also been found. That is, human CTL kill only target cells with both virus antigens and similar HLA antigens on their surface. This HLA-matching can be for a single antigen, and the target cells and effector cells do not need to be syngeneic. However, in the absence of any HLA-matching, no killing by cytotoxic T cells occurs [1, 3]. Two other types of lymphocyte-mediated cytotoxicity can be detected in these assays. NK cells can kill virus-infected target cells, oftentimes, but not necessarily, to a greater degree than they kill uninfected target cells. They do not bind to viral antigens on the cell surface, but bind to an undefined cell-surface structure. If they kill the infected cells preferentially, it is probably because they are activated by the virus to be more cytotoxic or because the target cells themselves are more easily killed nonspecifically when infected. There is no evidence that CMV infection of target cells increases the number of NK-cell recognition sites on their surface, although this mechanism is at least a theoretic possibility in the case of other viruses. The third type of cytotoxic cell depicted in this figure

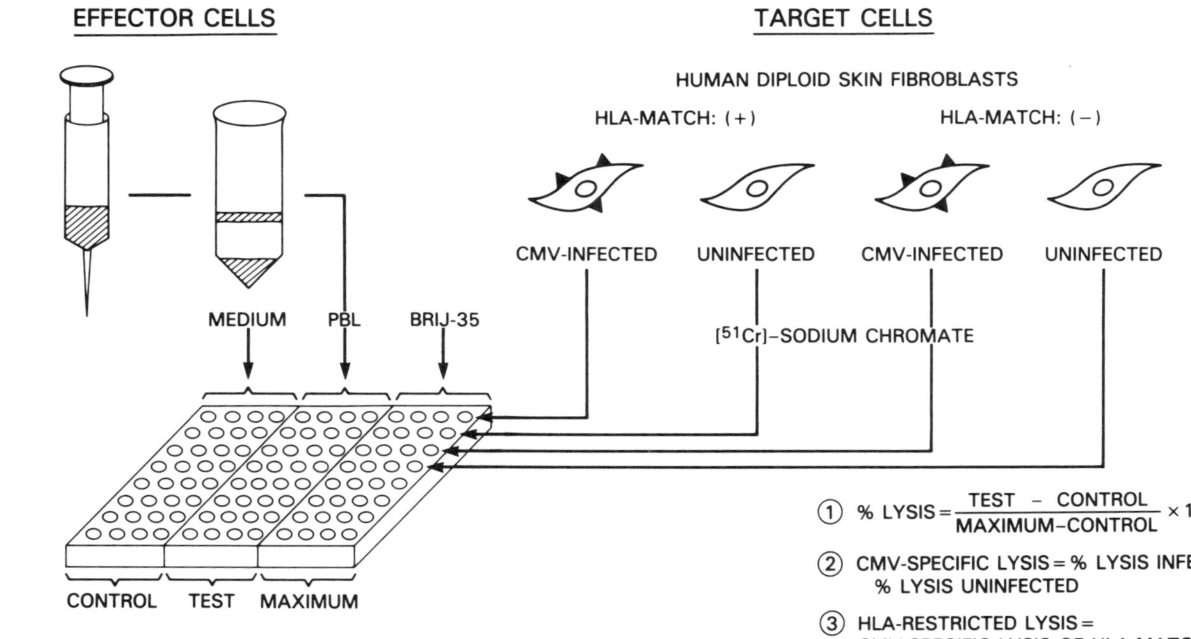

Fig. 1. The cytotoxicity assay for CMV-specific cytotoxic lymphocytes is a [^{51}Cr] release assay. Effector cells are separated from heparinized peripheral blood specimens by Ficoll-Hypaque density centrifugation; then varying concentrations of cells in 0.1 ml aliquots are added to 96 well round-bottom microtiter plates. Aliquots of 0.1 ml of [^{51}Cr]-labeled CMV-infected and uninfected human diploid skin fibroblasts which are either HLA-matched with the effector cells at one or more HLA-A or B loci, or completely HLA-mismatched, are added to the effector cells as targets and incubated for 6 hr at 37°C. The supernatants are harvested and [^{51}Cr] release counted on a gamma counter. Percent lysis of target cells is determined by the formula denoted (1) where Test is [^{51}Cr] CPM released from targets in the presence of effector cells, Control is [^{51}Cr] CPM released in the presence of medium alone, and Maximum is CPM released in the presence of 10% Brij-35 solution, a detergent.

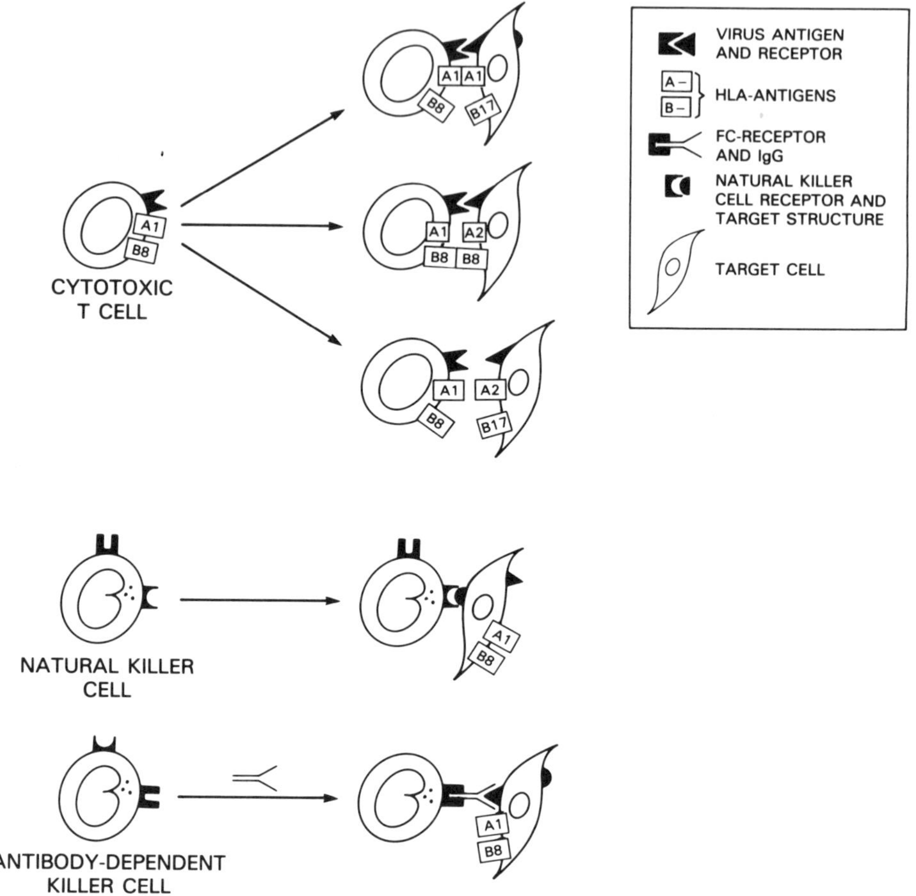

Fig. 2. See text for discussion.

is the antibody-dependent killer cell. These cells recognize viral antigens on target cells specifically by virtue of the ability of Fc receptors on the surface of these effectors to bind specific IgG. Cells which can mediate this antibody-dependent effect include both macrophages and NK cells. Although both NK cells and ADCC activity can be reflected in results of cytotoxicity assays using CMV-infected fibroblasts, other types of target cells are more sensitive for measuring these types of effector cells. In the case of NK cells, certain continuous tumor cell lines have large numbers of recognition structures and are better target cells. The most commonly used target cell for NK cell assays are K562 cells, a continuous myeloid cell line. ADCC is best measured using HLA-mismatched cells that lack NK-cell recognition structures. The target cells we usually use are Chang liver cells sensitized with antibodies. In practice, it is difficult to differentiate NK cell-mediated and ADCC-mediated killing if CMV-infected fibroblast target cells are used, since the effector cells have similar properties in both cases. The differentiation which usually we can make fairly easily is between T cell- and non-T cell-mediated killing. Based on results that will be summarized below, this differentiation is most easily done by demonstrating that killing is HLA-restricted. It can also be accomplished by separating PBL into T-cell and non-T-cell fractions and using these fractions as effector cells [1–3].

Before proceeding with a discussion of results of clinical studies that demonstrate the importance of these cytotoxic functions, some common features of chromium-release microcytotoxicity assays are worth noting. Release of chromium from target cells completely lysed by detergent is compared to release from target cells cultured with effector cells and to spontaneous release in the presence of medium alone. At time zero, spontaneous release is slightly greater than zero depending on the leakiness of the target cells, and subsequent release is generally linear over time. Specific killing by lymphocytes also tends to be linear, but at a more rapid rate. The assay should be harvested when the spontaneous release is still low enough to yield meaningful results, generally less than 30% of maximum, and when the difference between spontaneous- and lymphocyte-mediated release is greatest. Conversely, target cells should be used which give reasonable spontaneous release and adequate sensitivity to lymphocyte-mediated killing at the time the assay is harvested. With careful attention to the methods used for propagating, infecting, freezing, and thawing of skin fibroblast target cells, about two-thirds of skin biopsies we have processed have yielded target cells that are eventually useful in terms of low spontaneous chromium release and adequate sensitivity to virus-specific killing. Each lot of target cells is tested to prove their suitability by determining that they are killed by cytotoxic T cells in an HLA-restricted fashion.

Several characteristics of the human cytotoxic T-cell response to CMV infection in BMT recipients are demonstrated in Figure 3. These results are from a collaborative study performed with the Johns Hopkins Oncology Center Bone Marrow Transplant Unit. Eighty-eight patients were studied prospectively [4]. Virus cultures of throat washings, urine, and blood buffy coats were performed twice weekly. Serum anti-CMV complement-fixing antibodies were measured weekly, and CMV-specific cytotoxicity tests were performed approximately at one to three week intervals. Sixty-one of the 88

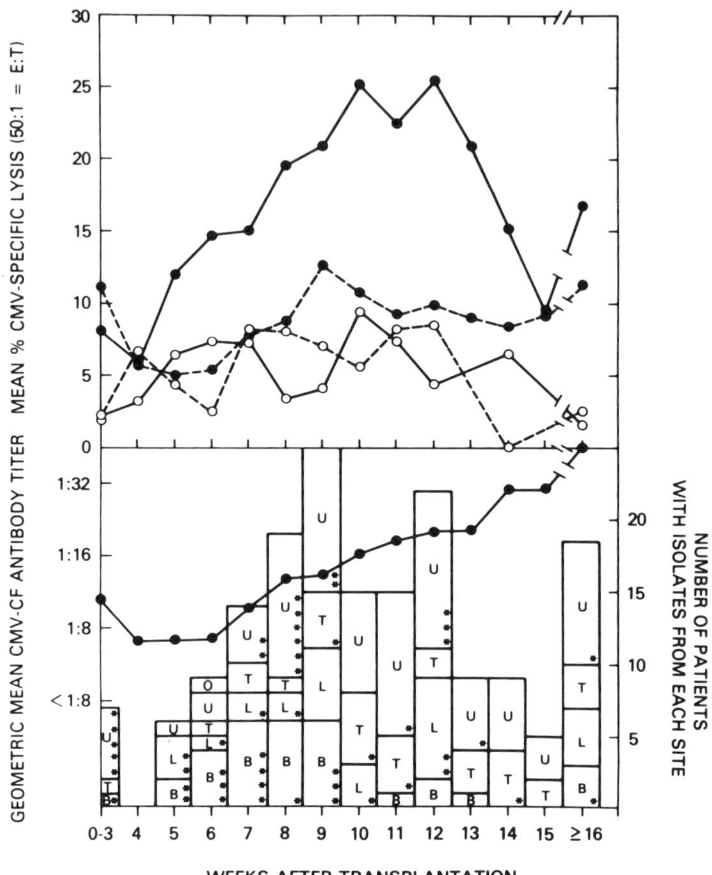

Fig. 3. CMV-specific cytotoxic responses of BMT recipients. Upper panel) Mean results of assays using HLA-matched (solid lines) and mismatched (dashed lines) target cells and lymphocytes from infected (solid circles) and uninfected (open circles) patients are shown by week after transplantation. Lower panel) Geometric mean antibody responses (solid line) are shown for all patients compared to numbers of virus isolates obtained from buffy coat or bone marrow (B), lung or liver (L), throat (T), urine (U), or other (O) sites. Asterisks (*) indicate the first CMV isolates obtained from individual patients.

patients developed CMV infection. The results of virus isolations and antibody testing are consistent with those reported by others indicating that most CMV infections occurring after transplantation occur between four and 12 weeks posttransplant [5]. The results of CMV-specific cytotoxicity tests are summarized in the upper panel. Killing of HLA-matched and mismatched target cells by lymphocytes from infected and uninfected patients is shown.

During the period of four to 12 weeks posttransplant, there was significantly greater killing by lymphocytes from infected patients of HLA-matched than mismatched target cells, demonstrating graphically the HLA-restricted nature of this response. It should be noted also that this response is short lived, and corresponds to the acute phase of infection, or approximately to that time period when symptoms or viremia are likely to occur. Finally, it should be noted that this HLA-restricted cytotoxicity is superimposed on a background of nonrestricted cytotoxicity. Prior to onset of infection, after resolution of acute infection, and continuously in uninfected patients, there is killing which is greater against infected than uninfected target cells, but is not HLA-restricted. Similar nonrestricted activity is typically found in healthy, uninfected individuals, whether previously immune or not, and is mediated by cells with characteristics of NK cells and/or antibody-dependent killer cells [6].

Results of experiments which exemplify the methods that were used to demonstrate that the HLA-restricted cytotoxic cells were T cells, and the nonrestricted cytotoxic cells were non-T, NK-like cells are shown in Table 1. The results shown here depict the same sequence just discussed, with HLA-restricted killing during acute infection (days 39 and 46) and nonrestricted killing later on (day 69). We fractionated the lymphocytes into T-cell enriched, NK-cell depleted [E-Ros(+) or Fc (−)], or T-cell depleted, NK-cell enriched [E-Ros (−)] fractions before using them as effector cells. The T cells kill only HLA-matched target cells and the non-T, NK-like cells kill

TABLE 1. CMV-Specific T- and Non-T-Cell-Mediated Cytotoxicity Early and Late During Infection*

Day Past Transplant	Effector	% CMV-Specific Lysis	
		HLA-Matched	HLA-Mismatched
39	PBL	7.3	0.0
	E-Ros (+)	22.3	0.0
	E-Ros (−)	0.0	0.0
46	PBL	25.3	0.0
	Fc (−)	27.1	0.0
69	PBL	15.7	11.5
	E-Ros (+)	0.2	0.0
	E-Ros (−)	5.3	7.0
	Fc (−)	0.0	0.0

*E-Ros (+) indicates cells that have receptors for sheep erythrocytes; Fc (−) indicates cells that have been depleted of Fc-receptor bearing cells.

both matched and mismatched cells. We have tested lymphocyte fractions from more than 30 patients with HLA-restricted and/or nonrestricted killing [1, 4]. In each case HLA-restricted killing was mediated by T cells, and nonrestricted killing was mediated by NK-like cells. Consequently, our current practice is to assume that HLA-restriction is definitive of a cytotoxic T-cell response. We define HLA-restriction as significantly greater lysis of two or more matched target cells than of mismatched target cells.

The time at which the CTL response first develops in relation to other indications of onset of infection is indicated by the results shown in Figure 4. The results shown relate to 34 patients with cytotoxic responses and CMV infection as evidenced by virus isolation, antibody responses, or both. The time of onset of cytotoxic responses is compared to onset of virus excretion, antibody response, or interstitial pneumonitis. The results demonstrate that cytotoxic lymphocyte responses occur as a very early manifestation. In most cases, CTL activity was detected before, or coincident with, virus culture positivity, seroconversion, and interstitial pneumonitis [4]. This finding is important since it indicates that this effector cell function is present early enough that it could be the immune function primarily responsible for determining the outcome of infection.

The type of evidence that indicates that CTL probably is the immune response which determines the outcome of infection is shown in Table 2. The absence of a CTL response in CMV-infected BMT patients is uniformly associated with a fatal outcome; all patients who survived infection developed specific cytotoxic responses [1]. In most cases, these responses are CTL-mediated, although in an occasional patient there is a significant increase in non-T-cell cytotoxicity only, with the same implications with respect to survival. In these same patients, numerous other factors were examined for correlation with outcome of infection, and in most cases none were found. The factors which did not correlate with survival included lymphocyte proliferation responses to T-cell mitogens and CMV antigens, serum antibodies to CMV in donor or recipient pretransplant, and in the patient during infection, graft rejection, GVHD, and underlying disease for which the transplantation was performed [1]. The only two other tests yielding results which did correlate with survival were NK-cell assays using uninfected K562 tumor cells as target cells, and ADCC assays using antibody-sensitized Chang liver cells as target cells [1]. For reasons that will be discussed subsequently, it is likely that these correlations of survival with NK cell and ADCC activity were secondary correlates of the CMV-specific cytotoxic responses. The implications of these secondary correlates will also be discussed subsequently.

Similar results have been obtained in various other study groups as summarized in Table 3. Among 20 CMV-infected renal transplant recipients, six

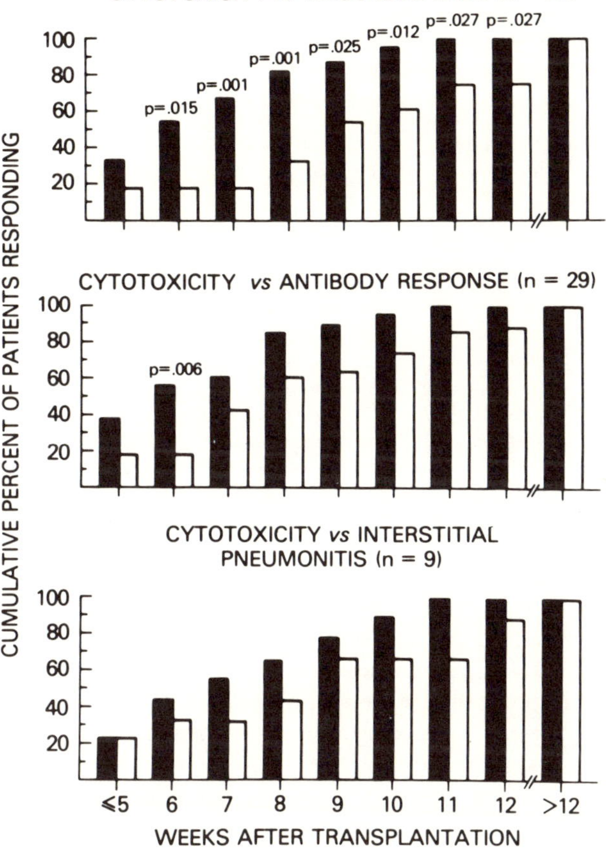

Fig. 4. Comparison of times of CMV-specific cytotoxic lymphocyte responses in infected patients (shaded areas) to times of other responses (unshaded areas). Upper panel) The responses compared are diagnosis of virus shedding or viremia by identification of cytopathic effect in tissue culture. Middle panel) Development of fourfold antibody rises. Lower panel) Interstitial pneumonitis. Patients were considered to have had cytotoxic responses if cytotoxicity were HLA-restricted, or if sequential increases in cytotoxicity $> 15\%$ CMV-specific lysis were seen. The number of patients available for each comparison are indicated by n. Significant differences between response rates by χ^2 analysis are indicated by p.

failed to develop cytotoxic responses [7]. The 14 responders were asymptomatic, with a few having mild laboratory abnormalities. The six nonresponders had significant symptoms, persistent viremia, and numerous complications. Although most nonresponding renal transplant recipients survived, several nonresponding patients we have studied eventually lost their grafts, after which their chemotherapy was discontinued, responses devel-

TABLE 2. Occurrence of CMV-Specific Cytotoxic Responses in Relation to Outcome of CMV Infection

Outcome of Infection	Frequency of Occurrence of Effector Cell Response		
	Cytotoxic T Cells*	Other†	Fraction Responding
Nonfatal	9	9	18/18
Fatal	0	2	2/10
Death from other causes	0	3	3/6

*Includes all patients proven to have cytotoxic T-cell responses by testing of fractionated lymphocytes, with or without concurrent non-T-cell responses.

†Includes patients with responses mediated by non-T lymphocytes only, and those whose effector cells were not fully characterized by fractionation studies.

oped, and they recovered from infection. The third high-risk group we have studied is homosexual men with immunodeficiency. CTL responses did not occur in patients with AIDS, or in some patients with chronic asymptomatic lymphadenopathy [8]. These results contrast with the uniform occurrence of CMV-specific cytotoxic responses in otherwise healthy individuals with CMV infection [9]. In homosexual men with mild or asymptomatic infection, and in nine healthy volunteers undergoing experimental infection, CMV-specific cytotoxic responses developed in all cases. It is noteworthy that serum antibodies did not correlate with outcome of infection in renal transplant recipients or in homosexual men, and in the study involving experimental infection of healthy volunteers, that the cytotoxic responses preceded antibody responses. However, like BMT recipients, depressed NK-cell activity was seen in homosexual men and renal transplant recipients who were unable to develop CTL responses [7, 8]. The evidence that CTL develop during naturally acquired infection, the early nature of the CTL response, and the extremely consistent correlation of the response by comparison to other responses with recovery, provide strong evidence that this immune function is an important determinant of recovery.

Since the CTL response appears to be of great significance in CMV infection, it is important to understand why some patients fail to respond. A current conceptualization of the cytotoxic T-cell maturation process is shown in Figure 5. Cytotoxic cell precursors go through three stages: activation, proliferation, and differentiation. Each stage involves soluble mediators produced by accessory cells. For example, IL-1 is produced by monocytes or

TABLE 3. Relationship of CMV-Specific Cytotoxic Lymphocyte Responses to Outcome of Infection in High-Risk Groups and Healthy Volunteers

Study Group	CMV-Specific Cytotoxicity	% in Group	Outcome of CMV Infection
BMT recipients	responders	59%	survived
	nonresponders	41%	died
Renal transplant recipients	responders	70%	asymptomatic or minimally symptomatic
	nonresponders	30%	severe symptoms and complications, graft loss, death
Homosexual men	responders	unknown	asymptomatic or minimally symptomatic; lymphadenopathy
	nonresponders	unknown	progressive infection and death (AIDS)
Experimentally infected healthy volunteers	responders	100%	asymptomatic or minimally symptomatic
(Towne or Toledo Strain)	nonresponders	0%	not applicable

macrophages, IL-2 is produced by small T cells and large granular lymphocytes, and γ-IFN is produced by small T cells. Precursor cells must be specifically activated by IL-1 and antigen, during which process the antigen-specific activated intermediates develop IL-2 receptors. Once receptors have developed, the cells are capable of proliferating in response to IL-2. The expanded pool of intermediates can then differentiate under the influence of γ-IFN, and probably another differentiation factor, into cytotoxic cells. γ-IFN production is induced by IL-2 in this process [10]. The role of α-IFN in this process is not well understood, although it is probably important. It may act early in the activation process or indirectly by stimulation of accessory cells. The accessory cells which produce α-IFN are large granular lymphocytes (LGL) [11], which are the subset of lymphocytes that includes NK cells. In addition to α-IFN production, however, these LGL produce many lymphokines including IL-2 [12]. They are absolutely required for development of cytotoxic T-cell responses [13]. Thus, they are very critical accessory cells for T cells, and it may be that the frequent correlation we have seen between NK-cell activity and CTL responses reflects this required accessory function. There is another possible reason for this relationship that should also be considered, however. The lymphokines produced by LGL not only affect T cells, but autoregulate LGL function [11]. Thus, coincident defects in NK cells and CTL could reflect either an accessory cell defect or a

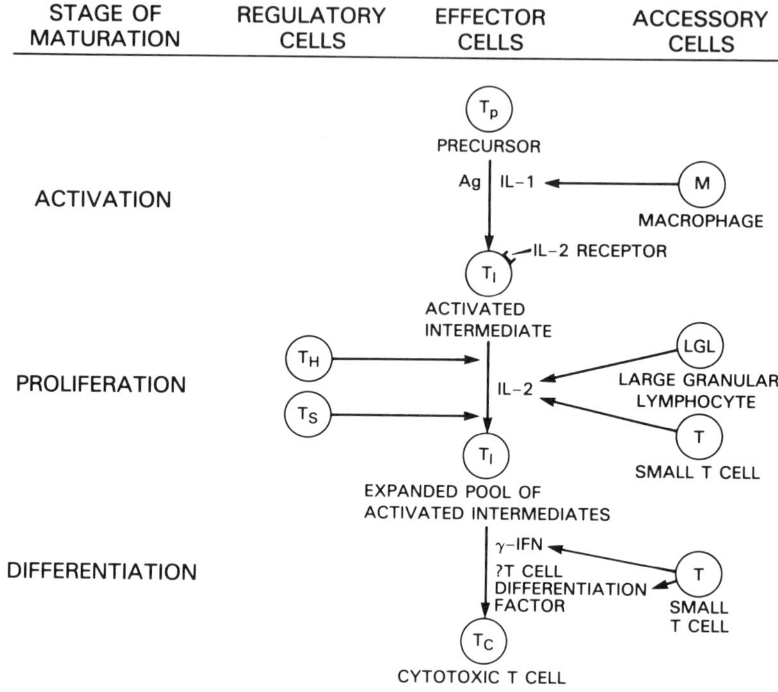

Fig. 5.   See text for discussion.

common defect in the similar maturation pathways of both cells. In general, then, for CTL responses to occur, precursors must be present in adequate numbers, and accessory cell functions must be intact. If these processes are intact, then the entire process is modulated by immunoregulatory helper and suppressor T cells.

With respect to the issue at hand, namely the determination of the causes of deficient CTL responses in high-risk patients infected with CMV, it is important to recognize that there are simple assays that can be used to evaluate the integrity of various components of this process. For example, accessory cell function can be evaluated by testing of macrophage activation or activities of LGL,such as NK-cell cytotoxicity, responsiveness of NK cells to IFN in vitro and production of α-IFN in vitro. T-cell mitogens are useful for evaluating the maturation pathway. If lymphocytes proliferate in response to T-cell mitogens, then adequate precursors are present and production of and, proliferation responses to, IL-2 are intact. γ-IFN production in response to T-cell mitogens reflects the integrity of the differentiation step. One other test of the maturation process important for this discussion is that of IL-2 on cytotoxicity in vitro. The addition of IL-2 by itself to lymphocyte cultures sometimes enhances their cytotoxicity. When this occurs, it implies that adequate precursors are present and that activation of precursors by macrophage accessory cell-produced IL-1 is intact and has already occurred. The immunoregulatory arm of the process now can be assessed easily using monoclonal antibodies to enumerate helper and suppressor cell numbers, or can be tested using conventional assays for these cells which are somewhat more cumbersome. Results of assays, such as these hypotheses, can be presented to explain deficient responses in the high-risk populations discussed above.

The results of experiments which form the basis for these hypotheses are summarized in Table 4. The first general comment to be made is that abnormalities in immunoregulatory cells occur in all three groups, but in no group have we found that these changes correlate with cytotoxic T-cell responsiveness (Quinnan et al, unpublished data). Thus, the principal defects must be in either the cytotoxic precursors, or the accessory cells. The second general point is that in all three high-risk populations studied deficient CTL responsiveness is associated with depressed NK-cell activity. As just discussed, there are two likely explanations for this consistent relationship. One is that deficient NK-cell activity may reflect a depression of LGL [14], including their important accessory functions for CTL responses [13]. The other is that NK-cell cytotoxicity is itself dependent on both IL-2 and IFN, indicating that they autoregulate their own activity through a maturation

TABLE 4. Immune Dysfunctions Associated With Deficient Cytotoxic T-Cell Responses

Study Group	Cytotoxic Cell Precursors	Accessory Cells	Immunoregulatory Cells
BMT recipients	decreased γ-IFN production a) proliferation intact b) proliferation depressed	decreased NK cells, responsive to IFN	T4/T8 inversion not correlated with responsiveness
Renal transplant recipients	steroid-related deficiency in nonactivated precursors	decreased NK cells	$\pm$ T4/T8 inversion
AIDS	activated precursors present and reponsive to IL-2 proliferation intact implying in vivo block in IL-2 production	decreased NK cells responsive to IL-2 but not IFN decreased α-IFN production	decreased in T4 cells

process similar to that for cytotoxic T cells. The other abnormalities listed in this table are just highlights of many different types of testing that were done in the process of trying to map these defects.

In BMT patients with deficient CTL responses the activation stage is deficient, since γ-IFN is not produced [15]. In some patients, there is a defect in the proliferation stage as well.

In renal transplant patients the results of this type of testing were similar, and there was evidence that the underlying defect was a deficiency of precursor cells induced by high-dose steroids used to treat graft rejection. The evidence for this effect will be summarized below.

In homosexual men with AIDS, the basic immune defect is apparently different than in transplant patients. Unlike the transplant patients, their NK cells are poorly responsive to IFN in vitro, but they are highly responsive to IL-2 [16]. The implication of this finding is that the cytotoxic cells have gone through the activation stage and have IL-2 receptors, but are not exposed to IL-2 in vivo. However, their lymphocytes proliferate in vitro in response to T-cell mitogens. As discussed above, the proliferation response implied that IL-2 was produced when their cells were removed from their serum. In AIDS, therefore, there was deficient cytotoxicity that was responsive to IL-2 even though the lymphocytes could produce IL-2 in vitro. The most likely explanation for these findings is the existence of a serum factor that blocks IL-2 activity.

The results referred to indicating a steroid effect in renal transplant patients are summarized in Table 5. Included here are results of only those studies performed during documented active infection. An important relationship was found between high-dose methylprednisolone treatment and cytotoxicity [7]. The steroids did have a depressive effect on CTL activity, but the effect was not immediate and took about five days to occur. These findings indicate that the effect is not on mature cytotoxic cells, but is one of blocking

TABLE 5. Time-Dependent Effect of Methylprednisolone Administration on the Development of CMV-Specific Cytotoxic Responses*

Interval Between Administration of Methyl- prednisolone and Assay Date †	Detectable CMV-Specific Cytotoxic Response (Assays with a Response/Total Number of Assays)
None given	10/12
0–4 days	4/4
5–14 days	5/20
> 14 days	5/6

*IV methylprednisolone dosage consisted of 1 gm boluses to treat acute allograft rejection.
†Assays include some patients tested at different times after methylprednisolone.

development of precursors into cytotoxic cells. The lag period required for this effect to be seen is remarkably consistent with the time required in animal models and in in vitro testing for cytotoxic responses to develop [17, 18]. The precursor cells that are being induced on the day the steroids are given would ordinarily be expected to appear in the circulation as effector cells about five days later. The other important finding demonstrated in this table is that recovery from the depressive effect of the steroids may take two weeks, thus defining the time period during which patients given high-dose steroid treatment are likely to be at risk of serious complications of CMV infection. Another implication of these results is that cytotoxicity testing might be used prior to initiation of treatment as a means of defining which patients would be at greatest risk of adverse effects. Using the model outlined in Figure 5, we have been able to design experiments intended to define precisely what are the causes of susceptibility to infection in each of these high-risk groups. Using this approach, it should be possible to define targeted use of lymphokines to correct these immunologic deficits. Although these suggestions are at present only speculative potential applications, they do exemplify the very likely possibility that precise definition of immunologic defects in high-risk patients should provide important clues regarding optimum management of CMV infections.

In Table 3, reference was made to data that have thus far only been published in abstract form on CTL responses in experimental CMV infection [19]. Normal volunteers were inoculated either with Towne strain vaccine CMV or a low-passage isolate of CMV, called the Toledo-1 strain. Both of these viruses induced cytotoxic T cells in the volunteers, giving assurance that the experimental vaccine induces this particular important response. However, there was a difference in the responses in that the cytotoxicity induced by the low-passage virus persisted much longer than that induced by the Towne strain. We did not test to see whether this difference in persistence of the response to infection also indicated a difference in persistence of immunologic memory for cytotoxic T-cell responses that might be important on subsequent exposure to CMV. On the other hand, we do not know whether cytotoxic T cells are important in protective immunity against reinfection or in prevention of reactivation of latent infection. These are important questions that need further study.

In summary, the experimental results outlined here are the findings available to date from study of HCMV infection that relate to the importance of CTL in determining recovery from CMV infection. Although numerous other in vitro parameters of immune function have been measured, and various abnormalities in these functions occur in different situations, it appears that they probably relate directly or indirectly to CTL responsiveness. The importance of NK-cell activity as a reflection of their critical role as accessory cells in cytotoxic T-cell responses has also become apparent. Using current technology, it is now possible to dissect the workings of the immune system and define precisely what the causes of susceptibility to CMV infection are in high-risk groups. Other CMV-specific immune functions, such as serum and secretory antibodies, probably contribute to recovery, but to a lesser extent than do CTL. These findings do not define which immune functions are responsible for the two other important effects: after recovery from infection occurs, what prevents latent virus from becoming reactivated, and what protects the individual from reinfection. Perhaps the simplest possibility is that these functions are mediated by serum or secretory antibodies. However, such is not likely the case. It has recently been well established that homosexual men undergo frequent reinfection despite very high levels of serum antibodies [20], and reactivation of latent CMV infection is known to occur in seropositive individuals [21]. It appears, therefore, that these effects too are mediated by the nebulous group of functions referred to collectively as CMI. Now is the time to design experiments that will yield the facts needed to understand these events. This type of information should improve the prospects for developing effective methods for immunization and for successful management of high-risk patients.

REFERENCES

1. Quinnan GV, Kirmani N, Rook AH, Manischewitz JF, Jackson L, Moreschi G, Santos GW, Saral R, Burns WH: Cytotoxic T cells in cytomegalovirus infection: HLA-restricted T lymphocyte and non-T lymphocyte cytotoxic responses correlate with recovery from cytomegalovirus infection in bone marrow transplant recipients. N Engl J Med 307:7–13, 1982.
2. Quinnan GV, Kirmani N, Esber E, Saral R, Manischewitz JF, Rogers JL, Rook AH, Santos GW, Burns WH: HLA-restricted cytotoxic T lymphocyte and nonthymic cytotoxic lymphocyte responses to cytomegalovirus infection of bone marrow transplant recipients. J Immunol 126:2036–2041, 1981.
3. Zinkernagel RM, Doherty PC: Restriction of in vitro T cell-mediated cytotoxicity in lymphocytic choriomeningitis within a syngeneic or semiallogeneic system. Nature 248:701–702, 1974.
4. Quinnan GV, Burns WH, Kirmani N, Rook AH, Manischewitz JF, Jackson L: HLA-restricted cytotoxic T lymphocytes are an early immune response and important defense mechanism in cytomegalovirus infections. Rev Infect Dis (In press).
5. Elfenbein GJ, Saral R: Infectious disease during immune recovery after bone marrow transplantation. In Allen JC (ed): "Infection in the Compromised Host." Baltimore: Williams & Wilkins, 1981, pp 157–196.

6. Kirmani N, Ginn RK, Mittal KK, Manischewitz JF, Quinnan GV: Cytomegalovirus-specific cytotoxicity mediated by non-T lymphocytes from peripheral blood of normal volunteers. Infect Immun 34:441–447, 1981.
7. Rook AH, Frederick W, Manischewitz JF, Epstein JE, Jackson L, Lee BB, Currier CB, Quinnan GV: Correlation of clinical outcome of CMV infection and immunosuppression with virus-specific cytotoxic lymphocyte responses in renal transplant recipients. This volume (abstract)
8. Frederick W, Quinnan GV, Rook AH, Fauci AS, Epstein J, Ames J, Manischewitz JF, Jackson L, Lane HC, Masur H: Cell-mediated immunity during cytomegalovirus infection in healthy and immunodeficient homosexual men. (Submitted for publication)
9. Rook AH, Quinnan GV: Cell-mediated immunity to human cytomegalovirus. In Ennis FA (ed): "Human Immunity to Viruses." New York: Academic Press. (In press)
10. Farrar JJ, Benjamin WR, Hilfiker ML, Howard M, Farrar WL, Fuller-Farrar J: The biochemistry, biology, and role of interleukin-2 in the induction of cytotoxic T cell and antibody forming B cell responses. Immunol Rev 63:129–166, 1982.
11. Djeu JY, Stocks N, Zoon K, Stanton GJ, Timonen T, Herberman RB: Positive self-regulation of cytotoxicity in human natural killer cells by production of interferon upon exposure to influenza and herpes viruses. J Exp Med 156:1222–1234, 1982.
12. Kasahara T, Djeu JY, Dougherty SF, Oppenheim JJ: Capacity of human large granular lymphocytes to produce multiple lymphokines: Interleukin-2, interferon and colony stimulating factor. J Immunol (In press)
13. Burlington DB, Djeu JY, Wells M, Quinnan GV: Large granular lymphocytes provide an accessory function in the in vitro development of influenza A virus-specific cytotoxic T cells. (Submitted for publication)
14. Rook AH, Ramsey KM, Djeu JY, Manischewitz JF, Quinnan GV: Mechanism of depressed natural killer cell activity in renal transplant recipients. Fed Proc 41:602, 1982.
15. Rook AH, Frederick WRJ, Burns WH, Kirmani N, Jackson LB, Manischewitz JF, Saral R, Djeu JY, Santos GW, Quinnan GV: Natural killer cell activity and immune interferon release predict survival from viral infection in bone marrow transplant recipients. Transplant Proc 15:1773–1776, 1983.
16. Rook AH, Masur H, Lane HC, Frederick W, Kasahara T, Macher AM, Djeu JY, Manischewitz JF, Jackson L, Fauci AS, Quinnan GV: Interleukin-2 enhances the depressed natural killer and cytomegalovirus-specific cytotoxic activities of lymphocytes from patients with the acquired immunodeficiency syndrome. J Clin Invest 72:398–403, 1983.
17. Daisy JA, Tolpin MD, Quinnan GV, Rook AH, Murphy BR, Mittal K, Clements ML, Mullinix MG, Kiley SC, Ennis FA: Cytotoxic cellular immune responses during influenza A infection of human volunteers. In Compans RW (ed): "The Replication of Negative Strand Viruses." New York: Elsevier-North Holland, 1981, pp 443–448.
18. Quinnan GV, Manischewitz JF, Ennis FA: Cytotoxic T lymphocyte response to murine cytomegalovirus infection. Nature 273:541–543, 1978.
19. Frederick W, Rook AH, Delery M, Epstein J, Ramsey K, Manischewitz J, Jackson L, Quinnan GV: Comparison of virulence and immunogenicity of Towne strain and low passage Toledo-1 strain isolate of human CMV. Proc 22nd Interscience Conference on Antimicrobial Agents and Chemotherapy, Miami FL, 1982.
20. Drew WL, Vintz L, Miner RC, Sands M, Ketterer B: Prevalence of cytomegalovirus infections in homosexual men. J Infect Dis 143:188–192, 1981.
21. Reynolds DW, Stagno S, Hostz TS, Tiller M, Alford CA: Maternal cytomegalovirus excretion and perinatal infection. N Engl J Med 289:1–5, 1973.

Live Cytomegalovirus Vaccination of Healthy Volunteers: Eight-Year Follow-up Studies

Harold Stern, MB, ChB, PhD, FRCPath

Department of Virology, St. George's Hospital Medical School, London SW17 ORE, England

Justification for the development of a CMV vaccine rests essentially on the incidence of brain damage caused by congenital infection. There is a case also for vaccination in organ transplantation but there are, here, other possible methods of prevention of CMV infection. In the United Kingdom, the incidence of congenital CMV infection is 0.3% to 0.4% [1, 2]. At least 80% of these are the result of primary infection in the mother during pregnancy (C. Peckham, personal communication and [3, 4]), and there is now convincing evidence that it is primary infection that carries the major risk of both fetal infection and fetal damage [5, 6]. There can be little doubt that CMV has displaced congenital rubella as the major cause of virus-induced fetal damage.

The initial investigations of CMV vaccination in man have been with live vaccines, which accepts the likelihood of persisting latent infection with the vaccine virus itself and its possible reactivation in subsequent pregnancies [7, 8]. On the other hand, a killed or subunit vaccine would be expensive and, almost certainly, repeated doses would be needed to maintain immunity through the main childbearing years. Moreover, in guinea pigs, which are a good model for HCMV infection, live vaccine is clearly superior to killed vaccine for preventing infection with virulent strains [9].

VACCINATION OF HEALTHY VOLUNTEERS

These studies were carried out with a live vaccine derived from the AD169 strain of CMV by 56 passages in human embryonic lung fibroblast tissue

Birth Defects: Original Article Series, Volume 20, Number 1, pages 263–269

cultures [7]. This vaccine has proved to be effectively immunogenic when given by the subcutaneous route in a standard dosage of 10,000 TCD50 (Table 1) [7, 10]. Seroconversion occurred in 68 of 69 seronegative volunteers, producing, within two to four weeks good levels of CF and neutralizing antibodies, without significant side effects and without detectable virus excretion or viremia. There was little evidence of strain specificity in the immune response, as the volunteers developed neutralizing antibodies not only against the vaccine virus but also against the other prototype strains, Davis and Kerr [7, 11]. These early volunteers were not examined, in the immediate postvaccination period, for CMV-specific cell-mediated immune (CMI) responses, but there is no doubt that the vaccine stimulates such activity, as CMI responses, detectable by the lymphocyte transformation test, were obtained both in vaccinated patients and in the healthy volunteers in subsequent follow-up studies, as described below.

Despite the initially favorable serologic response to vaccination, within one year most of the volunteers had lost their CF antibody, while retaining the neutralizing antibody (Table 2). This differs from what occurs after natural infection with CMV, where both CF and neutralizing antibodies persist indefinitely [12]. The situation resembles that seen with viruses that do not normally establish long-term latent infection, and provided the first hint that the vaccine virus also may not do so.

TABLE 1. CF-Antibody Response in Susceptible Volunteers Given CMV-AD169 Vaccine (10^4 TCD50 Subcutaneously)

	No. of Volunteers	No. With Ab Response
Elek and Stern [7]	26	25
Neff et al [10]	43	43
Total	69	68

TABLE 2. Persistence of Immune Responses in CMV-Vaccinated Volunteers

	Interval After Vaccination			
Test for	1 mo	1 yr	3 yr	8 yr
CF-Ab	36/36	11/31	7/30	5/22
N-Ab	36/36	28/28	23/23	10/22
ELISA IgG-Ab	—	—	—	12/22
CMI response*	—	—	—	12/22

*Lymphocyte transformation.

VACCINATION OF PATIENTS AWAITING RENAL TRANSPLANTATION

Further evidence regarding latent infection and the vaccine virus was obtained from the use of the vaccine in renal transplantation, although the present studies are limited compared with those under way in the United States [13, 14]. Five seronegative patients were vaccinated while on long-term hemodialysis for chronic renal disease. Seroconversion occurred in all five, without significant side effects other than a mild, transient local reaction at the site of vaccination, and without detectable virus excretion or viremia during the immediate follow-up period of three to four months. CF and immunofluorescent-IgG antibodies appeared within two to five weeks, and all five patients developed CMI responses. Figure 1 shows the development of these CMI responses, as demonstrated by the lymphocyte transformation technique. This was carried out by the method described by Møller-Larsen et al [15], using a crude CMV antigen prepared by alkaline extraction of infected tissue culture cells [16], 15% autologous plasma and labeling with tritiated thymidine (2 Ci/mmol) for the final 24 hr of incubation of the test; the results are expressed as a stimulation index, values of 2.4 or greater being regarded as positive. Despite the general depression of immunity in

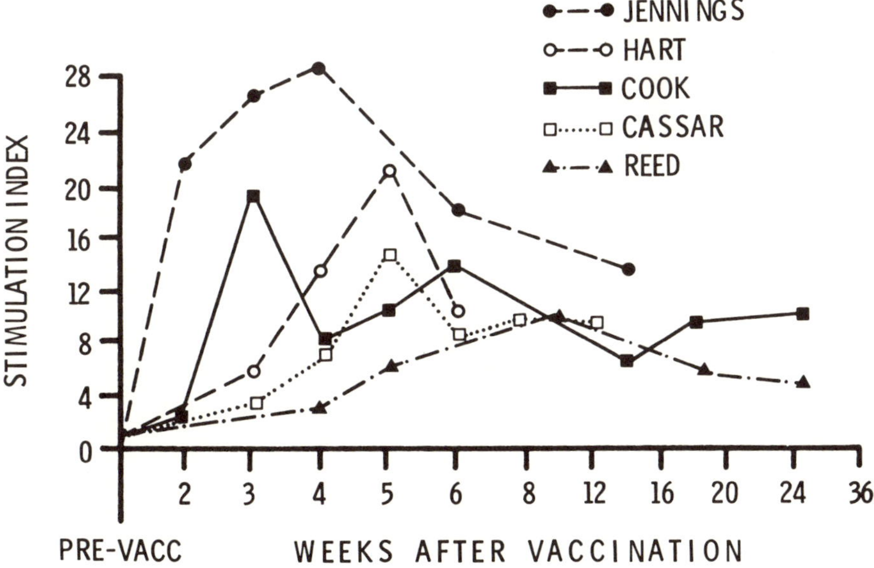

Fig. 1. Lymphocyte transformation responses in hemodialysis patients after CMV vaccination.

such patients, because of the renal disease, positive activity was obtained in all five, although the peak responses were somewhat delayed, when compared with those seen in healthy volunteers [17, 18]. Again, there was little evidence of strain specificity, as the patients also demonstrated comparable CMI responses against the Davis strain and against two other strains of CMV recently isolated in the London area.

Figure 2 illustrates, in more detail, the immune responses of one of these patients, subsequently given a kidney transplant from a seronegative donor. After vaccination, neutralizing antibody appeared at about four weeks, CF antibody a little later, and the CMI response at about three weeks. The CF antibody response was very transient, becoming undetectable within three to four months, while neutralizing antibody and CMI reactivity persisted. At the time of transplantation, the patient was put onto immunosuppressive therapy. This caused the immediate marked depression of the CMV-specific CMI response which lasted until the immunosuppression was reduced to maintenance levels, at about three months after transplantation. The reduction in dosage of the drugs was followed by a striking upsurge of CMI reactivity, but after a further three to four months it again fell to levels that were essentially negative over the next two years. A return to low-level activity then took place which has persisted for more than three years after transplantation and almost four years after vaccination. Specific antibody became undetectable about three months after transplantation, with a small and transient reappearance at the time of reestablishment of CMI response. Throughout this time, the patient has been in good health, with good kidney function, and, despite the long-term immunosuppression, has shown no evidence of reactivation, ie, no detectable virus excretion or viremia or significant rises in antibody levels.

Two other vaccinated patients have been closely followed for three to five years, one with a kidney from a seronegative donor and the other still without a kidney but who has undergone several major operations for hip bone

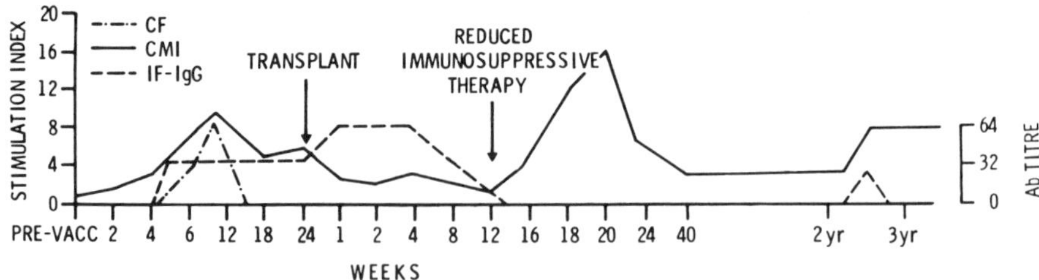

Fig. 2. Antibody and CMI (lymphocyte transformation) responses in a CMV-vaccinated patient before and after renal transplantation.

necrosis. Neither has given any evidence of reactivation. On the other hand, another patient, given a kidney from a seropositive donor, four months after vaccination, did begin to excrete CMV in the throat and urine, and developed not only striking rises in his CF and neutralizing antibody titers but also produced high levels of CMV-specific IgM antibody. This was associated with a febrile upper respiratory illness but when the immunosuppression was reduced he quickly recovered. He has remained well, with good kidney function, some three years after transplantation, despite continuing virus excretion and continuing high levels of both IgG and IgM antibodies, but with persistently negative CMI responses. His virus is slow-growing in tissue culture and, by restriction endonuclease analysis, is quite clearly not the vaccine virus.

This failure to recover vaccine virus from vaccinated patients on long-term immunosuppressive therapy provides convincing evidence that the vaccine virus does not establish persisting latent infection.

FOLLOW-UP STUDIES ON THE VACCINATED HEALTHY VOLUNTEERS

The original volunteers have now been followed for some eight years after vaccination (Table 2). At three years, only about a quarter of them had CF antibody although they all still possessed neutralizing antibody. However, by eight years only about half those followed up now had detectable antibody, either by the neutralization method or by the more sensitive ELISA technique; the latter, as developed in our laboratory, is as reliable as RIA for detecting CMV IgG antibody [16]. Similarly, only about half the volunteers had observable CMI responses after eight years. Eight volunteers had lost both antibody and CMI activity, two had detectable antibody but negative CMI activity, and two had positive CMI activity but were without detectable antibody.

Three of the volunteers became pregnant 6 yr, 4 and 6 yr and 8 yr, respectively, after vaccination. Their immune responses at three and eight years after vaccination are shown in Table 3. None of the four infants demonstrated any evidence of either congenital or perinatal CMV infections. All four are healthy and have been followed for six months to one year after birth; they have not excreted CMV, and they have remained seronegative for CMV antibody. There was, therefore, no evidence for reactivation of the vaccine virus in these mothers.

CONCLUSIONS

The failure of renal transplant patients to demonstrate reactivation of the vaccine virus, despite long-term immunosuppression, and the gradual loss of

TABLE 3. Volunteers Given CMV-AD169 Vaccine Who Subsequently Became Pregnant

Volunteer	Immune Status After Vaccination		Pregnant
	at 3 yr	at 8 yr	
1	N-Ab +ve	N-Ab −ve, ELISA-Ab −ve CMI +ve	at 6 yr
2	N-Ab +ve	N-Ab −ve, ELISA-Ab −ve CMI −ve	at 4 yr at 6 yr
3*	N-Ab +ve	N-Ab +ve, ELISA-Ab +ve CMI +ve	at 8 yr

All four infants are sero −ve and are not excreting CMV at 6 mo-1 yr.
*N-Ab, ELISA-Ab and CMI −ve when reexamined at 10 yr.
Ab = antibody.
N-Ab = neutralizing antibody.
+ve = positive.
−ve = negative.

immune responses in the healthy volunteers, over three to eight years, are both most likely due to the absence of latent infection with the vaccine virus. Similar findings have been reported by others in vaccinated renal transplant patients [13, 14]. Persisting immunity to herpesviruses may well be dependent on continuing latent infection. The absence of virus excretion and viremia after vaccination suggests that the tissue culture-adapted virus, given subcutaneously, can cause only a localized infection; it is unable, therefore, to reach those sites of the body where latent infection is normally established. More lasting immunity might be achieved by administering the vaccine by other, more natural routes; for example, by mouth, perhaps using less attenuated virus. Alternatively, a second dose of the vaccine, given subcutaneously, perhaps after three to five years, might be sufficient. Thus, five of the volunteers continued to show good levels of CF antibody, as well as neutralizing antibody and CMI responses, eight years after vaccination; this could be because of a booster infection with circulating wild virus. Revaccination remains to be tried and, of course, the inability of the vaccine virus to establish latent infection removes any problems of reactivation and oncogenicity [11].

REFERENCES

1. Stern H: Cytomegalovirus infection in the neonate and its prevention. Postgrad Med J 53:588–591, 1977.
2. McDonald H, Tobin JO: Congenital cytomegalovirus infection: A collaborative study on epidemiological, clinical and laboratory findings. Dev Med Child Neurol 20:471–482, 1978.

3. Stern H, Tucker SM: Prospective study of cytomegalovirus infection in pregnancy. Br Med J 1:268–270, 1973.
4. Grant S, Edmond E, Syme J: A prospective study of cytomegalovirus infection in pregnancy. I. Laboratory evidence of congenital infection following maternal primary and reactivated infection. J Infect 3:24–31, 1981.
5. Stagno S, Pass RF, Dworsky ME, Henderson RE, Moore EG, Walton PD, Alford CA: Congenital cytomegalovirus infection. The relative importance of primary and recurrent maternal infection. N Engl J Med 306:945–949, 1982.
6. Stagno S, Dworsky ME, Torres J, Mesa T, Hirsh T: Prevalence and importance of congenital cytomegalovirus infection in three different populations. J Pediatr 101:897–900, 1982.
7. Elek SD, Stern H: Development of a vaccine against mental retardation caused by cytomegalovirus infection in utero. Lancet 1:1–5, 1974.
8. Just M, Buergin-Wolff A, Emoedi G, Hernandez R: Immunisation trials with live attenuated cytomegalovirus Towne 125. Infection 3:111–114, 1975.
9. Bia FJ, Griffith BP, Tarsio M, Hsiung GD: Vaccination for the prevention of maternal and fetal infection with guinea pig cytomegalovirus. J Infect Dis 142:732–738, 1980.
10. Neff BJ, Weibel RE, Buynak EB, McLean AA, Hilleman MR: Clinical and laboratory studies of live cytomegalovirus vaccine AD169. Proc Soc Exp Biol Med 160:32–37, 1979.
11. Stern H: Cytomegalovirus vaccine: Justification and problems. Rec Adv Clin Virol 1:118–134, 1977.
12. Rowe WP, Hartley JW, Waterman S, Turner HC, Huebner RJ: Cytopathogenic agent resembling human salivary gland virus recovered from tissue cultures of human adenoids. Proc Soc Exp Biol Med 92:418–424, 1956.
13. Glazer JP, Friedman HM, Grossman RA, Starr SE, Barker CF, Persoff LJ, Huang S-E, Plotkin SA: Live cytomegalovirus vaccination of renal transplant candidates. A preliminary trial. Ann Intern Med 91:676–683, 1979.
14. Marker SC, Simmons RL, Balfour HH Jr: Cytomegalovirus vaccine in renal allograft recipients. Transplant Proc 13:117–119, 1981.
15. Møller-Larsen A, Anderson HK, Heron I, Sarov I: In vitro stimulation of human lymphocytes by purified cytomegalovirus. Intervirology 6:249–257, 1976.
16. Booth JC, Hannington G, Bakir TMF, Stern H, Kangro H, Griffiths PD, Heath RB: Comparison of enzyme-linked immunosorbent assay, radioimmunoassay, complement fixation, anticomplement immunofluoresence and passive haemagglutination techniques for detecting cytomegalovirus IgG antibody. J Clin Pathol 35:1345–1348, 1982.
17. Starr SE, Glazer JP, Friedman HM, Farquar JD, Plotkin SA: Specific cellular and humoral immunity after immunization with live Towne strain cytomegalovirus vaccine. J Infect Dis 143:585–589, 1981.
18. Gehrz RC, Christianson WR, Linner KM, Groth KE, Balfour HH: Cytomegalovirus vaccine. Specific humoral and cellular immune responses in human volunteers. Arch Intern Med 140:936–939, 1980.

Prevention of Cytomegalovirus Disease by Towne Strain Live Attenuated Vaccine*

Stanley A. Plotkin, MD, M. Lynn Smiley, MD, Harvey M. Friedman, MD, Stuart E. Starr, MD, Gary R. Fleisher, MD, Cliff Wlodaver, MD, Donald C. Dafoe, MD, Allan D. Friedman, MD, Robert A. Grossman, MD, and Clyde F. Barker, MD

The Children's Hospital of Philadelphia and the Department of Pediatrics, University of Pennsylvania (S.A.P., S.E.S., G.R.F., A.D.F.), The Wistar Institute, (S.A.P., S.E.S.), the Department of Medicine (M.L.S., H.M.F., R.A.G., C.W.), and the Department of Surgery (C.F.B., D.C.D.), University of Pennsylvania, Philadelphia, PA 19104

The previous articles in this book have provided ample reasons for the development of a vaccine against HCMV. Briefly summarized, the justifications include the frequent damage that intrauterine CMV causes to the fetal CNS [1,2], and the toll exacted by acquired CMV in organ transplantation and in other situations in which patients are immunosuppressed [3–5].

The rationale for vaccination is that a vaccine might provide nonimmune individuals with the same protection afforded by previous natural infection [6–8].

As with other virus diseases, both killed and live vaccine strategies have been considered for CMV [7]. A live vaccine was chosen for our studies because of the greater likelihood that by replication in the host a live virus would generate sufficient antigen for immunologic stimulation of humans and that the immunologic stimulation so produced would be longlasting.

DEVELOPMENT OF LIVE ATTENUATED CMV VACCINE

Accordingly, a virus isolated in WI-38 human embryo fibroblasts from the urine of a congenitally infected infant named Towne was passaged in W1-38

*This work was supported in part by NIH grant AI14927 and the Hassel Foundation.

Birth Defects: Original Article Series, Volume 20, Number 1, pages 271–287

(Fig. 1) [9]. The infant, incidentally, later proved to be mentally retarded. Towne virus was passaged 125 times with three clonings by plaque isolation before experimental pools were prepared. Two pools have been used in man, one made by RIT (Genval, Belgium) and the other by Merck Sharpe & Dohme (West Point, PA): the two pools have given identical results.

A question frequently posed is, "why do we believe that Towne virus is attenuated?" Although the vaccine virus is different from the parent virus in certain in vitro characteristics such as increased resistance to trypsin and increased release of cell-free virus, these appear to be indications of high passage in tissue culture rather than of attenuation. However, the study reported by Quinnan and Rook [10], and our own unpublished studies, show that a low-passage "wild" CMV tested in tandem with Towne produced illness and virus excretion after subcutaneous inoculation of volunteers, whereas Towne did not.

VACCINATION OF NORMAL VOLUNTEERS

Studies of vaccination in normal volunteers have been reported previously [11–14]. The results of these studies carried out by us and by others are consistent and may be summarized as follows:

DERIVATION OF TOWNE CMV VACCINE STRAIN

Isolation – 2 mos infant with cytomegalic inclusion disease (CID)

Urine --> WI-38

WI-38 50 passages cell to cell

WI-38 75 passages cell-free virus with 3 clonings

WI-38 125 passage – test pools

Fig. 1.   Derivation of Towne vaccine strain. CID = cytomegalic inclusion disease.

1) Serologic responses typical for primary infection appear by the fourth week postvaccination, including ACIF, CF, and neutralizing antibodies. Figure 2 depicts the responses graphically, and Table 1 gives the typical evolution of antibodies in two normal volunteers.

Table 2 gives data on neutralizing antibody. The antibodies that are elicited by Towne vaccine neutralize AD169 as well as Towne, but Towne is neutralized to the greater degree.

2) Specific in vitro lymphocyte proliferation (LP) responses to CMV antigen develop in all vaccinees (Table 3). These responses are not strain-specific, ie, antigens prepared from all laboratory and wild strains tested elicit LP.

3) So far no CMV has been isolated from urine, throat secretions, buffy coat, semen, or cervical secretions after vaccination of any normal subject.

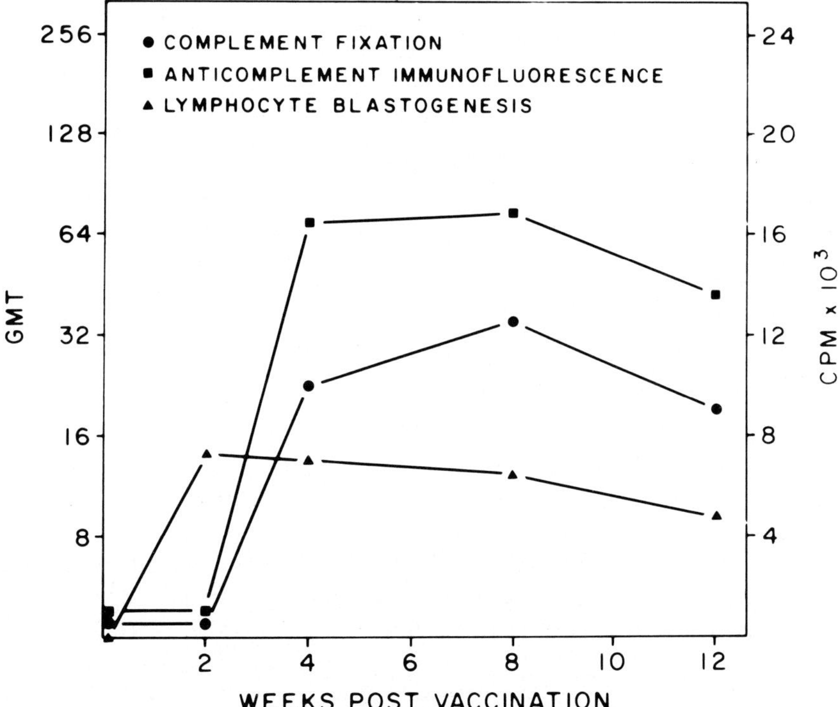

Fig. 2. Mean responses to Towne vaccine of 4 normal volunteers measured by CF, ACIF, and LP to Towne antigen.

TABLE 1. Serologic Responses of Volunteers to Subcutaneous Inoculations of $10^{4.7}$ PFU of the Towne Strain of HCMV

Volunteer	Test	Reciprocal Titers of Antibody at Indicated Week After Inoculation							
		0	1	2	3	4	5	6	8
0	CF	< 8	< 8	ND	8	ND	32	± 64	64
	IgG (IFA)	< 5	< 5	10	160	80	160	320	640
	IgM (IFA)	< 10	< 10	< 10	10	< 10	10	< 10	< 10
	EA	−	−	−	+	+	+	+	ND
P	CF	< 8	< 8	< 8	16	16	± 32	± 64	32
	IgG (IFA)	< 5	< 5	5	20	40	20	40	40
	IgM (IFA)	< 10	< 10	< 10	10	20	2	< 10	< 10
	EA	−	−	−	−	−	+	+	ND

CF = Complement-fixation.
IFA = Indirect fluorescent antibody.
EA = Antibodies to early CMV antigens in ara-C-treated infected cells.

TABLE 2. Towne and AD169 Neutralizing Antibody Titers Following Towne Vaccination of Seronegative Uremic and Normal Patients

	No. Pts	Months Postvaccination			
		0	1	2	3–6
Normals: anti-Towne	10	< 2	13.9(90)	27.5(100)	14.8(100)
Normals: anti-AD169	6	< 2	—	16.0(100)	—
Uremics: anti-Towne	15	< 2	2.3(40)	12.1 (87)	9.8 (86)
Uremics: anti-AD169	14	< 2	1.2(11)	2.6 (50)	2.5 (50)

( ) = Percent of patients with antibody response.

4) The only clinical reaction has been a local erythema and induration at the injection site developing during the second week postvaccination, and then disappearing. (See below.)

5) In collaboration with Dr. M. Hirsch, we studied the lymphocyte subsets after vaccination of normal volunteers. Altered T-cell helper/suppressor ratios or diminished Con A responses, which occur commonly in natural CMV infection [15], did not develop (Table 4).

6) Persistence of immunity to Towne vaccine was evaluated in normal volunteers from 1 to 3-1/2 years postvaccination, and in renal transplantation candidates (RTC) 12 to 18 months postvaccination. Only those RTC who received a kidney from a seronegative donor were included in this analysis.

TABLE 3. Lymphocyte Proliferation Responses to Several CMV Strains in Two Normal Vaccinees

Weeks Postimmunization	Net CPM Using Antigen Prepared From Strain		
	Towne	AD169	Davis
A)			
1	4,187	4,345	2,521
2	36,428	37,500	32,000
8	20,950	18,071	24,618
B)			
4	13,445	12,720	13,098
8	10,754	5,264	5,678

TABLE 4. T-Lymphocyte Subsets in Six Recipients of CMV Vaccine and in CMV Mononucleosis Patients

Weeks Postvaccination	OKT4 / OKT8	Con A Responses CPM $\pm$ Standard Error
0	1.8 ± 0.9	$180,322 \pm 11,254$
1	2.3 ± 0.6	$166,893 \pm 23,153$
2	2.0 ± 0.8	$156,979 \pm 19,710$
3	2.1 ± 0.7	$161,817 \pm 26,992$
4	2.2 ± 1.0	$154,285 \pm 30,903$
6	1.7 ± 0.8	$148,444 \pm 27,677$
8	2.9 ± 0.9	$111,545 \pm 19,041$
Control donors	1.9 ± 0.8	$166,877 \pm 10,856$
Acute CMV-mononucleosis patients	0.3 ± 0.2	$33,472 \pm 10,081$

TABLE 5. Persistence of Antibody to CMV After Towne Vaccine

Subjects	Interval	Ratio Pos.			
		CF	ACIF	SN	LPR
Normals	12–42 mo	2/7	14/18	9/10*	11/12
RTC	12–18 mo	2/5	4/5	5/5	ND

CF = Complement fixation
ACIF = Anticomplement immunofluorescence
SN = Serum neutralization
LPR = Lymphocyte proliferation responses to CMV antigen
*Single negative by SN was positive by ELISA
RTC = Renal transplant candidates

As shown in Table 5, CF antibodies were lost relatively rapidly, and were absent after a year in most vaccinees. ACIF antibodies, on the other hand, were lost in only a few individuals. In one case, neutralizing antibodies had also disappeared, but antibodies detectable by ELISA remained. Cellular immunity, as detected by CMV-specific LP, continued to be present in the subjects who had lost antibody.

We have attempted to determine whether the immune responses of vaccinees or the local reaction could be solely due to nonliving antigen in the vaccine rather than to the replication of live virus. Two experiments were performed. First, three volunteers received doses of Towne that had been exposed to 56°C for 60 min in order to inactivate virus. None of them developed either a local reaction or a detectable antibody response, but interestingly, all developed LP responses to CMV antigen (Table 6).

In the second experiment, graded dilutions of Towne were given to volunteers. As few as 50 PFU elicited uniform antibody responses, consistent with the inoculation of a replicating virus which generates new antigen. However, as shown in Table 7, the local reaction diminished with decreasing virus dose. This fact suggests that inoculation of less antigen reduced the

TABLE 6. Responses of Vaccinees to Inactivated Towne

	Responses					
	Prevacc.			Postvacc.		
Vaccinee	CF	ACIF	SI	CF	ACIF	SI
A	< 8	< 8	1.0	< 8	< 8	7.2
B	< 8	< 8	1.1	< 8	< 8	6.4
C	< 8	< 8	2.0	< 8	< 8	13.0

CF = Complement fixation.
ACIF = Anticomplement immunofluorescence.
SI = Stimulation index of lymphocyte cultures against CMV antigen.

TABLE 7. Relationship Between Vaccine Virus Dose and Local Reaction Size

	Median Antibody Response (8 wk)		Reaction Size
Dose (PFU)	CF	ACIF	(cm)
5,000	32	128	7.25
2,500	8	64	5.70
1,000	16	32	4.90
500	16	32	3.10
50	16	64	0.75

degree of local reaction expressed at the injection site. Thus, the local reaction is dose-dependent.

RENAL TRANSPLANT TRIAL

Among the many questions that arise in the consideration of a live virus vaccine against CMV, there are two that can be answered by trials in RTCs. One question is related to safety: does the vaccine virus persist in the vaccinee in some latent form? The fact that these patients are iatrogenically immuno-suppressed at the time of transplantation allows us to determine whether or not reactivation of vaccine virus occurs, in the same way as reactivation of naturally acquired virus. The second question is related to efficacy: does Towne vaccine prevent or modify CMV disease?

Of course, the justification for the trial was to see if vaccination could help prevent CMV disease in the RTC, although as we shall see, RTC are not the ideal patients in whom to attempt immunologic stimulation, as they are immunodebilitated.

The trial was organized on a controlled basis. RTC were randomly distributed to receive either vaccine or placebo eight weeks or more prior to transplantation. The patients were followed clinically by individuals who did not know to which group they belonged. Illnesses that occurred posttrans-plant were scored according to a rating scheme developed for this purpose, shown concomitant with laboratory evidence of CMV infection in Table 8. Each manifestation of CMV-associated disease was given a point score. The standard regimen for both placebo and vaccinated patients consisted of steroids and azathioprine. Antithymocyte globulin (ATG) was also adminis-tered during rejection crises.

Up to this time, 250 patients have been entered in the trial, of whom 146 have been transplanted, but this analysis is based on 91 patients who, in February 1983, had been transplanted for at least six months. As shown in Table 9, serologic responses in vaccinated RTC did not occur as uniformly

TABLE 8. Scoring System for CMV Disease

Manifestation	Points	Manifestation	Points
Fever	1–3	Glomerulonephritis	1–3
Leukopenia	1	Arthritis	2
Thrombocytopenia	1	Muscle wasting	2
Hepatitis	1–3	Superinfection	3
Pneumonia	1–3	GI bleed	3
CNS changes	1–3	Death	4

TABLE 9. Serologic Responses to Towne at 8 Weeks Postvaccine

Subjects	CF	ACIF
Normals		
Ratio	39/41 (95%)	41/41 (100%)
GMT	25	54
Renal Transplant Candidates		
Ratio	28/37 (76%)	31/37 (83%)
GMT	9	19

GMT = Geometric mean titer.

as in normal subjects, and the responses that did occur were weaker. This was also true for neutralizing antibody responses, shown in Table 2.

CMV-specific LP stimulated by Towne strain CMV antigen was determined at the time of immunization and eight weeks later. The responses of seronegative placebo recipients did not change, as indicated by calculation of stimulation indices (SIs) (Fig. 3). Since the mean plus two standard deviations for this group was 2.8, we considered a SI >2.8 a positive response. About half of the seronegative recipients of vaccine developed positive responses by eight weeks postimmunization. The failure of the other half to respond was quite different from results obtained with immunized normal adults, all of whom responded by eight weeks.

Plasma suppressive factors may provide an explanation for at least some of the impairment noted in the responses of RTCs to Towne vaccine. We recently compared the eight-week postimmunization responses of several vaccinees in autologous and pooled human plasma. All of the responses were higher in pooled plasma, and in two instances the differences were particularly striking (Fig. 4).

A number of the vaccinees were also tested for LP with CMV antigens prepared from wild strains isolated from congenitally infected infants. Both normal adults, and four RTCs, who responded well to Towne antigen, also responded to all of the wild strain antigens tested, although there were differences in the magnitudes among the responses (Table 10).

Following transplantation, LP responses were depressed regardless of whether immunity was natural or vaccine-induced. Although the number of patients for whom data are available is still small, there appeared to be no correlation between the magnitude of CMV-specific LP before transplantation and the likelihood of developing severe CMV disease. Of course, other lymphocyte functions were also depressed posttransplant, such as NK activity against CMV-infected targets, depicted on Figure 5. These deficits may contribute to the severity of CMV infections in transplant recipients.

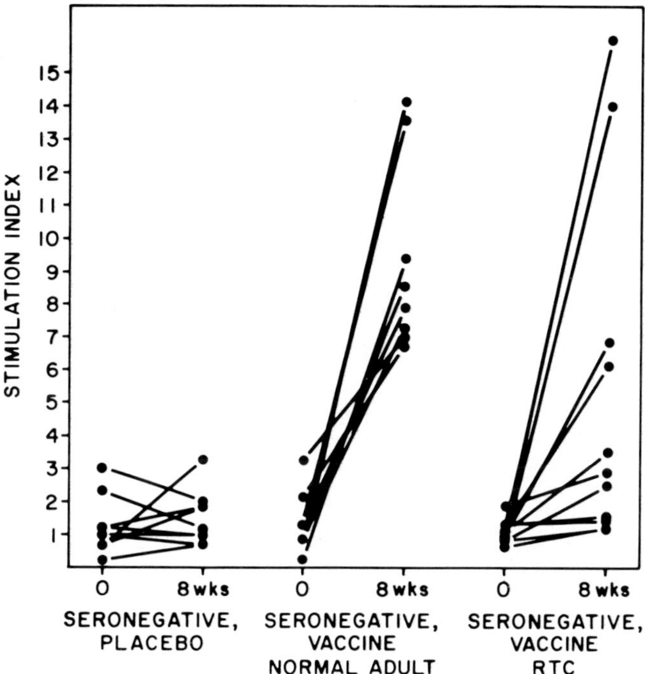

Fig. 3. SI for lymphocyte cultures made from the blood of placebo recipients, vaccinated normal volunteers, and vaccinated RTCs. The indices are calculated by dividing the thymidine uptake in the presence of CMV antigen by the uptake in the presence of control antigen.

In Table 11 the 91 patients are analyzed by the original serologic status of donors and recipients prior to vaccination, and whether the recipients received vaccine or placebo. From these data we can discern several points. First, CMV infections and diseases are almost absent in the $D- R-$ group, the only exception being a single placebo recipient, who may have been infected through blood transfusion.

Second, the overall infection rate is almost 100% in the recipients who received a kidney from a seropositive donor, regardless of the recipients' serologic status. However, as shown in Table 12, illness was less frequent in recipients who were originally naturally seropositive than those who were seronegative, indicating a strong protective effect of natural immunity.

Thus, the only group with a high rate of CMV disease consists of the originally seronegative patients who received a kidney from a seropositive donor ($D+ R-$ group).

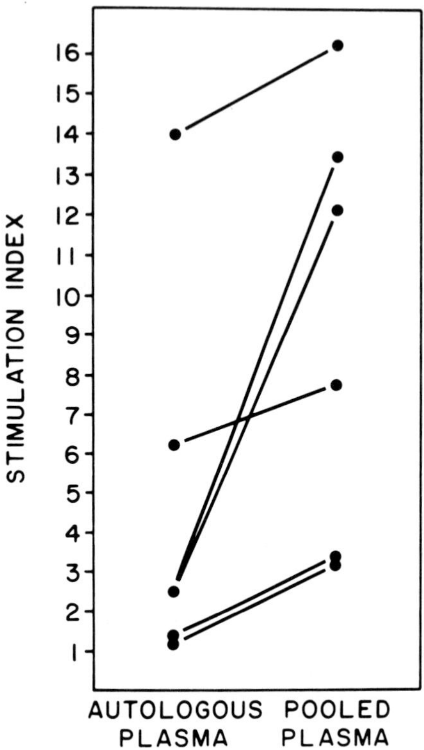

Fig. 4. SI for lymphocyte cultures of vaccinees suspended either in autologous serum or in pooled plasma from normal individuals.

As shown in Table 13, the vaccination status in this group of 30 patients had no effect on virus excretion posttransplant. The disease rate was slightly lower in vaccinees (56% *v* 71%), but the difference was not statistically significant. However, infected placebo patients were almost always ill (91%), compared to 60% illness in vaccinees (P = 0.07 by χ^2). We examined the clinical symptoms among these patients, displayed in Table 14. Thrombocytopenia, hepatitis, pneumonia, and superinfections with bacteria and fungi were seen less frequently in vaccine recipients.

If we add two seronegative patients whose donors' serologic status was unknown, but who became infected and who, therefore, probably received a CMV-bearing kidney, there are 32 patients in the D+ R− group. The distribution of clinical scores among these patients is shown on Table 15. In contrast to the scores of the placebo recipients, the vaccinees' scores are skewed to the lower end of the scale. The mean scores for the placebo group

TABLE 10. Strain-Specific Lymphocyte Proliferation Responses in Recipients of Towne Vaccine

Vaccinee		Weeks After Immunization	Stimulation Indices When Tested Against						
				Wild Strains					
			Towne	1	2	3	4	5	6
Normal	A	4	28.1	ND	44.0	18.6	25.6	ND	32.1
		8	11.6	13.6	11.0	13.8	14.0	11.3	8.6
	B	4	50.9	43.0	22.9	31.7	21.4	58.1	28.4
		8	10.6	17.0	17.6	12.9	6.9	9.1	8.7
	C	4	29.8	31.5	23.2	17.2	23.2	5.6	28.5
		8	30.5	25.3	23.8	20.8	32.2	9.3	28.6
	D	4	14.1	20.3	17.7	12.9	14.7	6.1	8.6
RTCs	E	8	14.2	ND	ND	11.1	14.9	14.7	ND
	F	14	5.0	5.0	4.5	26.9	9.3	21.3	6.6
	G	8	2.5	8.3	4.5	26.9	9.3	18.8	6.6
	H	8	4.7	7.9	4.0	ND	5.1	5.3	11.6

revealed an average of more than twice the clinical severity compared to the vaccine group (Table 16) (5.67 v 2.70, respectively). Application of the rank sum test of the difference in illness severity reveals a P value at the < 0.05 level, or at the 0.005 level if uninfected patients are excluded.

If the patients in the D+ R− group are grouped into those who were asymptomatic after transplant, those who had mild or moderate illnesses scoring 1–6 and those who had more severe illnesses with scores of 7 or greater, we see (Table 17) a different distribution in the vaccinees and placebo recipients. Whereas about half of the placebo recipients had scores of 7 or greater, only one of the vaccinees fell in this group. This difference was significant at the $P = 0.05$ level.

The single severe case of CMV in the vaccine group is worth further comment. This patient had to wait longer than a year for a kidney transplant and by that time his positive antibody response had fallen to undetectable levels by CF and ACIF, though he still had neutralizing antibodies. In fact, of 12 vaccinees transplanted within six months of vaccination, six had no CMV illness, whereas only one of five transplanted after six months escaped CMV illness.

Thus Towne vaccine did not prevent infection with CMV, but did mitigate the disease that resulted from the infection. Natural immunity may have been more protective than vaccine-induced immunity, but taking into account the low immune responses of the RTC, the difference in protection may be related only to the quantity of antibody.

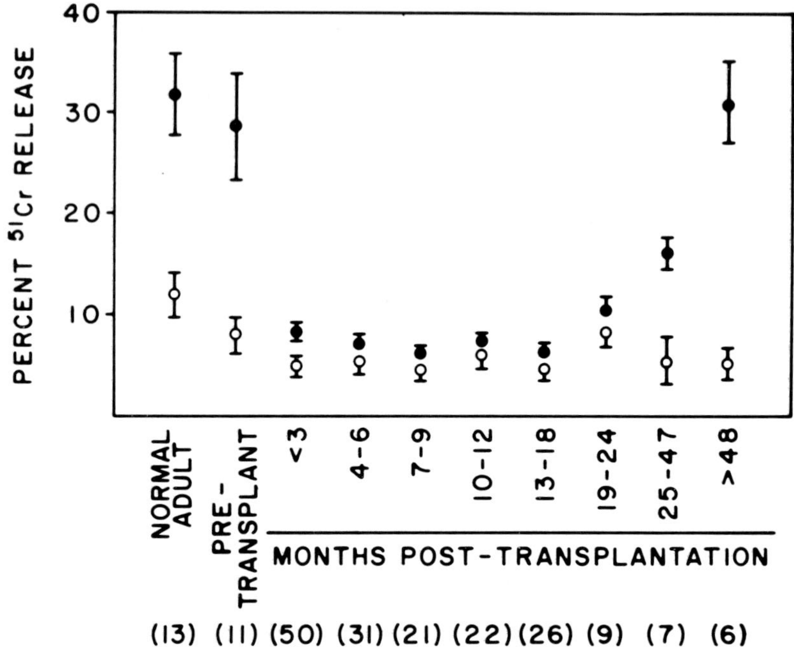

Fig. 5. NK activity against CMV-infected target fibroblasts or uninfected fibroblasts before and after transplantation. Mean values ± 1 SEM are shown for killing of uninfected (○) and CMV-infected (●) targets. Numbers of individuals studied are shown in parentheses.

TABLE 11. CMV Illness and Infection Posttransplant

	Vaccinees				Placebo			
	Donor +		Donor −		Donor +		Donor −	
Recipients	Sick	Inf.	Sick	Inf.	Sick	Inf.	Sick	Inf.
Seroneg*	9/16	15/16	0/20	0/20	10/14	11/14	1/12	1/12
Seropos	2/8	6/7	1/9	3/9	2/7	6/7	0/5	2/5

*Original serologic status prevaccination.
+ = Seropositive.
− = Seronegative.

TABLE 12. CMV Illness and Infection Rates in Recipients Who Received D+ Kidneys

Recipients	Sick	Infected
Seronegative*	19/30 (63%)	21/30 (87%)
Seropositive	4/15 (27%)	12/14 (86%)

*Original serologic status irrespective of vaccination.

TABLE 13. CMV Illness and Infection Posttransplant in D+ R− Group

	Vaccine	Placebo
Sick	9/16	10/14
Infected	15/16	11/14
Sick/Infected	9/15(60%)	10/11(91%)

TABLE 14. Clinical Symptoms of D+ R− Group

	Vaccinees (17)	Placebo (15)
WBC ↓	8	11
Plat ↓	3	6
LFT ↑	5	9
Creat ↑	5	6
Nephrec.	1	2
Pneumonia	0	2
CNS changes	1	3
Superinfection	0	3
Death	1	1

TABLE 15. Clinical Scores in D+ R− Group

	0	1	2	3	4	5	6	7	8	9	10	11	12	13	14	15
Vaccinees (N = 17)	7	1	1	2	2	1	2						1			
Placebo recipients (N = 15)	4				3	1		2		3			1			1

TABLE 16. Mean Clinical Scores

Vaccinees	2.70
Placebo recipients	5.67

TABLE 17. Grouping of Clinical Scores in D+ R− Group

	Score		
	0	1–6	⩾ 7
Vaccine	7	9	1
Placebo	4	4	7

LATENCY OF VACCINE VIRUS

The fact that vaccinees who received a kidney from seronegative donors never excreted virus posttransplant provided strong evidence that the vaccine virus was not latent. Nevertheless, it was important to examine the viruses excreted after transplantation with a kidney from seropositive donors to see if the strains isolated were identical to Towne or if they were wild viruses. Dr. E.-S. Huang performed endonuclease restriction analysis on these viruses [16,17].

At the time of writing, 44 isolates obtained posttransplant from 23 vaccinated RTC have been analyzed by R-E gels, using ECOR-1, Xba, or BAMH-1 enzymes. Figure 6 provides a photograph of a typical pattern. The pattern of the vaccine virus itself was well conserved after in vitro passage and from run to run. All 44 isolates were different from Towne in their patterns.

Also interesting is the fact that not all of the CMV strains excreted after transplantation by the same patient were identical: two patients excreted viruses from different sites with different patterns. Examples are strains 1097 and 1132, which were isolated from the same patient. It is possible that exogenous reinfection from the donor kidney may occur with more than one strain, which also suggests that infection with multiple strains may occur in nature.

CONCLUSIONS

The interim conclusions we draw from these data are as follows: The Towne vaccine virus is attenuated, and after subcutaneous injection has little or no ability to become latent in the vaccinee, at least in a complete genomic form. Replication of the vaccine virus appears to be limited to the subcutaneous tissue.

The immune responses elicited by Towne in normal volunteers are similar to those observed in individuals who have had previous natural infection.

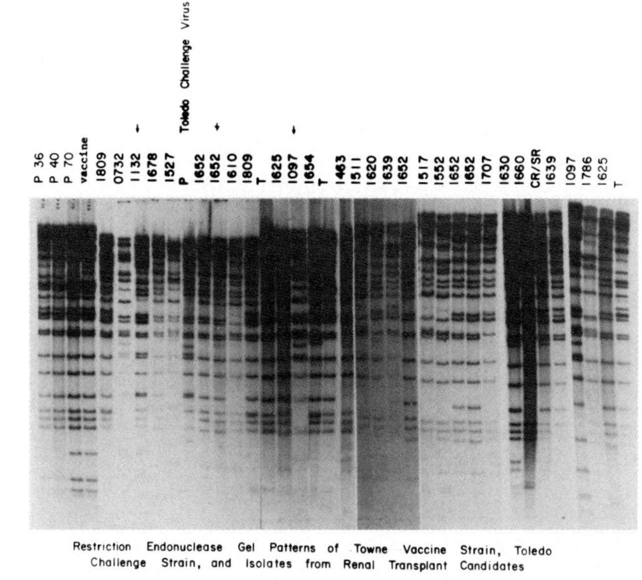

A

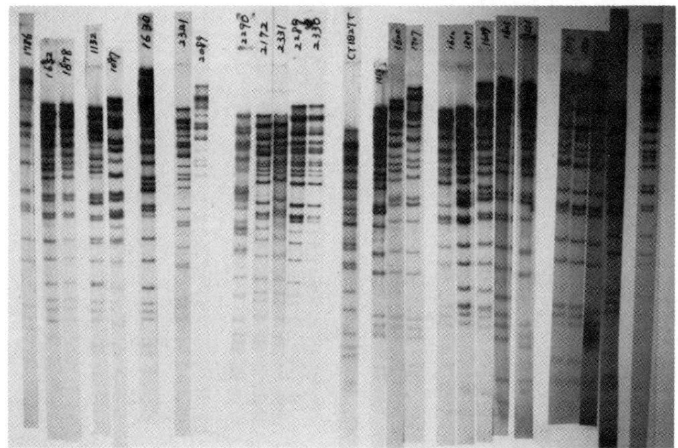

B

Fig. 6. Restriction gels of CMV DNA with ECO-RI. Each lane represents a different isolate. A) Towne vaccine virus on left. Strain P is wild isolate unrelated to study. B) Other isolates.

Vaccination prior to renal transplantation partly protects patients without previous experience of CMV. They are no less likely to be infected, but their chance of developing serious disease is significantly reduced. This protection is achieved despite the poor or mediocre immune responses to CMV vaccine in the RTC compared to healthy volunteers. Would normal pregnant women also be protected by Towne vaccine against viremic infection by wild CMV? This is the question that remains to be answered.

REFERENCES

1. Stagno S, Pass RF, Alford CA: Perinatal infections and maldevelopment. In Bloom AD, James LS (eds): "The Fetus and The Newborn." New York: Alan R Liss for The March of Dimes Birth Defects Foundation, BD:OAS 17(1):31–50, 1981.
2. Stagno S, Pass RF, Dworsky ME, Henderson RE, Moore EG, Walton PD, Alford CA: Congenital cytomegalovirus infection: The relative importance of primary and recurrent maternal infection. N Engl J Med 306:945–949, 1982.
3. Glenn J: Cytomegalovirus infections following renal transplantation. Rev Infect Dis 3:1151–1178, 1981.
4. Peterson PK, Balfour HH, Marker SC, Fryd DS, Howard RJ, Simmons RL: Cytomegalovirus disease in renal allograft recipients; a prospective study of the clinical features, risk factors and impact on renal transplantation. Medicine 59:283–300, 1980.
5. Balfour HH Jr: Cytomegalovirus: The troll of transplantation (Editorial). Arch Intern Med 139:279–280, 1979.
6. Plotkin SA: Is it possible to vaccinate against herpes virus infections and their effects? Behring Inst Mitt 63:123–134, 1979.
7. Plotkin SA, Friedman HM, Starr SE, Arbeter AM, Furukawa T, Fleisher GR: Prevention and treatment of cytomegalovirus infection. In Nahmias AJ, Dowdle WR, Schinazi RF (eds): "The Human Herpesviruses: An Interdisciplinary Perspective." New York: Elsevier, 1981, pp 401–413.
8. Elek SD, Stern H: Development of a vaccine against mental retardation caused by cytomegalovirus infection in utero. Lancet 1:1–5, 1974.
9. Plotkin SA, Furukawa T, Zygraich N, Huygelen C: Candidate cytomegalovirus strain for human vaccination. Infect Immun 12:521–527, 1975.
10. Quinnan GV Jr, Rook AH: The importance of cytotoxic cellular immunity in the protection from CMV infection. This volume.
11. Plotkin SA, Farquhar J, Hornberger E: Clinical trials of immunization with the Towne 125 strain of human cytomegalovirus. J Infect Dis 134:470–475, 1976.
12. Starr SE, Glazer JP, Friedman HM, Farquhar JD, Plotkin SA: Specific cellular and humoral immunity following immunization with live Towne strain cytomegalovirus vaccine. J Infect Dis 143:585, 1981.
13. Gehrz RC, Christianson WR, Linner KM, Groth KE, Balfour HH Jr: Cytomegalovirus vaccine: Specific humoral and cellular immune responses in human volunteers. Arch Intern Med 140:936–939, 1980.
14. Fleisher GR, Starr SE, Friedman HM, Plotkin SA: Vaccination of pediatric nurses with live attenuated cytomegalovirus. Am J Dis Child 136:294–296, 1982.
15. Carney WP, Rubin RH, Hoffman RA, Hansen WP, Healey K, Hirsch MS: Analysis of T lymphocyte subsets in cytomegalovirus mononucleosis. J Immunol 126:2114–2116, 1981.

16. Kilpatrick A, Huang E-S, Pagano JS: Analysis of cytomegalovirus genomes with restriction endonucleases HinD III and EcoR-1. J Virol 18:1095–1105, 1976.
17. Huang E-S, Alford CA, Reynolds DW, Stagno S, Pass RF: Molecular epidemiology of cytomegalovirus infections in women and their infants. N Engl J Med 303:958–962, 1980.

Cytomegalovirus Vaccine in Renal Transplant Candidates: Progress Report of a Randomized, Placebo-Controlled, Double-Blind Trial*

Henry H. Balfour, Jr., MD, Gregory W. Sachs, MS, Patricia Welo, BSN, Richard C. Gehrz, MD, Richard L. Simmons, MD, and John S. Najarian, MD

Departments of Laboratory Medicine and Pathology, and Pediatrics (H.H.B., G.W.S., P.W.), Department of Surgery (R.L.S., J.S.N.), University of Minnesota Health Sciences Center, Minneapolis, MN 55455; Department of Pediatrics, St. Paul Children's Hospital, St. Paul, MN 55102 (R.C.G.)

The role of CMV in organ transplantation first was appreciated in 1964 when Hill and associates [1] reported autopsy findings suggesting that CMV was a major posttransplant pathogen. These observations were extended in subsequent retrospective surveys of renal allograft recipients [2–11]. Prospective studies now have confirmed that CMV is an important pathogen for renal allograft recipients. Investigations from at least 12 renal transplant centers have provided convincing evidence that CMV is a major posttransplant problem, causing fever, leukopenia, arthralgia, pneumonitis, hepatitis, GI bleeding, encephalitis, retinitis, graft loss, and mortality [12–28]. In our prospective study of 272 renal allograft recipients, CMV infection occurred after 181 (57%) transplants [29]. Using a multivariate analysis that employed an exponential survival model, CMV was a significant risk factor (P < 0.05) for posttransplant fever, leukopenia, graft failure, and mortality. Overall,

*Supported in part by research grants AM13083 and AM18883 from NIH, and by a grant from Merck, Sharp & Dohme.

Birth Defects: Original Article Series, Volume 20, Number 1, pages 289–304

CMV was responsible for 20% of graft failure, 25% of mortality, 30% of fever, and 35% of episodes of leukopenia.

Effective antiviral therapy for CMV disease has not yet been developed and thus a method of prevention is desperately needed. Because the success of live, attenuated viral vaccines in general has been excellent, a rational approach would be to immunize patients with live vaccine before renal transplantation. Plotkin and associates [30, 31] developed Towne strain CMV live, attenuated vaccine and showed it to be safe and immunogenic in normal volunteers. We confirmed their findings and observed that Towne vaccine elicited CMV-specific humoral and CMI responses in a small group of adult volunteers [32]. A preliminary study of 12 RTCs inoculated with Towne vaccine has been published [33]. We are now conducting a randomized, placebo-controlled, double-blind study of Towne vaccine in RTCs and our results to date are the subject of this progress report.

SUBJECTS AND METHODS

Patients for the placebo-controlled vaccine trial were RTCs of at least 12 years of age. This study was approved by the University of Minnesota Committee on the Use of Human Subjects in Research, and informed consent was obtained from all subjects before participation. Patients were told verbally of possible side effects at the time of enrollment and also were given written information that included a description of potential reactions. Patients were telephoned six to 12 weeks after inoculation of vaccine or placebo and any adverse reactions that they experienced were recorded.

Towne live, attenuated CMV vaccine, 129th passage, lot 726/C-F189, and placebo (sterile buffered cell culture medium, lot 315) were supplied by Merck, Sharp and Dohme Research Laboratories, West Point, PA. The infectivity titer of the lyophilized vaccine was 6.6×10^3 plaques per ml in MRC 5 fibroblast cells. Vaccine was sterility and safety tested at the Merck, Sharp and Dohme Research Laboratories. Subjects were given either 1.0 ml of vaccine or placebo sc.

Our standard procedures for immunosuppression and renal transplantation have been described [34, 35]. Since September 1980, patients were randomized to receive either our conventional immunosuppression (antilymphoblast globulin, azathioprine, and prednisone) or cyclosporine and prednisone [36]. Since July 1979, patients have been transfused approximately two months before transplantation with 5 to 10 units (average volume 75 ml of each) of packed RBCs from different donors.

All patients transplanted at the University of Minnesota since 1974 have been studied prospectively before, during, and after transplantation for the occurrence of CMV infection. Specimens for virus isolation and sera for CMV antibody titers were collected from all patients regardless of symptoms. Urine, throat swabs, and blood were obtained pretransplant, weekly for 2 to 6 wk and at clinic visits thereafter at approximately monthly intervals. Bronchoscopy, biopsy, and autopsy tissue were also cultured when appropriate. Whenever possible, an isolate from each culture-positive patient was frozen at $-70°C$ in 10% dimethyl sulfoxide for future laboratory studies. Methods of CMV isolation, CF, and indirect immunofluorescent (IF) antibody titer determinations have been previously described [37–39]. Antibody titers are expressed as reciprocals of serum dilutions. On enrollment, patients were categorized as seronegative or seropositive. Seropositive patients had a CMV CF titer $\geqslant 8$ or an IF titer $\geqslant 40$. Patients with a CF titer of 4 and an IF titer of 20 were also considered seropositive. All others were defined as seronegative. CMV-specific CMI responses were measured using an in vitro lymphocyte proliferation assay as previously described [32]. The antigen employed was partially purified, concentrated AD169 strain CMV. The data are expressed as net counts per minute (proliferative response to CMV antigen minus response to uninfected cell control antigen). Counts $\geqslant 5,000/$ min were considered positive.

Laboratory diagnosis of CMV infection after transplantation was based on isolation of CMV from any clinical specimen and/or a fourfold or greater rise in CMV CF or IF antibody titers posttransplant. Patients considered to have CMV disease were hospitalized and had laboratory confirmation of CMV infection. To define the degree of clinical illness due to CMV, a disease scoring system was devised by the groups at Children's Hospital of Philadelphia and the University of Minnesota. Points were assigned according to the scheme outlined in Table 1. For example, if a patient had CMV isolated from urine, a fever above 101°F for 4 days, and a peripheral WBC count of 2500/ mm^3 for 3 days, that patient would be scored as having CMV disease with 2 points. Severity of CMV disease was categorized as follows: mild, 1 to 3 points; moderate, 4 to 6 points; severe, $\geqslant 7$ points; lethal, death occurred during the course of laboratory-documented CMV infection.

Restriction endonuclease enzyme digestion analyses of viral DNA from CMV strains shed posttransplant were performed by Dr. E.-S. Huang [40], Dr. S.A. Spector [41], or ourselves. In our laboratory, CMV isolates from study subjects were grown in MRC 5 cells, DNA was isolated by phenol extraction, and viral DNA was separated from eukaryotic DNA by isopyknic CsCl density gradient ultracentrifugation. Gradient fractions containing viral DNA, as determined by refractive indices, were collected, dialyzed to remove CsCl, and digested with the enzymes HindIII and EcoRI. Cleaved

TABLE 1. System for Scoring Severity of CMV Disease

I. Laboratory documentation of CMV infection required. No points.
II. Fever > 101 °F either orally or rectally
   Mild: 2–4 days = 1 point
   Moderate: 5–20 days = 2 points
   Severe: >21 days = 3 points
III. Additional findings during the febrile illness:
  1. Respiratory
     Mild: infiltrate on chest x-ray = 1 point
     Moderate: infiltrate and symptoms (cough, shortness of breath) = 2 points
     Severe: assisted ventilation = 3 points
  2. Central nervous system
     Mild: lethargy = 1 point
     Moderate: stupor or semicoma = 2 points
     Severe: coma = 3 points
  3. Renal
     Mild: 2- to 4-fold increase above the lowest posttransplant serum creatinine = 1 point
     Moderate: >4-fold increase above the lowest posttransplant creatinine = 2 points
     Severe: nephrectomy or return to permanent dialysis = 3 points
  4. Hepatic
     Mild: liver function tests 2-fold above baseline and into the abnormal range = 1 point
     Severe: clinical hepatitis manifested by jaundice = 3 points
  5. Hematologic
     Mild: WRC count <4000/mm^3 = 1 point
     Platelet count < 100,000/mm^3 = 1 point
  6. Gastrointestinal
     Severe: overt GI bleeding = 3 points
  7. Musculoskeletal
     Moderate: muscle wasting or arthritis = 2 points
  8. Superinfection (bacterial or fungal)
     Severe: deep organ or bloodstream involvement = 3 points
  9. Death
     Death occurring at any time during CMV disease regardless of the cause = 4 points

fragments were electrophoresed in a 0.8% agarose gel and the gel was stained with the intercalating dye ethidium bromide. DNA fragment bands were visualized by ultraviolet transillumination and photographed.

Since 95% of all symptomatic CMV infections in our patients occur within six months after transplantation [42], subjects were entered in the efficacy analysis after they had been transplanted and followed for six months. The randomization code was broken for interim data analysis in June 1980, September 1981, and March 1983. The code remains unknown to the clinical staff and only aggregate information has been disclosed. Therefore, interim data analyses have not affected the management and outcome of individual subjects. Differences in proportions were evaluated by the chi-square test with continuity correction. P values <0.05 were considered significant.

RESULTS

From January 15, 1979 through March 1, 1983, 332 RTCs were enrolled in our placebo-controlled, double-blind trial of Towne vaccine: 162 received vaccine and 170 were given placebo.

Reactions

Of the 332 subjects enrolled, 270 (81%) had sufficient follow-up to be included in an analysis of side effects. No serious untoward reactions were reported. Table 2 displays reaction rates in vaccinees and placebo recipients. Subjects were divided into those seronegative and those seropositive for CMV at enrollment. Reactions were most frequent among seronegative subjects given Towne vaccine. The most common side effect was erythema and swelling at the injection site that was often accompanied by pain. This reaction developed 1 to 21 days after inoculation (mean time of onset, 7.2 days) and lasted a mean of 6.3 days (median, 4.5 days). Fever occurred between the 1 and 21st days postinoculation with a mean time of onset of 7.1 days postinoculation. Fever lasted a mean of 5.1 days (median, 3.0 days). The proportion of vaccinees experiencing any reaction was significantly higher than that of the placebo group (corrected χ^2 = 50.7, P <0.001). Rates of local reactions were significantly different for seronegative vaccinees compared with seronegative placebo subjects (corrected χ^2 = 29.44, P <0.001), as were rates for seropositive vaccinees compared with seropositive placebo subjects (corrected χ^2 = 16.95, P <0.001). Rates of local reactions were also significantly higher for seronegative vaccinees compared with seropositive vaccinees (corrected χ^2 = 6.84, P <0.01). Frequency of fever after inoculation was significantly higher for seronegative vaccinees

TABLE 2. Reactions After Inoculation

	CMV Vaccinees		Placebo Recipients	
	Seroneg. N = 63	Seropos. N = 67	Seroneg. N = 54	Seropos. N = 86
Any reaction	35 (56%)	23 (34%)	3 (6%)	6 (7%)
Local reaction*	33 (52%)	19 (28%)	2 (4%)	3 (3%)
Fever	11 (17%)	7 (10%)	2 (4%)	1 (1%)
Chills	0	0	0	2 (2%)

*Includes erythema, swelling, and pain at injection site.

compared with seronegative placebo recipients (corrected χ^2 = 4.27, P <0.05). The frequency of fever in seropositive vaccinees compared with seropositive placebo recipients was not quite significant (corrected χ^2 = 3.54, P = 0.06). Although the incidence of fever after immunization was higher in the seronegative vaccinees compared with the seropositive vaccinated group, this difference was not significant (corrected χ^2 = 0.82, P >0.1).

Immunogenicity

Of the 332 study subjects, 174 (52%) have been transplanted and followed for at least six months. Immunogenicity, safety, and efficacy evaluations were based on data from these 174 patients. The sex ratios, ages, number of HLA-identical subjects, presence of CMV antibody at enrollment, number of patients given cyclosporine instead of our conventional immunosuppression, and time from enrollment to transplant were nearly identical for the vaccinees and the placebo recipients (Table 3). The proportion of vaccinees who received kidneys from living, related donors was larger than that of the placebo group, but the difference was not significant (corrected χ^2 = 2.06, P >0.1).

Humoral immune responses measured by CMV IF antibody titers are shown in Table 4. Overall, 78.6% of seronegative vaccinees seroconverted by IF testing before transplantation. The geometric mean IF titer of seronegative vaccinees peaked at 3 mo postimmunization. At transplantation, which

TABLE 3. Characteristics of Subjects Followed at Least Six Months' Posttransplant

	Study Group	
	Vaccinees	Placebo
No. of patients	83	91
Male	59	64
Female	24	27
Age at enrollment (yrs)		
Mean	34.5	36.5
Median	33.5	34.0
Proportion with living related donor	64%	51%
No. HLA-identical	13	11
Proportion CMV seropositive at enrollment	48.2%	51.6%
No. given cyclosporine	18	19
Months from enrollment to transplant		
Mean	6.2	6.3
Median	4.3	4.6

TABLE 4. CMV Immunofluorescence Antibody Titers in Study Subjects

| | | | Geometric Mean Titer | |
Group	No. Tested	Prestudy	Three-month Follow-up	At Transplant
Vaccine				
Seronegative	43	<20	68.4	39.2 (5.7)*
Seropositive	40	37.8	62.2	59.7 (6.6)
Placebo				
Seronegative	44	<20	1.3	1.9 (7.7)
Seropositive	47	52.2	51.7	49.4 (5.0)

*In parentheses are mean months from enrollment to transplant.

was accomplished a mean of 5.7 mo after immunization, their geometric mean titer had fallen from 68.4 to 39.2. The geometric mean titer of seronegative vaccinees at transplant was somewhat lower than the geometric mean titer of subjects naturally immune (the seropositive placebo recipients). Vaccinees who were seropositive before immunization experienced a boost in their geometric mean IF titer from 37.8 on enrollment to 62.2 at the three-month follow-up. Their geometric mean IF titer was still substantially above the prestudy level when these subjects were transplanted a mean of 6.6 mo after enrollment. One of the seronegative placebo patients seroconverted at three-month follow-up and six (13.6%) of the seronegative placebo recipients had seroconverted at the time of transplantation, which was an average of 7.7 mo after enrollment. There was no appreciable change in the geometric mean IF titer of the seropositive placebo recipients from enrollment in the study to transplantation.

CMV-specific CMI responses as measured by in vitro lymphocyte proliferation to CMV antigen for subjects seronegative at enrollment are shown in Table 5. Eighteen patients had lymphocyte proliferative responses to CMV measured before inoculation and again at transplant. Eleven of these subjects received Towne vaccine and nine (82%) developed positive lymphocyte proliferative responses to CMV by the time of transplantation. Vaccinees had positive lymphocyte proliferative responses as early as 1 mo postimmunization and two had positive responses when tested 20 months' postimmunization. All 11 seronegative vaccinees appropriately tested at transplant either had seroconverted or had positive lymphocyte proliferative responses to CMV antigen. Three subjects, one of whom was transplanted 5 mo after immunization and two of whom were transplanted 20 mo after immunization did not have documented seroconversion but did have positive lymphocyte proliferative responses. One of the seven seronegative placebo recipients

TABLE 5. Lymphocyte Proliferation to CMV (AD169 Strain) Antigen in Seronegative Subjects

	Vaccinees		Placebo Recipients	
	Prestudy	At Transplant (mos)	Prestudy	At Transplant (mos)
1.	1360*	13,560 (1)†	342	360 (1.5)
2.	0	210 (1)	−6611	−27 (2.5)
3.	1320	18,450 (1.5)	2870	110 (3)
4.	459	22,900 (1.5)	100	1361 (5)
5.	833	42,820 (2.5)	109	1080 (5)
6.	340	860 (5)	4551	−2206 (6)
7.	2100	25,860 (5)‡	1580	59,070 (6)§
8.	1180	23,620 (6)		
9.	0	9,740 (10)		
10.	836	11,861 (20)‡		
11.	1231	44,320 (20)‡		

*Net counts per minute; counts ≥ 5000 are considered positive.
†In parentheses are months from enrollment to transplant.
‡These subjects did not have documented seroconversion.
§Patient seroconverted before transplant.

tested for CMV-specific CMI seroconverted pretransplant and developed the highest positive lymphocyte proliferative response of the 18 patients studied. This patient undoubtedly acquired a primary CMV infection between the time of enrollment in the study and the day of transplantation. He did not have CMV disease before or after transplantation.

Safety

CMV strains from 17 patients who shed virus posttransplant have been examined by restriction endonuclease digestion analysis to learn if the DNA of these isolates resembled Towne. Nine CMV strains were recovered from vaccinees and eight from placebo recipients. Seven of the viruses tested were isolated from PBMCs, nine came from the urine, and one was recovered from the throat. All of the isolates examined by restriction endonuclease digestion analysis had DNA fragment band patterns that differed from each other and from Towne. Fragment band patterns of four patient isolates and Towne strain CMV are compared in Figure 1.

Efficacy

During the period covered by this progress report, 113 (65%) of 174 patients had CMV infections during the first 6 mo posttransplant (Table 6). Infection rates were significantly higher for patients who had CMV antibody (seropositive) at the time of enrollment (corrected $\chi^2 = 19.8$, P < 0.001).

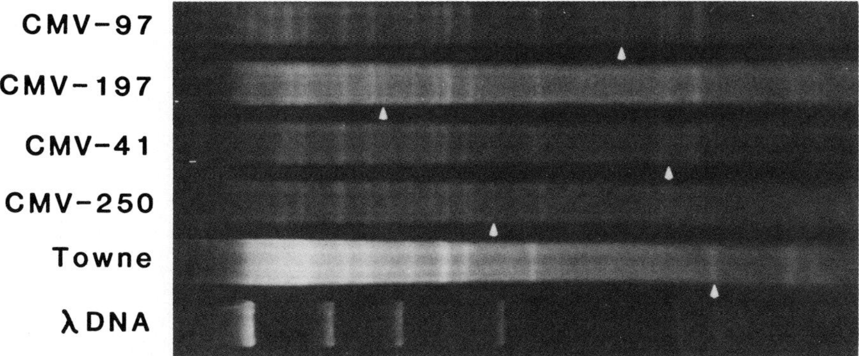

Fig. 1. HindIII restriction endonuclease cleavage patterns of 4 CMV patient isolates (Strains 97, 197, 41, and 250), Towne vaccine, and lambda bacteriophage. Arrows point to DNA fragments that distinguish strains of CMV from each other.

TABLE 6. CMV Infection After Transplantation in All Patients

	No. Studied	No. With CMV Infection
Vaccine recipients		
Seronegative	43	21 (49%)
Seropositive	40	29 (73%)
Total	83	50 (60%)
Placebo recipients		
Seronegative	44	21 (48%)
Seropositive	47	42 (89%)
Total	91	63 (69%)

However, rates of CMV infection after transplantation were similar for vaccinees and placebo recipients (60% v 69%).

CMV disease occurred in 31 (17.8%) of the 174 transplant patients. The distribution of all patients by disease score (Fig. 2) showed that more placebo recipients had CMV disease than vaccinees and the illness in placebo subjects tended to be more severe.

In Table 7, the data are grouped by degree of CMV disease (mild, moderate, severe, or lethal) and arranged according to the CMV serology of the recipients before entry to the study and that of the donors at the time of transplant. When all subjects were considered, the frequency of symptomatic CMV disease was higher in the placebo group than in the vaccinated subjects but the rates were not significantly different (corrected $\chi^2 = 0.27$, P > 0.1). If only the patients who were seronegative at the onset of the study were considered, the proportion of vaccinees who developed severe or lethal CMV

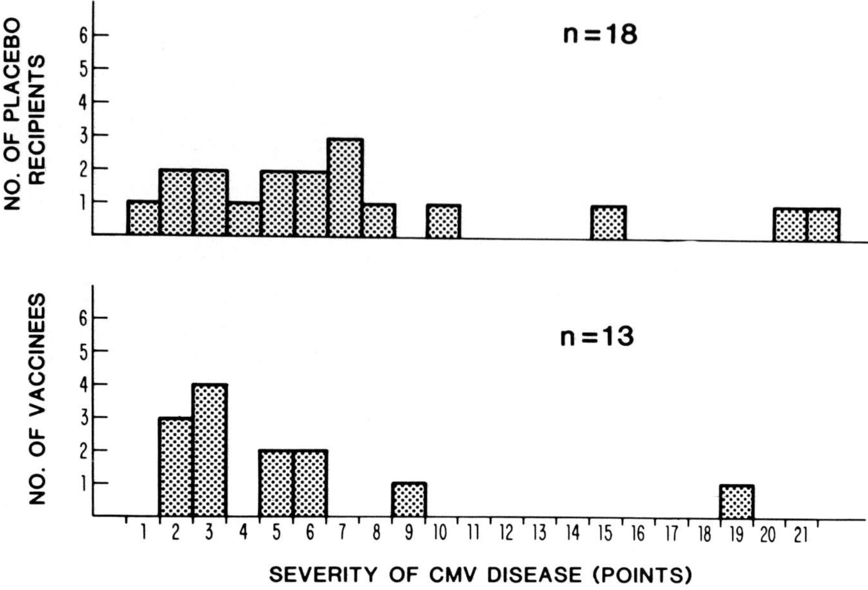

Fig. 2. Distribution of all study patients both seronegative and seropositive with CMV disease by disease score.

disease was lower than that of the placebo recipients but the difference was not quite significant (corrected χ^2 = 3.32, P = 0.07). When seronegative subjects with CMV disease were compared, a significantly higher proportion of placebo recipients had severe or lethal CMV disease than did vaccinees (corrected χ^2 = 7.34, P = 0.007). Seronegative patients whose donors were seropositive are of special interest because they are challenged with virus transmitted by donor renal tissue or by leukocytes trapped in the transplanted kidney (Table 8). Here, the rates of CMV infection were similar for both groups, but significantly fewer vaccinees developed severe or lethal CMV disease (corrected χ^2 = 4.76, P = 0.03). All three cases of lethal CMV disease occurred in patients who were seronegative, received placebo, and were given a kidney from a seropositive donor.

Effect of Cyclosporine Immunosuppression on Posttransplant CMV Infections

Thirty-seven (21%) of the 174 study subjects received cyclosporine and prednisone (Table 9). The frequency of CMV infection among cyclosporine recipients, 24/37 or 65%, was not different from the total study group nor were rates of CMV disease (6/37, 16.2%). Numbers were too small for a

TABLE 7. CMV Disease After Transplantation in All Subjects

CMV Serology*		No. Studied	No. of Patients With CMV Disease			
Donor	Recipient		Mild	Moderate	Severe	Lethal
Vaccine recipients						
−	−	21	1	0	0	0
+	−	14	3	1	0	0
?	−	8	1	0	0	0
−	+	19	2	1	1	0
+	+	14	0	1	1	0
?	+	7	0	1	0	0
	Total	83	7	4	2	0
Placebo subjects						
−	−	19	0	0	0	0
+	−	9	0	0	1	3
?	−	16	0	0	1	0
−	+	17	1	2	1	0
+	+	15	2	1	1	0
?	+	15	2	2	1	0
	Total	91	5	5	5	3

*− = seronegative; + = seropositive; ? = antibody titers not available.

TABLE 8. CMV Disease in Seronegative Recipients Whose Kidney Donor Was Seropositive

	No. Studied	No. HLA Identical	No. Infected	CMV Disease		
				Mild-to-Moderate	Severe	Lethal
Vaccine	14	3	12	4	0	0
Placebo	9	2	7	0	1	3

valid comparison of severity of CMV disease in patients given cyclosporine versus patients receiving antilymphoblast globulin and azathioprine. The cyclosporine recipients were evenly divided among the vaccinee and placebo study groups.

DISCUSSION

Although the frequency of CMV infection was similar among vaccinated and placebo subjects, Towne CMV vaccine protected seronegative patients from severe or lethal CMV disease. While the ideal vaccine might be one that completely prevents CMV infection, the goal of the immunization program is to decrease morbidity and mortality due to CMV disease after renal transplantation.

TABLE 9. CMV Infection and Disease After Transplantation in Patients Receiving Cyclosporine

Group	No. Studied	No. Infected	No. of Patients With CMV Disease			
			Mild	Moderate	Severe	Lethal
Vaccine						
Seronegative	7	5	2	0	0	0
Seropositive	11	8	1	0	1	0
Total	18	13	3	0	1	0
Placebo						
Seronegative	9	3	0	0	0	1
Seropositive	10	8	0	1	0	0
Total	19	11	0	1	0	1

The clinical benefit of Towne vaccine was most apparent in subjects who were seronegative when they entered the trial and who subsequently received kidneys from seropositive donors (Table 8). In this patient category, four placebo subjects had severe CMV disease and three of the four died. None of the vaccinees in this category had severe or lethal CMV disease, but one was moderately ill with a disease score of five points. This man was transplanted 49 days after immunization. Since humoral and cellular immune responses to CMV vaccine develop relatively slowly in RTCs [43], it is possible that if his transplantation had been delayed for several months he might have had a milder CMV infection.

Towne live, attenuated CMV vaccine elicited both humoral antibody responses and CMV-specific CMI in the majority of RTCs. Rates of seroconversion measured by IF antibody testing were 78.6%. Development of positive lymphocyte proliferative responses occurred in 82% of seronegative vaccinees tested. Although Towne vaccine boosted humoral antibody titers in subjects seropositive before immunization and also boosted lymphocyte proliferative responses in approximately half of seropositive subjects (data not shown), this immunologic effect was not accompanied by a clinical benefit since the proportion of patients infected and the severity of CMV disease was not different for seropositive vaccinees and seropositive placebo patients. Indeed, the vaccinee who had the most severe CMV disease with a total score of 19 was a seropositive recipient whose donor was seronegative. He had been immunized 10 mo before transplantation but developed CMV disease in the immediate posttransplant period and nearly died.

If patients in the vaccine trial represent a truly unselected portion of all our RTCs, the frequency of CMV disease in placebo subjects should be similar to that found in patients enrolled in a prospective study of posttransplant infectious diseases conducted here between October 1977 and September

1981 [42]. That was the case: 18 (19.8%) of 91 placebo subjects in the vaccine trial had CMV disease, while 111 (21%) of 518 renal allograft recipients in the infectious disease study developed CMV disease.

A number of factors, especially the immunosuppressive regimen, determine the frequency and severity of CMV disease. In a recent study we found that there was a decreased risk of CMV pneumonia in patients given cyclosporine compared with those given our conventional immunosuppression [44]. However, patients immunosuppressed with cyclosporine in the vaccine trial did not have appreciably lower frequencies of CMV infection and disease than those given antilymphoblast globulin, azathioprine, and prednisone.

We have reported that HLA-identical recipients have a significantly lower risk of CMV disease than do patients who are transplanted with non-HLA-matched cadaver kidneys [42]. Therefore, an uneven distribution of HLA-identical recipients could influence the outcome of a controlled vaccine trial. Twenty-four (13.8%) of 174 subjects in our vaccine trial had HLA-identical donors and none developed CMV disease. Recipients of HLA-identical kidneys were randomly distributed among the total vaccine and placebo study groups (Table 3) and also evenly distributed among seronegative vaccine and placebo recipients who were transplanted with kidneys from seropositive donors (Table 8).

Do multiple small volume RBC transfusions cause patients to acquire CMV before transplantation? This may occur in a few instances because six (13.6%) of 44 seronegative placebo subjects seroconverted between the time of enrollment in the vaccine trial and transplantation. These six subjects could have been infected by virus transmitted in the "mini-transfusions," but it is also possible that they acquired CMV from an infected relative, patient, or health-care worker. A longitudinal serosurvey is in progress in our renal transplant and dialysis wards to determine if in-hospital person-to-person transmission of CMV is a problem.

Reactions at the injection site were quite common, occurring in 56% of seronegative and 34% of seropositive vaccinees. The main systemic complication, fever, was not as frequent as injection site reactions. Fever was reported in 17% of seronegative and 10% of seropositive vaccinees. Both the local reactions and fever lasted for no more than a week in most subjects and none of the patients required medical attention for these side effects. Natural immunity protected against the side effects of CMV vaccine. Viral replication with resultant inflammatory reaction at the injection site probably caused the sore arms and perhaps fever as well. We speculate that viral replication was shut off so rapidly in many seropositive subjects that the inflammatory response was insufficient to produce symptoms.

Although many more patients need to be studied in order to demonstrate conclusively that CMV vaccine does not reactivate and cause disease after renal transplantation, data from nine of our vaccinees combined with that already published [33] and currently being collected by Dr. Plotkin's group in Philadelphia indicate that CMV strains shed posttransplant resemble wild viruses rather than Towne. Vaccine-strain CMV has not been recovered from any recipient of Towne vaccine studied to date.

How long should our vaccine trial continue? We have decided to terminate the study when 200 patients have been transplanted and followed for at least six months. At that point we should be able to discover, with an alpha error of 0.05 and a beta error of 0.20, whether there is a significant difference in incidence of severe or lethal CMV disease between the entire vaccine and placebo groups.

ACKNOWLEDGMENTS

We thank E.-S. Huang, Stephen A. Spector, and Donald M. Mattsson for performing restriction endonuclease digestion analyses of CMV DNA, Dorothee Aeppli for biostatistical consultation, Charlene K. Edelman for clinical virology procedures, and Connie Lindberg for assistance in collection of clinical data.

REFERENCES

1. Hill RB Jr, Rowlands DT, Rifkind D: Infectious pulmonary disease in patients receiving immunosuppressive therapy for organ transplantation. N Engl J Med 271:1021–1027, 1964.
2. Hedley-Whyte ET, Craighead JE: Generalized cytomegalic inclusion disease after renal homotransplantation: Report of a case with isolation of virus. N Engl J Med 272:473–475, 1965.
3. Kanich RE, Craighead JE: Cytomegalovirus infection and cytomegalic inclusion disease in renal homotransplant recipients. Am J Med 40:874–882, 1966.
4. Craighead JE, Hanshaw JB, Carpenter CB: Cytomegalovirus infection after renal allotransplantation. JAMA 201:99–102, 1967.
5. Rifkind D, Goodman N, Hill RB Jr: The clinical significance of cytomegalovirus infection in renal transplant recipients. Ann Intern Med 66:1116–1128, 1967.
6. Andersen HK, Spencer ES: Cytomegalovirus infection among renal allograft recipients. Acta Med Scand 186:7–19, 1969.
7. Fine RN, Grushkin CM, Anand S, Lieberman E, Wright HT Jr: Cytomegalovirus in children: Postrenal transplantation. Am J Dis Child 120:197–202, 1970.
8. Fine RN, Grushkin CM, Malekzadeh M, Wright HT Jr: Cytomegalovirus syndrome following renal transplantation. Arch Surg 105:564–570, 1972.
9. Armstrong D, Balakrishnan SL, Steger L, Yu B, Stenzel KH: Cytomegalovirus infections with viremia following renal transplantation. Arch Intern Med 127:111–115, 1971.

10. Lopez C, Simmons RL, Mauer SM, Najarian JS, Good RA, Gentry S: Association of renal allograft rejection with virus infections. Am J Med 56:280–289, 1974.

11. Simmons RL, Lopez C, Balfour HH Jr, Kalis J, Rattazzi LC, Najarian JS: Cytomegalovirus: Clinical virological correlations in renal transplant recipients. Ann Surg 180:623–634, 1974.

12. Pien FD, Smith TF, Anderson CF, Webel ML, Taswell HF: Herpesviruses in renal transplant patients. Transplantation 16:489–495, 1973.

13. Luby JP, Burnett W, Hull AR, Ware AJ, Shorey JW, Peters PC: Relationship between cytomegalovirus and hepatic function abnormalities in the period after renal transplant. J Infect Dis 129:511–518, 1974.

14. Fiala M, Payne JE, Berne TV, Moore TC, Henle W, Montgomerie JZ, Chatterjee SN, Guze LB: Epidemiology of cytomegalovirus infection after transplantation and immunosuppression. J Infect Dis 132:421–433, 1975.

15. Ho M, Suwansirikul S, Dowling JN, Youngblood LA, Armstrong JA: The transplanted kidney as a source of cytomegalovirus infections. N Engl J Med 293:1109–1112, 1975.

16. Armstrong JA, Evans AS, Rao N, Ho M: Viral infections in renal transplant recipients. Infect Immun 14:970–975, 1976.

17. Betts RF, Freeman RB, Douglas RG Jr, Talley TE, Rundell B: Transmission of cytomegalovirus infection with renal allograft. Kidney Int 8:387–394, 1975.

18. Nankervis GA: Comments on CMV infections in renal transplant patients. Yale J Biol Med 49:27–28, 1976.

19. Betts RF, Freeman RB, Douglas RG Jr, Talley TE: Clinical manifestations of renal allograft derived primary cytomegalovirus infection. Am J Dis Child 131:759–763, 1977.

20. Rytel MW, Balay J: Cytomegalovirus infection and immunity in renal allograft recipients: Assessment of the competence of humoral immunity. Infect Immun 13:1633–1637, 1976.

21. Rytel MW, Aguilar-Torres FG, Balay J, Heim LR: Assessment of the status of cell-mediated immunity in cytomegalovirus-infected renal allograft recipients. Cell Immunol 37:31–40, 1978.

22. Linnemann CC Jr, Kauffman CA, First MR, Schiff GM, Phair JP: Cellular immune response to cytomegalovirus infection after renal transplantation. Infect Immun 22:176–180, 1978.

23. Naraqi S, Jackson GG, Jonasson O, Yamashiroya HM: Prospective study of prevalence, incidence, and source of herpesvirus infections in patients with renal allografts. J Infect Dis 136:531–540, 1977.

24. Naraqi S, Jonasson O, Jackson GG, Yamashiroya HM: Clinical manifestations of infections with herpesviruses after kidney transplantation: A prospective study of various syndromes. Ann Surg 188:234–239, 1978.

25. Rubin RH, Cosimi B, Tolkoff-Rubin NE, Russell PS, Hirsch MS: Infectious disease syndromes attributable to cytomegalovirus and their significance among renal transplant recipients. Transplantation 24:458–464, 1977.

26. Pass RF, Long WK, Whitley RJ, Soong SJ, Diethelm AG, Reynolds DW, Alford CA Jr: Productive infection with cytomegalovirus and herpes simplex virus in renal transplant recipients: Role of source of kidney. J Infect Dis 137:556–563, 1978.

27. Whelchel JD, Pass RF, Diethelm AG, Whitley RJ, Alford CA Jr: Effect of primary and recurrent cytomegalovirus infections upon graft and patient survival after renal transplantation. Transplantation 28:443–446, 1979.

28. Chatterjee SN, Jordan GW: Prospective study of the prevalence and symptomatology of cytomegalovirus infection in renal transplant recipients. Transplantation 28:457–460, 1979.

29. Marker SC, Howard RJ, Simmons RL, Kalis JM, Connelly DP, Najarian JS, Balfour HH Jr: Cytomegalovirus infection: A quantitative prospective study of three-hundred-twenty consecutive renal transplants. Surgery 89:660–671, 1981.

30. Plotkin SA, Furukawa T, Zygraich N, Huygelen C: Candidate cytomegalovirus strain for human vaccination. Infect Immun 12:521–527, 1975.

31. Plotkin SA, Farquhar J, Hornberger E: Clinical trials of immunization with the Towne 125 strain of human cytomegalovirus. J Infect Dis 134:470–475, 1976.

32. Gehrz RC, Christianson WR, Linner KM, Groth KE, Balfour HH Jr: Cytomegalovirus vaccine: Specific humoral and cellular immune responses in human volunteers. Arch Intern Med 140:936–939, 1980.

33. Glazer JP, Friedman HM, Grossman RA, Starr SE, Barker CF, Perloff LJ, Huang ES, Plotkin SA: Live cytomegalovirus vaccination of renal transplant candidates: A preliminary trial. Ann Intern Med 91:676–683, 1979.

34. Najarian JS, Simmons RL: The clinical use of antilymphocyte globulin. N Engl J Med 285:158–166, 1971.

35. Simmons RL, Kjellstrand CM, Najarian JS: Kidney transplantation: Technique, complications and results. In Najarian JS, Simmons RL (eds): "Transplantation." Philadelphia: Lea & Febiger, 1972, p 445.

36. Sutherland DER, Goetz FC, Elick BA, Najarian JS: Experience with 49 segmental pancreas transplants in 45 diabetic patients. Transplantation 34:330–338, 1982.

37. Balfour HH Jr, Slade MS, Kalis JM, Howard RJ, Simmons RL, Najarian JS: Viral infections in renal transplant donors and their recipients: A prospective study. Surgery 81:487–492, 1977.

38. Lee MS, Balfour HH Jr: Optimal method for recovery of cytomegalovirus from urine of renal transplant patients. Transplantation 24:228–230, 1977.

39. Peterson PK, Balfour HH Jr, Marker SC, Fryd DS, Howard RJ, Simmons RL: Cytomegalovirus disease in renal allograft recipients: A prospective study of the clinical features, risk factors and impact on renal transplantation. Medicine 59:283–300, 1980.

40. Huang E-S, Kilpatrick B, Lakeman A, Alford CA: Genetic analysis of a cytomegalovirus-like agent isolated from human brain. J Virol 26:718–723, 1978.

41. Spector SA, Spector DH: Molecular epidemiology of cytomegalovirus infections in premature twin infants and their mother. Pediatr Infect Dis 1:405–409, 1982.

42. Peterson PK, Ferguson R, Fryd DS, Balfour HH Jr, Rynasiewicz J, Simmons RL: Infectious diseases in hospitalized renal transplant recipients: A prospective study of a complex and evolving problem. Medicine 61:360–372, 1982.

43. Starr SE, Glazer JP, Friedman HM, Farquhar JD, Plotkin SA: Specific cellular and humoral immunity after immunization with live Towne strain cytomegalovirus vaccine. J Infect Dis 143:585–589, 1981.

44. Peterson PK, Balfour HH Jr, Fryd DS, Ferguson R, Kronenberg R, Simmons RL: Decreased risk of pneumonia in renal transplant recipients receiving cyclosporin A. (Submitted for publication.)

Selection of Particles and Proteins for Use as Human Cytomegalovirus Subunit Vaccines*

Wade Gibson and Alice Irmiere[†]

Department of Pharmacology and Experimental Therapeutics, The Johns Hopkins School of Medicine, Baltimore, MD 21205

Since their introduction nearly two centuries ago [1], vaccines have played a central role in the control of viral diseases. Recently, their use in limiting the biologic effects of HCMV has been explored [2–5]. In the absence of suitable noninfectious material, live strains of HCMV were used, following their "attenuation" by long-term passage in tissue culture [2, 6]. In view of potential complications arising from the introduction of viral DNA in this or even killed whole virus preparations, the possibility of using biochemically defined "subunit" preparations which do not contain DNA is attractive. With the application of new techniques for isolating virus particles and proteins from the infected cell, and the advent of new approaches to synthesizing defined proteins and peptides able to elicit protective immunity, this objective seems attainable. Moreover, until effective antiviral drugs become readily available, it is likely that vaccination will remain an important antiviral approach for many years to come.

In this paper we discuss 1) the isolation of an unusual noninfectious virus particle having properties which make it an attractive subunit vaccine candidate, and 2) information concerning a few specific viral proteins that show

*Supported by research grants AI 13718, AI 16959 and AI 19373 from the National Institute for Allergy and Infectious Diseases.

†A.I. is a predoctoral fellow in the Biochemistry, Cellular and Molecular Biology Training Program and was supported by Training Grant GM 07445 from NIH.

Birth Defects: Original Article Series, Volume 20, Number 1, pages 305–324
© **1984 March of Dimes Birth Defects Foundation**

promise for the development of additional diagnostic and therapeutic approaches to CMV-related diseases.

RESULTS AND DISCUSSION
Noninfectious HCMV Particles Are Subunit Vaccine Candidates

Two types of noninfectious particles are shed from human foreskin fibroblast cells infected with HCMV. These have been designated as "dense bodies" and "noninfectious enveloped particles" (NIEPs), respectively. Dense bodies are routinely observed in infected cells [7–11] and their biochemical properties have been examined by others [11–15]. NIEPs, whose existence was suggested by electron microscopy [8, 10, 16], have only recently been recovered and characterized [17].

These two noninfectious particles can be cleanly separated from virions by the negative viscosity-positive density gradient system described by Barzilai et al [18], and first adapted to HCMV by Talbot and Almeida [19] (Fig. 1:1A,B). Electron microscopy revealed that NIEPs and virions are distinguished by the appearance of their core structure, but otherwise are architecturally very similar (Fig. 1:2A,B). Dense bodies were observed to be solid spheres generally larger in diameter than virions (Fig. 1:2C) [7–11]. All three particles are bound by an outer envelope. When assayed for DNA content and infectivity, it was found that the virion band contained 99% of the DNA and infectivity present in the gradient (Fig. 2). The NIEP and dense body bands contained only background levels of DNA and < 0.1% of the virion infectivity. When subjected to additional rate-velocity and equilibrium centrifugation steps, the specific infectivity (ie, infectivity/protein mass) of these two particles was further reduced but not eliminated.

NIEPs Contain Full Complement of Virion Proteins

Analyses of the protein constituents of these three HCMV particles showed that the architectural similarities between virions and NIEPs were reflected by their protein compositions (Fig. 3A). Only two differences between these patterns were noted. First, NIEPs contain a 35,000 dalton (35K) protein not present in virions. This 35K species is referred to as the "assembly protein," based on properties shared with its counterpart in the B-capsid putative assembly intermediates of herpes simplex [20–22] and strain Colburn CMV [23] and is thought to contribute to the NIEPs altered core appearance (Fig. 1:2A). The second difference between the NIEP and virion protein compositions is that NIEPs contain significantly less of the two "matrix proteins," relative to virions. We have suggested [17] that this discrepancy could be

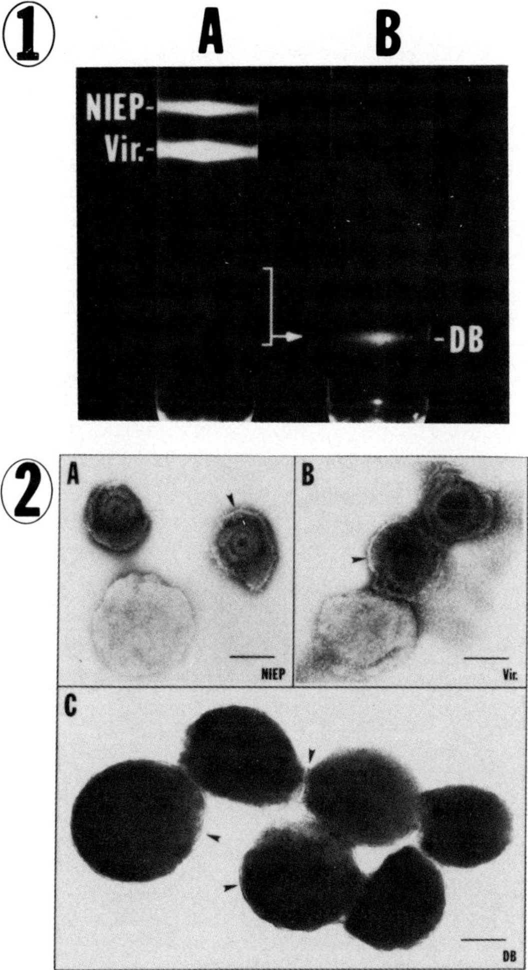

Fig. 1. Extracellular virus particles from HCMV-infected cells. Medium from AD169-infected human foreskin fibroblast (HFF) cells was clarified and subjected to rate-velocity centrifugation using glycerol-tartrate gradients [19]. Noninfectious enveloped particles (NIEPs) and virions (Vir.) are seen in the upper half of the tube (Panel 1A). Dense bodies (DB) are more easily seen after rebanding to equilibrium (Panel 1B). Aliquots of NIEPs (Panel 2A), Vir. (Panel 2B) and DBs (Panel 2C) were negatively stained with uranyl formate and photographed using an electron microscope. Arrows point to membrane structure; bars represent 100 nm. (Data are from Irmiere and Gibson [17].)

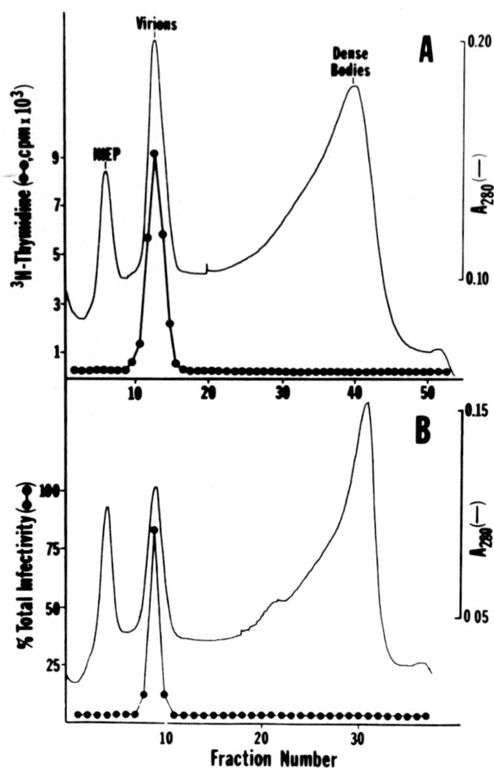

Fig. 2. NIEPs (noninfectious enveloped particles) and dense bodies lack DNA and infectivity. Media from cells infected with AD169 and either radiolabeled with ^{3}H-thymidine (Panel A), or not labeled (Panel B), were layered above glycerol-tartrate gradients; subjected to centrifugation; and monitored at 280 nm during fractionation. Panel A shows the amount of trichloroacetic acid (TCA) precipitable ^{3}H-thymidine present in each fraction; Panel B shows the amount of infectivity present in each fraction of the second gradient. Further details of these experiments are presented elsewhere [17]. (Data are from Irmiere and Gibson [17].)

explained if additional matrix protein were associated with the viral DNA or otherwise required for its incorporation into the particle. It could also be accounted for by volumetric considerations if the NIEP assembly protein occupies space in the particle that would otherwise contain matrix protein.

Consistent with their apparently simpler architectural organization (Fig. 1:2C), and earlier reports of an altered protein composition compared with virions [13–15], at least 90% of the dense body protein mass was accounted for by the lower (69K) matrix protein (Fig. 3A).

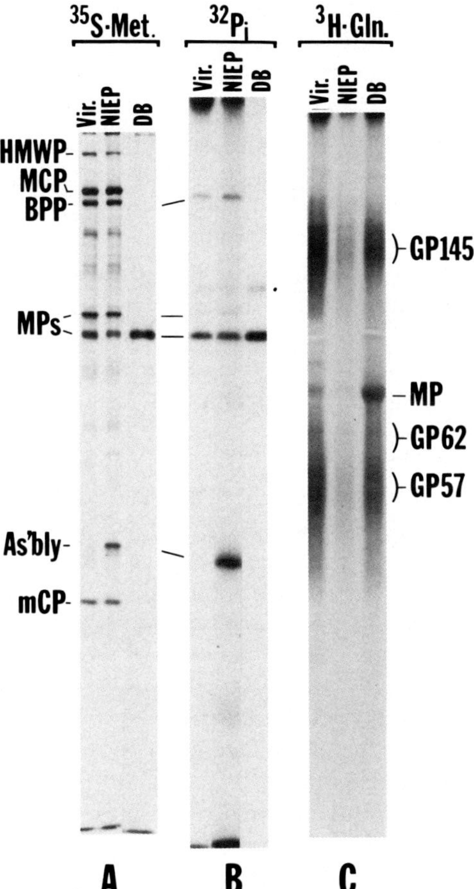

Fig. 3. Protein constituents of HCMV virions (Vir.), NIEPs, and dense bodies (DB) were recovered from the media [19] of infected cultures radiolabeled using 35S-methionine (Panel A), 32P-orthophosphate (Panel B), or 3H-glucosamine (Panel C). Shown here are fluorographic images of 10% polyacrylamide gels (Panels B and C) containing the protein constituents of these particles. The gel in Panel A was cross-linked with a higher-than-usual amount of bis-acrylamide to resolve the MCP and BPP [17]. Abbreviations and estimated molecular weights are as follows: high molecular weight protein (HMWP, 212K), major capsid protein (MCP, 153K), basic phosphoprotein (BPP, 150K), matrix proteins (MPs, 74K and 69K), assembly protein (As'bly, 35K), minor capsid protein (mCP, 34K) and three glycoproteins (GP). Dot in the margin adjacent to Panel B indicates the position of the 80K protein. (Data in Panel A are from Irmiere and Gibson [17].)

NIEP and Dense Body Proteins Modified Like Virion Proteins

We have also determined that NIEP and dense body proteins are phosphorylated and glycosylated similarly to their virion counterparts (Fig. 3B,C). Virions contain two predominant (ie, 150K basic phosphoprotein and 69K matrix protein) and at least two minor (ie, 80K protein, see dot Panel B, and 74K matrix protein) phosphorylated proteins [17, 24, 25]. The NIEP phosphoprotein pattern is similar to that of virions but distinguished by the presence of the highly labeled assembly protein band. Dense bodies contain only two of these four protein species (ie, 80K and 69K matrix protein), and both are phosphorylated. No differences were detected in the pattern of phosphorylation of counterpart proteins from NIEPs, virions and dense bodies, when their tryptic peptides were compared by two-dimensional (electrophoresis-chromatography) separation (Stader and Gibson, unpublished observations).

NIEPs and dense bodies were also found to contain all of the glycosylated species present in virions (Fig. 3C). These have broad size ranges centering around 145,000 (GP145), 62,000 (GP62) and 57,000 (GP57). This similarity in glycoprotein content is compatible with the fact that all three particle types are enveloped (Fig. 1:2A-C), and the likelihood that these glycoproteins are envelope constituents. It is noteworthy that the glycoprotein pattern of HCMV virions is much less well defined than those of many other enveloped viruses, including herpes simplex [26, 27] and strain Colburn CMV [24]. This observation has been made by others [13, 14] but, while suggestive of a comparatively greater degree of heterogeneity in the carbohydrates added, remains unexplained. Parenthetically, it should be emphasized that the size heterogeneity of HCMV glycoproteins can present a complicating factor in their purification or separation from other proteins based on sizing techniques alone (eg, gel filtration chromatography; SDS-polyacrylamide gel electrophoresis). Additionally, long-term radiolabeling with ^{3}H-glucosamine (eg, 5 days) frequently results in the incorporation of the radioisotope into other proteins. We suspect that such radiolabeling is due to metabolism and reutilization of the ^{3}H-glucosamine since: 1) the specific activities (radioactivity/staining) of these other proteins are much lower than those of the three bands provisionally designated as glycoproteins (ie, GP145, GP62, GP57). 2) The radiographic intensities of these additional bands closely parallel the amount of protein present, as would be expected if the radioisotope were present in the form of amino acids. And, 3) most prominent among the additional labeled bands are the highly abundant major capsid protein and the two matrix proteins, all of which are structurally internal, nonenvelope constituents (Fig. 7).

NIEPs and Dense Bodies Contain Protein Kinase Activity

Although NIEPs and dense bodies lack DNA, and consequently infectivity, they may contain other biologically active components. Since we and others have found a protein kinase activity present in HCMV virions [25], it was of interest to establish whether the two noninfectious particles also contained this activity. For this purpose, preparations of highly purified particles were disrupted using NP40 and incubated in the presence of γ-^{32}P-ATP, as described in the legend to Figure 4. Results of this experiment demonstrate that all three particles contain the phosphorylating activity. Further, with the notable exception of the NIEP assembly protein, the protein species phosphorylated biosynthetically (Fig. 3B) were also the principal phosphate acceptors in vitro. The presence of this enzyme in dense bodies, which lack a nucleocapsid and at least two of the tegument proteins (ie, 150K basic phosphoprotein and 74K matrix protein), suggests that it is an envelope or tegument constituent (Roby and Gibson, manuscript in preparation).

Enrichment for NIEPs

NIEPs are produced by all HCMV strains tested, including laboratory prototypes and fresh isolates, and are usually present in about 5% to 10% the amount of virions. Strain AD169 is an exception in that it produces nearly tenfold more NIEPs than the other strains (Fig. 5). The reason for this overproduction is not established, but the altered assembly protein of AD169 offers an attractive explanation [17].

Since NIEPs lack DNA, it was reasoned that inhibitors of DNA synthesis might have a comparatively greater inhibitory effect on the biogenesis of virions. This possibility was tested as follows. Three days after infection with HCMV (after the onset of viral DNA synthesis), the medium in three cultures was replaced with fresh medium containing either no drug, hydroxyurea (50 μg/ml), or phosphonoformate (200 μg/ml). Five days later, the culture media were analyzed for their virus particle content by rate-velocity sedimentation. Results of this experiment are shown in Figure 6 and demonstrate that hydroxyurea, while reducing the amount of virions and dense bodies by over 95%, had no negative effect on NIEP production. Results using phosphonoformate were similar, but less dramatic in the sense that some reduction in NIEP production was also noted. We have not investigated the effect that varying these drug concentrations, or the time of their addition, may have on the relative virus particle yields.

Surface Proteins of the Virion

As interest and technology move toward the isolation or synthesis of specific proteins or peptides for use as vaccines against CMV, it will be

Fig. 4. HCMV virions (Vir.), NIEPs, and dense bodies (DB) contain protein kinase activity. Virions, NIEPs, and dense bodies were recovered from the medium [19] of cells infected with AD169, and assayed in vitro for protein kinase activity. Reaction conditions were: 0.1% NP40, 10 mM DTT, 20 mM $MgCl_2$, 1-5 μCi γ-^{32}P-ATP, 50 mM Tris, pH 8.0; 24°C × 60 min. Shown here is a fluorogram prepared from a 10% polyacrylamide gel containing the electrophoretically separated proteins. Abbreviations are as in Fig. 3.

increasingly important to identify biologically relevant viral antigens. Among the first to be considered in this regard are the virion envelope proteins. Efforts to define them by direct analysis of the architectural organization of the HCMV virion, however, have been hampered by two factors. First, when mild nonionic detergents (ie, 0.5% NP40) were used in an attempt to strip away the envelope structure — a procedure used successfully with other herpesviruses (eg, HSV, EBV) — it was observed that the virion nucleocapsid was also disrupted ([23] and Irmiere and Gibson, unpublished observations,

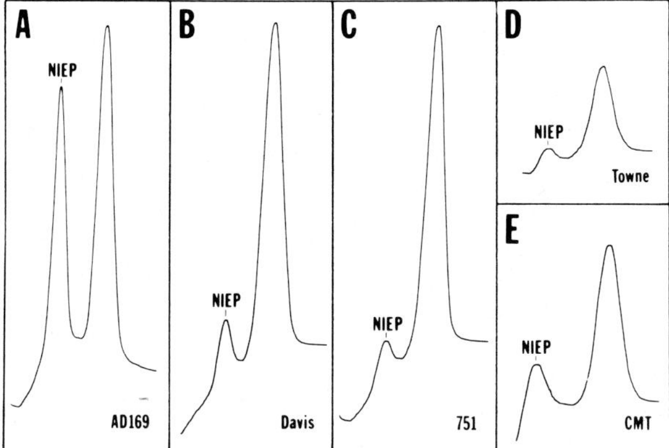

Fig. 5. AD169 overproduces NIEPs. Media from cultures infected with HCMV strain AD169, Davis, Towne, 751, or CMT-6 were subjected to rate-velocity sedimentation and the gradients scanned at 280 nm. Shown here are the resulting absorbance profiles. (Data are from Irmiere and Gibson [17].)

using HCMV virions and NIEPs). Second, we have not had good success in obtaining nonenveloped intracellular capsids in good yield and purity from HCMV-infected human foreskin fibroblast (HFF) cells. Since such subvirion particles can be recovered from Colburn (simian-like isolate)-infected cells, we have studied its structural organization as an alternative [23]. These findings were subsequently extended to HCMV by establishing counterpart proteins in the two systems [24]. Figure 7 summarizes aspects of that work pertinent to this paper. It shows that HCMV virions contain 1) two capsid proteins which are neither phosphorylated nor glycosylated, 2) at least four tegument proteins, three of which are phosphorylated (ie, BPP, MP74, MP69), and 3) several envelope proteins, at least three of which are glycosylated (ie, GP145, GP62 and GP57). This figure also demonstrates that the protein patterns of five HCMV strains, including three laboratory prototypes (ie, Towne, Davis, AD169) and two recent isolates (ie, 751, CMT-6) were very similar. Only two consistent variations in mobility were noted. One of these was in the glycoprotein designated GP62, and the other was in a diffuse band designated as the 39K protein.

Since the surface glycoproteins of enveloped viruses are commonly important targets of the immune response, they are of particular interest. We have found, however, that two of the principal HCMV glycoproteins are not easily detected in preparations radiolabeled with amino acids and separated by size alone (ie, GP145, GP57, Fig. 7). Therefore, we further examined

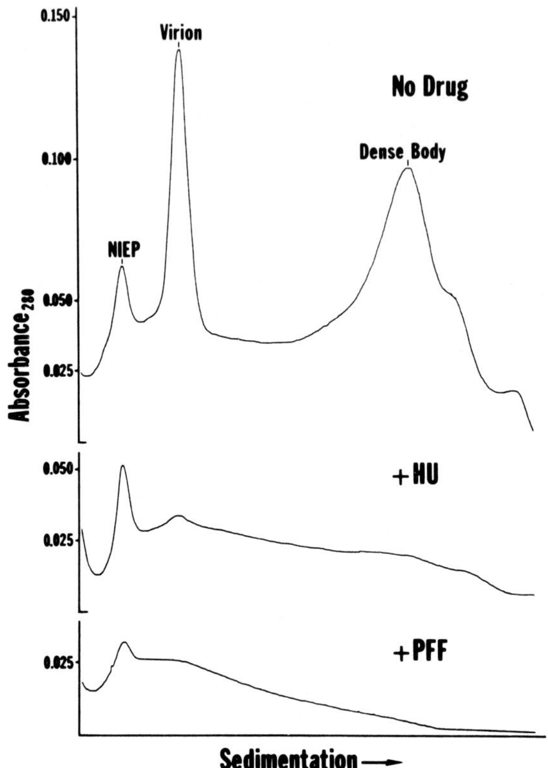

Fig. 6. Selective enrichment for NIEPs using inhibitors of DNA synthesis. Cultures were infected with AD169 and treated with hydroxyurea (HU) or phosphonoformate (PFF) as described in the text. Shown here are optical absorbance (280 nm) profiles of gradients [19] containing the virus particles shed into the media.

these proteins using ^{3}H-glucosamine as the label and two-dimensional (charge-size) separation for their resolution. Figure 8 presents the results of such an experiment and shows more clearly that HCMV virions contain one comparatively narrow glycosylated band (ie, GP62, channel "b") which resolved into a series of six discrete spots following two-dimensional separation, and two very broad zones (ie, GP145, GP57). It can be seen that GP145 and GP57, in addition to being more heterogeneous in size than GP62, are more acidic in net charge. Further, the relative fluorographic intensities of the ^{3}H-glucosamine and ^{35}S-methionine labeled proteins indicate that GP145 and GP57 have a higher ratio of carbohydrate to protein mass than GP62 (compare left- and right-hand panels).

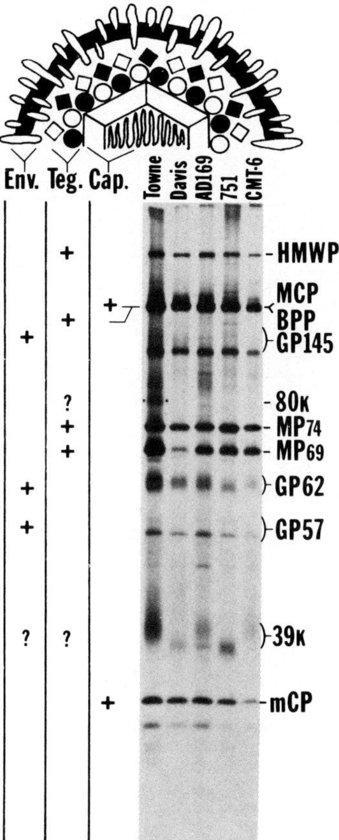

Fig. 7. Strain comparison and hypothetical organization of major HCMV virion proteins. Virions labeled with ^{14}C-amino acids were recovered from the medium of cells infected with HCMV strains Towne, Davis, AD169, 751, or CMT-6. Shown here is a fluorogram prepared from a 10% polyacrylamide gel (MCP and BPP not resolved as in Fig. 3A). Architectural locations are assigned based on comparative studies using strain Colburn [23, 24]. Protein abbreviations are as in Fig. 3; others are envelope (Env.), tegument (Teg.) and capsid (Cap.).

While logic and precedent with other enveloped viruses suggest that the CMV virion glycoproteins will play an important role in eliciting the immune response, the involvement of additional virion and nonvirion proteins and antigens must also be evaluated. In particular, it will be important to better define the role of CMI in limiting CMV disease, and determine which antigens serve to establish and maintain this response. Of interest in this regard is the observation by Middeldorp et al (this volume, abstract) that

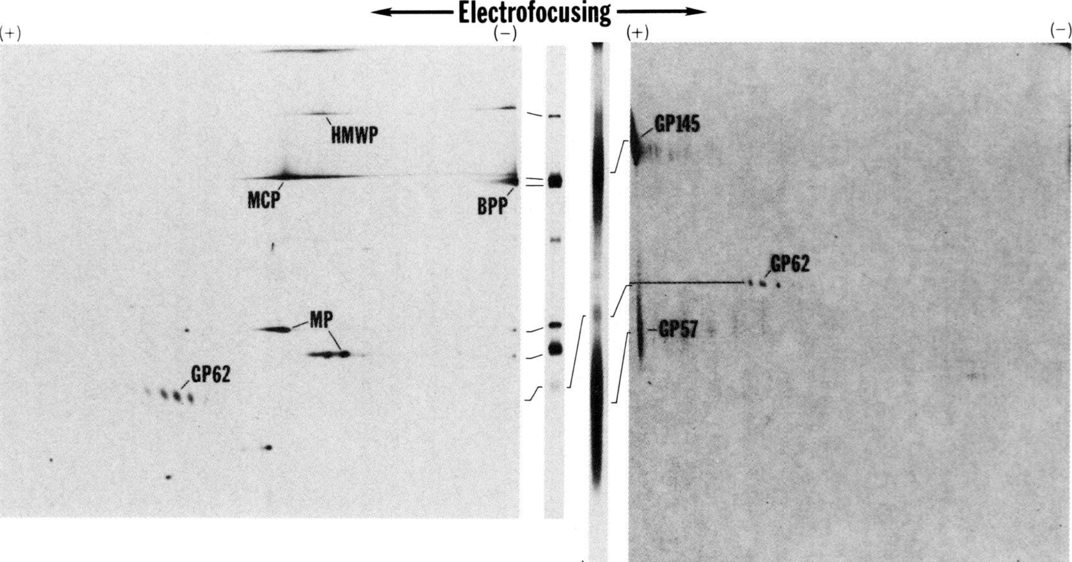

Fig. 8.   Virion glycoproteins of HCMV. Strain 751 HCMV virions, radiolabeled with either ^{35}S-methionine or ^{3}H-glucosamine, were subjected to one- and two- dimensional separation in denaturing polyacrylamide gels. Shown here are the resulting fluorographic images. The center channels "a" (^{35}S-methionine) and "b" (^{3}H-glucosamine) were from 7.5% and 10% polyacrylamide gels, respectively. Abbreviations are as in Fig. 3. (Data are from Gibson [24].)

immune memory to "early membrane antigen(s)" of HCMV can be demonstrated using lymphocytes from some seronegative donors. In addition, we have found that, whereas the highly abundant 69K matrix protein is a comparatively poor immunogen in the humoral response (Weiner and Gibson, unpublished observations), it appears to serve as a potent mitogen in eliciting a secondary CMI response in vitro (Converse, Donnenberg, Sheridan and Gibson, unpublished observations). And finally, we have recently found that the virion basic phosphoprotein, a putative tegument constituent, is immunologically highly reactive when electrotransferred to nitrocellulose and assayed using plasma from individuals with AIDS (Fig. 9). This reactivity is present at a greatly reduced level in other CMV seropositive individuals (eg, Fig. 9, "Uganda"; bone marrow transplant recipients, not shown), and absent from CMV seronegative individuals (eg, Fig. 9, "Norm."). We do not yet know whether the specificity and magnitude of this particular response is peculiar to AIDS patients. However, the observation does emphasize the importance of using a variety of assay procedures and sources of antigen in attempting to assess which CMV proteins are immunologically relevant.

Other Proteins of Potential Diagnostic and Therapeutic Interest

Within the infected cell only a small number of virus-specific proteins are present in comparatively large amounts (Fig. 10). Among these 1) the 153K "major capsid protein" is the principal structural element of the virion's icosahedral capsid; 2) the 69K matrix protein appears to interface the virion capsid structure with the outer envelope, and accounts for over 90% of the dense body protein mass, 3) the 53K DNA-binding protein is synthesized earlier than most other viral proteins, binds to DNA, is basic in net charge and phosphorylated, 4) the 35K assembly protein is a constituent of the B-capsid putative assembly intermediate, and is thought to play a role in DNA packaging and/or nucleocapsid envelopment, and 5) the 34K minor capsid protein is the second of three proteins that form the elementary capsid structure. (For details, see [23, 24, 28, 29]).

An antiserum prepared to "detergent-stripped" nuclei that contained these proteins, such as shown in Figure 10, was found to be highly reactive with infected cells (Fig. 11A) and without reactivity toward noninfected cells. The pattern of fluorescence was coincident with the intranuclear inclusions which are pathognomic for HCMV infection. Immunoprecipitation and electrotransfer-nitrocellulose immunoassays [30] showed that this serum reacted primarily with the major capsid and DNA-binding proteins (Weiner and Gibson, unpublished observations). Development of immunodiagnostic reagents with

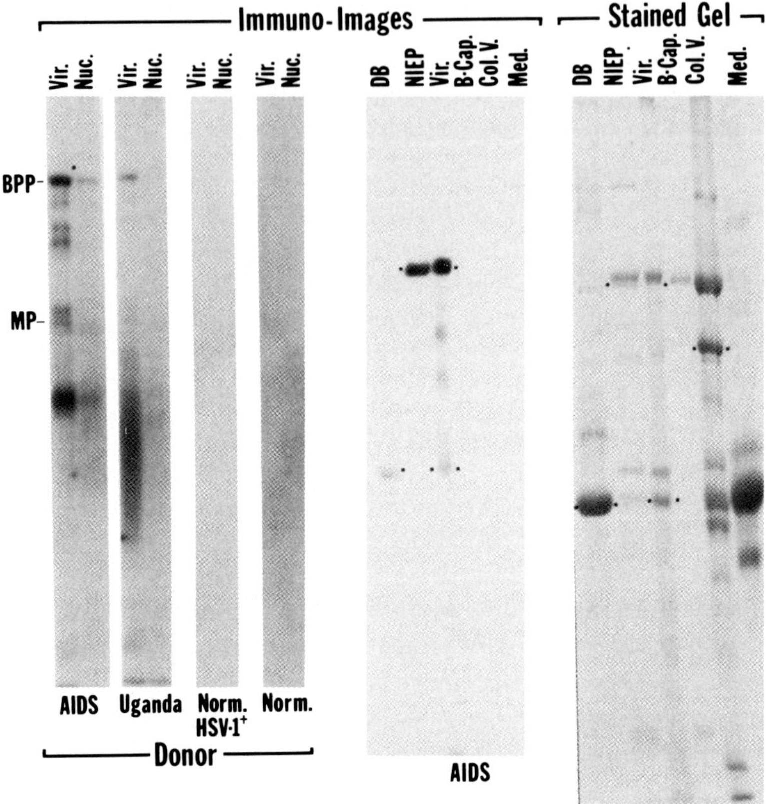

Fig. 9. Immunoassay of HCMV virion proteins following electrotransfer to nitrocellulose. Left-Hand Panel: HCMV virions (Vir.) and the nuclear fraction (Nuc.) of infected cells were subjected to electrophoresis in a 10% polyacrylamide gel; electrotransferred to nitrocellulose [30, 33]; and immunoassayed [34] using plasma from an AIDS patient and sera from 1) a seropositive male from Uganda, 2) a known HSV 1-seropositive male, and 3) a CMV-seronegative male. Abbreviations are as in Fig. 3; dot above BPP indicates position of MCP. Middle Panel: Six preparations were subjected to electrophoresis in a 7.5% polyacrylamide gel; electrotransferred to nitrocellulose; and immunoassayed using plasma from an AIDS patient. Dots indicate the positions of corresponding BPP (top) and MP (lower) bands in this and the right-hand panel. Abbreviations: AD169 dense bodies (DB), NIEPs and virions (Vir.); strain Colburn B-capsids (B-Cap.) and virions (Col. V); and medium from noninfected cells (Med.) Right-Hand Panel: A replicate set (same gel) of the preparations subjected to immunoassay in the middle panel was stained with Coomassie brilliant blue. Dots beside DB, NIEP and Vir. channels indicate the positions of the BPP and MP (69K) revealed by immunoassay; dots beside Col. V. channel indicate position of Colburn BPP (ie, 119K). Abbreviations are as in middle panel. Left-hand and middle panels show fluorographic images; right-hand panel shows proteins present in preparations immunoassayed in adjacent panel.

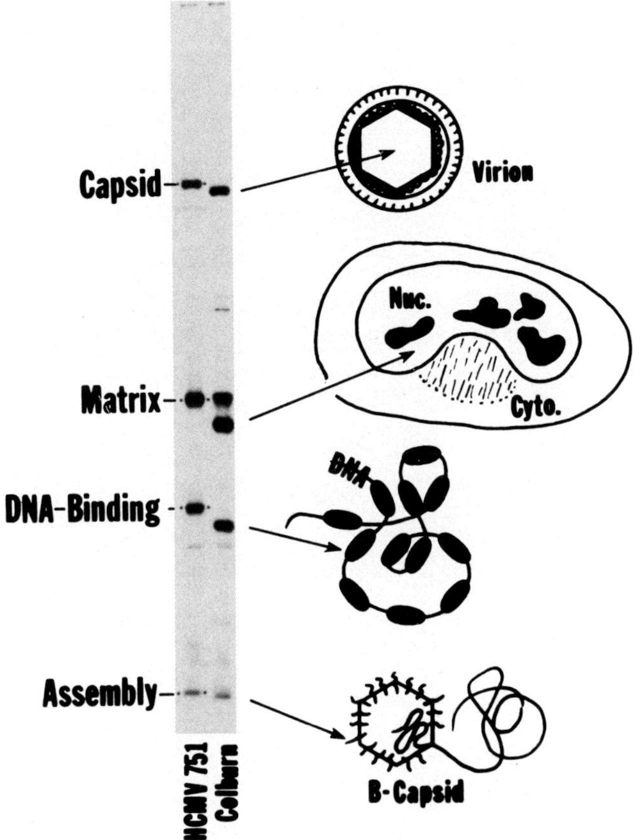

Fig. 10. Predominant intracellular CMV proteins. Cells were infected with either strain Colburn or HCMV strain 751; radiolabeled using ^{35}S-methionine; and separated into nuclear and cytoplasmic fractions using 0.5% NP40 [23]. The resulting "NP40 nuclei" were further treated with a mixture of deoxycholate and Tween 40 [35] to remove cytoplasmic "tags," and the proteins were separated in a 7.5% polyacrylamide gel. Shown here is a fluorographic image of the resulting gel. The functional designations indicated for these proteins in the left-hand margin, and their hypothetical involvement during infection shown on the right, are based on comparative studies of different HCMV isolates, two simian CMV isolates, and strain Colburn, as described elsewhere [24].

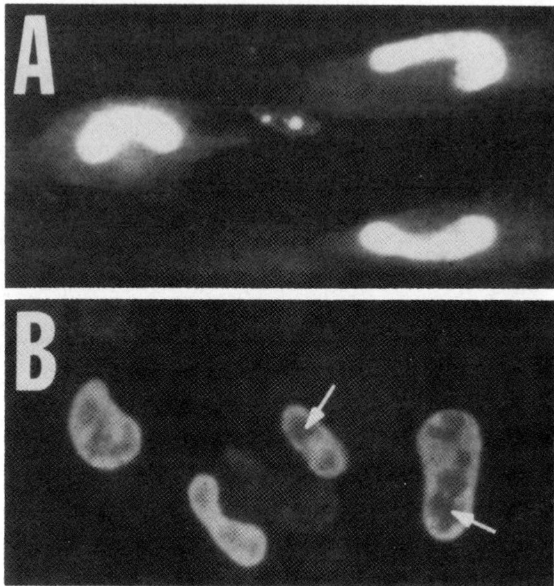

Fig. 11. Localization of viral proteins by anti-complement immune fluorescence. Three days following infection with HCMV strain 751, cells were fixed with acetone (-20°) and incubated with guinea pig antiserum prepared using 1) infected-cell nuclei that had been prepared by sequential treatment using NP40 and deoxycholate/Tween-40 as described in the legend to Fig. 10 (Panel A), or 2) SDS gel-purified HCMV 69K matrix protein, obtained from nuclei treated as above to eliminate comigrating glycoprotein contaminants (Panel B). To avoid the problem of nonspecific Fc receptor binding, the distribution of bound antibody was visualized by subsequently treating the slides with guinea pig complement followed by fluorescein-conjugated goat anti-guinea pig complement (ACIF [36]). Arrows point to nonstained intranuclear inclusions.

specificity for these two proteins would seem promising for the following reasons. 1) Both are present in large amounts in the cell and, therefore, should be easier to detect than low abundance species. 2) Synthesis of the DNA-binding protein requires preceding viral protein and DNA synthesis, but begins prior to that of many other CMV proteins. Thus, it provides a marker for the expression of a temporally more intermediate function that may also appear in nonlytic infections (eg, latency). And, 3) based on the results of studies using monospecific antisera to the counterpart proteins of strain Colburn (Roby and Gibson, unpublished observations, and [29]), it is probable that antisera to these HCMV proteins will be both CMV group-specific, and broadly cross-reactive among the primate CMVs.

Another antiserum prepared using purified HCMV matrix protein (69K) proved useful in demonstrating the nuclear compartmentalization of this species (Fig. 11B). However, the fact that this protein is less immunogenic than the others (Weiner and Gibson, unpublished observations), and appears to be localized in the nucleoplasm rather than the pathognomic nuclear inclusions (see arrows), suggests that it has less potential for immunodiagnosis than the two mentioned above. On the other hand, since there is immunologic evidence that the amino acid sequence of the matrix protein may be evolutionarily less well conserved than that of some of the other viral proteins (Zaia et al, this volume, abstract; Weiner and Gibson, unpublished observations, and [29]), it may be of value in further evaluating the antigenic relatedness of different HCMV isolates.

SUMMARY

Uncertainties about the ultimate biologic consequences of using live virus vaccines to confer immunologic protection against CMV have focused attention on the use of noninfectious subunit vaccines. At least two classes of such preparations have been demonstrated to be effective in other systems. The first is virus particles bearing the relevant antigens but lacking nucleic acid (eg, hepatitis vaccine [31]). And the second class is biologically or chemically synthesized proteins or peptides with appropriate immunogenicity (eg, foot and mouth disease virus vaccine [32]). In this paper, two noninfectious CMV particles and several viral proteins have been discussed in view of their potential for use as such a vaccine.

The two noninfectious virus particles discussed are referred to as dense bodies and NIEPs. The use of dense bodies for vaccine purposes has been suggested by others [14], but the simplicity of their composition has only recently been established [17]. Two characteristics of these particles make them attractive prospects for vaccine purposes. First, neither contains more than trace amounts of DNA or infectivity (ie, $\leqslant 0.1\%$ that of virions). Thus, the concerns about possible adverse consequences of introducing DNA with the vaccine are greatly reduced. Second, both NIEPs and dense bodies contain all of the glycoprotein species present in virions and in approximately the same relative amounts. If, as anticipated, these proteins are important in eliciting the immune response to CMV, then NIEPs and dense bodies may be as effective as virions in that capacity. The fact that NIEPs contain the full complement of virion proteins, and in approximately the same relative amounts, suggests that they may produce a more complete immunologic response than dense bodies, which lack all of the capsid and most of the tegument proteins of the virion.

Although NIEPs normally represent only a small percentage of the extra-cellular particles (eg, < 1%), we have found that strain AD169 produces them in amounts nearly equivalent to virions. More importantly, we have shown here that NIEP production is essentially unaffected following treatment of infected cells with a concentration of hydroxyurea that reduced virion and dense body production by more than 90% (Fig. 6). Thus, by using strain AD169 to infect cells and hydroxyurea treatment for selective enrichment, it is possible to produce NIEPs in relatively large amounts and with theoretically very low levels of contaminating virions (ie, ≤ 0.01% infectivity of equivalent amount of virions). Such preparations of NIEPs (or dense bodies) could be treated subsequently to eliminate this trace contamination with viral DNA. And finally, in assessing the suitability of these particles for vaccination purposes, the significance of the fact that they contain other biologically active molecules (eg, protein kinase [25]; Fig. 4; Roby and Gibson, manuscript in preparation) must be evaluated.

Studies to better define the role of specific CMV proteins during infection, and establish which ones are immunologically relevant, should aid efforts to produce purified protein and synthetic peptide subunit vaccines. Perhaps foremost among the proteins of interest in this connection are the glycosylated species. While it is feasible to use monospecific sera (eg, monoclonal antibodies) to recover such proteins directly from infected cells, the problem of contaminating virions and viral DNA will again have to be eliminated. The production of viral glycoproteins in bacteria transfected with appropriate viral genes would avoid this difficulty, and be a logical beginning for the application of recent technology to CMV vaccine production. Compatible with previous descriptions of HCMV virion glycoproteins [13, 37], our results show three major glycosylated protein species, two of which behaved as if their carbohydrate moieties were very heterogeneous in number and/or structure [24] (Fig. 8). If this interpretation is correct and if their carbohydrate side chains play a significant immunogenic role, then production of immunologically active forms of these glycoproteins may require the use of eukaryotic cells rather than bacteria or some other system lacking the appropriate glycosylation pathway. Nevertheless, these procedures, in conjunction with further developments in the area of in vitro protein modification, offer the promise of biologically safe, chemically well-defined vaccines.

ACKNOWLEDGMENTS

We thank our colleagues Clint Roby and Diana Weiner for the use of their unpublished data shown in Figures 4 and 11; Bill Burns, Tom Quinn, and

Laure Aurelian for supplying human serum and plasma samples used in the experiment summarized in Figure 9; and Louise Flannery for typing the manuscript.

REFERENCES

1. Jenner E (1978): An inquiry into the causes and effects of the variolae vaccinae, a disease discovered in some of the western counties of England, particularly Gloucestershire, and known by the name of cow pox', reprinted by Cassel, 1896 (Pamphlet Vol. 4232, Army Med. Lib., Wash., D.C.).

2. Elek SD, Stern H: Development of a vaccine against mental retardation caused by cytomegalovirus infection *in utero*. Lancet 1:1-5, 1974.

3. Plotkin SA, Farquhar J, Hornberger E: Clinical trials of immunization with the Towne 125 strain of human cytomegalovirus. J Infect Dis 134:470, 1976.

4. Plotkin SA: 1979. Vaccination against herpes group viruses, in particular cytomegalovirus. In Falkner F, Kretchmer N, Rossi E (eds): "Monographs in Paediatrics." Basel: Karger, 1979, vol 11, pp 58-74.

5. Gehrz RC, Christianson WR, Linner KM, Groth KE, Balfour HH: Cytomegalovirus vaccine: Specific humoral and cellular immune responses in human volunteers. Arch Intern Med 140:936-939, 1980.

6. Plotkin SA, Furukawa T, Zygraich N, Huygelen C: Candidate cytomegalovirus strain for human vaccination. Infect Immun 12:521-527, 1975.

7. Luse SA, Smith MG: Electron microscopy of salivary gland viruses. J Exp Med 107:623-632, 1958.

8. McGavran MH, Smith MG: Ultrastructural, cytochemical, and microchemical observations on cytomegalovirus (salivary gland virus) infection of human cells in tissue culture. Exp Mol Pathol 4:1-10, 1965.

9. Patrizi G, Middlecamp JN, Herweg JC, Thornton HK: Human cytomegalovirus. Electron microscopy of a primary viral isolate. J Lab Clin Med 65:825-838, 1965.

10. Ruebner BH, Hirano T, Slusser RJ, Medearis DN Jr: Human cytomegalovirus infection. Electron microscopic and histochemical changes in cultures of human fibroblasts. Am J Pathol 46:477-496, 1965.

11. Craighead JE, Kanich RE Almeida JD: Nonviral microbodies with viral antigenicity produced in cytomegalovirus-infected cells. J Virol 10:766-775, 1972.

12. Stinski MF: Human cytomegalovirus: Glycoproteins associated with virions and dense bodies. J Virol 19:594-609, 1976.

13. Kim KS, Sapienza RI, Carp RI, Moon HM: Analysis of structural polypeptides of purified human cytomegalovirus. J Virol 20:604-611, 1976.

14. Sarov I, Abady I: The morphogenesis of human cytomegalovirus. Isolation and polypeptide characterization of cytomegalovirions and dense bodies. Virology 66:464-473, 1975.

15. Fiala M, Honess RW, Heiner DC, Heine JW Jr, Murnane J, Wallace R, Guze LB: Cytomegalovirus proteins. I. Polypeptides of virions and dense bodies. J Virol 19:243-254, 1976.

16. Kanich RE, Craighead JE: Human cytomegalovirus infection of cultured fibroblasts. II. Viral replicative sequence of a wild and an adapted strain. Lab Invest 27:273-282, 1972.

17. Irmiere AF, Gibson W: Isolation and characterization of a noninfectious virion-like particle released from cells infected with human strains of cytomegalovirus. Virology 130:118-133, 1983.

18. Barzilai R, Lazarus LH, Goldblum N: Viscosity-density gradient for purification of foot-and-mouth disease virus. Arch Ges Virusforsch 36:141-146, 1972.

19. Talbot P, Almeida JD: Human cytomegalovirus: Purification of enveloped virions and dense bodies. J Gen Virol 36:345-349, 1977.

20. Gibson W, Roizman B: Proteins specified by herpes simplex virus. VIII. Characterization and composition of multiple capsid forms of subtypes 1 and 2. J Virol 10:1044-1052, 1972.

21. Gibson W, Roizman B: Proteins specified by herpes simplex virus. X. Staining and radiolabeling properties of B-capsid and virion proteins in polyacrylamide gels. J Virol 13:155-165, 1974.

22. Heilman C Jr, Zweig M, Hampar B: Herpes simplex virus type 1 and 2 intracellular p40: Type-specific and cross-reactive antigenic determinants on peptides generated by partial proteolysis. J Virol 40:508-515, 1981.

23. Gibson W: Structural and nonstructural proteins of strain Colburn cytomegalovirus. Virology 111:516-537, 1981.

24. Gibson W: Protein counterparts of human and simian cytomegaloviruses. Virology 128:391-406, 1983.

25. Mar E -C, Patel PC, Huang E -S: Human cytomegalovirus-associated DNA polymerase and protein kinase activities. J Gen Virol 57:149-156, 1981.

26. Heine JW, Honess RW, Cassai E, Roizman B: Proteins specified by herpes simplex virus. XII. The virion polypeptides of type 1 strains. J Virol 14:640-651, 1974.

27. Norrild B: Immunochemistry of herpes simplex virus glycoproteins. In Arber W et al (eds): "Current Topics in Microbiology and Immunology." New York: Springer-Verlag, 1980, vol 90, pp 67-106.

28. Gibson W, Murphy TL, Roby C: Cytomegalovirus-infected cells contain a DNA-binding protein. Virology 111:251-262, 1981.

29. Weiner D, Gibson W: Identification of a primate CMV group-common protein antigen. Virology 115:182-191, 1981.

30. Towbin H, Staehelin T, Gordon J: Electrophoretic transfer of proteins from polyacrylamide gels to nitrocellulose sheets: Procedure and some applications. Proc Natl Acad Sci USA 76:4350-4354, 1979.

31. Buynak EB, Roehm RR, Tytell AA, Bertland AU II, Lampson GP, Hilleman MR: Vaccine against human hepatitis B. JAMA 235:2832, 1976.

32. Bittle JL, Houghton RA, Alexander H, Shinnick TM, Sutcliffe JG, Lerner RA, Rowlands DJ, Brown F: Protection against foot-and-mouth disease by immunization with a chemically synthesized peptide predicted from the viral nucleotide sequence. Nature 298:30, 1982.

33. Gibson W: Protease-facilitated transfer of high-molecular-weight proteins during electrotransfer to nitrocellulose. Anal Biochem 118:1-3, 1981.

34. Burnette WN: "Western blotting": Electrophoretic transfer of proteins from SDS-polyacrylamide gels to unmodified nitrocellulose and radiographic detection with antibody and radioiodinated protein A. Anal Biochem 112:195-203, 1981.

35. Penman S: RNA metabolism in the HeLa cell nucleus. J Mol Biol 17:131-135, 1966.

36. Kettering JD, Schmidt NJ, Gallo D, Lennette E: Anti-complement immunofluorescence test for antibodies to human cytomegalovirus. J Clin Microbiol 6:627-632, 1977.

37. Stinski M: Synthesis of proteins and glycoproteins in cells infected with human cytomegalovirus. J Virol 23:751-767, 1977.

SECTION 5:
PASSIVE IMMUNIZATION AND ANTIVIRALS

Prevention of Cytomegalovirus Infection in Bone Marrow Transplant Recipients by Prophylaxis With an Intravenous, Hyperimmune Cytomegalovirus Globulin

Richard M. Condie, PhD,* and Richard J. O'Reilly, MD[†]

Department of Surgery, University of Minnesota School of Medicine, Minneapolis, MN 55455 (R.M.C.); The Memorial Sloan-Kettering Cancer Center, New York, NY 10021 (R.J.O'R.)

CMV infection and related disease are the most serious infectious problems in patients receiving allogeneic marrow transplants as treatment for leukemia. Interstitial pneumonia constitutes the most devastating complication of marrow transplantation and is the principal contributor to the 40% early mortality in this patient group [1–3]. CMV is the most frequently isolated pathogen, accounting for more than 50% of cases in published studies [2]. This means that prevention of CMV infection would markedly alter the prospects for a more successful outcome of BMT.

Strategies for both treatment and prevention have included prophylactic administration of IFN [4], ara-A [5], ara-C [6], acyclovir (H. Balfour, personal communication, and [7]), and transfer factor (TF) [8]. All have failed to alter the incidence or severity of CMV infections in marrow transplant recipients. Since CMV infection in this population not only results from reactivation of latent virus [9], but also from exogenous infections from blood products [9], the use of blood products from antibody-negative donors has been used to reduce transmission of CMV in newborns [10] and could

*Supported by USPHS grant AM 13083.

†Supported by USPHS grants, CA-08748, CA-23766.

Birth Defects: Original Article Series, Volume 20, Number 1, pages 327–344
© **1984 March of Dimes Birth Defects Foundation**

well reduce the incidence in BMT recipients. CMV vaccine has been considered and studies are in progress with renal transplant recipients. The use of vaccine in BMT is not feasible since the conditioning regimen of whole body irradiation creates an "immunologic virgin"; thus, the vaccine would probably be of questionable benefit.

Prevention or modification of what would otherwise be a lethal CMV infection in immunosuppressed patients by passive administration of specific CMV antibodies was considered by us [11–13] and others [14, 15] to be an approach worth developing, particularly in light of the failures of other strategies.

The clinical history of CMV infections in the immunocompetent, immunologically mature individuals poses no problems, and, in fact, goes unnoticed; virtually all human beings become infected with CMV at some point in their lives. However, in the allograft recipient, treatments designed to promote graft acceptance, prevent graft rejection, and treat GVHD do so by virtue of suppression of cellular immunity. All these treatments clearly predispose to CMV infections. CMV-related mortality in the transplant recipient is directly related to the degree of immunosuppression required with the lowest mortality in renal transplant recipients (2%) and the highest (40%) in the BMT recipient.

It is clear that T-cell immunity is the major host defense in CMV infection in the immunologically mature, immunocompetent individual [16, 17]. The role of humoral immunity has been considered to be of minor importance [18, 19]. However, in the BMT recipient, passive anti-CMV antibodies might well tip the balance in favor of survival and are worth careful consideration and evaluation.

If a case for passive seroprophylaxis were to be made, it must also deal with a certain body of nonsupportive clinical observations. These include the possibility that passive antibodies could play a potentiating role in CMV disease [20] in the presence of depressed cellular immunity. Fragmentation or reduction and alkylation of neutralizing antibody can result in an antibody-coated virus protected against neutralizing antibody [21–23]. These modifications of the antibody molecule also significantly reduce the circulatory half-life of passive Igs and would therefore be contraindicated [24]. Finally, recent reports indicate the IgG subclass composition to be important. These studies show that of the four human IgG subclasses, the anti-herpesvirus neutralizing activity resides predominantly, if not exclusively, in the IgG_3 subclass [25, 26].

In BMT recipients, CMV-related mortality correlates significantly with a negative or fall in posttransplant CMV CF antibody titer [27]. Patients with a rise in CF antibody posttransplant have a more favorable outcome [27, 28]. Clinical experience at three BMT centers corroborates the positive role for CMV antibody rise (unpublished observations). It is, therefore, reasonable to suggest that while CMV antibody may not prevent CMV infection, it could hopefully reduce both the severity and CMV-related mortality. Animal studies likewise support a protective role for antibody. These reports clearly demonstrate that passive CMV antibody protects against otherwise lethal doses of CMV [29, 30]. Finally, there are single case reports where passive serotherapy has been utilized to treat CMV infections in immunocompromised individuals. These include administration of hyperimmune CMV plasma to a renal transplant recipient [31], IM immune serum globulin (ISG) to a hypogammaglobulinemic with CMV infection [32], and ISG to a patient with chronic CMV bowel disease [33]. We, in an early noncontrolled trial, treated renal transplant recipients in the terminal stages of CMV disease with intravenous IgG made from pooled normal human plasma, and observed a temporal relationship between IgG administration and clinical improvement [11].

During the planning for this trial we defined properties that would be required of suitable clinical hyperimmune globulin preparations [12, 24]. These specifically included: 1) safety for IV administration at high dosage—low anticomplementary activity, less than 1% aggregates, negative for plasmin activity, negative for hepatitis B antigen, and positive for hepatitis B antibody; 2) native, unmodified, intact IgG molecules including all four subclasses—less than 1% fragments; 3) the same circulatory half-life as native IgG—18 days; and 4) a preparation in which the biologic neutralizing activity had been isolated and significantly concentrated over the starting plasma. We were successful in achieving all but the subclass composition. The IV hyperimmune CMV IgG used in our controlled, randomized trial lacked the IgG_3 subclass [12, 24].

Since that time, there have been three controlled trials evaluating seroprophylaxis in BMT recipients. All have concluded that this approach has resulted in significant benefits to the patient. The UCLA group used hyperimmune CMV plasma obtained primarily from renal transplant recipients with high CMV antibody titers [14]. The Seattle group utilized an IM globulin purified from the normal volunteer blood donor population with high CMV antibody titers [15]. Our own trial used a hyperimmune intravenous IgG prepared from normal volunteer blood donors with high CMV antibody levels to prevent CMV infection in BMT recipients [12, 24].

The directions seroprophylaxis should now take, as well as the safest and most effective preparation, will be considered in this presentation. We raise the following questions: 1) Who should be the source for the hyperimmune CMV plasma; renal transplant recipients recovered from severe CMV infections with extremely high CMV antibody titers, or paid or volunteer blood donors with high CMV antibody titers? 2) What should be the preferred preparation—hyperimmune plasma or hyperimmune globulin? 3) If it is a hyperimmune globulin, should it be an IM or IV preparation? 4) Should the IV globulin be a modified or a native, unmodified globulin preparation?

We will present evidence that the most effective preparation is an IV, native, unmodified, hyperimmune IgG prepared from volunteer donor plasma with high CMV antibody titer by a new ion exchange chromatographic method [24].

SOURCE OF HYPERIMMUNE CMV PLASMA

The incidence of CMV infection in renal transplant recipients can be over 30% [34–36]. In those individuals who have recovered from particularly severe infections, antibody levels to CMV can be extremely high, and it is not uncommon to see CF titers > 8,096. These patients, therefore, constitute a possible source of high titer plasma. In preliminary studies to determine the feasibility of utilizing this as a source of plasma for the hyperimmune CMV IgG, we compared a group of such individuals with volunteer donors with CF CMV antibody titers of 256. The purpose was to determine if the distribution of antibody activity in the two groups was comparable, as well as the relative distribution of antibody in the various IgG subclasses. The CF CMV antibody titer, the plasma, and the IgG subclass distribution are compared in Table 1. The renal transplant group has higher IgG levels than the donor pool of high titer CMV plasma and low CMV antibody-deficient pool. One possible explanation could be that repeated plasmapheresis lowers IgG levels in the normal donors. There also is a shift in the relative distribution of the various IgG subclasses. In the renal transplant group, the relative concentration of the IgG_3 subclass now becomes greater than the IgG_2 subclass. Whether the extremely high CMV antibody titer in this group is a reflection of the presence of high CMV antibody levels in the IgG_3 subclass, as has been suggested by others [2, 26], was of interest. To determine whether such was the case, the various pools were fractionated on QAE Sephadex, the IgG concentrated, the IgG_3 isolated on Protein A Sepharose, and the specific antibody titers determined. Table 2 summarizes the results. There was no detectable CMV antibody in the IgG_3 isolated from the IgG of normal donor high titer plasma, while the titer in the high titer renal transplant IgG_3 was 400. This does not reflect the activity reported by others

TABLE 1. Comparison of IgG Subclass Distribution and CF Antibody to CMV in Renal Transplant Recipients Following Severe CMV Infection

Patient	CF Titer	IgG	% IgG by Subclass			
			1	2	3	4
A	8,192	8.8	82.3	4.6	13.0	0.1
B	8,192	9.7	73.0	6.6	20.0	0.4
C	4,096	13.6	97.3	0.8	1.3	0.6
D	2,048	10.5	71.1	4.1	24.4	0.5
E	1,024	6.9	66.9	10.2	21.4	1.5
F	1,024	4.2	65.2	11.2	21.7	1.9
G	1,024	5.5	79.4	4.2	20.6	0.8
Average	2,496	9.3	78.7	4.8	15.7	0.8
Normal high titer plasma- pheresis pool	>128	6.2	77.6	9.5	7.6	5.3
Normal low titer plasma- pheresis pool	<8	5.4	72.7	20.0	6.0	5.2

where it was shown that over 90% of antibodies to herpesvirus was contained in the IgG_3 subclass. From these studies, we concluded that while the antibody levels were higher because of the marked shifts in IgG subclass distribution, there was relatively little to be gained by utilizing the renal transplant group as donors; therefore, we focused on identifying, within the volunteer donor population, those with high CMV antibody titers.

CMV HYPERIMMUNE PLASMA POOLS AND CMV ANTIBODY-DEFICIENT PLASMA POOLS

The CMV hyperimmune globulin and CMV antibody-deficient globulins used in this study were derived from separate single plasma pools collected from normal volunteer donors at Memorial Sloan-Kettering Cancer Center (MSKCC). The hyperimmune plasma was derived from ten volunteer blood donors at MSKCC, repeatedly plasmapheresed at 3 to 6 wk intervals. Each donor for the pool of hyperimmune plasma was pretested and selected on the basis of an anti-CMV CF antibody titer in the serum of at least 256. The antibody-deficient plasma pool was similarly derived by serial plasma- phereses of ten normal volunteer blood donors who were seronegative for antibody to CMV both in ELISA and CF tests. All donors were repeatedly screened and their blood shown to be free of hepatitis antigen or antibody, antinuclear antibody, rheumatoid factors, or VDRL reactivity.

TABLE 2. Comparison of CMV IgG Antibody Isolated by Methods Including IgG$_3$ Subclass

	CMV IgG + IgG$_3$ ELISA Titer

Volunteer donor
  high titer plasma
  protein 50 mg/ml
	1,600

Final product protein 10 mg/ml	9,500
IgG$_3$ protein 10 mg/ml	< 100

High titer CMV
  renal Tx recipients' plasma
  protein 50 mg/ml
	12,800

Final product protein 10 mg/ml	12,800
IgG$_3$ protein 10 mg/ml	400

The intravenous IgG was prepared by methods previously described [24]. The preparation of each IgG fraction may be briefly described as follows: citrated hyperimmune plasma was stabilized with synthetic silica dioxide to remove lipoproteins, plasminogen, fibrinogen, and the plasma esterases and kallikreins. The stabilized plasma was then fractionated on sterile QAE Sephadex gel, an ion exchange resin which, under the conditions of the procedures developed, yields pure monomeric unfragmented and undenatured human IgG. Repeated analyses of the MW of the purified fraction on MW sieves (Biogel A1.5) have demonstrated < 1% high MW components, < 1% fragments, and a single peak consistent with monomeric 7S IgG. The approximate yield per liter of plasma was 6 gm of purified IgG. The product was tested and found to be free of viral or microbial contaminants. The CMV antibody levels and the subclass content of the IgG preparations used in this study are presented in Table 3. The CMV antibody titer by ELISA assay of the CMV antibody-deficient pool was < 100, while the titer in the hyperimmune pool was 1,600. The CMV antibody titer in the IgG preparations was 100 for the CMV antibody-deficient IgG and 9,500 for the hyperimmune CMV IgG.

PLAN OF STUDY

Initially, this trial was planned as a two-armed study comparing the incidence and severity of CMV infections in patients infused with Ig prepa-

TABLE 3. CMV Antibody Levels and Subclass Composition in the Starting Plasma and Final Product Intravenous IgG Used in the Study

Population	ELISA CMV Antibody	IgG	IgG Subclass			
			1	2	3	4
Volunteer donor high titer CMV CF > 128	1,600	6.2	77.6	9.5	7.6	5.3
Hyperimmune CMV IgG	9,500	10.0	94.7	5.2	0.06	0.13
Volunteer donor CMV antibody-deficient CF < 16	< 100	5.4	72.7	20.0	6.0	1.3
CMV antibody-deficient IgG	100	10.0	94.7	5.1	6.04	0.15

TABLE 4. Leukemia Patients Receiving Bone Marrow Transplants

Days Posttransplant	Stratified		
	Hyperimmune CMV Globulin	No Globulin	CMV Negative Globulin
25	200 mg/kg IV	None	200 mg/kg IV
50	200 mg/kg IV	None	200 mg/kg IV
75	200 mg/kg IV	None	200 mg/kg IV

rations containing or lacking antibody to CMV. Patients were randomized on day 24 posttransplant. Prior to randomization, patients were stratified on the basis of pretransplant CF antibody titer to CMV, and the type and stage of their leukemia. A third arm, the no treatment group, was drawn from matched, concurrently transplanted individuals, who, for reasons of unavailable globulin, did not receive this prophylactic treatment. An outline of the study is presented in Table 4. The globulin preparations were administered in three separate IV infusions each at a dose of 200 mg/kg/BW, on days 25, 50, and 75 posttransplant. During and following the three hour infusions, patients were closely monitored for untoward reactions.

Dose intervals and timing were chosen in accordance with the biologic half-life of the globulin and to span the period of maximal susceptibility to CMV-induced interstitial pneumonia [2]. The dose of CMV hyperimmune globulin used in this trial, 200 mg/kg/infusion, was based on globulin availability and preliminary dose escalation studies conducted in consenting seronegative transplant recipients. At doses of 200 and 300 mg/kg, seroconversions to CF antibody titers of 1:8 and 1:32 and IgG titers of 1:64 to 1:256 by ELISA test were regularly observed. CF antibody titers returned to preinfusion levels within seven days. However, antibody could still be detected 14 days after infusion by the ELISA test.

VIRAL SURVEILLANCE

All patients were monitored for evidence of CMV infection by weekly cultures of urine and throat washings. In addition, patients developing interstitial pneumonia were biopsied to determine its etiology. Cultures for CMV were performed using WI38 monolayers for virus propagation. Isolates were identified by growth characteristics and reactivity with specific antibody. Patients were also monitored with CMV-specific IgM and IgG antibody titers using an ELISA assay developed as a modification of the technique of Voller [37]. CMV infection was diagnosed on the basis of either a positive culture from urine, throat, or biopsy specimens, or a fourfold increment in the titer of IgM antibody to CMV.

PATIENTS

Candidates for this trial were exclusively patients admitted for transplantation for acute leukemia. The characteristics of each patient group are summarized in Table 5. Prior to transplantation, patients were treated with 1320r total body irradiation administered at a dose rate of 15 to 20r/min in 11 doses of 120r over 4 days, with partial lung shielding and testicular and thoracic cage intensification, followed by cyclophosphamide, 60 mg/kg/2

TABLE 5. Patient Population

	Control Supportive Therapy	CMV Antibody-Deficient IgG	Hyperimmune CMV IV IgG
Number	20	18	17
Mean age	17 ± 6 yrs	12 ± 8 yrs	13 ± 7 yrs
Underlying disease			
AML	12	8	8
ALL	8	10	9
Remission	16	14	13
Relapse	4	4	4
Pretransplant CMV CF antibody titer			
negative (< 1/8)	12	12	13
positive (1/8–1/32)	8	6	4

AML = acute myelocytic leukemia.
ALL = acute lymphoblastic leukemia.

days, as previously described [38]. Patients transplanted in late remission or relapse were maintained in laminar flow isolation with skin and mucosal decontamination, as previously described [39]. Patients transplanted in early remission were maintained in single room reverse isolation without decontamination. Neither prophylactic nor therapeutic granulocyte transfusions were used in the study patients. All patients received standard methotrexate prophylaxis [40] against GVHD. GVHD was diagnosed on the basis of clinical manifestations, confirmed by skin biopsy [41] and graded according to the criteria of Glucksberg et al [42]. GVHD of grade 2 to 4 severity was treated with prednisone, 2 mg/kg/day. Patients or their parents were informed of the nature of the trial and agreed to participate in the trial and to the globulin infusions by written consent.

BIOSTATISTICS

Patient groups were compared to assess differences in the distribution of patients and in the incidences of CMV infection and interstitial pneumonia using the Fisher exact test. Differences between groups exceeding the 95% confidence (P < 0.05) intervals were considered significant.

PREVENTION OF CMV INFECTION AND INTERSTITIAL PNEUMONIA BY IV HYPERIMMUNE CMV IgG

The age, disease characteristics, and the pretransplant CMV antibody status of the three patient groups are presented in Table 4. As can be seen, the distribution of patients by disease and disease status was comparable in each group. Patients in the untreated group were slightly older.

Patients found to be seropositive for antibody to CMV have been found to be at increased risk for infections caused by this agent [2]. In Table 5, the patients in each group are compared for pretransplant CMV antibody titers. While the geometric mean of titers of antibody detected in each patient group was quite comparable, and uniformly low, the proportion of seropositive patients was slightly increased in the no treatment group, as compared to the group receiving hyperimmune globulin. However, this difference in proportional representation was not statistically significant (P > 0.25).

The infusions of globulin were well tolerated. Of the 38 patients treated, three developed fever (38° to 40°C) during initial infusions; two developed transient chills, rigors, and mild tachycardia, which resolved after administration of an antihistamine. No other untoward reactions were detected.

The incidences of CMV infection, interstitial pneumonia, and mortality in the three patient groups are recorded in Table 6. Of the 20 patients who

TABLE 6. Incidence of CMV Infection, Interstitial Pneumonia, and Mortality in all Patients Over 120 Days

	Deficient IgG	Supportive Therapy Control	Hyperimmune CMV IV IgG
Number patients	18	20	17
CMV infection	6	10	0
Interstitial pneumonia	3	6	0*
GVHD	11	12	7
Mortality	NA	6	0

CMV infection: $P = 0.009$; $P = 0.001$
Interstitial pneumonia: $P = 0.014$
Mortality: $P = 0.014$

*Three patients developed interstitial pneumonia 140, 210, and 286 days posttransplant.

received no globulin prophylaxis, ten developed CMV infection documented by culture or serologic conversion during the period from 25 to 100 days postgrafting. Six patients developed interstitial pneumonia attributable to CMV (four), VZ (one), or unknown (one) causes.

Of the 18 patients treated wtih globulin derived from the seronegative plasma pool, none developed CMV antibody titers detectable by CF or ELISA IgG tests immediately following the globulin infusions. Six developed CMV infection during the test observation period (25 to 100 days), documented by culture (two), or IgM antibody titer rise (four). Three developed interstitial pneumonia. Only one case was clearly attributable to CMV infection; for the other two episodes all cultures were negative.

None of the 17 patients treated with hyperimmune globulin developed CMV infection or interstitial pneumonia during the period of prophylaxis (day 25 to 100). Ten of the 14 experienced significant increments in CMV antibody restricted to the IgG class immediately following infusion of the globulin, which fell to preinfusion levels 14 days thereafter. One patient was found by culture to be viruric three days before her first globulin infusion. All subsequent cultures, however, were negative. Three of the 17 patients ultimately experienced episodes of interstitial pneumonia 140, 210, and 286 days posttransplant, well beyond the period of prophylaxis. One of these patients died with severe hepatic and pulmonary disease secondary to GVHD and prior chemotherapy. No pathogen was found. The other two patients (one pneumocystis carinii and one idiopathic pneumonia) cleared their infections and are well over two years postgrafting.

Analysis of the results of the prophylactic study indicates a dramatic and highly significant reduction in the incidence of CMV infections in recipients of hyperimmune globulin, in comparison with either the group infused with globulin from seronegative donors (P = 0.009) or the no treatment group (P = 0.001). The incidence of interstitial pneumonia was significantly greater in the no treatment group as compared to that in the hyperimmune globulin prophylaxis group (P = 0.014). While three patients receiving the CMV antibody-deficient IgG developed interstitial pneumonia and none in the hyperimmune IgG group, the differences were not significant. Mortality was also significantly different when comparing the hyperimmune CMV IgG group with the no treatment group (P = 0.014).

DISCUSSION

The prevention of detectable CMV infection and disease in BMT recipients receiving high doses of IV hyperimmune CMV IgG was striking and not expected.

Our findings in this trial of an IV hyperimmune CMV IgG differ from those recently reported [14] in a trial of heat-inactivated hyperimmune plasma for prevention of CMV infections and in another trial with an intramuscular CMV immune globulin in BMT recipients [15]. Both groups document a decrease in the incidence of interstitial pneumonia and symptomatic CMV infections. Even though both started treatment approximately one week before marrow transplantation and we started 25 days posttransplant, they failed to document the decrease in the overall incidence of CMV infection in the treated group which we found in our study. In part, this may reflect a greater sensitivity of their virus surveillance procedure which incorporates buffy coat cultures for CMV in addition to culture of urine, throat washings, and biopsy material. However, the results may also reflect differences in the antiviral activity of the antibody preparations used and the route of administration. The pooled immune plasma from which the IgG was isolated for our study had an exceedingly high initial titer of CF antibody, and was drawn exclusively from normal seropositive blood donors, whereas the hyperimmune plasma used by the UCLA group was largely derived from immunosuppressed transplant recipients [14]. The dose of globulin used (200 mg/kg) IV provides a plasma equivalent dose of almost 20 ml/kg of IgG, slightly increased over the IV plasma dose used by the UCLA group.

In the trial involving the intramuscular CMV immune globulin, treatment was started four days prior to transplantation and continued weekly through 77 days after transplantation. The total dose of globulin was one third that used in our trial. While their results show significantly fewer infections in the globulin-treated group, they did not document the striking benefit observed with our preparation. An apparent explanation for the differences with IV and IM hyperimmune IgG preparations is the increased vascular levels of antibody achieved and the rapid delivery action by IV over the IM routes.

Other variables, such as differences in cytoreductive techniques, our very limited use of therapeutic as well as prophylactic granulocytes, and the patient populations themselves could also be cited to explain this disparity.

Passive seroprophylaxis with specific human Igs has been effective in the "normal" immunocompetent individual in preventing measles, hepatitis A, hepatitis B, polio, and zoster. Small doses of hepatitis A and measles immune globulin are effective even when given by the IM route. However, to achieve the degree of protection we demonstrated for CMV in highly immunosuppressed BMT patients, much higher doses of antibody were required, plus administration by the IV route. It is also to be noted that the immunosuppressive conditioning treatments these patients received, while directed toward CMI, also depress the humoral side.

Why then have passive Igs for CMV prevention been overlooked? Perhaps the belief that T-cell immunity is all that was important. There is a large body of research in animal models and in clinical settings which indicates that passive immunization with hyperimmune serum or plasma will prevent or abort subsequent disseminated infection following inoculation with HSV or VZV [38–42]. While the data for CMV infections are much more fragmentary, a number of observations would support the concept that antibody to CMV may prevent subsequent development of symptomatic disease. Early studies in mice have indicated that the offspring of previously immunized mice were protected from lethal disseminated infection due to CMV [37]. These studies also suggested that passive transfer through milk might be protective [43]. Subsequent studies [29], demonstrated that serum derived from mice within three to five days of CMV infection contained a complement-dependent neutralizing antibody of IgG type which, when passively transferred, protected mice from a subsequent lethal infection challenge with CMV.

In man, it has been repeatedly demonstrated that congenital CMV infection occurs almost exclusively in infants born to women primarily infected with CMV during the course of pregnancy. Seropositive women, who experience reactivation of CMV infections with persistent viruria during pregnancy, give birth to normal offspring without evidence of infection in the vast majority of cases [32, 33, 44–46]. Although Alford [46] has demonstrated viruria in such neonates in up to 1% of cases, the infections that have been seen have been invariably asymptomatic. The fetus in utero is presumed to lack antecedent experience with CMV. The protection afforded to neonates of secondarily infected mothers would appear to be based exclusively on transplacental passage of maternal antibody of the IgG class.

Other evidence suggesting a possible protective role for antibody is suggested by the studies on marrow transplant recipients [2]. These investigators observed that although the incidence of CMV-induced interstitial pneumonia is high in individuals who are seropositive prior to transplant (suggesting latent virus infection in the pathogenesis of this disease), the severity of these infections in seropositive individuals is somewhat reduced. Most importantly, patients with titers of CF CMV antibody $> 1{:}64$ prior to transplantation have a very low incidence of infection [2].

Between 1964 and 1979, there were at least three case reports of life-threatening infections due to CMV occurring in immunosuppressed patients in whom administration of pooled gamma globulin or immune plasma was associated with clinical improvement [31–33]. Subsequently, we reported results of an uncontrolled trial in which an IV preparation of gamma globulin derived from a normal pool of individuals without attention to their serologic status was used for the treatment of life-threatening interstitial pneumonia in renal allograft recipients [11]. Eighteen of the 42 patients receiving these infusions completely cleared the interstitial pneumonia; an additional 12 patients were not affected by this therapy and died. Patients who improved or who had complete resolution of this process were treated earlier in the disease course, suggesting that early therapy was potentially more effective, and that prophylactic administration of gamma globulin might be particularly effective in preventing subsequent development of disease [11].

Based on the above information, we initiated our prospective randomized trial of intravenous CMV hyperimmune globulin for prevention of CMV infections following marrow transplantation. A control group receiving globulin from seronegative donors was used in this study in an attempt to better characterize the importance of CMV antibody if protection were indeed documented. The results show that the incidence of CMV infections may be eliminated by passive immunization with specifically hyperimmune globulin preparations. The fact that the incidence of interstitial pneumonia in recipients of hyperimmune globulin was not significantly reduced from that observed in recipients of globulin from seronegative donors, while clearly reduced from that observed in the no treatment group, may reflect either the presence of low levels of CMV antibody in the seronegative pool, or more likely, administration of other antibodies potentially useful for preventing this complication. The IV hyperimmune CMV IgG used successfully in this trial specifically lacks the IgG_3 subclass. The ion exchange method used for its preparation has been used by us over the past ten years to isolate biologically active IgG antibody from human hyperimmune antibotulinal plasma [47], from human Lassa fever convalescent plasma [48], and from equine antilymphoblast plasma [49]. In each case, the biologic activity has been isolated with an increase in specific activity of from threefold to fivefold over that in the starting plasma. The contribution of specific antibodies in the IgG_3 subclass to the overall activity of an IgG preparation is, from our studies, extremely limited. In fact, in the high CMV titers in volunteer donor plasma used in this trial, no CMV antibody could be detected in IgG_3. Even in the renal transplant recipient, with high CMV titer plasma where IgG_3 content made up over 15% of the IgG, the CMV antibody titer was low, ie, an ELISA titer of 400 compared to 12,800 of the total IgG.

What is the ultimate preparation and how should it be used? Dosage, high circulating antibody levels, and the rapid delivery achieved by the IV route appear to explain the increased effectiveness observed by us when compared with the trial using an intramuscular CMV globulin preparation. With an unmodified intravenous IgG preparation having a circulatory half-life approaching three weeks, monthly administration over the period of greatest risk (100 days) is effective, but additional administrations are indicated when GVHD therapy is initiated. There are also indications that IV CMV globulin would be effective in treating ongoing CMV infection and definitely should be considered. Finally, the use of IV hyperimmune CMV IgG should be considered in prophylaxis of newborns at high risk to CMV infection.

THE FUTURE DIRECTION OF SEROPROPHYLAXIS—HUMAN MONOCLONAL ANTIBODIES TO CMV

In the excitement and rush of identifying the intricate network of T cells involved in viral immunity, we may have ignored and neglected those earlier studies demonstrating the effectiveness of seroprophylaxis in prevention of virus infection. Today, with the amazing progress being made in the elucidation of the structural functional relationships of the CMV genome, we should, in the not too distant future, know the structure and have synthesized the CMV glycoproteins associated with viral absorption, membrane fusion, penetration and latency. These surface relationships are illustrated in Figure 1. It should then be possible to prepare human monoclonal antibodies with potent neutralizing activity to each of these specific glycoproteins. By proper formulation, a monoclonal antibody preparation could be prepared that should be effective in treatment of ongoing CMV infections. This form of therapy would very likely not result in a resistant virus, as will probably be the case with antivirals.

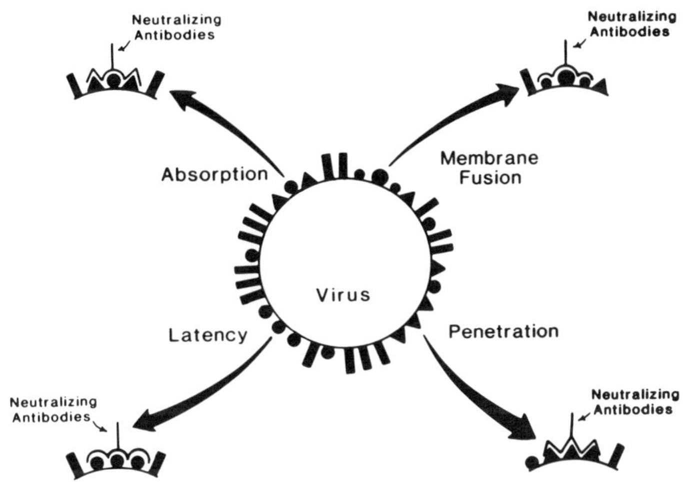

CMV surface glycoproteins and neutralizing human monoclonal antibodies

Fig. 1.   Future prospects for CMV seroprophylaxis.

CONCLUSION

Large IV doses of hyperimmune CMV IgG prepared from high CMV titer plasma obtained from volunteer donors were found to be safe and highly effective in prophylaxis of CMV infection in BMT recipients. While the group receiving the hyperimmune CMV IgG was small, 18 in number, there were no CMV infections, interstitial pneumonia, and mortality during the period of treatment and extending 130 days beyond transplantation. The significant benefits of this form of treatment in preventing CMV infection and disease would indicate its use in newborns at high risk as well as for treatment of ongoing CMV infections.

ACKNOWLEDGMENTS

We thank Chris Drayton, Gerri Baglien, Norm Will, Meredith Falley, Pam Vaughan, Debbie Bresina, Ted Taylor, and Kris Waskosky for their excellent contributions to this effort.

REFERENCES

1. Thomas ED, Buckner CD, Banaji M, Clift RA, Fefer A, Flournoy N, Goodell BW, Hickman RO, Lerner KG, Neiman PE, Sale GE, Sanders JE, Singer J, Stevens M, Storb R, Weiden PL: One hundred patients with acute leukemia treated by chemotherapy, total body irradiation, and allogeneic marrow transplantation. Blood 49:511–533, 1977.

2. Neiman PE, Reeves W, Ray G, Flournoy N, Lerner KG, Sale GE, Thomas ED: A prospective analysis of interstitial pneumonia and opportunistic viral infection among recipients of allogeneic bone marrow grafts. J Infect Dis 136:754–767, 1977.

3. Neiman P, Wasserman PB, Wentworth BB, Kao GF, Lerner KG, Storb R, Buckner CD, Clift RA, Fefer A, Fass L, Glucksberg H, Thomas ED: Interstitial pneumonia and cytomegalovirus infection as complications of human marrow transplantation. Transplantation 15:478–485, 1973.

4. Meyers JD, McGuffin RW, Bryson YJ, Cantell K, Thomas ED: Treatment of cytomegalovirus pneumonia after marrow transplant with combined vibarabine and human leukocyte interferon. J Infect Dis 146:1, 1982.

5. Ch'ien LT, Cannon NJ, Whitley RJ, Diethelm AG, Dismukes WE, Scott CW, Buchanan RA, Alford CA: Effect of adenine arabinoside on cytomegalovirus infections. J Infect Dis 130:32–39, 1974.

6. McCracken GH, Luby JP: Cytosine arabinoside in the treatment of congenital cytomegalic inclusion disease. J Pediatr 80:488–495, 1975.

7. Saral R, Burns WH, Laskin OL, Santos GW, Lietman PS: Acyclovir prophylaxis of herpes-simplex-virus infections. N Engl J Med 305:63–67, 1981.

8. Jones JF, Jeter WS, Fulginiti VA, Minnich LL, Pritchett RF, Wedgwood RJ: Treatment of childhood combined Epstein-Barr virus/cytomegalovirus infection with oral bovine transfer factor. Lancet 1:122–124, 1981.

9. Hersman J, Meyers JD, Thomas ED, Buckner CD, Clift R: The effect of granulocyte transfusions on the incidence of cytomegalovirus infection after allogeneic marrow transplantation. Ann Intern Med 96:149–152, 1982.

10. Yeager AS, Grumet FC, Hafleigh EB, Arvin AM, Bradley JS, Prober CG: Prevention of transfusion-acquired cytomegalovirus infections in newborn infants. J Pediatr 8:281–287, 1981.

11. Condie RM, Hall BL, Howard RJ, Fryd D, Simmons RL, Najarian JS: Treatment of life-threatening infections in renal transplant recipients with high dose intravenous human IgG. Transplant Proc 1:66–68, 1979.

12. Condie RM, O'Reilly RJ: Prophylaxis of CMV infection in bone marrow transplant recipients by hyperimmune CMV gamma-globulin. Dev Biol Scand 52:501–513, 1982.

13. O'Reilly RJ, Reich L, Gold J, Condie RM: A randomized trial of intravenous, hyperimmune globulin for the prevention of CMV infections following marrow transplantation: Preliminary results. Transplant Proc 15:1405–1411, 1983.

14. Winston DJ, Pollard RB, Ho WG, Gallagher JG, Rasmussen LE, Huang SNY, Lin C-H, Gossett TG, Merigan TC, Gale RP: Cytomegalovirus immune plasma in bone marrow transplant recipients. Ann Intern Med 97:11–18, 1982.

15. Meyers JD, Leszczynski J, Zaia JA, Flournoy N, Newton B, Snydman DR, Wright GG, Levin MJ, Thomas ED: Prevention of cytomegalovirus infection by cytomegalovirus immune globulin after marrow transplantation. Ann Intern Med 98:442–446, 1983.

16. Meyers JD, Flournoy N, Thomas ED: Cytomegalovirus infection and specific cell-mediated immunity after marrow transplant. J Infect Dis 142:816–824, 1980.

17. Rubin RH, Wolfson JS, Cosimi AB, Tolkoff-Rubin NE: Infection in the renal transplant recipient. Am J Med 70:405–411, 1981.

18. Osborn JE: Cytomegalovirus: Pathogenicity, immunology, and vaccine initiatives. J Infect Dis 143:618–630, 1981.

19. Zaia JA, Levin MJ, Leszczynski J, Wright GG, Grady GF: Cytomegalovirus immune globulin: Production from selected normal donor blood. Transplantation 27:66–67, 1979.
20. Mandel B: Neutralization of animal viruses. Adv Virus Res 23:205–268, 1978.
21. Philipson L, Killander J, Albertsson PA: Interaction between poliovirus and immunoglobulins: I. Detection of virus antibodies by partition in aqueous polymer phase systems. Virology 28:22–34, 1965.
22. Philipson L: Interaction between poliovirus and immunoglobulins. II. Basic aspects of virus-antibody interaction. Virology 28:35–46, 1965.
23. Philipson L, Bennich H: Interaction between poliovirus and immunoglobulins: III. The effect of cleavage products of rabbit IgG-globulin on infectivity and distribution of virus in polymer phase systems. Virology 29:330–338.
24. Condie RM: Preparation and intravenous use of undenatured human IgG. In Alving B, Finlayson J (eds): "Immunoglobulins: Characteristics and Uses of Intravenous Preparations." Washington, DC: US Government Printing Office, 1980.
25. Beck ED: Distribution of virus antibody activity among human IgG subclasses. Clin Exp Immunol 43:626–632, 1981.
26. Immunohemotherapy Workshop in Immunopathological Aspects of Immunoglobulin Infusions, Interlaken, Switzerland, August 1981.
27. Winston DJ, Pollard RB, Ho WG, Gallagher JG, Rasmussen LE, Haung SN, Lin CH, Gossett TG, Merigan TC, Gale RP: A controlled trial of cytomegalovirus immune plasma in bone marrow transplant recipients. Ann Intern Med 7:11–18, 1982.
28. Neiman PE, Thomas ED, Reeves WC, Ray CG, Sale G, Lerner KG, Buckner CD, Clift RA, Storb R, Weiden PL, Fefer A: Opportunistic infection and interstitial pneumonia following marrow transplantation for aplastic anemia and hematologic malignancy. Transplant Proc 8:663, 1976.
29. Araullo-Cruz TP, Ho M, Armstrong JA: Protective effect of early serum from mice after cytomegalovirus infection. Infect Immun 21:840–842, 1978.
30. Shanley JD, Jordan MC, Stevens JG: Modification by adoptive humoral immunity of murine cytomegalovirus infection. J Infect Dis 143:231–237, 1981.
31. Dijkmans BAC, Versteeg J, Kauffmann RH, van den Broek PJ, Eternisse JG, van Zanten JJ, Bakker W, Kalff MW, van Hooff JP: Treatment of cytomegalovirus pneumonitis with hyperimmune plasma. Lancet 1:820–821, 1979.
32. Jacox RF, Mongan ES, Hanshaw JB, Leddy JP: Hypogammaglobulinemia with thymoma and probable pulmonary infection with cytomegalovirus. N Engl J Med 271:1091–1096, 1964.
33. Levine RS, Warner NE, Johnson CF: Cytomegalic inclusion disease in the gastro-intestinal tract of adults. Ann Surg 159:37–48, 1964.
34. Simmons RL, Lopez C, Balfour HH Jr et al: Cytomegalovirus: Clinical virological correlations in renal transplant recipients. Ann Surg 180:623–634, 1974.
35. Simmons RL, Matas AJ, Rattazzi LC et al: Clinical characteristics of the lethal cytomegalovirus infection following renal transplantation. Surgery 82:537–546, 1977.
36. Peterson PK, Balfour HH Jr, Marker SC et al: Cytomegalovirus disease in renal allograft recipients: A prospective study of the clinical features, risk factors and impact on renal transplantation. Medicine (Baltimore) 59:283–300, 1980.
37. Voller A, Bidwell D, Bartlett A: Microplate enzyme immunoassays for the immunodiagnosis of virus infections. In Rose N, Friedman H (eds): "Manual of Clinical Immunology." Washington, DC: American Society of Microbiology, 1976.
38. Shank B, Hopfan S, Kim JH, Chu FCH, Grossbard E, Kapoor N, Kirkpatrick D, Dinsmore R, Simpson L, Reid A, Chui C, Mohan R, Finegen D, O'Reilly RJ: Hyper-

fractionated total body irradiation for bone marrow transplantation: I. Early results in leukemia patients. Radiat Onc Biol Phys 7:1109–1115, 1981.

39. O'Reilly RJ, Dupont B, Pahwa S, Grimes E, Smithwick EM, Pahwa R, Schwartz S, Hansen JA, Siegel FP, Sorell M, Svejgaard A, Jersild C, Thomsen M, Platz P, L'Esperance P, Good RA: Reconstruction in severe combined immune deficiency by transplantation of marrow from an unrelated donor. N Engl J Med 297:1311–1318, 1977.

40. Storb R, Epstein RB, Graham TC, Thomas ED: Methotrexate regimens for control of graft-versus-host disease in dogs with allogeneic marrow grafts. Transplantation 9:240–246, 1970.

41. Woodruff J, Hansen JA, Good RA et al: The pathology of the graft-versus-host reaction (GVHR) in adults receiving bone marrow transplants. Transplant Proc 8:675–684, 1976.

42. Glucksberg H, Storb R, Fefer A, Buckner CD, Neiman PE, Clift RA, Lerner KG, Thomas ED: Clinical manifestations of graft-versus-host disease in human recipients of marrow from HL-A matched sibling donors. Transplantation 18:295–304, 1974.

43. Medearis DN Jr, Prokay SL: Effect of immunization of mothers on cytomegalovirus infection in suckling mice. Proc Soc Exp Biol Med 157:523–527, 1978.

44. Berenberg W: Letter to the editor. Pediatrics 45:891, 1970.

45. Yaeger AS, Martin HP, Stewart JA: Congenital cytomegalovirus infection outcome for the subsequent sibling. Clin Pediatr 16:455–458, 1977.

46. Stagno S, Reynolds DW, Tsiantos A, Fuccillo DA, Long W, Alford CA: Comparative serial virologic and serologic studies of symptomatic and subclinical congenitally and natally acquired cytomegalovirus infections. J Infect Dis 132:568–577, 1975.

47. Lewis GE, Condie RM: Preparation of an intravenous, human, pentavalent botulinal, immune globulin. (In preparation)

48. Jahrling PB, Lewis GE Jr, Condie RM: An intravenous, human, anti-Lassa immune globulin: Protection of guinea pigs and monkeys against Lassa fever infection. (In preparation)

49. Najarian JS, Simmons RL, Condie RM, Thompson EJ, Fryd DF, Howard RJ, Matas AJ, Sutherland DER, Ferguson RM, Schmidtke JR: Seven years experience with anti-lymphoblast globulin for renal transplantation from cadaver donors. Ann Surg 184:352–367, 1976.

Therapeutic Approaches to the Control of Cytomegalovirus Infections*

Meyer Dworsky,[†] MD, Robert F. Pass, MD, Sergio Stagno, MD, and Richard J. Whitley, MD

The Department of Pediatrics, The University of Alabama School of Medicine, Birmingham, AL 35294

INTRODUCTION

The proceedings of this meeting have documented the acute need for the development of rational and specific measures to prevent and treat CMV infections in humans. While developments of treatment modalities for other herpesvirus infections, particularly those caused by HSV and VZV, are proceeding along expedient lines, therapeutic advances in the area of CMV infections in humans remain woefully lacking. As has already been delineated from prior presentations, the HCMVs are capable of producing a broad spectrum of clinical diseases, ranging from infections in the newborn to life-threatening diseases in the immunocompromised host. Worldwide, HCMVs cause congenital infection in approximately 0.5%–2% of all live births [1–3]. Although the majority of these children are born completely without symptoms, upwards of 5%–15% will ultimately develop significant hearing, developmental, and/or visual impairment. Furthermore, 5%–10% of chil-

*Supported by grants from the National Cancer Institute (NCI-13148), the Division of Research Resources (RR-032).

[†]M.D. held a fellowship from the Johnson and Johnson Foundation.

Birth Defects: Original Article Series, Volume 20, Number 1, pages 345–352
© 1984 March of Dimes Birth Defects Foundation

dren, depending upon circumstances, will acquire CMV in the period immediately surrounding birth by contact with infected genital secretions, through ingestion of infected breast milk, or via blood products [4–6]. The consequences of these infections are less apparent, although it has been learned that pneumonia in the young infant or even acute perinatal morbidity can result from these agents [6–8]. CMV infections in children and adults are most frequently asymptomatic; however, in the presence of immunosuppression, infection can be of clinical significance. Individuals receiving organ transplants, including renal, bone marrow, and cardiac transplant recipients, are all at risk for severe and even life-threatening CMV infections, particularly pneumonitis [9,10]. It has been reported that mortality from CMV pneumonia in the BMT recipient ranges between 45% and 90%. Furthermore, CMVs have been associated with the development of AIDS as well as Kaposi sarcoma [11]. Clearly, the association of CMV with mortality and morbidity underscores the need for the development of preventive and therapeutic modalities for these viral infections.

CMVs, as members of the herpesvirus family, possess unique characteristics which have thwarted the development of antivirals specific for their inhibition. These viruses can establish latency, be chronically excreted, and recur at periodic intervals later in life. This latter characteristic, the ability to recur, is of particular importance in those individuals receiving immunosuppressive therapy. Moreover, during replication, the CMVs do not code for a viral specific thymidine kinase, as do HSV and VZV. As a consequence, the design of antiviral agents becomes more difficult as events unique to viral replication are more limited, namely to the DNA polymerase of CMV. Likely, future attention will be directed to the inhibition of: 1) generation of messenger RNA and events of transcription, and 2) regulation of RNA polymerases as processes specific for inhibition of viral replication. The lack of unique sites of viral inhibition early in the replicative process would suggest a narrow range between safety and efficacy for existing antiviral agents.

In spite of these stumbling blocks, a variety of therapies have been attempted for the management of patients with CMV infections. These approaches can be classified according to the medication administered: 1) IFN, either leukocyte or recombinant DNA IFN, has been utilized in an attempt to induce an antiviral state; or 2) antiviral drugs. The focus of this review, then, will be on the status of therapy for the major disease states caused by CMV via relevant data from prior clinical trials. Ig studies will be deferred for other reports.

THERAPY

Congenital Infection

Human leukocyte IFN, and IFN inducers have all been administered to infants with symptomatic congenital CMV infections. These immunotherapeutic approaches have been based upon the observation that congenitally infected infants have little circulating IFN and that their lymphocytes have a decreased ability to produce IFN in vitro [12]. IFN inducers have been administered to a limited number of infants with no obvious success [13]. The administration of leukocyte IFN, at dosages between $1.5-10 \times 10^5$ reference units, has been given to nine infants with congenital infection either as single doses or by repeated courses of therapy over seven to ten days. No clinical benefit can be determined from the administration of IFN by these regimens; yet, a variable effect was demonstrable on viral excretion. In two infants, viruria was suppressed for months; in three infants, there was a transitory effect on viral excretion; while in the remaining four infants, there was no apparent effect on the excretion of virus in the urine [14,15]. The spectrum of disease in the treated newborns and the lack of long-term follow-up prevented the rigorous evaluation of these data from an efficacy standpoint. Thus, no conclusion can be reached regarding the value of this therapeutic approach.

Adverse effects of high-dose leukocyte IFN are common and include poor weight gain, transient elevation of SGOT, and fever [15]. It is unlikely that a therapeutic effect would be achieved in the absence of significant alteration of the viral excretion patterns for prolonged periods of time, as occurred in two of these children. It would be necessary to perform a therapeutic controlled follow-up study to further assess any theoretic value of this treatment approach. The purity and potency of IFN preparations are improving because of the availability of recombinant DNA IFN. Perhaps these preparations, either alone or in combination with other antivirals, will prove useful, as noted below.

A more extensive experience has been gained with utilization of nucleoside analogs for the treatment of congenital CMV infection. Treatment of subclinical intrauterine CMV infection is not justifiable because of the incomplete definition of this infection regarding outcome. For the most part, then, chemotherapeutic trials have been offered to the symptomatically infected child at birth or shortly thereafter [16,17]. Obviously, such a treatment strategy requires administration of a chemotherapeutic agent after the fact, since these infections began at some unknown time in utero and multiple organ system disease of a highly variable nature has become well established. Treatment efforts have employed the purine and pyrimidine nucleoside analogs, idoxuridine, ara-C, vidarabine, and fluorodeoxyuridine [18]. These studies taken together demonstrate a seemingly transitory but variable reduction in urinary virus excretion in most cases, with some reduction in pharyngeal shedding and viremia.

For several years, we have studied the effects of vidarabine therapy for congenital CMV infection. With evidence of low toxicity of this medication at 30 mg/kg/day, and with the goal of reducing acute organ disease, we initiated a new uncontrolled trial. For comparative purposes, symptomatically congenitally infected babies were employed. Summarizing data from an ongoing study at the University of Alabama School of Medicine, we have evaluated and treated nine congenitally infected children who suffered from growth retardation, microcephaly, petechiae, thrombocytopenia, and/or direct hyperbilirubinemia. All nine infants were hospitalized for at least two weeks. A dosage of 30 mg/kg of vidarabine was administered daily over 12 hr for a total of 14 days. Drug was reconstituted in a solution such that the solubility would not exceed 0.5 mg/ml of standard IV solution. Routine clinical and laboratory toxicity assessments were performed to assess potential toxicity. Urine and throat washes were obtained for quantitation of virus during and after the treatment course. Patients were followed longitudinally to determine long-term outcome. Interestingly, six of the nine infants were of low birthweight ranging from 1.2–2.5 kg. Five of these infants were small for dates or were premature; three of the five small-for-gestational-age infants were also microcephalic. Aside from growth parameters, these infants manifested the usual constellation of signs and symptoms of babies with congenital CMV inclusion disease: thrombocytopenia (9), direct hyperbilirubinemia (8), and hepatosplenopathy (9). Two children died, resulting in a mortality no different from historical controls. As shown in Figure 1, vidar-

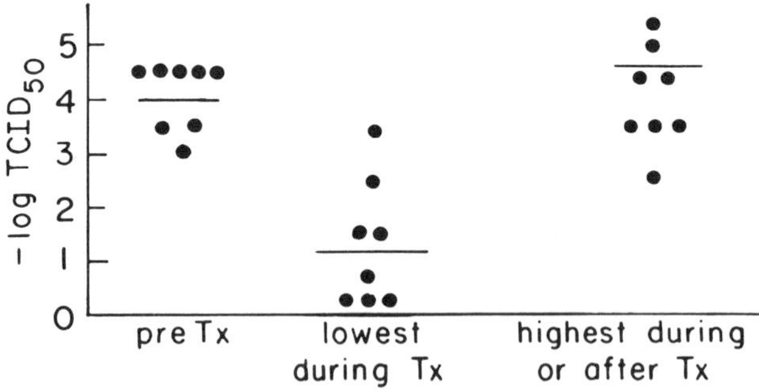

Fig. 1.   Effect of vidarabine therapy (30 mg/kg/day × 14 days) on reduction of the quantity of virus excreted in the urine.

abine administration resulted in a significant decrease in the titratable quantity of virus in the urine. This decrease was not sustained and, in a few cases, virus increased during the period of therapy. Although the numbers remain too small for conclusions regarding the salutary effects of therapy on hepatic and bone marrow function, liver function tended to normalize as did bone marrow function in seven of the nine children.

Clearly, longitudinal follow-up of many years is required to assess hearing and psychomotor development. Although it is preliminary, we have observed the preservation of normal head growth in the treated infants who were normocephalic at birth. This is in contrast with a previous group of 12 untreated infants, five of whom, who were initially normocephalic, ultimately developed microcephaly (Fig. 2). Should this observation be borne out with time, a suggestion for clinical usefulness would become apparent.

With all other nucleoside analogs, the unpredictable reduction in replication of virus occurred in the presence of bone marrow toxicity. This occurrence is not surprising since each of these compounds affects both viral and cellular DNA metabolism to different degrees and by different mechanisms. The use of toxic or potentially toxic compounds can be justified only for symptomatic congenital CMV infection on the grounds that it may reduce prolonged illness as well as permanently debilitating brain, eye, and auditory damage. The hope of elimination of viral replication and its consequence on decreasing organ involvement remains a goal for future studies, as it was not achieved in the current trial. The antiviral effects noted, particularly with

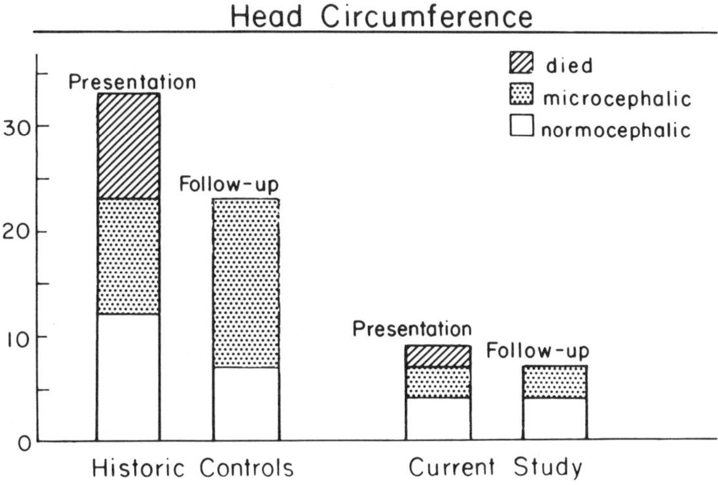

Fig. 2. Follow-up of head circumference in historical controls and vidarabine-treated infants (current study). The ordinate denotes the number of children evaluated.

vidarabine, were transitory and with severe disease so inadequate as not to be able to reverse lethality in those patients. It remains impossible to ascribe any clinical efficacy in these studies because of the enormous spectrum of disease resulting from congenital CMV infection and the unpredictable nature of its progression. Thus, although an antiviral effect can be demonstrated, the clinical usefulness of this antiviral effect is dubious at best.

ORGAN TRANSPLANTATION

With the advent of organ transplantation, particularly renal allograft, heart, and bone marrow, and the requisite immunosuppressive therapy to maintain the transplanted graft, a high incidence of herpesvirus infections has been noted posttransplantation. This is particularly true for CMV infections, both primary and recurrent. Of particular concern is the high mortality rate associated with CMV pneumonia in the BMT recipients. Thus, even with successful transplantation, the viral complication may be of such severity as to lead to early demise or loss of the transplanted organ.

Because of the high mortality in these patient populations, IFN and nucleoside analogs have been used both alone and in combination. Meyers and colleagues [19] have attempted to establish successful therapeutics for biopsy-proven CMV pneumonia, but to no avail. Human leukocyte IFN, at dosages of $0.2–6.4 \times 10^5$ U/kg/day administered at the time of diagnosis, failed to alter the clinical expression of CMV pneumonia in these patient populations. Similarly, vidarabine and acyclovir alone or administered with IFN were also of no value [20]. Importantly, the lung biopsies from these patients contained large quantities of virus. Thus, as a therapeutic for existing disease, IFN, vidarabine, and acyclovir do not appear to be useful.

Renal transplant recipients often suffer from CMV infections. Beginning initially with vidarabine administration, Chien and colleagues [16] were able to demonstrate that vidarabine therapy decreased viruria coincident with administration of study medication. Nevertheless, in many of these patients virus was persistently found in organs at autopsy. Similar studies by Rytel and Kauffman [21] drew an analogous conclusion. Vidarabine is ineffective in eliminating CMV from the immunosuppressed host and, at best, has a transient effect on decreasing the quantity of virus excreted in the urine, but without clinical benefit. Furthermore, Marker et al [22] noted significant neurotoxicity of this drug in patients with poor renal function.

In the heart transplant patient, CMV retinitis is a grave consequence in a few patients. Pollard and colleagues [23] have shown that high-dose vidarabine is helpful in the prevention of this progressive disease.

More recently, a controlled study utilizing the drug acyclovir [24] has been reported in the immunocompromised host principally suffering from CMV viremia. This compound is most useful for herpes simplex infections. The controlled studies of Balfour et al [24] suggested an earlier time to defervescence and resolution of clinical symptomatology in patients receiving 1,500 mg/m^2 of acyclovir intravenously. These studies are being further assessed in an ongoing trial.

CONCLUSION

Therapeutic trials using IFN, nucleoside analogs, or a combination of these two preparations have not provided encouragement for the treatment of CMV infections. The nature of the replicative cycle of CMV, as well as our inability to define processes specific for inhibition of viral replication, pose problems of significant magnitude at the present time. Furthermore, the need for early diagnosis and early intervention with a chemotherapeutic agent remain of paramount importance in the therapy of viral infection. Trifluorothymidine is active at low concentrations against CMV in vitro; but, our ability to use this drug in human disease remains to be established. Future therapeutic trials should take the form of combination chemotherapy or attempt to assess drugs acting at sites different in the replicative cycle than those currently available.

REFERENCES

1. Hanshaw JB, Scheiner AP, Moxley AW et al: School failure and deafness after "silent" cytomegalovirus infection. N Engl J Med 295:468, 1976.
2. Stagno S, Reynolds DW, Tsiantos A et al: Comparative serial virologic and serologic studies of symptomatic and subclinical congenitally and natally acquired cytomegalovirus infections. J Infect Dis 132:568, 1975.
3. Lang DJ: The epidemiology of cytomegalovirus infections: Interpretation of recent observations. In Krugman S, Gershon AA (eds): "Infections of the Fetus and the Newborn Infant." New York: Alan R Liss, 1975, pp 35–45.
4. Stagno S, Reynolds DW, Pass RF et al: Breast milk and the risk of cytomegalovirus infection. N Engl J Med 302:1073–1076, 1980.
5. Reynolds DW, Stagno S, Hosty TS, Tiller M, Alford CA Jr: Maternal cytomegalovirus excretion and perinatal infections. N Engl J Med 289:1–5, 1973.
6. Yeager AS: Transfusion acquired cytomegalovirus infection in newborn infants. Am J Dis Child 128:478–483, 1974.
7. Stagno S, Brasfield DM, Brown MB, Cassell GH, Pifer LL, Whitley RJ, Tiller RE: Infant pneumonitis associated with cytomegalovirus, chlamydia, pneumocystis, and ureaplasma: A prospective study. Pediatrics 68:322–329, 1981.
8. Yeager AS, Palumbo PE: Symptomatic cytomegalovirus infections in premature infants following transmission of virus from mother to infant. This volume (abstract).

9. Rubin RJ, Russell PS, Levin M et al: Summary of a workshop on cytomegalovirus infections during organ transplantation. J Infect Dis 139:728–734, 1979.
10. Meyers JD, Spencer HC Jr, Watts JC et al: Cytomegalovirus pneumonia after human marrow transplantation. Ann Intern Med 82:181–182, 1975.
11. Drew WL, Mintz L, Miner RC, Sands M, Ketterer B: Prevalence of cytomegalovirus infection in homosexual men. J Infect Dis 143:188–192, 1981.
12. Glasgow L, Hanshaw JB, Merigan TC et al: Interferon and cytomegalovirus in vivo and in vitro. Proc Soc Exp Biol Med 125:843–849, 1967.
13. Falcoff E, Falcoff R, Foumier F, Chany C: Production en masse, purification partielle et caracterisation d'un interferon destiné à des essais therapeutiques humains. Ann Inst Pasteur 111:562–584, 1966.
14. Emodi G, O'Reilly R, Miller A et al: Effect of exogenous interferon in cytomegalovirus infections. J Infect Dis 133:A199–A204, 1976.
15. Arvin AM, Yeager AS, Merigan T: Effect of leukocyte interferon on urinary excretion of cytomegalovirus by infants. J Infect Dis 133:A205–A209, 1976.
16. Chien LT, Cannon NJ, Whitley RJ: Effect of adenine arabinoside on cytomegalovirus infections. J Infect Dis 130:32–39, 1974.
17. Whitley RJ, Chien LT, Buchanan RA, Alford CA Jr: Studies on adenine arabinoside—A model for antiviral chemotherapeutics. In Pollard M (ed): "Antiviral Mechanisms— Perspectives in Virology IX." New York: Academic Press, 1975, pp 315–335.
18. Whitley RJ, Alford CA Jr: Chronic intrauterine and perinatal infections. In Galasso GJ, Merigan TC, Buchanan RA (eds): "Antiviral Agents and Viral Diseases of Man." New York: Raven Press, 1978, pp 541–604.
19. Meyers JD, McGuffin RW, Neiman PE et al: Toxicity and efficacy of human leukocyte interferon for treatment of cytomegalovirus pneumonia after marrow transplantation. J Infect Dis 141:555–562, 1980.
20. Meyers JD: Cytomegalovirus infection following marrow transplantation: Risk, treatment and prevention. This volume.
21. Rytel MW, Kauffman HM: Clinical efficacy of adenine arabinoside in therapy of cytomegalovirus infections in renal allograft recipients. J Infect Dis 133:202–205, 1976.
22. Marker SG, Howard RJ, Groth KE et al: A trial of vidarabine for cytomegalovirus infection in renal transplant patients. Arch Intern Med 140:1441–1444, 1980.
23. Pollard RB, Egbert PR, Gallagher JG et al: Cytomegalovirus retinitis in immunosuppressed hosts. I. Natural history and effects of treatment with adenine arabinoside. Ann Intern Med 93:655–660, 1980.
24. Balfour HH Jr, Bean B, Mitchell CD et al: Acyclovir in immunocompromised patients with cytomegalovirus disease. A controlled trial at one institution. Am J Med 73(1A):241–248, 1982.

ABSTRACTS

HOSPITAL-ACQUIRED CYTOMEGALOVIRUS INFECTIONS IN NEONATES

S.P. Adler, T. Chandrika, L. Lawrence, J. Baggett, and V. Biro

Children's Medical Center, The Medical College of Virginia, Richmond, VA 23298

The purpose of this study was to determine the incidence of hospital-acquired CMV infections in neonates in a 60-bed intensive care unit and to determine whether the mode of acquisition of these infections was from blood products, maternal sources, or hospital personnel. The clinical significance of these infections was assessed.

METHODS

During a 32-month period (August 1980 until April 1983) all newborns admitted to the neonatal intensive care unit had urines cultured for CMV on admission, and weekly after 4 weeks of age until hospital discharge. Two flasks of freshly voided urine were cultured on confluent MRC-5 or WI-38 human fibroblast cells. The presence or absence of CMV antibody in infants and blood donor sera was determined using an EIA assay (M.A. Bioproducts). No infant was fed nonmaternal breast milk.

RESULTS

During the first 20 months of the study 8 of 178 infants hospitalized for over 30 days developed viruria. Acquired CMV infection in these infants was significantly associated with:

A) *Birthweight:* All CMV-infected infants had birthweights of 1,050 gm or less. Twenty-nine infants with birthweights < 1,050 gm survived to over 30 days of age. Thus, the risk of CMV acquisition was 27.5% (8/29) for these premature infants. There was no correlation between birthweight and duration of hospitalization for any infants hospitalized for over 30 days.

Birth Defects: Original Article Series, Volume 20, Number 1, pages 355–499
© **1984 March of Dimes Birth Defects Foundation**

B) *Maternal Antibody to CMV:* At least 7 of the 8 infected infants lacked maternal antibody to CMV (sera were unavailable from one infant). Fifty-nine percent of all infants and 50% of all low-birthweight infants ($<1,250$ gm) lacked maternal antibody to CMV.

C) *Blood Donors:* The correlation between the number of blood donors for an infant and the acquisition of CMV was highly significant ($P < 0.0001$). Every infected infant received blood from 8 or more donors prior to developing viruria (mean of 15 donors). Uninfected infants, all birthweights, received blood from a mean of 3 different donors. Uninfected low-birthweight infants ($<1,250$ gm) received blood from a mean of 10 different donors ($P > 0.05$, Student's t test, when compared to infected infants).

D) *CMV Seropositive Blood Donors:* The presence or absence of antibody to CMV (CMV EIA) was determined for donor sera for 7 seronegative infants with acquired CMV infection and for 36 uninfected low-birthweight infants ($< 1,250$ gm). Infected infants received blood from a mean of 6.5 donors with antibody to CMV, while the 36 uninfected infants received transfusions from a mean of 3.1 donors with antibody to CMV ($t = 3.31$, $P = 0.002$). Eighteen uninfected low-birthweight infants lacking maternal antibody to CMV received transfusions from a mean of 3.4 seropositive donors ($t = 2.58$, $P = 0.02$).

During the last 12 months of the study, 23 low-birthweight infants ($< 1,250$ gm) lacking maternal antibody against CMV have been transfused with frozen deglycerolized red cells from seronegative donors for all non-emergency transfusions. This group of infants was similar to the previous group of 25 seronegative low-birthweight infants (Table 1), yet none acquired CMV infections.

MANIFESTATIONS OF ACQUIRED CMV

After acquiring CMV, 3 infants died. An autopsy performed on one infant revealed extensive disseminated CMV and *Candida albicans*. Each of the infants who died developed CMV viruria in the 2nd or 3rd month of life after ventilatory assistance was no longer required and significant weight gain had occurred. Each of these infants developed one or more of the following problems: ascites, pneumonia, hepatosplenomegaly, respiratory and renal failure, and shock.

Five of the infants who acquired CMV while hospitalized survived. After they began excreting CMV, 2 of the infants developed hepatitis characterized by hepatosplenomegaly, elevated liver enzymes (SCOT and SGPT), and hyperbilirubinemia. At 13 months of age, one of these infants had a profound bilateral sensorineural hearing deficit. A third infant developed only hepatosplenomegaly without hepatitis. Two infants remained asymptomatic.

During the last 12 months of the study, 9 of 137 infants born to seropositive mothers acquired CMV. Of 73 infants with birthweights $> 1,250$ gm born to seropositive mothers, 4 acquired CMV infections (mean birthweight 2,200 gm) and all 4 remained asymptomatic. Of 40 infants with birthweights $< 1,250$ gm, born to seropositive mothers, 5 (mean birthweight of 900 gm) acquired CMV infection in the 2nd or 3rd month of life. Of these, 2 infants developed severe thrombocytopenia, and one infant developed fever. One of the infants with thrombocytopenia also developed pneumonia, hepatospleno-megaly, and ascites in the week following the onset of viral excretion. This infant survived although all of the symptoms were similar to those observed in the 3 fatal cases of CMV disease which occurred in the low-birthweight infants born to seronegative mothers.

CONCLUSIONS

Acquired CMV infections are a significant cause of morbidity and mortality to low-birthweight infants ($< 1,250$ gm) born to mothers lacking passively acquired antibody against CMV. The source of these infections is seropositive blood donors. The infection can be prevented by appropriate donor selection (seronegative donors) and/or blood processing (frozen deglycerolized red cells).

Infants born to seropositive mothers probably acquired CMV from maternal sources. No fatalities associated with CMV infection occurred in these

TABLE 1. **Acquired CMV Infection Among Low-Birthweight CMV Seronegative Infants Receiving Either Liquid Packed Red Cells From Random Donors (Group A), or Frozen Deglycerolized Red Cells From CMV Seronegative Donors (Group B)**

	Group A	Group B	P Value
No. of infants	25	23	
Mean birthweight (gm ± SD)	952 ± 209	1,052 ± 200	$P > 0.1$*
Mean length of hospitalization (day ± SD)	71 ± 26	74 ± 46	$P > 0.1$*
Mean no. of total donors ± SD	11 ± 6	10 ± 10	$P > 0.1$*
Mean no. of seropositive donors ± SD	4 ± 3	0.47 ± .84	$P < 0.001$*
No. infants acquiring CMV	7	0	$P < 0.01$[†]

*Student's t test.
[†]$\chi^2 = 7.53$, 1 df.

infants; the CMV-associated morbidity in these infants requires additional evaluation.

REFERENCES

1. Adler SP, Chandrika T, Lawrence L, Baggett J: Cytomegalovirus infections in neonates acquired by blood transfusions. Pediatr Infect Dis 2:114–118, 1983.
2. Yeager AS, Grumet FC, Hafleigh EB, Arvin AM, Bradley JS, Prober CG: Prevention of transfusion-acquired cytomegalovirus infections in newborn infants. J Pediatr 98:281–287, 1981.

EPIDEMIOLOGIC STUDIES OF CONGENITAL CMV INFECTION

K. Ahlfors, S. Ivarsson, S. Harris, L. Svanberg, R. Holmqvist, B. Lernmark, G. Theander, and M. Forsgren

University of Lund, Malmö General Hospital, Malmö, Sweden and General Laboratory of Stockholm County Council, Stockholm, Sweden

A prospective study of maternal and congenital CMV infections was started in 1977 in Malmö, a city in Sweden with 225,000 inhabitants. The study is in progress. In principle, serum or urine samples were obtained from all pregnant women and their live-born infants. The women were usually enrolled before the 16th week of pregnancy. Repeat blood specimens were obtained from each of them from the first antenatal visit until delivery. In several cases sera had also been obtained and frozen before conception. ELISA, indirect immunofluorescence, and CF were used for the demonstration of CMV IgG, IgM, and IgG+IgM, respectively. The serologic studies of the mothers were performed retrospectively. The infants were studied for CMV excretion in urine within one week of age by virus isolation in human embryonic lung cells.

In 1977–1979 all mothers were investigated for CMV IgG in sera obtained in early pregnancy. Seronegatives were also tested in sera obtained at delivery. In case of seroconversion, the point of time was more precisely determined by studies of intermediate sera. In the whole study period, mothers of congenitally infected infants and control infants were investigated for CMV IgG and IgM activities in all serum specimens obtained. All samples from each woman were tested simultaneously.

According to the ELISA, 72% of the 4,382 women studied in the 1977–1979 period had CMV IgG antibodies at their first antenatal visit. Seroconversion was shown in 14 (1.2%) of the 1,175 seronegatives retested at delivery. Of the seroconverters 6 (43%) transmitted the infection to the fetus as shown by a positive virus isolation test at birth. Transmission occurred both in early and late pregnancy.

Of 12,243 live-born infants in the period 1977–1982, 10,328 (84%) were studied by virus isolation. The remaining 16% were lost mainly because of shortage of good cell cultures. Fifty (0.5%) separate or pooled urine samples (pools used for a short time) were positive for CMV. Three isolates in pools could not be reisolated from individual samples. Of the 47 congenitally infected infants identified, none had neurologic symptoms but 9 (19%) had mild or moderate symptoms from the reticuloendothelial system (RES) such as hepatomegaly, splenomegaly, icterus and/or thrombocytopenic purpura. Thirty-eight (81%) of the infants had no symptoms typical of congenital CMV infection.

The infants congenitally infected, as well as 51 control infants, were followed up at 3, 6 and 9 months of age, and thereafter at 1, 1.5, 2, 2.5 and 4 years of age. Final examination will be performed when the infants are 6 years old. The examinations were done by specialists at the pediatric, audiologic, ophthalmologic, roentgenologic, and virologic clinics and laboratories, respectively, and by psychologists.

Of the 9 infants with RES symptoms at birth 2 (22%) have neurologic sequelae. One of them is gravely psychomotor retarded and deaf, and the other is deaf. Of the 37 infants asymptomatic at birth and followed up, 3 (8%) are neurologically injured. One of them is moderately psychomotor retarded, and 2 are deaf. Altogether 5 (11%) of the 46 infants followed up have neurologic disturbances at an age ranging from 3 months to 4 years. Of all 10,328 children studied 5 (0.05%) have neurologic sequelae.

Of 51 control infants studied, 16 (31%) had acquired a postnatal CMV infection by 6 months of age. At the age of 18 months, 23 (45%) were infected. None of them had any neurologic complications.

Of the 47 mothers of the infants congenitally infected, 21 (45%) had a primary CMV infection as shown by seroconversion. Ten women had a secondary infection verified by a positive CMV IgG test in sera from the preconceptional period. Three of the 10 secondary infections were accompanied by an IgG titer rise. In the remaining 16 cases, the infection was nontypable with a positive CMV IgG test in the first postconceptional serum. Of the 21 mothers with a primary infection, 18 had CMV IgM in one or several sera. In mothers with secondary or nontypable infections, only 1 had a low IgM titer. Because of serologic similarities in the postconceptional sera of the latter 2 groups it was suggested that most of the nontypable infections were of a secondary type. All 47 maternal infections were asymptomatic.

Of the 21 primary infections, 3 occurred in the 1st trimester. In all 3 cases the infants had RES symptoms at birth but only 1 has neurologic sequelae (grave psychomotor retardation and deafness). Primary infections in the 2nd or 3rd trimester in 4 cases were followed by neonatal symptoms in the infants but in no case by permanent illness.

Of the 10 secondary maternal infections, 2 were followed by permanent symptoms in the infant. One of these infants had moderate RES symptoms at birth. Because of suspected bacterial infection the infant was treated for 3 days with a moderate dosage of gentamycin. The child was later found to be deaf. The 2nd infant, born in bad social conditions, was small for gestational age. At 3 years of age his psychomotor development is comparable with that of a 1.5-year-old infant. In neither of the 2 cases was the time of the maternal infection indicated.

Of 16 nontypable maternal infections, 2 resulted in deafness in the child. Both infants were born asymptomatic. One of the mothers had CMV IgG but no IgM in the 3rd month of pregnancy, and thereafter a stable IgG activity. The other had a positive IgG and a negative IgM test in the 4th month but an IgG titer rise by the 6th month of pregnancy. The latter serologic pattern is compatible with a secondary infection.

One infant with suspected congenital CMV infection, born in 1983, in the 37th gestational week had microcephaly and intracerebral calcifications at birth. Repeat virus isolation tests on urine, throat secretions, blood, and cerebrospinal fluid were negative. No CMV IgM was found in cord serum. However, the mother had a CMV IgG seroconversion in the period 8 months before—4 months after conception. Also CMV IgM was demonstrated at the latter point of time suggesting a recent infection. As in the other cases of neurologic disease, syphilis, rubella, and toxoplasmosis were excluded.

Only 1 case of neurologic injury (grave psychomotor retardation and deafness) could have been predicted by prospective CMV IgM and IgG studies of maternal sera in the period 1977–1982. However, in such a study an unknown number of pregnancies resulting in noninfected or infected/asymptomatic infants had also been considered at risk.

In a separate study, performed in collaboration with Dr. Marianne Forsgren, Stockholm, infants referred because of severe, often neurologic symptoms of CMV infection at birth were investigated. In these cases, primary maternal infection in the 1st and 2nd trimesters predominated. However, one fatal case might have been due to a secondary maternal infection. Severe symptoms at birth were generally combined with a bad prognosis but there were exceptions.

Evidently, the prospective study detected more cases of congenital CMV infection with mild neonatal symptoms compared to routine diagnosis. This fact has implications on prognostic figures. In the prospective study, only 2 of 9 infants with symptoms at birth, compared to 6 of 9 detected in routine diagnosis, had neurologic sequelae. In routine diagnosis severe neurologic disease could mainly be referred to primary maternal infections in the 1st and 2nd trimesters. However, according to the prospective study secondary maternal CMV infection might be more than an exceptional cause of neurologic disease. Attention is also called to a case of possible congenital CMV disease without CMV excretion.

EPSTEIN-BARR VIRUS ESTABLISHED HUMAN B-LYMPHOCYTE CELL LINES SECRETING HUMAN CYTOMEGALOVIRUS SPECIFIC NEUTRALIZING ANTIBODIES

Claire Amadei, Susan Michelson, and André Boué

Unité 73 of INSERM, Chateau de Longchamp, 75016 Paris, and Unité de Virologie Médicale, Institut Pasteur, 75724 Paris Cedex 15, France

The production of human anti-CMV Ig in vitro is of critical importance. So far, hybridoma techniques used to prepare mouse monoclonal antibodies [1] have not been successful in making human antibody secreting hybridomas. Another approach is to establish B-lymphoblastoid cell lines by immortalization with EBV [2–5]. We have used this approach to establish lines secreting antibodies that neutralize HCMV infectivity.

Two cell lines were established from PBMLs. Line LL80 was established from a 30-year-old male who developed a posttransfusional CMV syndrome following splenectomy and multiple surgery for trauma. It was initiated at a time when this patient's IHA titer had increased from 1/80 (day 27 after surgery) to 2,560 (day 82). Cell line LL83 was established from a 20-year-old male renal transplant patient who, since grafting 6 years previously, has continuously shed CMV and maintained an IHA titer of $> 1/5,120$.

Cell line supernatant fluids were regularly tested for the presence of neutralizing and immunofluorescent antibodies, class of Ig production, and presence of mycoplasma.

Table 1 summarizes the detection of neutralizing HCMV antibodies secreted by the two cell lines as a function of cell passage. Table 2 summarizes the analyses of Ig secretion by these cultures.

TABLE 1. Neutralizing HCMV Antibodies (Percentage of Plaque Reduction)

	LL80				LL83		
Passages	AD169	Davis	Towne	Passages	AD169	Davis	Towne
7	72.4%	92.7%	NT	1	93.2%	NT	NT
16	63.9%	64.9%	63.8%	8	54.5%	45.4%	39.8%
18	58.6%	62.7%	63.5%	9	39.4%	63.2%	NT
19	54%	61.2%	NT	11	66.2%	59.9%	NT
21	59.3%	71.7%	NT	14	57.5%	NT	NT
24	71%	NT	NT				

TABLE 2. Production of Globulins by Cell Lines as a Function of Time by Immunonephelometry

Passages	Time in Culture (months)	Human Globulin (μg/ml)		
		γ	μ	α
LL80				
7	1.5	8.9	30	< 5
15	4.0	15.8	14.5	< 5
18	4.5	10.6	< 5	< 5
21	5.2	10.2	< 5	< 5
23	5.7	10.5	< 5	< 5
25	6.2	9.3	< 5	< 2
LL83				
8	3.6	14.7	5	< 2
11	4.5	15.7	5	< 5
13	5.0	9	< 5	< 5
15	5.5	10.7	6	< 5
18	6.0	8.3	< 2	< 3
Culture medium average values		4.5	< 4	< 2

Both cell lines, after more than 6 months in culture, continue to secrete neutralizing HCMV antibodies. In some instances (line LL83), the degree of neutralization fluctuates with time. This may be attributable to sampling irregularities since, within one passage, the production of IgG is itself bimodal. Both lines secrete only IgG, though line LL80 produced both IgG and IgM for the first 15 passages.

Both lines produce antibodies which give a cytoplasmic fluorescence. However, in light of the induction of Fc-receptors [6] by the virus, confirmation of the presence of antigens recognized by LL80 and LL83 antibodies will have to fluoresce using purified Fab fragments.

Both cell lines have a normal diploid karyotype. They show EBV nuclear antigens in all cells with 2%–5% of the cells having viral capsid antigen.

We have thus obtained two B-lymphoblastoid cell lines which produce antibodies which neutralize HCMV infectivity. The presence of EBV capsid antigens in these cells may indicate EBV production, which would complicate use of these anti-HCMV antibodies for immunotherapy. However, it is hoped that upon cloning of producer cells, now underway, antibody production can be improved and any eventual EBV production eliminated.

REFERENCES

1. Köhler G, Milstein C: Continuous cultures of fused cells secreting antibody of predefined specificity. Nature 256:495, 1975.
2. Steinitz M: Human monoclonal antibodies produced by EBV immortalized cell lines. In Hämmerling GJ, Hämmerling U, Kearney JF (eds): "Monoclonal Antibodies and T Cell Hybridomas: Perspectives and Technical Advances." New York: Elsevier-North Holland, 1981, pp 447–452.
3. Sugden B: Epstein-Barr virus: A human pathogen inducing lymphoproliferation in vivo and in vitro. Rev Infect Dis 4:1048–1060, 1982.
4. Callard RE: Specific in vitro antibody response to influenza virus by human blood lymphocytes. Nature 282:734–736, 1979.
5. Crawford DH, Harrison JF, Barlow MJ, Winger L, Muehus ER: Production of human monoclonal antibody to rhesus D antigen. Lancet 1:386, 1983.
6. Furukawa T, Hornberger E, Saku S, Plotkin SA: Demonstration of immunoglobulin G receptors induced by human cytomegalovirus. J Clin Microbiol 2:332–336, 1975.

IMPAIRED MIGRATORY AND CHEMOTACTIC ACTIVITY OF NEUTROPHILS DURING CYTOMEGALOVIRUS INFECTION OF MICE

J.F. Bale, Jr., E.R. Kern, and J.C. Overall, Jr.

Department of Pediatrics, University of Iowa College of Medicine, Iowa City, IA, and Department of Pediatrics, University of Utah School of Medicine, Salt Lake City, UT

CMV infection has been associated with altered host defense and increased susceptibility to secondary infections with bacterial and fungal pathogens. In a mouse model, we have demonstrated that, during the acute stages of a 0–20% lethal murine CMV (MCMV) infection, there was enhanced mortality after an intranasal inoculation of *E coli* K1 and a diminished inflammatory response to a subcutaneous challenge with the same bacteria (Bale JF et al: J Infect Dis 145:525–531, 1982). To further investigate alterations in neutrophils during MCMV infection, we 1) examined absolute neutrophil counts in the peripheral blood; 2) determined the migration of neutrophils into a SC implanted sponge; and 3) measured the chemotactic activity of neutrophils harvested from the sponge. On days 2 and 4 of the MCMV infection, neutrophil migration into a SC sponge was reduced (1,300 to 2,000 cells/mm^3 of sponge fluid in MCMV-infected animals *v* 6,000 to 7,000 cells in controls, P < 0.01) (Fig. 1), and chemotaxis of neutrophils harvested from the sponge was markedly impaired (chemotactic index of 1.5 to 2.1 in infected animals *v* 4.5 to 5.7 in controls, P < 0.01) (Fig. 2). In contrast, the

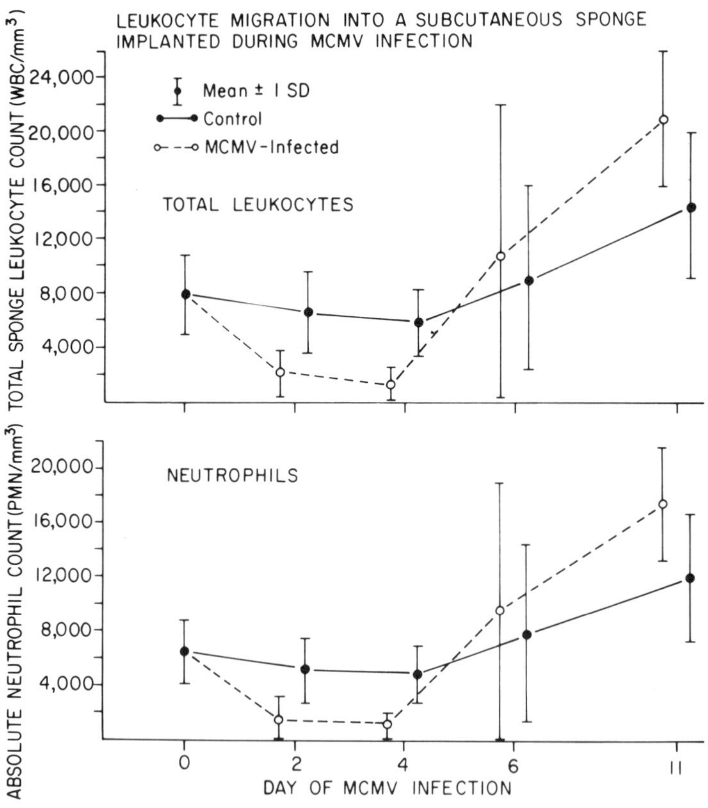

Fig. 1. Total leukocytes (top) and neutrophil (bottom) migration into a SC sponge. MCMV-infected mice were inoculated IP with 2 × 10^5 PFU of MCMV. Control mice were inoculated with a preparation of normal salivary gland. Each point represents the mean of data from 10 to 15 animals. Bars indicate the mean value ± 1 SD.

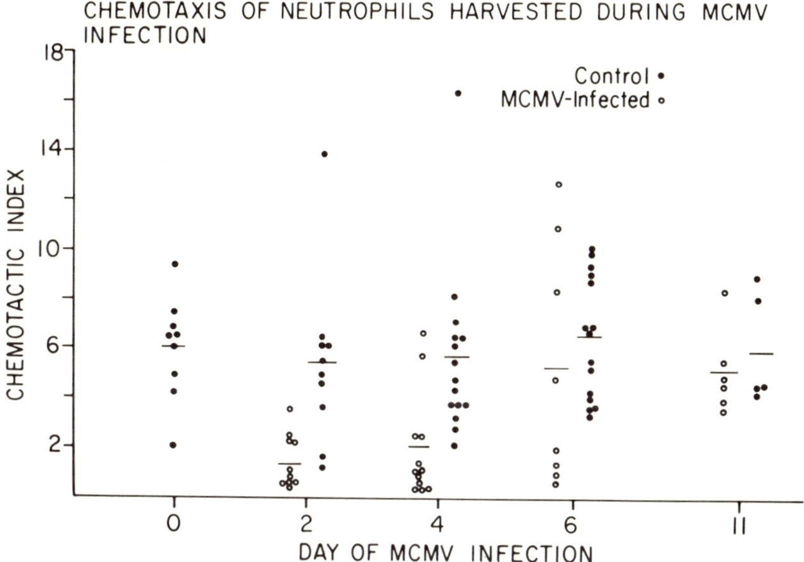

Fig. 2. Chemotaxis of neutrophils harvested from sponges implanted during MCMV infection. MCMV-infected mice were inoculated with 2×10^5 PFU MCMV; control mice were inoculated with a preparation of normal salivary gland. Each point represents data from a single animal. Bars indicate mean values.

number of neutrophils in the peripheral blood was not altered. For example, on day 2 the mean neutrophil count in peripheral blood was 732 in infected animals v 899 in controls (P = 0.3). Assay of peripheral blood demonstrated that MCMV was present in the neutrophil-rich fraction on days 4, 6, and 8 with peak titers of log 1.4 PFU per million leukocytes on day 4. MCMV was also present in plasma and in the mononuclear-rich fraction on days 2, 4, 5, and 8 with peak titers in the mononuclear-rich fraction of log 2.4 PFU per million cells on day 6. In contrast, assay of leukocytes from SC sponges demonstrated that MCMV could be recovered only on days 4 and 6 of MCMV infection with peak titers of only log 0.5 PFU per million cells on day 4. Despite impaired migratory and chemotactic activity of neutrophils on day 2 of MCMV infection, infectious virus was not detected in sponge leukocytes or in neutrophils from the peripheral blood. These results indicate that the migratory and chemotactic activity of neutrophils is impaired during acute MCMV infection, and these abnormalities may account for the diminished numbers of neutrophils in bacteria-infected tissues of mice infected with MCMV. These studies also indicate that the amount of infectious virus in neutrophils is small and that abnormal neutrophil function may occur in the absence of infectious virus. These observations suggest that other mechanisms, such as nonproductive infection of leukocytes or induction of soluble inhibitors, may be operative. Abnormalities in neutrophil function during acute CMV infection may contribute to the enhanced susceptibility to secondary bacterial and fungal infections that have been observed in experimental animals and humans.

EVALUATION OF CYTOLYTIC ANTI-CYTOMEGALOVIRUS (CMV) ANTIBODY AND/OR CERVICAL VIRUS SHEDDING IN PREDICTING CONGENITAL CMV INFECTION

F. Betts, E. Warner, G. Cutris, S. Erb, S. Schmidt, and M. Menegus
University of Rochester School of Medicine, Rochester, NY 14642

In the obstetric clinic of Strong Memorial Hospital, we evaluated 676 pregnant women [410 Black (B) and 266 White (W)] at first visit for IgG antibody to CMV as measured by CF using glycine extracted antigen. Antibody frequency was greater in B (71%) compared to W (42%). Cervical cultures for CMV were obtained at 36–38 wk [a time previously shown by Stagno et al (JID 131:522, 1975) to be equivalent to nonpregnant women] from 252 of the antibody-positive patients (181 B, 71 W), representing 62% and 63% of the antibody-positive women in each race, and from 93 antibody-negative women. Of the 252 women, 21 B (11.6%) and 13 W (18.5%) were shedding CMV *v* 2 antibody-negative women who were undergoing primary infection. Percentage of seropositive subjects shedding was greater in women less than 19 years of age (18%) than those over 25 years of age (7%). Measurement of virus excretion at birth was carried out in 166 of the babies of these 252 seropositive women. Seven (4.2%) were shedding virus. These results were evaluated in relation to maternal virologic (cervical shedding) and serologic (cytolytic antibody) characteristics. Among 24 CMV shedders, 2 babies (9%) were infected *v* 5 babies (3.5%) of the nonshedders. Cytolytic antibody is an IgM antibody that lyses CMV infected cells in the presence of rabbit or human but not guinea pig complement. It first appears following primary CMV infection just after IgG is detectable and persists for only 3–18 mo. Among the 5 women whose first visit sera contained both CF and cytolytic anti-CMV antibody, 4 had babies with congenital infection. This contrasts with the 151 women whose first visit sera contained CF but not cytolytic antibody. Only 3 of these babies had congenital infection. The only other baby identified in this study with congenital infection was delivered by 1 of 3 women who developed primary CMV infection after their first visit.

Thus, cytolytic antibody measured early in pregnancy identified more women who would deliver children with congenital infection than did evaluation of cervical virus shedding late in pregnancy. The majority of women in this study who delivered children with congenital infection either had acquired infection in the few months prior to conception or had developed primary infection after conception. Measurement of cytolytic antibody in the 1st trimester women may help in the management of pregnant women.

VIRAL LYTIC ANTIBODY RESPONSE TO CYTOMEGALOVIRUS INFECTION AND VACCINATION

K.R. Beutner, S.G. Schmidt, and R.F. Betts
University of Rochester School of Medicine, Rochester, NY 14642

Employing assays for CMV viral lytic antibody (VLAb), cytolytic antibody (CyAb), and CF antibody, sera from normal and CMV-infected subjects were tested. VLAb is a neutralizing antibody which, in the presence of complement, renders the CMV DNA susceptible to exogenous DNase. CyAb is an IgM antibody capable of mediating complement dependent lysis of CMV-infected cells. Samples tested included sera from normal subjects (50), patients with acute CMV-infectious mononucleosis (16), renal transplant patients (10), recipients of the Towne strain CMV vaccine (6), congenitally infected infants (15) and their mothers (9), and uninfected infant-mother pairs (13).

All 50 sera tested from healthy donors were CyAb negative, while 25 and 29 of these sera were seropositive by CF and VLAb, respectively. CyAb was detected in 21/26 subjects with acute CMV infection, 3/6 CMV vaccinees, 5/15 congenitally infected infants and in 5/9 of their mothers. CMV CF antibody was observed in all infected or vaccinated subjects. VLAb was detected in 12/16 patients with acute primary CMV infections. The 4 VLAb seronegative CyAb seropositive subjects were very early in the acute phase and seroconverted for VLAb during convalescence. VLAb was observed in 10/10 renal transplants, 15/15 congenitally infected infants, and in 9/9 of their mothers, as well as 13/13 uninfected CF-positive mother-infant pairs. VLAb titers of $\geqslant 1024$ were observed in 1/13 uninfected and 11/15 infected infants. VLAb was detectable in 3/6 CMV vaccinees. Selected sera were fractionated on a Sephadex G-200 column to determine the isotype of VLAb. VLAb activity was only present in the IgG fractions. This study demonstrates the formation of CMV VLAb in response to primary CMV infection and vaccination. This antibody is predominantly of the IgG isotype and high titers of VLAb are observed in congenitally infected infants. This assay provides a simple, rapid (one day) method of measuring complement-dependent CMV neutralizing antibody.

TRANSFORMING ACTIVITY OF CELLULAR DNA AFTER HCMV INFECTION

I. Boldogh, E. Gönczöl, E.-S. Huang, and L. Váczi
Department of Microbiology, School of Medicine, Debrecen, Hungary, and Cancer Research Center, School of Medicine, Chapel Hill, NC 27514

HCMV has been implicated as a possible oncogenic agent. The ability of HCMV to stimulate the synthesis of macromolecules of infected cells is supported by several publications. The oncogenic transformation of normal cells by HCMV and its DNA fragments has been documented also. The common characteristic of the transformed cells is that the presence of viral DNA, RNA, and antigen(s) are related only to early events of cell transformation. It seems to us that HCMV has no role in the maintenance of the transformed state since after the initial events the HCMV markers are eliminated from the cells without altering the transformed phenotypes. In our experiments, the DNAs of HCMV infected human embryo fibroblasts were tested for the ability to transform hamster embryo fibroblast cells. After insertion of cellular DNA originated from HCMV-infected cells showed transforming activity. The pilled up cell foci were isolated and 6 cell lines were established. The cell lines show continuous growth and biologic properties typical of transformed cells. The transformed cells are oncogenic in syrian newborn hamsters. The tumors were identified as poorly differentiated fibrous sarcomas. In the cell lines or in the tumor cells there was no evidence for HCMV specific antigens or nucleic acids.

These findings suggest that HCMV might induce dominant mutations or gene rearrangements in cellular DNA which possibly may be related to the transforming ("onc") gene(s) of human cells.

ANALYSIS OF THE HUMAN CYTOTOXIC AND HELPER T-CELL RESPONSE TO CYTOMEGALOVIRUS IN VITRO

L.K. Borysiewicz, S. Morris, J. Page, and J.G.P. Sissons

Departments of Medicine and Virology, Royal Postgraduate Medical School, London W12 OHS, England

The cellular immune response is widely assumed to play a major role in limiting reactivation of human herpesviruses, but the precise nature of this response is unclear. In individuals who are seropositive for EBV there is a high precursor frequency of EBV-specific cytotoxic T-cell (Tc) precursors that limit outgrowth of autologous EBV-transformed B cells in vitro. The evidence for a similar response to herpesviruses with different sites of latency is less well-established. Although Quinnan and colleagues have presented evidence for a similar response to herpesviruses with different sites of latency is less well established. Although Quinnan and colleagues have presented evidence by direct examination of PBMCs that Tc may be present during

In order to approach the problem of the nature and specificity of any T cells which might be involved in controlling HCMV reactivation, we have studied the T-cell response to HCMV in vitro using PBMC of normal seropositive subjects who have had no clinically overt HCMV infection. The responding lymphocytes were maintained in culture with lectin-free IL2, to ultimately permit their clonal analysis.

PBM of HCMV seropositive individuals proliferated in response to live, UV-inactivated or heat-inactivated AD169 strain CMV. Similar proliferative responses were observed with free HCMV, 4d HCMV-infected, or 4d HCMV-infected phosphonoformate-blocked fibroblasts expressing HCMV early antigens. In order to determine whether T cells were present among the proliferating cells, we cultured lymphocytes with live or UV-inactivated HCMV (MOI 5:1) for 5 days. IL2 and autologous irradiated PBMCs were added and cultures were maintained for 7 to 43 days. The lymphocytes were used as effector cells in a 6-hr ^{51}Cr release assay using autologous or HLA-matched and HLA-mismatched, HCMV-infected and uninfected fibroblast lines as target cells. No virus-specific cytotoxicity was observed in 18 such short-term T-cell lines, and the surface phenotype of the effector cells was Leu 3a, and Leu 4a positive.

When free HCMV was presented on autologous irradiated feeder cells in the absence of exogenous IL2, the T-cell lines continued to proliferate. This proliferation correlated with release of IL2 by the lymphocyte line. These T-cell lines were cloned by limiting dilution, and the Leu 3 positive clones continued to proliferate to gradient purified HCMV.

Some nonstructural HCMV antigens may only be expressed in HCMV-infected cells. We cocultured HCMV-infected autologous fibroblasts with PBMC, and 5 days later, IL2 and autologous feeder cells were added. After 7 days, infected autologous fibroblasts were again added. The lymphocytes were assayed on day 14 against autologous and HLA-mismatched target cells as previously described. No evidence of virus-specific lysis was observed after 5 or 7 days' coculture, but by 14 days, virus-specific lysis of HCMV-infected autologous target cells, but not HLA-mismatched targets,was observed. The results obtained from 13 such short-term T-cell lines are shown in Figure 1. T-cell lines from seronegative subjects were difficult to establish using this protocol and showed no evidence of virus-specific lysis. Nine of 10 lines from seropositive subjects showed virus-specific lysis, and 8 of these 9 lysed autologous HCMV-infected target cells only.

The surface phenotype of these lines was Leu 2a and Leu 4a positive. Figure 2 shows that these Tc were HLA-A and -B restricted, as there was equal lysis of HCMV-infected, HLA-matched target cells; cytotoxicity was also HCMV specific as herpes simplex-infected HLA-matched and mismatched cells were not lysed. In addition, target cells that were infected with HCMV for 6 hr prior to the 6 hr ^{51}Cr release assay were lysed as readily as

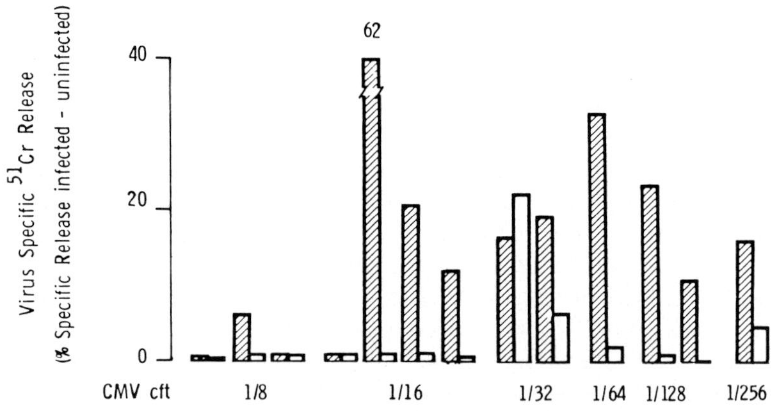

Fig. 1. Cytotoxicity of 13 short-term T-cell lines established after coculture with autologous HCMV-infected fibroblasts, against autologous (▨) and HLA mismatched (☐) HCMV infected target cells. Specific ^{51}Cr release of uninfected target cells has been subtracted in each case (E:T 20:1).

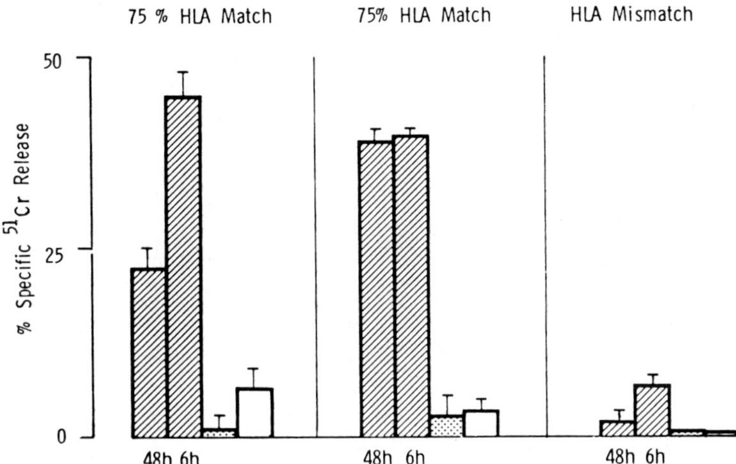

Fig. 2. HCMV-specific cytotoxicity expressed by a T-cell line against HCMV (▨) or herpes simplex (▧) infected or uninfected (□) targets. There was equivalent lysis of target cells infected with HCMV for 6 hr and 48 hr (E:T 20:1).

target cells infected for 48 hr, suggesting that at least some Tc were able to recognize and lyse target cells expressing HCMV early antigens. We have also observed that in order to generate HCMV-specific Tc, exposure to HCMV-infected fibroblasts is required through the 14-day culture period. If there were no reexposure to antigen after 5 days, Leu 3a positive, noncytotoxic lines were obtained.

CONCLUSIONS

We examined the T-cell response of normal latently infected subjects to HCMV in vitro. The nature of the HCMV antigen used for secondary in vitro stimulation in part determined the T-cell response observed.

1. Leu 3a-positive T-cell lines were established using free HCMV, and these lines continued to proliferate and release IL2 to free antigen. Similar Leu 3a-positive T-cell lines could be established using infected autologous fibroblasts as stimulator cells.

2. The only condition under which Leu 2a-positive HCMV-specific cytotoxic T-cell lines could be generated was by continued secondary in vitro stimulation with infected autologous fibroblasts.

Hence, we have demonstrated the presence of HCMV-specific Tc-precursors in PBMC of normal HCMV-seropositive subjects without preceding clinically overt HCMV infection. The requirement for infected fibroblasts to be present as stimulator cells and the lysis of 6 hr infected target cells suggests that at least some of the Tc precursors show specificity for HCMV-induced early antigens.

SEROEPIDEMIOLOGY OF CMV INFECTIONS: A BASIS FOR THE STRATEGIES OF PREVENTION

A. Boué and N. Cabau

Unité de Recherches de Biologie Prénatale, Château de Longchamp, Bois de Boulogne, 75016 Paris, France

Wide variations in the incidence of infections by CMV have been reported. Epidemiologic analyses of these variations are needed in order to establish the basis for strategies of prevention.

MATERIALS AND METHODS

During the last decade, epidemiologic surveys based on the prevalence of CMV antibodies have been undertaken in different groups (children from 1 to 4 years of age, their mothers, pregnant women, blood donors), in the French population and in migrant mothers from Spain, Portugal, French Antilles and North Africa.

In most of these surveys, blood samples were collected on blotting cards requiring a few drops of blood obtained by puncture of the finger.

The IHA has been used throughout this study.

RESULTS

Seroepidemiology in the First Years of Life

A follow-up serologic study was done on 207 mothers and their children at the ages of 10 months, 2 years, and 4 years during health check-ups; 117 mothers were seropositive, and 42 (35.9%) had a child who was seropositive at the age of 4; 29 children were already seropositive at 10 months of age. In the group of 90 seronegative mothers, only 3 (3.3%) had a CMV-seropositive child by the age of 4 (all 3 were seronegative at 10 mo of age).

CMV-seropositive mothers were the most important sources of infection during the first years of life.

Different surveys compared the prevalence of CMV infections from sero-positive mothers during the first year of life, in relation to the socioeconomic conditions. Table 1 shows the results. If seropositive mothers represented potential sources of CMV infection, the transmission of the infection was highly correlated with the socioeconomic conditions and could vary from 10%–40% in the same country.

As the prevalence of seropositive mothers varied in the same direction (Table 2), at one year of age in the total infant population, the number of seropositive infants varied from 4%–35% in relation to the socioeconomic conditions.

Prevalence of CMV Antibodies in Adults

Different surveys were done in 18 to 40-year-old women belonging to different socioeconomic groups in France (Table 2).

The prevalence of CMV antibodies varied with: the socioeconomic class of the French couples; the place of birth: migrant women had arrived in France during the last 10 years and had been infected during their infancy. Thus, about 90% were seropositive, their present socioeconomic class having no effect upon the prevalence. The time: with the general improvement of the socioeconomic conditions, a decrease in the prevalence of seropositive French women was observed during the last 10 years in the same socioeconomic class.

The prevalence of CMV-seropositive adult subjects in relation to age was studied in 604 French blood donors from the middle class. In the 20–30 year age group, 30.2% were seropositive; in the 30–50 year age group, 51.8%; and 68.3% in the 50–60 year age group. The increase in the prevalence of CMV-seropositive subjects in relation to age was not only a reflection of viral transmission, but that of a cohort effect, especially in the older group,

TABLE 1. Comparison of the Prevalence of CMV Infection in 1-Year-Old Infants Having a Seropositive Mother, In Relation to Socioeconomic Conditions

| | | CMV Antibodies in Their 1-Year-Old Infants | |
| | No. of | | |
Groups of Mothers	Seropositive Mothers	No.	%
Mozambique	36	29	80
France			
Migrant mothers			
Low socioeconomic class	43	18	42
Middle class	77	20	26
French mothers			
Low socioeconomic class	120	24	20
Middle-class urban	145	16	11
Middle-class rural	157	14	9

TABLE 2. Prevalence of CMV Antibodies in Different Groups of 18 to 40-Year-Old French Women

	French Women		Migrant Women	
	No. Tested	% Seropositive	No. Tested	% Seropositive
Paris and suburbs				
Low socioeconomic class				
Mothers of 1-year-old infants (1974–1975)	182	66%	47	91%
Pregnant women (1978–1979)	194	59.8%	225	94.2%
Low and middle class				
Pregnant women (1978–1979)	698	51.1%	309	84.8%
Middle class				
Mothers of 1-year-old infants (1974–1975)	310	47%	89	89%
Pregnant women (1978–1979)	445	41.1%	128	85.9%
Rural areas. Alsace				
Mothers of 1-year-old infants (1972–1973)	339	46%	26	96.2%
Pregnant women (1982)	303	39.6%		

who were born at a time when the socioeconomic conditions were generally low, breast-feeding was usual, and thus the risk of viral transmission during the perinatal period was high.

CONCLUSIONS

Perinatal Transmission of CMV

Due to the decreasing prevalence of CMV-seropositive mothers and the decreasing transmission of the infection, the incidence of CMV-perinatal infection will reach very low levels in the major part of the population in countries with good socioeconomic conditions.

Natural Transmission in Adults

Are the socioeconomic factors, which have been evidenced in perinatal transmission, also influencing the incidence of CMV transmission between adults?

The decreasing prevalence of CMV-seropositive young adults in the general population supports this hypothesis. It can be expected that in these groups the risk of intrauterine infection will spontaneously decrease.

Iatrogenic Transmission

There is presently an increasing number of CMV-seropositive patients receiving transfusions or organ transplants. This situation will require a policy of prevention in these highly susceptible groups.

HUMAN AND MURINE MHC-RESTRICTED CYTOTOXIC LYMPHOCYTE RESPONSES TO CMV INFECTION

M.K. Breinig, P. Camp, S. Dummer, and M. Ho
University of Pittsburgh, Pittsburgh, PA 15261

CMI is presumed to be important in host defenses against CMV infection. H-2 restricted CTLs against murine CMV have been demonstrated in vivo [1] and generated in vitro [2]. Recent evidence suggests HLA-restricted CTLs develop in vivo in BMT recipients with CMV infection [3]. The present studies were performed to determine the effect of cyclosporine (cyA), an immunosuppressant that acts selectively within subsets of T lymphocytes, on human and murine CMV-restricted CTL responses.

METHODS
Human Studies

Six male kidney transplant recipients were studied prospectively for CMV-specific CTL responses. Four received cyA, one received azathioprine (AZ), and one received cyA except for a 16-day period during which he received AZ. All patients also received prednisone. Serum was assayed for antibody against CMV using the anticomplementary immunofluorescent test. Isolation of CMV from throat wash, urine, and buffy coat was performed using human skin fibroblasts.

CMV-specific cytotoxic responses were tested using one or more target cells with which the patient shared at least one HLA antigen at the A or B locus (matched target cell) and one or more target cells which were completely mismatched at the A and B locus. Briefly, fibroblasts cultured from skin biopsies from patients with known HLA haplotype were infected at an MOI of 0.1–0.2:1 with CMV (strain AD169), harvested when 100% of the cells demonstrated cytopathic effect, and stored in liquid nitrogen. Uninfected fibroblasts were prepared in a similar manner. For use in the cytotoxicity assay, CMV-infected and uninfected target cells were thawed quickly, added to medium, centrifuged, resuspended, labeled with 50 μCi of ^{51}Cr and incubated for 1 hr at 37°C. The cells were then washed two times and 100 μl of labeled target cells (5×10^3) were added to each well of a 96-well U-bottomed microassay plate. Effector (PBM) cells at various dilutions were added to replicate wells, 100 μl/well. Results presented here are those obtained at a 50:1 effector-to-target ratio. After 16–18 hr incubation at 37°C in humidified 5% CO_2, supernatant fluids were harvested and counted in a gamma counter. Specific release (SR) was calculated as follows:

$$\%SR = \frac{\text{test CPM} - \text{control CPM}}{\text{maximum CPM} - \text{control CPM}} \times 100,$$

where test CPM = ^{51}Cr release in presence of effector cells, control CPM = spontaneous ^{51}Cr release in presence of unlabeled K562 cells, and maximum CPM = ^{51}Cr release in 0.5% Triton X-100. To determine CMV-specific lysis, %SR of uninfected fibroblasts was subtracted from %SR of the homologous CMV-infected fibroblasts.

Mouse Studies

Effector splenic lymphocytes were obtained from Balb/c mice 9 days after IP infection with 4×10^5 PFU of MCMV. CyA-treated mice received 50 mg/kg each day after infection. Thioglycolate stimulated peritoneal macrophages, obtained from Balb/c mice and infected with MCMV, were used as targets. Briefly, macrophages were dispensed ($1–2 \times 10^5$/well) into 96-well flat-bottomed plates and incubated for 4 hr at 37°C in humidified 5% CO_2. Plates were then decanted and 0.05 ml of medium was added to half the wells. To the other half, 0.05 ml of MCMV was added at an MOI of 2:1. Plates were centrifuged for 30 min at 2,000 rpm, incubated at 37°C for 1 hr, then 0.1 ml of medium was added to each well. After overnight incubation, the macrophages were labeled with 1 μCi of ^{51}Cr/well, incubated for 1–1½ hr at 37°C, washed twice, and 0.1 ml of medium was added to each well. After this procedure, approximately $0.5–1 \times 10^5$ macrophages remained in each well. Serial twofold dilutions of effector cells were made and added to replicate wells, 0.1 ml/well. After 18 hr incubation at 37°C in humidified 5% CO_2, 1 ml of supernatant fluid was harvested from each well and counted in a gamma counter. Specific release and virus-specific lysis were calculated, as previously described.

RESULTS

CMV infection was documented by virus isolation in all patients (Fig. 1). Infection was reactivated in patients 1 to 5; none had symptomatic disease. Patient 6 had primary CMV infection and symptomatic disease. Patient 1 was on AZ and demonstrated CMV-specific, HLA-restricted lysis on the four occasions tested. The levels of lysis ranged from 9% to 34%. Patient 2 demonstrated a high level (49%) of CMV-specific, HLA-restricted lysis when receiving AZ and a lower level when receiving cyA. Patient 3, who received the lowest dose of cyA (mean 300 mg/day), demonstrated CMV-

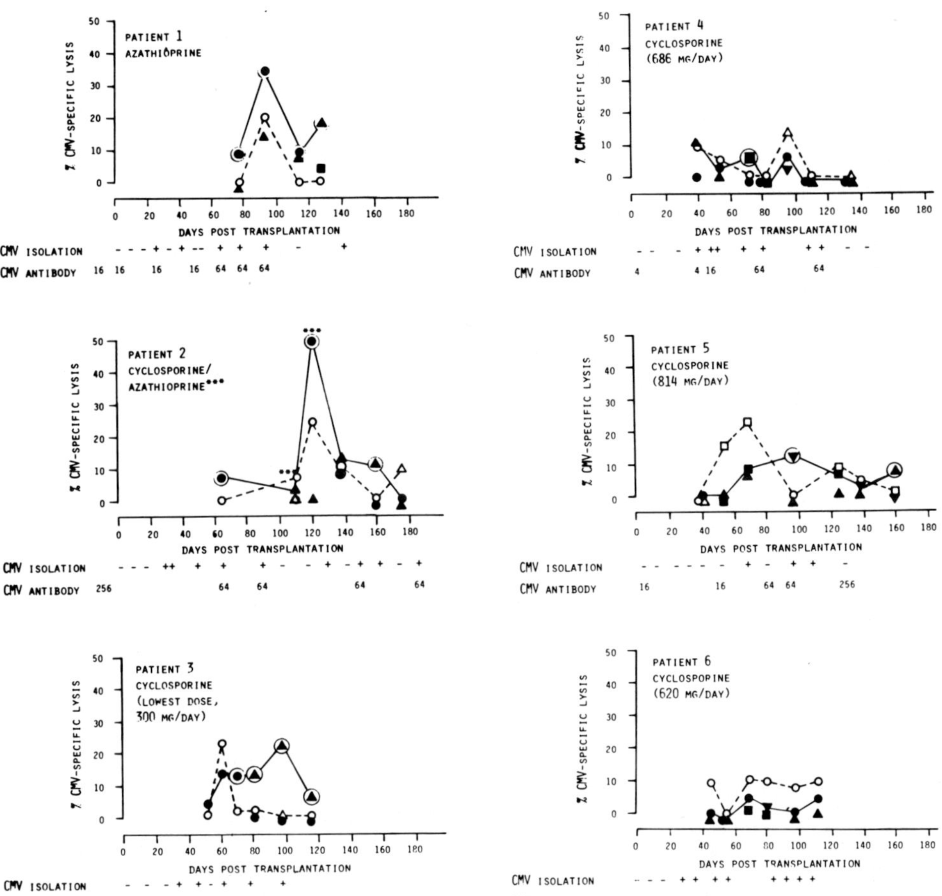

Fig. 1. CMV-specific CTL responses, CMV isolation, and CMV antibody titer of 6 kidney transplant recipients. Lysis of HLA-matched target cells is represented by a solid line connecting closed symbols (●, ▲, ■, ▼, each symbol representing a different matched target cell); lysis of mismatched target cells is represented by a dashed line connecting open symbols (○, △, each symbol representing a different mismatched target cell). Encircled closed symbols ⊙ represent HLA-restricted lysis. CMV isolation (± = positive, − = negative) and antibody titer (expressed as reciprocals of serum dilutions) are presented on the lower portion of the figure.

specific, HLA-restricted lysis on four of six occasions tested, with levels ranging from 6% to 22%. Patients 4 and 5, who received mean doses of 686 and 814 mg cyA/day, respectively, occasionally demonstrated low levels (< 12%) of specific lysis. Patient 6, who received a mean dose of 620 mg cyA/ day, developed primary CMV infection and pneumonia due to pneumocystis

TABLE 1. Effect of Cyclosporine (cyA) on Specific Cytotoxicity of MCMV Infected Mice

Exp. No.	Treatment[a]	% Virus-Specific Lysis at Effector:Target Ratios of					
		25	20	12.5	10	6.25	5
1	MCMV	13.8 ± 3.3	ND[b]	4.1 ± 2.5	ND	5.1 ± 2.0	ND
	MCMV + CyA	10.7 ± 2.4	ND	9.8 ± 3.0	ND	15.4 ± 4.5	ND
2	MCMV	9.9 ± 2.6	ND	9.8 ± 1.9	ND	8.1 ± 2.4	ND
	MCMV + CyA	13.8 ± 1.9	ND	5.1 ± 3.2	ND	6.4 ± 2.1	ND
3	MCMV	ND	ND	ND	8.3 ± 1.9	ND	10.0 ± 2.0
	MCMV + CyA	ND	ND	ND	10.8 ± 1.4	ND	5.8 ± 3.1
4	MCMV	ND	ND	ND	21.3 ± 2.3	ND	10.9 ± 2.3
	MCMV + CyA	ND	ND	ND	19.4 ± 2.7	ND	14.3 ± 2.4
5	MCMV	ND	16.4 ± 3.7	ND	13.2 ± 3.0	ND	6.9 ± 2.3
	MCMV + CyA	ND	11.7 ± 2.9	ND	2.2 ± 2.8	ND	3.9 ± 3.3
6	MCMV	ND	9.4 ± 3.8	ND	13.4 ± 3.7	ND	9.0 ± 5.0
	MCMV + CyA	ND	7.3 ± 2.9	ND	4.6 ± 2.4	ND	−1.4 ± 3.4

[a]Balb/c mice were infected IP with 4×10^5 PFU of MCMV (day 0), then either treated daily (starting with day 0) with 50 mg/kg cyA, IP, or not treated. Spleens were harvested on day 9. No significant difference between MCMV and MCMV + cyA group as measured by paired *t*-test.
[b]Not done.

and CMV. This patient did not develop CMV-specific, HLA-restricted lysis. The presence or lack of cytotoxic response was not related to morbidity. The cytotoxic responses (mean ± SE) of the 5 patients when receiving cyA was 3.5 ± 0.7 against matched, and 5.6 ± 1.2 against mismatched targets, whereas the responses of the 2 patients when receiving AZ was 13.5 ± 4.6 against matched, and 7.4 ± 3.9 against mismatched targets. The preceding results suggest that cyA may prevent the development of virus-specific, HLA-restricted CTL in kidney transplant patients with CMV infection. We then tested directly the effect of cyA on the development of CTL against murine CMV in Balb/c mice. Table 1 shows the results of 6 separate experiments. Overall, there was no significant difference between the cyA-treated and untreated groups (P > 0.05; paired *t* test). Within individual experiments, occasional depressions of cytotoxicity by cyA are noted; at the same time, there are instances where it appears cyA enhances cytotoxicity.

CONCLUSIONS

When the CMV-specific cytotoxic responses of 4 patients on cyA were tested, one patient had no HLA-restricted lysis, two occasionally demonstrated low levels of lysis, and one demonstrated HLA-restricted lysis. This patient was receiving the lowest dose of cyA. In contrast, patient 1, receiving AZ, developed HLA-restricted lysis, as did patient 2 tested when receiving AZ. The mean levels of lysis of the 5 patients when receiving cyA were comparable against matched and mismatched target cells, whereas the mean levels of lysis of the patients tested when receiving AZ were greater against matched than mismatched targets. These results suggest that cyA may prevent the development of HLA-restricted lysis. However, caution must be used in interpreting these results. First, the presence of HLA-restricted lysis was interpreted as evidence of presence of CTL, although it is probably unlikely that non-T lymphocytes would be truly HLA-restricted. The nature of the effector cells was not confirmed by fractionation procedures. Second, only one patient not receiving cyA was tested. Third, the levels of lysis are low. Fourth, when the effect of cyA on the development of primary CTL was directly tested in mice, no inhibition was demonstrated.

It should also be noted that we were successful in assaying mouse CTL against MCMV using infected stimulated macrophages, which in our hands produced more consistent results than infected fibroblasts [1]. The responsible cells were shown to be T cells using anti-theta serum and complement.

REFERENCES

1. Quinnan GJ, Manischewitz JE, Ennis FA: Cytotoxic T lymphocyte response to murine cytomegalovirus infection. Nature 273:541–543, 1978.
2. Ho M, Ashman RB: Development in vitro of cytotoxic lymphocytes against murine cytomegalovirus. Aust J Exp Biol Med Sci 57:425–428, 1979.
3. Quinnan GJ, Kirmani N, Esber E et al: HLA-restricted cytotoxic T lymphocytes and nonthymic cytotoxic lymphocyte responses to cytomegalovirus infection of bone marrow transplant recipients. J Immunol 126:2036–2041, 1981.

PREVENTION OF PRIMARY CMV INFECTION IN RENAL TRANSPLANT PATIENTS BY ANTIBODY SCREENING OF DONORS AND RECIPIENTS*

R.L. Burleson, H.V. Lamberson, C. Hubbel, and A. Burleson

State University of New York, Upstate Medical Center and the American Red Cross Blood Services, Syracuse, NY 13210

Several centers have reported increased morbidity and mortality and decreased allograft survival in renal allograft recipients who develop 1° CMV infection in the posttransplantation period. We have retrospectively reviewed

* Supported in part by American Red Cross funds.

CMV serology of donors and recipients transplanted at our center from 1974–1980. During this period, all patients received renal allografts irrespective of the serologic status (IHA or CF) of the donor or the recipient. One hundred and thirteen recipients lacked detectable anti-CMV prior to transplantation and were assumed to be at risk for 1° CMV infection. Forty (35%) of these patients developed serologic evidence of 1° CMV and 10 (25%) of these died. Seventy-three CMV(−) recipients failed to develop detectable anti-CMV and 6 of these died (9.0%) (P = < 0.05). During this period, the antibody status of 48 donors was known. Fifteen of 20 CMV(−) recipients of kidneys from CMV(+) donors developed 1° CMV, whereas 3/28 recipients of kidneys from CMV(−) donors developed 1° CMV (P < 0.005).

Since January 1981, we have determined the CMV status of donors and recipients (ELISA) prior to transplantation. During this time, 21 CMV(−) recipients received kidneys from 17 CMV(−) donors and 4 CMV(+) donors. None of the 17 recipients of CMV(−) kidneys has developed serologic evidence of CMV infection and none has died (6 months minimum follow-up). All 4 CMV(−) recipients of CMV(+) kidneys developed serologic evidence of CMV and 2 have died. Thirteen of the 17 CMV(−) recipients of CMV(−) kidneys received perioperative transfusions of red blood cells from donors of undetermined serologic status. Forty-five percent of blood donors from the region are CMV(+). Four CMV(−) potential recipients of kidneys from CMV(+) live, related donors have each received 3 transfusions of 100 ml RBC within 24 hr of collection from the prospective donors. These potential recipients were receiving azathioprine in conjunction with a donor-specific transfusion (DST) protocol. None of these 4 patients developed clinical CMV infection or serologic evidence of 1° CMV infection.

We conclude that the transplantation of a CMV(+) kidney to a CMV(−) recipient carries a risk of 1° CMV infection which approaches 100%. In our center, CMV infection is associated with increased mortality. The practice of transplanting only CMV(−) kidneys to CMV(−) donors has greatly decreased the risk of 1° CMV infection. The risk of developing primary CMV infection from blood products and other sources is small in the patients studied, since none of the 17 CMV(−) recipients of CMV(−) kidneys and none of the 4 recipients of CMV(+) DST have developed CMV.

COMMON ANTIGEN ON HUMAN CYTOMEGALOVIRUS-TRANSFORMED CELLS AND UROGENITAL TUMORS

A.E. Campbell, J.J. Starling, M.L. Beckett, and
G.L. Wright, Jr.
Eastern Virginia Medical School, Norfolk, VA 23501

Cancer of the prostate is the second most common form of malignant neoplasia among males in the United States and results in nearly 20,000 deaths each year. Although various sociologic factors have been associated with this disease, the etiology remains unknown. One possibility, however, is HCMV, which has several properties of an oncogenic virus [1]. Infection of human fibroblasts with HCMV isolated from normal prostate tissue can lead to transformation in vitro, and these transformed cells are tumorigenic in mice [2]. Primary prostate cancer cell lines passaged in vitro express HCMV antigens in the nucleus and membrane [2]. Furthermore, serologic studies indicate that significantly more prostate cancer patients have higher HCMV antibody titers than control patients [3]. Because of the associations between HCMV and prostate cancer, this laboratory tested the reactivity of a prostate-associated monoclonal antibody with HCMV-transformed cells. This mouse monoclonal antibody, designated 83.21, reacts specifically with a

TABLE 1. Binding of 83.21 Monoclonal Antibody to HCMV-Transformed Cells

Cell Line	Transforming Agent	RIA B.R.	Immunofluorescence % Positive	CDC % Specific Lysis
CMV-transformed*				
CMV-Mj-HEL-1	HCMV isolate, prostate	21	17	48
BH-19	Towne strain HCMV, fragmented	8	17	46
BH-21		16	33	52
BH-47		10	36	44
LH-1	Towne strain HCMV	8	14	34
LH-2		11	33	28
LH-5		14	27	22
6H	BT1757 strain HCMV	7	17	16
5B		9	20	18
7E		11	17	34
Herpesvirus-transformed				
333.8.9	HSV 2	3	0	0
EB-3	EBV	1	0	0
SV40-transformed				
SV80	SV40	2	0	0
Nontransformed				
HEL-299	—	2	0	0
WI-38	—	1	0	0

*The CMV-Mj-HEL-1 cell line [2] was kindly provided by Dr. Fred Rapp. The remaining HCMV-transformed cells were a generous gift of Dr. E.-S. Huang.

membrane antigen on prostate and bladder tumor cells and does not bind to a variety of other malignant or normal cells [4]. The HCMV-transformed cells used were human fibroblasts transformed by human isolates of the virus or Towne strain HCMV. The results indicated that the prostate-associated antibody bound to a membrane antigen on all 10 HCMV-transformed cell lines, as detected by RIA (reported as binding ratio, B.R.), immunofluorescence, and complement-dependent cytotoxicity (CDC) (Table 1). This cross-reactivity appeared to be specific for HCMV, as uninfected fibroblasts and cells transformed by other viruses did not react with 83.21. The antibody also did not react with viral coded proteins in the nucleus, cytoplasm, or membranes of HCMV (AD169)-infected human fibroblasts at the IE, early, or late stages of infection. The HCMV-transformed cells were found to express surface Fc receptors, much like HCMV-infected cells, and bond human IgG but not IgM. The 83.21 antibody was not able to block this Fc-mediated reaction which was inhibited by rabbit IgG. We therefore conclude that 83.21 does not react with a viral-coded protein and does not bind to an Fc receptor. These results suggest that the antibody reacts with a host cell surface protein expressed on HCMV-transformed cells and urogenital tumors. Identification of this common antigen on prostate tumor, bladder tumor, and HCMV-transformed cells requires further investigation and may contribute to the understanding of the development of urogenital tumors.

REFERENCES

1. Geder L: In Rapp F (ed): "Oncogenic Herpesviruses." Boca Raton, Florida: CRC Press, Inc, 1980, vol 2, pp 47–60.
2. Geder L, Sanford EJ, Rohner TJ, Rapp F: Cancer Treat Rep 61:139, 1977.
3. Laychock AM, Geder L, Sanford EJ, Rapp F: Cancer 42:766, 1978.
4. Starling JJ, Sieg SM, Beckett ML, Schellhammer PF, Ladaga LE, Wright GL: Cancer Res 42:3084, 1982.

STUDIES OF CYTOMEGALOVIRUS ACQUISITION IN A NEWBORN INTENSIVE CARE UNIT

S.H. Cheeseman, E.E. Rosquette, B.R. McGraw, and F.J. Bednarek

University of Massachusetts Medical School, Worcester, MA 01605

In recent years CMV has been recognized as a frequent nosocomial infection and a possible cause of clinically significant deterioration among premature infants receiving intensive care. It has thus become important to define the sources and routes of transmission of CMV in this setting, as well as to determine which infants are at risk. Yeager et al have amply documented that blood transfusion may transmit CMV to infants of seronegative mothers, when the total quantity exceeds 50 ml and at least one donor is seropositive (J Pediatr 98:281–287, 1981). One of us (E.E.R.) has been studying quantitative Igs in multiply transfused, sick premature infants, and we decided to look at a specific antibody, that of CMV, with three questions in mind:

1. Do any infants of seropositive mothers lose all traces of their transplacentally-acquired CMV antibody (and presumably become more vulnerable to exogenous CMV infection)?
2. What is the CMV acquisition rate in our nursery (where routine viral culturing is not performed), and what factors determine the risk?
3. Does our use of banked breast milk provide an additional nosocomial source of CMV?

Newborns of < 36 weeks' gestational age admitted to the neonatal intensive care unit are being studied at 0, 1, 2, and 4 weeks and 2, 4, and 6 months for serum antibody to CMV. Forty-nine infants are now enrolled in this study, with a goal of 30 multiply transfused and 30 control prematures. Patient selection is entirely by parental willingness to participate. CMV antibody is determined by an RIA using iodinated staphylococcal protein A, which requires extremely small quantities of serum.

Thirty-six babies with an average ($\pm$SD) birthweight of 1,573 ($\pm$ 534 gm), and gestational age of 31.1 ($\pm$ 2.1) wk have been followed for 2 to 6 mo. Nine had CMV antibody in cord blood, which remained elevated throughout the hospital course, despite transfusion of red cells and plasma amounting to more than twice the calculated blood volume in 3 of the infants (Table 1).

Twenty-seven babies were seronegative in cord blood, of whom 12 (44%) developed CMV antibody. These seroconvertors are compared to those who remained seronegative in Table 2.

TABLE 1. Seropositive at Birth

BW gm	Vol Transfused Calc. Blood Vol	CMV Antibody by RIA–P/N Values			
		Cord	1–2 wk	4 wk	2 mo
2,100	2.26	3.66	6.24	6.12	4.07
1,640	0.07	15.65	16.26		
1,320	2.67	12.57	16.14	7.87	
1,700	0.12	6.30	13.99/13.20*	12.85	
1,880	0.51	27.75	21.47		
840	2.13		18.84/15.18*		
1,900	0.09	53.80	30.10	41.17	20.78
1,060	0.89		25.89	32.08	21.23
930	0.94	26.16	25.30	27.59	

*1 wk/2 wk

TABLE 2. Seronegative at Birth

	Developed CMV Antibody		
	Yes (N = 12)	No (N = 15)	P
Birthweight (gm)	1383 ± 396	1775 ± 627	0.06
Gestational age (wk)	29.8 ± 1.8	29.9 ± 7.9	NS*
RBC transfusions	10.2 ± 9.3	2.5 ± 2.3	0.017*
RBC donors	7.1 ± 4.4	2.4 ± 2.1	0.004*
Total blood product donors	10.5 ± 6.2	3.4 ± 3.3	0.003*
Milk donors	5.7 ± 6.1	8.2 ± 8.8	NS*
≥5 Blood product donors	11	4	0.009†
<5 Blood product donors	1	11	

*Student's *t* test
†Fisher's exact text

The 15 initially seronegative infants, who have not seroconverted, did not differ from those who did in gestational age, but were larger at birth (1,775 ± 627 gm *v* 1,383 ± 396 gm) and were exposed to significantly fewer red cell donors (2.4 ± 2.30, P = 0.004, Student's *t* test) and total donors of blood products (3.4 ± 3.3, P = 0.003). Eleven out of 15 infants who received blood products from 5 or more donors seroconverted, as compared to 1 out of 12 who were exposed to <5 donors (P = 0.0009, Fisher's exact test).

The CMV antibody appeared by the second week of life in all 12 seroconverting infants, and only one has so far proven to be actively infected with CMV by persistence of antibody to 6 months. Five cleared what appears to have been transfused antibody by the 4- or 6-month sample, and 6 are still being followed with antibody detectable at 2 months. This prolonged persistence of transfused antibody was unexpected. The titer, as estimated by P/N ratios (counts in CMV antigen-coated wells divided by counts in mock antigen-counted wells), was lower in most cases of transfused antibody (range 2.67–7.17) than in those seropositive at birth (range 3.66–53.8).

Many of the infants in our study received banked breast milk in addition to their own mother's milk. Banked milk from individual donors is stored at −20°C for a minimum of 3 days and usually more than a week before use. The baby who acquired CMV infection in the nursery received no breast milk. We have found no acquisition of CMV among 13 babies followed for 4 or more months who received banked milk from a minimum of 136 donors, or a mean of 10.5 (± 8.1, range 3–25) per infant. Nor have any of the 4 infants who did not require transfusion developed CMV infection or antibody. No infant has developed antibody late in the hospital course, as would be expected if infection occurred by a route other than that of administration of seropositive blood products.

CONCLUSION

1) Most of the CMV seroconversions detected in this study represent transfused antibody. 2) Using transfused antibody as a minimum estimate of the number of infants exposed to seropositive donors may permit calculation of a ratio of infection to exposure in the absence of serology on the blood units themselves. So far, 1 out of 6 infants with transfused antibody has proved to be truly infected. 3) The transfused CMV antibody persists for several months and complicates diagnosis of CMV acquisition by serologic means in this patient population. At present we would require persistence of antibody for 6 months to diagnose infection. The advantage of viral isolation over serology in such a situation is obvious. 4) Multiple transfusions do not seem to "wash out" transplacentally acquired CMV antibody. 5) Our data at present are insufficient to answer the question whether donor breast milk is a source of CMV infection.

NEOPLASTIC TRANSFORMATION BY A CLONED HUMAN CYTOMEGALOVIRUS DNA FRAGMENT UNIQUELY HOMOLOGOUS TO ONE OF THE TRANSFORMING REGIONS OF HERPES SIMPLEX VIRUS TYPE 2

D.J. Clanton,[†] R.J. Jariwalla,[*] C. Kress,[†] and L.J. Rosenthal[†]

[†]Departments of Microbiology and Pediatrics, Georgetown University Schools of Medicine and Dentistry, Washington, D.C. 20007; [*]Laboratory of Molecular Carcinogenesis, Linus Pauling Institute of Science and Medicine, Palo Alto, CA 94306

Specific DNA fragments of HCMV strain Towne exhibited sequence homology to the transforming regions of HSV-2 when examined by nitrocellulose filter hybridization under nonstringent conditions. Cloned Towne XbaI-B and C fragments were homologous to both BglII-N and BglII-C transforming fragments of HSV-2 DNA, whereas cloned Towne XbaI-E was uniquely homologous to the HSV-2 BGlII-C fragment. Furthermore, Towne XbaI-E exhibited homology to a unique fragment of HCMV strain AD169 (XbaI-C)

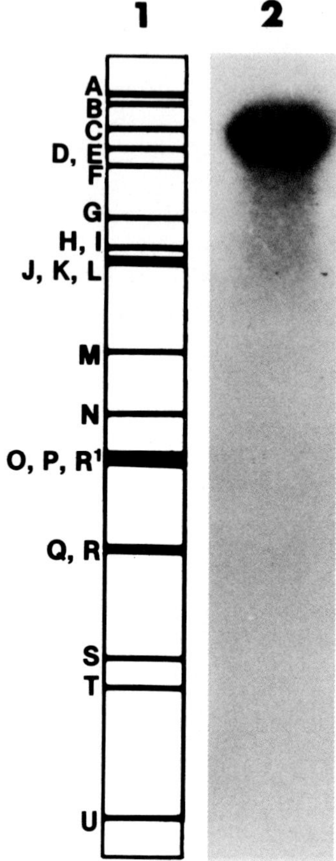

Fig. 1. Homology between HCMV strain AD169 and cloned Towne XbaI-E. Lane 1: guide strip showing fragments of XbaI-digested AD169 DNA as resolved on a 0.75% agarose gel. Lane 2: hybridization reaction between unlabeled XbaI fragments of AD169 DNA and ^{32}P-labeled Towne XbaI-E fragment. Hybridization was carried out at $T_m - 25°C$.

but lacked homology to the recently identified XbaI-N transforming (focus-forming) fragment (Fig. 1). Normal diploid Syrian hamster embryo (SHE) cells transfected with cloned Towne XbaI-E displayed colonies of refractile, rapid-dividing cells which escaped senescence to form immortal cell lines (Table 1). At early passages, these lines exhibited growth in 2% serum and formed small (< 0.1 mm) colonies in 0.3% agarose. Serial passaging resulted in the appearance of large (> 0.25 mm) colonies in agarose, indicating the involvement of more than one step in Towne XbaI-E-induced

TABLE 1. Phenotypic Characteristics of SHE Cells Transformed by Cloned Towne XbaI-E Fragment

Property	Normal SHE (P3–5)	SX (PTP[a])	SX-F1[c] (PIP[b])	SX-F2[c] (PIP)	SX-F3[c] (PIP)
% CE at low cell density					
in 10% serum	< 0.100	33	24	5.5	1.5
in 2% serum	< 0.100	31.5	8	2.5	< 0.1
% CE in 0.3% agarose[e]	< 0.001	8.7	6.5	8.3	6.2
Size[d] in agarose	—	S(14)	S(4)	S(4)	S(4)
		M,L(21)			
		L(30)			
% CE in 0.3% agar[e]	< 0.001	12.4	< 5	< 5	5.6

[a]PTP = Posttreatment passage.

[b]PIP = Postisolation passage.

[c] These lines were established from refractile colonies observed in SX cells at PTP 10.

[d]Definition of colony size as based on diameter: Small (S) $\leqslant$ 0.1 mm; Medium (M) $\leqslant$ 0.2 mm; Large (L) > 0.25 mm.

[e]For colonies of all 3 sizes counted at 3–4 wk.

transformation of diploid SHE cells. NIH 3T3 cells transfected with Towne XbaI-E rapidly displayed large colonies in agarose and tumors in vivo. The present study allows us to conclude that the genome of HCMV, like HSV-2, contains a unique class of DNA sequences capable of inducing progressive neoplastic transformation of normal diploid cells. This data, together with the observations of Nelson et al, indicate the presence of two distinct transforming regions in the genome of HCMV.

RAPID IDENTIFICATION OF CYTOMEGALOVIRUS (CMV) IN BREAST MILK BY "MICRODOT" MOLECULAR HYBRIDIZATION

D.J. Clanton, S.M. Peters, R. Wientzen, J.A. Bellanti, and L.J. Rosenthal

Georgetown University Schools of Medicine and Dentistry, Washington, D.C. 20007

It is now generally accepted that CMV is the most common cause of congenital and perinatal viral infection and the most common environmental cause of mental retardation in the United States. Although the major source of infection has been considered to be the genital tract of the mother during the birth process, recent evidence suggests that an important source of perinatal infection may occur through the ingestion of CMV-infected breast milk. In the present study, we have compared 2 methods for the identification of CMV in breast milk. Using a conventional tissue culture procedure and a newly developed "microdot" molecular hybridization assay, 32 breast milk samples were examined for the presence of CMV. By the tissue culture technique, CMV was identified by the appearance of typical CMV cytopathic effect. The "microdot" hybridization procedure was performed by phenol extraction of breast milk, alkaline denatured and neutralized, and spotted onto nitrocellulose filters. ^{32}P-labeled CMV DNA (Strain AD169) was nick translated to a specific activity of 1×10^8 cpm/μg, hybridized under stringent conditions (TM $-25°$C) to filters for 24 hr, and exposed to x-ray film for 24 hr. In reconstruction experiments, the limit of sensitivity of the "microdot"

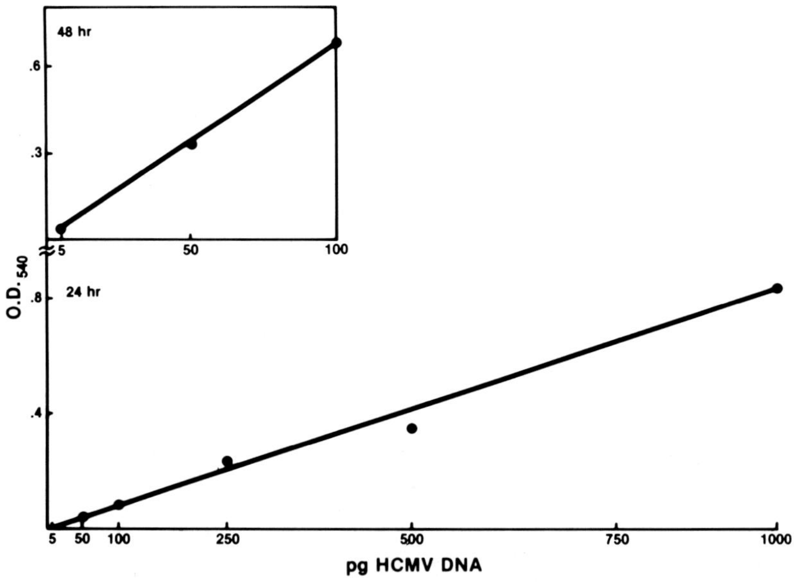

Fig. 1. Plot of intensity (O.D.$_{540}$) of "microdot" v concentration (pg) of CMV DNA added to breast milk. CMV DNA in amounts ranging from 5 to 1000 pg was added to breast milk, extracted as described, and spotted onto a nitrocellulose filter. After hybridization with ^{32}P-labeled AD169 DNA, filters were exposed for 24 hr or 48 hr (insert). Intensities of dots were determined by densitometry.

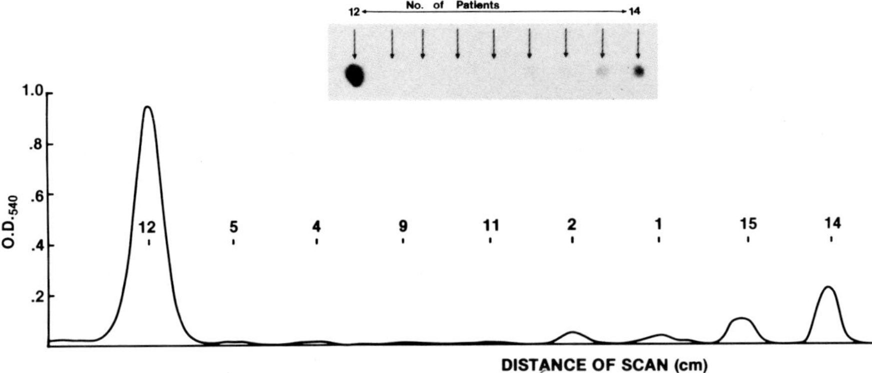

Fig. 2. Densitometer scan of autoradiogram illustrating the "microdot" molecular hybridization technique. Insert depicts the autoradiogram (arrows mark the location of patient's specimen) scanned by densitometry (O.D.$_{540}$).

procedure was found to be approximately 5 pg of CMV DNA which corresponds to 2×10^4 genome equivalents (Fig. 1). No hybridization was detected between ^{32}P-labeled AD169 DNA and human DNA (as much as 10 μg) indicating the viral-specificity of the probe (data not shown). By the tissue culture method, CMV was identified by cytopathic effect in 10 of 32 breast milk specimens during a time interval which ranged from 7 to 17 days. Using the "microdot" hybridization procedure, detection of CMV was obtained in 12 of 32 specimens in 48 hr. The results in Figure 2 show a typical densitometer scan of an autoradiogram of ^{32}P-labeled CMV probe hybridized to breast milk specimens. In our study comparing both techniques, concordance was found in 18 specimens; these included 4 positive and 14 negative specimens by both techniques. Discordance was found in 14 specimens; 6 specimens positive by tissue culture were negative by molecular hybridization, and 8 specimens negative by tissue culture were positive by molecular hybridization. The inability to detect virus by tissue in the 8 breast milk specimens that were positive by molecular hybridization may represent the presence of defective CMV which inhibited the replication of infectious virus. In the remaining 6 specimens, negative by molecular hybridization and positive by tissue culture, the amount of virus may be below the limit of sensitivity of detection of the molecular hybridization technique. These preliminary results indicate that the molecular hybridization technique provides a rapid method for the identification of CMV in breast milk.

MONOCLONAL ANTIBODIES (McAb): A NEW APPROACH TO THE DIAGNOSIS OF CMV INFECTIONS

R. Colimon,* M.C. Mazeron,* A. Roseto,** and Y. Perol*

*Laboratoire Central de Bactériologie–Virologie, **Oncologie Expérimentale–Unité INSERM 107 LOI CNRS, Hôpital Saint Louis, Paris, France

CMV is one of the most frequent causes of fever and pneumonia following BMT. At the Saint-Louis hospital BMT unit (Pr Gluckman, Paris, France), a study performed in 1982 showed that 27 of 43 (63%) allograft recipients became infected by CMV within 3 mo after grafting. Diagnosis was established by isolation of virus from the blood and/or a significant rise in antibody titers using CF and passive hemagglutination. Isolation of the virus from the blood in human embryonic fibroblasts necessitates a delay of 10–30 days. The rise of antibodies occurs in immunosuppressed patients on the average 15–20 days after detection of virus in the blood. Using monoclonal antibodies (McAb), we have developed a much more rapid diagnostic technique to confirm viremia.

MATERIAL AND METHODS

Forty-nine blood samples from bone marrow allograft recipients were studied.

Isolation of CMV From Peripheral Blood

Ten milliliters of heparinized blood was sedimented for 2 hr at 37°C, and plasma and buffy-coat layers removed. Plasma and buffy-coat were inoculated onto human embryonic fibroblasts in MEM containing 10% fetal calf serum and antibiotics. Flasks were kept at 37°C, and 4–5 hr later inoculation medium was changed. Flasks were observed daily for CMV cytopathic effect (CPE). If no CPE appeared after 2 wk, a blind passage was done and monolayers were kept for 2 more wk.

Diagnosis by IF Procedure Using McAb

Production of CMV McAb. SP 2/0 Ag 14 murine placytoma cells were fused with splenic lymphocytes from BALB/c mice immunized against CMV (AD169, ATCC VR 538). Clone E 13 McAb detected a CMV early nuclear antigen by indirect immunofluorescence. These McAb were tested on reference strains (Davis and Towne) and on different field isolates of CMV. Therefore, E 13 McAb was selected for the diagnostic tests.

IF test. Eight $\times$ 10^5 MRC–5 cells in 1 ml were seeded into flat-bottom tubes containing round (12 mm ∅) coverslips. Tubes were held at 37°C for 72 hr. Two tubes were inoculated with 1 ml of plasma and buffy-coat and centrifuged at 4,000 g for 1 hr at 36°C. After centrifugation, plasma were replaced with 1 ml of MEM containing 20% fetal calf serum and antibiotics. Tubes were kept at 37°C for 48 hr. One tube was then fixed in acetone. The other was trypsinized and cells were seeded into 2 new tubes which were kept at 37°C for an additional 48 hr before being fixed in acetone. The IF test was performed using the E 13 McAb and sheep antimouse IgG conjugated to fluorescein. The fluorescent nuclei were counted.

RESULTS

CMV was isolated by conventional culture techniques from 6 out of 49 (12%) blood specimens (Table 1). In all 6 cases, the IF test performed at the 96th hr was positive.

CONCLUSION

The IF-McAb test has advantages over conventional culture techniques. The diagnosis was performed within 96 hr after drawing blood, as opposed to an average of 14 days by virus isolation for positive cases, and 30 days for negative cases. We have a simultaneous antigenic confirmation of CMV viremia and 100% correlation with virus isolation (on this small number of cases).

TABLE 1.

Positive Case*	IIF With McAb Number Fluorescent Nuclei per Coverslip (96 H PI)	Virus Isolation Days of Detection of CMV CPE
1	Innumerable[†]	9
2	5	20
3	Innumerable[†]	15
4	25	12
5	18	14
6	Innumerable[†]	14

*Out of 49 blood specimens.
[†]Positive 48 hr postinoculation.

CYTOMEGALOVIRUS AND CHRONIC GENERALIZED LYMPHADENOPATHY IN HOMOSEXUAL MEN

A.C. Collier, J.D. Meyers, L. Corey, K.K. Holmes, and H.H. Handsfield
University of Washington and the Seattle–King County Health Dept., Seattle, WA 98104

To determine the virologic and immunologic characteristics of homosexually active men, we have compared 44 homosexual men who had chronic ($\geq$ 3 months) generalized lymphadenopathy (LA) with 46 homosexual and 12 heterosexual men randomly selected from our STD clinic population. CMV antibody was demonstrated by ELISA in 43 (98%) of the LA patients and 44 (96%) of the homosexual controls, compared with 2 (17%) of the heterosexual controls (P < 0.001). Among the LA patients, 23 (52%) shed CMV from at least one site, compared with 16 (35%) of the homosexual controls (P = NS); none of the heterosexual men shed CMV (P $\leq$ 0.01 v either group of homosexual men). Among the 39 culture-positive homosexual men, 22 (56%) shed CMV in semen alone, 8 (21%) in urine alone, 8 (21%) in both semen and urine, and 2 (5%) in the rectum. HSV was isolated from the rectums of 7 (16%) of 44 LA patients, all of whom lacked both signs and symptoms of proctitis or perianal skin lesions, compared with 0 of 46 homosexual controls (P < 0.025) and 0 of 12 heterosexual men. Fifteen (39%) of 38 LA patients failed to react to 4 skin test antigens, compared with 6 (14%) of 42 homosexual controls (P < 0.025) and none of 12 heterosexual controls (P < 0.05 v LA group). Among CMV-seropositive subjects, 7 (16%) of 43 LA patients and 5 (11%) of 44 homosexual controls had subnormal in vitro lymphocyte blastogenesis to CMV (P = NS). OKT4:OKT8 (helper:suppressor) T-cell subset ratios (mean $\pm$ 1 SD) were: LA patients, 0.84 $\pm$ 0.50; homosexual controls, 1.12 $\pm$ 0.79; and heterosexual controls, 1.71 $\pm$ 0.72 (P < 0.05 for each comparison). Skin test responses correlated better with presence or absence of LA than with OKT4:OKT8 ratios. Neoantigen immunization with bacteriophage ØX 174 and keyhole limpet hemocyanin demonstrated in vivo impairment of help and/or suppressor T-cell function in 4 of 7 men with LA. There was no correlation between isolation of CMV and OKT4:OKT8 ratios or cutaneous anergy. No study subjects have developed overt AIDS; only one such case has been documented in Seattle. Chronic LA and subclinical defects in CMI are common in homosexual men in a community where overt AIDS is thus far rare. The relationship of these syndromes to CMV infection requires further study.

TS$^+$ CMV STRAINS, AND VACCINE PRODUCTION

P. Diosi and L. Georgescu
The Medical Research Center, Timişoara, Romania

Disruption of the CMV particle is accompanied by a loss of antigenicity. The separated antigens appear to have less potential than does the same amount of material assembled in a viral structure. This problem could be overcome by using the CMV-associated tubular structures (TS) for vaccine production. TS formation appears to be an inherent property of CMV, shared by some human and rodent strains (TS$^+$ strains), permitting experimental work to be performed on rodents.

TS of up to three different calibers have been recognized by thin-section electron microscopy in various cell types infected with different CMVs. The small TS observed in mouse, guinea-pig, and ground-squirrel CMV-infected cells (7 to 13 nm in diameter), are restricted to the cell nucleus, tending to form palisades or lattice-like structures. The medium-sized TS encountered in human and guinea-pig CMV-infected cells are about the width of a core particle, measuring 55 to 60 nm in diameter, while the large TS found in human and ground-squirrel CMV-infected cells are the same diameter as viral capsids, about 100 nm. Both are rigid, capsomered structures, which acquire an envelope when extending from the perinuclear space into the nucleus. Moreover, they are often converted by terminal "budding" to spherical capsids reflecting an alternative pathway of CMV development, which appears characteristic for TS$^+$ strains.

The TS cannot be attributed either to cell associated factors, or to in vitro artifacts, since a variety of cell types used as substrates for CMV growth readily support the expression of TS of diverse calibers, and the same TS are also encountered in vivo, in different tissues. Thus, TS$^+$ appears to be a strain-related property under genetic control. However, the degree of its expression depends largely upon the cell type used as substrate, and upon other environmental factors inhibiting or delaying viral DNA replication, which are enhancing this kind of substructure assembly, or selecting morphologic variants from a mixed population of wild CMVs.

Chemical inhibition experiments suggest that TS development does not require DNA synthesis, but is dependent upon de novo protein synthesis, the TS probably being protein in nature. The medium-sized and large TS are believed to be built up from the subunits which normally form icosahedra.

PROSPECTIVE STUDY OF CYTOMEGALOVIRUS INFECTION IN PREGNANCY (EDINBURGH)

E. Edmond

University of Edinburgh Medical School, Teviot Place, Edinburgh, Scotland

For the last 6 years prospective studies have been carried out to determine the incidence and the effect on the fetus of primary infection with CMV during pregnancy. During the first 3 years of the survey, 4,446 women were screened for antibody to CMV by the CF technique. 2,026 women (45.5%) were found to be without antibody. In 1,841 seronegative women followed to term, 13 (0.7%) seroconverted. There was a higher risk of congenital infection in the offspring when the maternal infection occurred before the 20th week of pregnancy.

In the second prospective study, sera taken at booking from 2,741 women were screened for CMV IgG by ELISA using a glycine extract antigen.

So far, 1,229 completed pregnancies of seronegative women have been followed with 11 showing seroconversion. CMV was isolated from 2 babies, seroconversion having occurred between weeks 16–28 in one mother, and weeks 22–32 in another.

Two other mothers with seroconversions at almost exactly the same weeks did not produce infected infants, nor did 7 other mothers with later or untimed seroconversion.

Women who were seropositive for CMV were tested retrospectively for CMV IgM by enzyme linked immunoassay (ELA), by an indirect ELISA

TABLE 1. Results of Antibody Screening by ELISA

Age	No. Screened	No. Without a/b	% Seronegative
14–25	1,326	748	56%
26–35	1,321	661	50%
36–41	94	41	44%
Total	2,741	1,450	53%

system, and by RIA. Two percent of women were found to be positive for CMV IgM at booking.

This work is supported by a grant from the Scottish Home and Health Department.

CYTOMEGALOVIRUS (CMV) INFECTION IN SEXUALLY PROMISCUOUS POPULATIONS: COMPARISON WITH OTHER POPULATIONS AND ANALYSIS OF FACTORS RELATED TO SEXUAL TRANSMISSION

J.A. Embil, F.R. Manuel, J.B. Garner, L. Pereira, and F.M.M. White
Departments of Microbiology, Preventative Medicine, Pediatrics, Dalhousie University, Halifax, Nova Scotia, Canada B3J 3G9

We surveyed the prevalence of CMV and *Herpesvirus hominis* (HVH) in women attending nine different Halifax clinics: Sexually Transmitted Diseases (STD) Clinic, Family Planning Clinic, Prenatal Clinic (all uniformly attended by women of lower socioeconomic status), Women's Clinic (attended by women of middle socioeconomic status), Student Health Clinic, Infertility Clinic, Gynecology Tumor Clinic, Pediatric Gynecology Clinic, and a hospital gynecology ward. We cultured a total of 2,648 cervical specimens.

The data were statistically analyzed by the use of log-linear models. A statistical comparison of CMV and HVH culture results from these clinics suggests that the prevalence rates for CMV and HVH are directly proportional: the rate for HVH is 0.4 that for CMV in all clinics. We found that the rate of CMV infection was significantly higher in the STD clinic (12.3%) compared to all other clinics (2.0%).

We evaluated the possible factors associated with CMV infection separately for each clinic. At some but not all clinics, we found a statistically significant relationship between CMV and age (more common among younger age groups), pregnancy, use of oral contraceptives, unmarried status, and the presence of *Neisseria gonorrhoeae*.

In another study, we recovered CMV from the semen of 6 of 389 men. Nine of these men were homosexual, and 3 of the homosexuals were positive for CMV. STD-clinic patients and homosexuals tend to have multiple sexual partners. Our studies suggest that CMV is more common among such sexually promiscuous groups.

CMV can persist for many months in asymptomatic carriers. It has been reported to persist for 5 years in a woman's urine and for 2 years in a man's semen. The 3 homosexuals mentioned earlier all secreted CMV for at least 3 months (2 in their urine and semen and one in semen only). Three other men from the same study secreted CMV for 3, 9 (in urine and semen), and 12 (in semen only) months.

The potential for sexual transmission of CMV from an asymptomatic carrier and its potential for infecting the fetus of an asymptomatic mother make CMV a public health hazard.

CYTOMEGALOVIRUS (CMV)-SPECIFIC HUMORAL AND CELLULAR IMMUNE RESPONSES IN HEALTHY AND IMMUNODEFICIENT HOMOSEXUAL MEN

J.S. Epstein, W.J.R. Frederick, A.H. Rook,
H. Masur, W. Turner, J.F. Manischewitz, J. Ames,
A.S. Fauci, H.C. Lane, and G.V. Quinnan
Office of Biologics, NCDB, FDA, and NIH, Bethesda, MD 20205

A potential role of CMV in the pathogenesis of AIDS has been suggested by the high prevalence of active CMV infections in AIDS patients [1] and by the finding of CMV nucleic acids in KS biopsies [2]. To further study the possible role of CMV in AIDS, we studied 26 male homosexuals with AIDS, 9 with chronic lymphadenopathy syndrome (LS), and 8 asymptomatic subjects with normal physical examination.

LS and AIDS were diagnosed using the CDC criteria [3]. Patients were studied at the NIH Clinical Center. For each subject, CMV culture in MRC-5 human embryonic lung fibroblasts was performed at least twice on blood buffy coats, urine, and throat washings [4]. Biopsies were cultured when available. CMV serology was done by ACIF test [5] and by ELISA utilizing alkaline phosphatase-conjugated goat antiglobulins specific for human IgG or IgM (Dynatech Diagnostics, Inc., South Windham, ME) [6]. IgM detection was enhanced by pretreating serum on a DEAE Affi-Gel Blue Column (Bio-Rad Laboratories, Richmond, CA) to remove IgG [7]. Leukocyte counts were obtained by Coulter counter, and lymphocyte subsets were defined by complement-mediated lysis using monoclonal antibodies OKT4 and OKT8

(Ortho Diagnostics, Raritan, NJ) for specific helper and suppressor/cytotoxic cell markers, respectively. Virus-specific cytotoxicity was measured in ^{51}Cr release microassays using CMV-infected and uninfected, HLA-matched and mismatched target cells, as previously described [8].

Most of the laboratory findings are summarized in Table 1. The ages of the volunteers ranged from 18 to 52 years. The mean leukocyte and lymphocyte counts for the AIDS and LS patients were within the normal range. However, 10/22 AIDS patients had leukopenia with white cell counts < 3,000 per mm^3. Total serum IgG was elevated in patients with AIDS and LS compared to laboratory controls. The ratios of OKT4+/OKT8+ lymphocytes were depressed in patients with AIDS and some of the asymptomatic volunteers compared to the normal range. Table 2 summarizes the results of CMV culture and CMV-specific serology. CMV cultures were positive in 24 AIDS patients, 7 LS patients, and 3 of the asymptomatic homosexuals. All individuals had CMV-specific serum antibodies by ACIF and by ELISA test for IgG. Mean titers did not differ between the 3 groups. CMV-specific IgM was found on testing of whole serum from 4 AIDS patients. Sera from some subjects were tested after IgG removal. Titers $\geq$ 1:50 were detected in 13/ 15 patients with AIDS, 4/8 asymptomatic subjects with lymphadenopathy, and 0/5 asymptomatic subjects without lymphadenopathy. Titers of IgM in AIDS patients were highest in the first few months after diagnosis and declined progressively thereafter. One of the 2 AIDS patients from whom no virus was isolated had a CMV-specific IgM response. The other patient had CMV antigens identified by immunofluorescence in cells from a biopsy of

TABLE 1. Laboratory Studies in Homosexual Men With and Without AIDS

Study Group	No. Studied	Age (Mean ± SD)	Blood Leukocyte Count/mm^3 × 10^{-3}		Total Serum IgG, mg/dL (Mean ± SD)	OKT4/OKT8 GM (1 SD)
			Total (Mean ± SD)	Lymphocytes (Mean ± SD)		
AIDS	26	36.2 ± 7.7	4.1 ± 2.0	0.8 ± 0.7	2058 ± 1062	0.1 (0.05–0.3)
Chronic lymph-adenopathy syndrome	9	31.3 ± 7.0	5.2 ± 1.1	1.5 ± 0.5	2316 ± 1415	0.5 (0.4–0.6)
Asympto-matic	8	35.3 ± 5.9	Not done	Not done	Not done	0.6 (0.1–2.4)
Normal range			5.0–10.0	1.5–4.0	650–1650	1.0–2.4

TABLE 2. Frequency of CMV Infection and CMV-Specific Serology in Homosexual Men With and Without AIDS

| | CMV Isolations | | | CMV-Specific Serum Antibodies | | |
| | | | | ELISA | | |
Study Group (No.)	Blood No. Pos.	Total No. Pos.	ACIF GMT (1 SD)†	IgG GMT (1 SD)†	IgM No. Pos./ No. Tested*
AIDS (26)	12	24	205 (79–532)	2263 (1002–5108)	13/15
Chronic lymphadenopathy syndrome (9)	0	7	161 (69–377)	2016 (806–5043)	4/8
Asymptomatic (8)	0	3	235 (118–467)	1131 (373–3438)	0/5

*Tests for CMV-specific IgM were done after removal of IgG from sera of the number of individuals indicated. Sera from all individuals were tested before IgG removal and 4 AIDS patients were positive.

†Results shown are reciprocal geometric mean titers (GMT) with a range of 1 SD obtained by ELISA or ACIF tests.

KS. Thus, all AIDS patients, 7 of 9 patients with lymphadenopathy, and 3 of 8 asymptomatic volunteers had evidence of active CMV infection.

CMV-specific cytotoxicity of lymphocytes from these patients was compared (data not shown). The 3 infected asymptomatic volunteers, and 2 of 6 with lymphadenopathy, had HLA-restricted cytotoxic T-cell responses. Only one of the AIDS patients had HLA-restricted cytotoxicity, that being a patient with KS but no opportunistic infections. Nonrestricted cytotoxicity by NK cells against CMV-infected target cells was also depressed in AIDS patients.

Active CMV infection was detected by virus culture or IgM serology in 25/26 patients with AIDS and 7 of 9 patients with LS. Detection of CMV-specific IgM was dependent on removal of IgG from sera, presumably because there was competitive inhibition of binding by the high levels of IgG. The high frequency of CMV infection in these 2 syndromes is consistent with the possibility that CMV may be involved in their etiology. CMV infection may be immunosuppressive and is known to cause other symptoms which are typical of these syndromes. Since CMV-specific cytotoxic T-cell responses were deficient in AIDS patients, other factors must also be involved in causing the immunosuppression.

REFERENCES

1. Durack DT: Editorial: N Engl J Med, 305:1465–1467, 1981.
2. Drew WL et al: Lancet 2:125–127, 1982.

3. MMWR 31:507-508, 513-514, 1982.
4. Benyesh–Melnick M: "Diagnostic Procedures for Viral and Rickettsial Infections." New York: American Public Health Association, 701-732, 1969.
5. Rao N, Waruszewski DT, Armstrong JA: J Clin Microbiol 6:633-638, 1977.
6. Castellano GA, Hazzard GT, Madden DL, Sever JL: J Infect Dis 136, Suppl:5337-5339, 1977.
7. Bruck C, Portetelle D, Glineur C, Bollen A: J Immunol Methods 53:313-319, 1982.
8. Quinnan GV Jr et al: N Engl J Med 307:7-13, 1982.

CELL-MEDIATED IMMUNITY IN CONGENITAL AND ACQUIRED CMV INFECTION

M. Fiorilli, M.C. Sirianni, P. Iannetti, A. Pana, and F. Aiuti

University of Rome, Rome, Italy

CMV infection, either congenital or acquired during childhood, may be followed by chronic virus excretion. In the case of congenital infection, this phenomenon has been shown to be accompanied by a state of specific cellular immune unresponsiveness to CMV. In this study we examined specific CMI to CMV (as evaluated by a direct leukocyte migration inhibition test, CMV-LMIT) and NK activity against CMV-infected fibroblasts (CMV-IF) and K562 cells in a group of children with congenital or acquired infection. We found that: 1) of 9 children with a history of acquired CMV, 4 had viruria persisting for 5 to 21 mo (median 14), during which time all but one failed to develop CMV-LMIT responses; in contrast, all 5 patients who had resolved their viruria had restored CMV-LMIT reactivity; 2) one out of 2 children with congenital CMV had ceased to shed virus and had full CMV-LMIT reactivity at the age of 4 years 7 months, whereas the other continued to produce CMV and to have negative CMV-LMIT at the age of 7 yr; interestingly, the latter patient was also found to have a marked deficiency of NK activity against both CMV-IF and K562 cells.

These findings indicate that: 1) acquired CMV infection, like the congenital form, can induce a long-lasting cellular desensitization to the virus; 2) chronic infection following congenital CMV can be accompanied, and perhaps partially sustained, by a functional deficiency of NK cells. Overall, in our patients the persistence of viruria significantly correlated with the absence of CMV-LMIT reactivity and the recovery from infection coincided with the restoration of CMV-LMIT responses. Therefore, CMV-LMIT provides a useful and biologically relevant assay for specific cellular host responses to CMV. We are using this assay to investigate in vitro the effects of immunomodulating agents such as dialyzable transfer factor and thymic hormones on CMV immunity.

EFFECT OF 2′-FLUOROARABINOSIDES (FIAC, FIAU, AND FMAU) ON CMV INFECTION IN CELL CULTURES AND IN GUINEA PIGS*

C.K.Y. Fong, S. Cohen, S. McCormick, and G.D. Hsiung

Virology Laboratory, VA Medical Center, West Haven CT 06516, and Department of Laboratory Medicine, Yale University School of Medicine, New Haven, CT 06516

In previous studies, we reported that neither acyclovir nor phosphonoformate showed any positive therapeutic effect on the course of CMV infection in the guinea pig model [1]. Three 2′-fluoroarabinosyl pyrimidine nucleosides, potent antiviral agents, were evaluated against CMV infection in the present study: these included 2′-fluoro-5-iodoarabinosyl-cytosine (FIAC), 2′-fluoro-5-iodoarabinosyl-uracil (FIAU), and 2′-fluoro-5-methyl-arabinosyl-uracil (FMAU). In this study, the antiviral effect of FIAC, FIAU, and FMAU on GPCMV replication in cell cultures, and the therapeutic effect of FMAU on GPCMV infection in guinea pigs were investigated.

EXPERIMENTAL RESULTS
Effect of FIAC, FIAU, and FMAU on GPCMV Replication in Guinea Pig Embryo Cell Cultures

Virus yield and plaque formation. Guinea pig embryo (GPE) cells infected with GPCMV were treated with various concentrations of drug and incubated for 3–4 days. Virus yields were determined in GPE cells by cytopathic effect. Of the three compounds tested, only FMAU showed a significant inhibitory effect on GPCMV replication (Table 1). At a concentration of 10 μg/ml, FMAU inhibited virus yield up to 1.8 $\log_{10}$; at 40 μg/ml, virus yield was reduced by 4 $\log_{10}$ or greater as compared to the

*Study supported in part by contract no. A1-12665 from the NIH, grant no. HD 10609 from the National Institute of Child Health and Human Development, and the Medical Research Service of the Veterans Administration. This is publication no. 72 from the Cooperative Antiviral Testing Group of the Antiviral Substance Program, Development and Application Branch, NIAID, NIH, Bethesda, MD.

drug-free infected culture. Significant inhibition of GPCMV replication was obtained even when FMAU was added to the virus-infected cultures as late as 24 hr after infection. The continuous presence of the compound was necessary in order to achieve antiviral effect; when the drug was removed from the cultures, virus replication resumed. FMAU did not affect the growth of GPE cells at 10 μg/ml, although cell growth rates were slower at 20 μg/ml and even more reduced at 40 μg/ml of medium used.

Ultrastructural studies. Electron microscopic examination of GPCMV-infected GPE cells revealed a significant reduction of nucleocapsids in cells from cultures containing 10 μg/ml of FMAU and near absence of nucleocapsids in the infected cells taken from cultures containing 40 μg/ml of FMAU. However, the proteinaceous tubular structures associated with GPCMV infection were not affected by FMAU. It appeared that inhibition of viral nucleic acid synthesis was the basis for the antiviral effect of FMAU similar to that previously reported with GPCMV-infected cells in the presence of other known DNA inhibitors [2, 3].

Effect of FMAU on GPCMV Infection in Guinea Pigs

Randomly bred Hartley guinea pigs were inoculated subcutaneously with virulent GPCMV-SG passaged in salivary gland. Three days PI, half of the

TABLE 1. Effect of FMAU, FIAC, and FIAU on GPCMV Replication in Guinea Pig Embryo (GPE) Cells

Drug Concentration (μg/ml)		Virus Yield[†] ($\mathrm{Log_{10}}$ $\mathrm{TCID_{50}}$/0.1 ml)	Log Reduction of Virus Yield
FMAU	0	5.50	—
	10	3.66	1.84
	30	2.50	3.00
	40	1.00	4.50
FIAC	0	6.50	—
	10	>5.00	1.5
	30	4.50	2.0
	40	5.00	1.5
	80	4.33	2.2
FIAU	0	6.50	—
	10	>5.00	1.5
	30	5.00	1.5
	40	5.00	1.5
	80	4.50	2.0

[†]GPE cells were infected with GPCMV at an input multiplicity of one $\mathrm{TCID_{50}}$/cell. Virus adsorption = 1 hr. Infected cultures were harvested 4 days after virus inoculation. Virus yields were determined in GPE cells.

infected animals received intraperitoneal injection of FMAU dissolved in diluent (propylene glycol:ethanol:water = 20:20:60) at 50 mg/kg/dose in 0.5 ml, two times daily for 4–7 days. Sham-treated animals received the same amount of diluent alone. Animals were weighed daily or every other day; blood samples were taken on days 6 and 9 for virus isolation procedures; animals were sacrificed between days 7 and 13 for virus distribution and histopathology of various tissues.

Clinical evaluation. Control Hartley guinea pigs (uninfected, FMAU-treated or untreated) gained body weight at almost the same rate (Fig. 1). On the other hand, weight loss was evident in GPCMV-infected animals by day 3 and continued to day 7 or 10 PI. FMAU (100 mg/kg/day/7 days) failed to prevent the body weight loss in infected animals. In addition, FMAU-treated animals showed a slower rate of body weight recovery than the sham-treated animals.

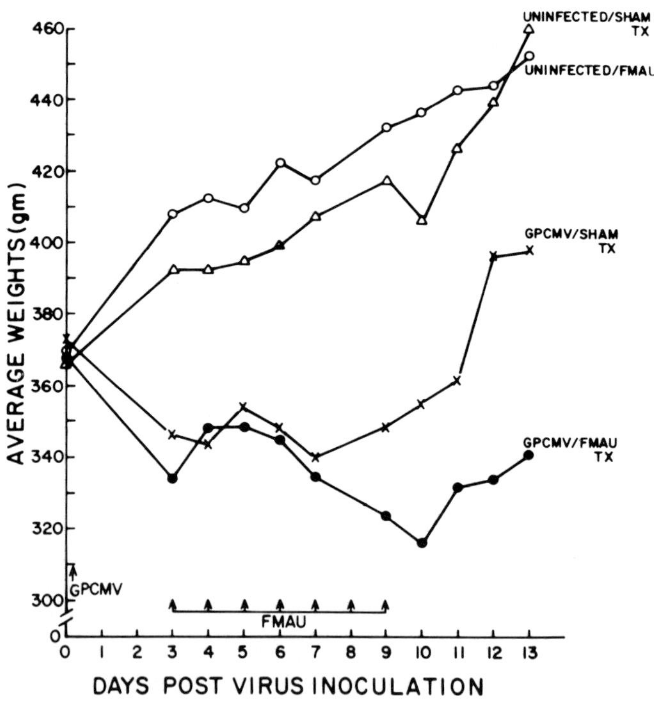

Fig. 1. Effect of FMAU on body weight of GPCMV-infected or uninfected guinea pigs. FMAU 100 mg/kg/day was given to guinea pigs daily from day 3 to day 9 post virus inoculation.

Virus distribution and histopathology. FMAU did not prevent viremia during acute GPCMV infection. Virus infectivity titers in various organs including spleen, lung, liver, and salivary gland of GPCMV-infected animals were not reduced as a result of FMAU treatment. The presence of viral inclusions in various tissues of GPCMV-infected guinea pigs was demonstrated in both the FMAU-treated animals and the sham-treated controls. Focal interstitial pneumonia was noted with similar degree of severity in both drug-treated and sham-treated infected animals but not in the drug-treated or sham-treated uninfected guinea pigs.

SUMMARY AND CONCLUSION

Among the three 2′-fluoroarabinosyl pyrimidine nucleosides tested, FMAU showed significant inhibition of GPCMV replication in cell culture. In the presence of FMAU at 40 μg/ml of medium, virus yields were significantly reduced and viral nucleocapsids were almost completely inhibited. However, comparable inhibition was not obtained when FMAU was administered to guinea pigs infected with GPCMV. In FMAU-treated animals with GPCMV infection, 100 mg/kg/day for 7 days, viremia was not prevented and infectious virus was found in various tissues including spleen, lung, liver, and salivary gland. Viral pneumonia was noted and viral inclusions were evident in many organs. In addition, body weight loss appeared to be more pronounced in the infected guinea pigs treated with FMAU than in the sham-treated ones.

Thus, FMAU, a highly potent antiviral agent against HSV infection in cell culture and in guinea pigs [4], is not effective for treatment of CMV infection in the guinea pig, although its inhibitory effect in cell culture was significant. Thus, the data would indicate that extensive testing of new antiviral agents is essential not only in cell cultures but also in animal models in order to ascertain their potency in vivo prior to application for human use.

REFERENCES

1. Lucia HL, Griffith B, Hsiung GD: Effect of acyclovir and phosphonoformate on cytomegalovirus infection in guinea pigs. (Submitted for publication)
2. Fong CKY, Bia F, Hsiung GD, Madore P, Chang PW: Ultrastructural development of guinea pig cytomegalovirus in cultured guinea pig embryo cells. J Gen Virol 42:127-140, 1979.
3. Fong CKY: Effect of acyclovir on guinea pig cytomegalovirus replication: An ultrastructural study. Abstract. Amer. Soc. Microbiol. Annual Meeting, 1982, p 237.
4. Mayo DR, Hsiung GD: Comparison of three fluoropyrimidines (FIAC, FIAU, FMAU), acyclovir and phosphonoformate in the treatment of genital herpes in guinea pigs. Abstract. 23rd Interscience Conference on Antimicrobial Agents and Chemotherapy, 1983.

CMV CELL-MEDIATED IMMUNITY IN PREGNANCY

Lawrence D. Frenkel
Medical College of Ohio, Toledo, OH 43699

Female health-care workers are a largely middle-class, young, and fertile group. Approximately half are CMV seronegative. Primary acquisition of CMV infection during pregnancy is now accepted as the main contributor to congenital affliction. A total of 212 pregnant subjects and nonpregnant controls were matched for age, gravidity, parity, number of abortions, history of genital HSV infection, number of sexual partners, age of first sexual activity, socioeconomic status, and race. The majority of the women in this study were middle-income patients referred from private practitioners, or were health-care workers who volunteered for the study directly. The participants were followed for up to 5 years with respect to CMV and HSV viral excretion, serologic status, and specific and nonspecific assays of CMI as measured by lymphocyte transformation. The suppression of CMV and HSV-specific CMI by serum factors and the presence of specific suppressor cell activity was also assayed in a subset of these populations. Pregnant women demonstrated significant suppression of specific CMI to CMV in all trimesters, particularly in the third. This specific suppression was not related to serum factors, but did seem to be related to a suppressor cell subpopulation. The study suggests that specific lymphocyte transformation can be used as a sensitive predictor of previous infection. The patterns of the suppression of specific and nonspecific CMI differed, suggesting different mechanisms.

CLINICAL AND IMMUNOLOGIC FOLLOW-UP OF 11 CHILDREN WITH MODERATE-TO-SEVERE CONGENITAL CYTOMEGALOVIRUS AFFLICTION

Lawrence D. Frenkel, Nasreen A. Bhumbra, and
Kytja K.S. Voeller
Medical College of Ohio, Toledo, OH 43699

Eleven infants between 1 day and 2 years of age were referred for evaluation of suspected intrauterine infection with CMV. These children and their mothers were followed at regular intervals for up to 3½ years with viral isolation, serology, assays of CMI, neutrophil and platelet counts, liver enzyme evaluation, quantitative immunoglobulins (QIG), developmental assessment, electroencephalogram (EEG), brain computerized tomography (CT) scan, audiologic, and ophthalmologic evaluation. Seven of the infants ceased viral excretion at an average age of 16 months (range: 9 mo to 24 mo); however, 2 patients have been persistent excretors for over 2½ years, and 2 others for a shorter period of time. All but 1 of the infants had persistently and significantly depressed CMV-specific CMI by the lymphocyte transformation assay, while they generally had low normal nonspecific T-cell function, as measured by mitogen stimulation. Eight of 10 mothers tested also had depressed CMV-specific CMI. The 2 exceptions were first assayed 2 years after the birth of the afflicted child. Although only 3 of the children had clinically recognized seizures, 6 children had a prominent seizure focus noted on EEG. Eight children were microcephalic, and 4 had periventricular calcification on CT scans. Five children developed severe psychomotor retardation. Five of the 10 who were completely evaluated had audiologic impairment with 2 showing progressive impairment over time. Significant ophthalmologic impairment was noted in 3 of 10 completely evaluated children. Mild hypogammaglobulinemia of several months' duration was noted in 4 of 10 children evaluated. Nine of these infants had mild-(1500 to 2000) to-moderate (500-1500) neutropenia, and 6 had mild elevations of SGPT, both conditions lasting for approximately 7 months. These findings would suggest that not all children diagnosed at birth, or even with microcephaly, develop severe psychomotor retardation. Children with congenital CMV affliction may present with seizures and delayed development. The damage of congenital CMV infection may be progressive, with the implications that early diagnosis may allow for therapeutic intervention.

MURINE CYTOMEGALOVIRUS (MCMV) ACUTE AND PERSISTENT INFECTION: RELATIONSHIP BETWEEN HUMORAL IMMUNE RESPONSE AND PRESENCE OF THE VIRUS IN VARIOUS ORGANS*

G. Furlini, P. Coppolecchia, M.C. Re, and M.P. Landini

Institute of Microbiology, University of Bologna Medical School, Bologna, Italy

*This work was partially supported by Italian Ministry of Education and C.N.R., grant no. 82.02405.52.

After a first acute infection, CMV like other herpesviruses, can induce persistent infection, both in humans and animals. Our previous results showed the primary MCMV infection evolved in two different phases: the first was characterized by a short interval of virus replication in parenchymal organs, followed by the second phase characterized by a persistent infection limited to the salivary glands. The transition from the first to the second phase coincided with the maximum level of specific humoral immune response [1].

Due to the relatively low accuracy of virus isolation procedures and the presence of discordant data in the literature, we have studied primary MCMV infection tracing the presence of virus-specific antigens in organ homogenates by ELISA. The Smith strain of MCMV propagated and harvested as previously described [1] was used in all the experiments.

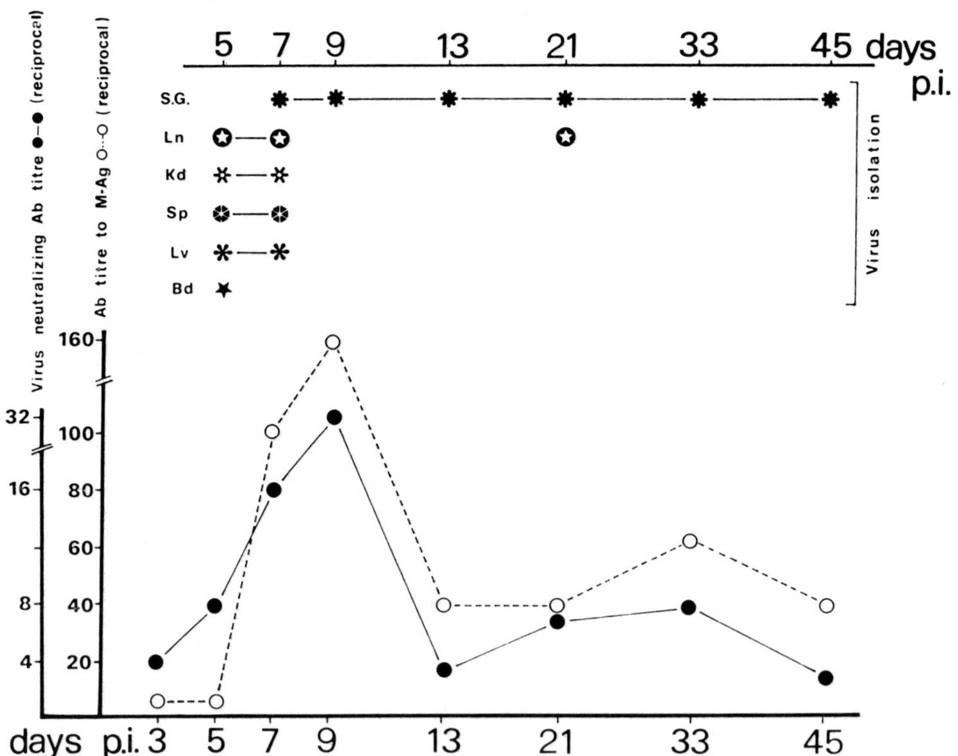

Fig. 1. Evolution of humoral immune response against MCMV-specific membrane antigen(s) detected by IIF (O---O) and specific viral neutralizing antibody titers (●—●) in relation to virus isolation from salivary glands (SG), lungs (Ln), kidney (Kd), spleen (Sp), liver (Lv), and blood (Bd).

Four-week-old female mice (Swiss strain) were inoculated IP and IM with a total amount of 0.5×10^5 PFU of MCMV and were sacrificed at predetermined intervals by exsanguination (under diazepam anesthesia) for collection of serum and tissue samples. Pooled sera were tested for the presence of neutralizing antibodies (Nt Ab) by the method described by Araullo-Cruz et al [2], and for the presence of antibodies against MCMV-specific cell membrane antigens (MCMV-CM Ab) by indirect immunofluorescence (IIF) in unfixed cells 48 hr PI. The presence of MCMV-specific Ab was also detected by indirect ELISA, using as antigen a homogenate of infected salivary glands ($50 \mu g$ of proteins in each well); uninfected salivary glands were processed in the same way and were used as negative controls.

Tissue homogenates were tested for the presence of infectious MCMV by inoculation in mouse embryo fibroblast cultures [1] and for the presence of MCMV-specific antigen by ELISA carried out as follows: lungs, salivary glands, and kidney suspensions, diluted in carbonate-bicarbonate buffer (pH 9.6) at a final concentration of $200 \mu g/ml$ of protein, were used to coat microplates (0.2 ml/well). ELISA was then carried out following the procedure described by Voller et al [3] with minor modifications.

MCMV was isolated from homogenates of spleen, liver, kidney, and lungs from 5 to 7 days PI, while viremia was detected only on the 5th day PI. The Virus was never isolated from urine. Virus was not isolated from spleen, liver, kidney, or blood at later times, but was isolated from lungs 21 days PI.

MCMV was continuously isolated from salivary glands beginning from 7 days PI to the end of the observation period (45 days PI). Virus titers in salivary glands ranged from 5×10^5 to 1.4×10^6 PFU/g (data not shown), reaching a maximum concentration on the 21st day PI.

Serum-neutralizing antibodies, and antibodies against MCMV-specific membrane antigen were observed early after infection, and both reached maximum concentrations 9 days PI, coinciding with the disappearance of the virus (detectable by virus isolation in tissue culture) from parenchymal organs and the beginning of virus recovery from salivary glands (Fig. 1).

Beginning 9 hr PI and for 7 days, a gradual decrease in the amount of MCMV-specific antigens detectable by ELISA was observed in all the organs tested. Starting 8 days PI, detectable antigenic material increased, and reached a maximum concentration 13 days PI in kidney and salivary glands; the maximum concentrations were detected in lung homogenates 21 days PI, coinciding with the second virus isolation from the organ (Fig. 2). The virus-specific antigens then showed a progressive decline until the end of the observation period.

MCMV-specific serum antibodies detected by indirect ELISA showed a peak 9 days PI followed by a rapid decline and a subsequent increase until the end of our observation period (Fig. 2).

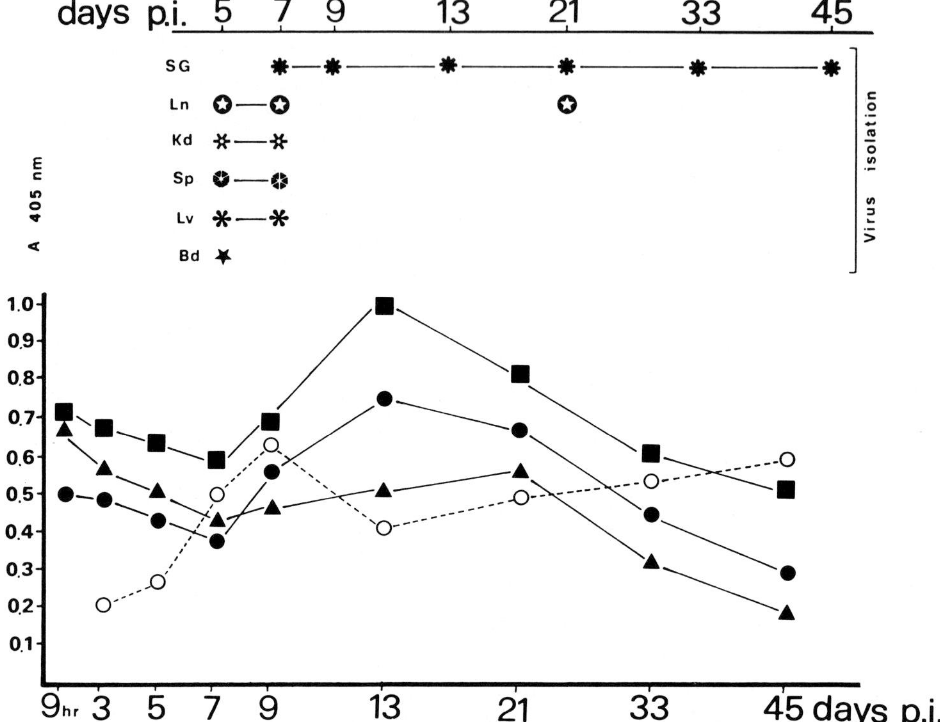

Fig. 2. Evolution of MCMV-specific humoral immune response detected by ELISA (○---○) and presence of viral antigens in kidney (■—■), lungs (▲—▲), and salivary glands (●—●) detected by the same method, in relation to virus isolation.

In contrast, viral-specific antigens were detected by ELISA for a much longer period of time, in spite of the absence of MCMV isolation in tissue culture. Moreover, viral antigens were detected by ELISA in urine 5 days PI, even though no infectious virus was ever recovered from this fluid (data not shown).

Therefore, in primary MCMV infection, the involvement of parenchymal organs seems to last much longer than what we and other authors thought on the basis of virus isolation [1,5]. The absence of MCMV isolation could be due either to MCMV neutralization by anti-MCMV antibodies or to the damage of virions by lytic enzymes present in organ homogenates, as suggested elsewhere [4]. Consequently, the detection of virus-specific antigens by ELISA seems to be a more sensitive indicator of the presence of MCMV infection.

REFERENCES

1. Coppolecchia P, Furlini G, Re MC, Landini MP: Evolution of serum antibodies against different classes of murine cytomegalovirus-induced antigens and virus isolation following a primary infection. Microbiologica 6:175–179, 1983.
2. Araullo-Cruz TP, Ho M, Armstrong JA: Protective effect of early serum from mice after cytomegalovirus infection. Infect Immun 21:840–842, 1978.
3. Voller A, Bidwell D, Bartlett A: Enzyme-linked immunosorbent assay. In Rose N, Friedman (eds): "Manual of Clinical Immunology." Washington, DC; Am Soc for Microbiology, 1980, pp 359–371.
4. Ruebner BH, Hirano T, Slusser R, Osborn J, Medearis DW: Cytomegalovirus infection: Viral ultrastructure with particular reference to the relationship of lysosomes to cytoplasmic inclusions. J Pathol 48:971–989, 1966.
5. Osborn JE, Walker DL: Virulence and attenuation of murine cytomegalovirus. Infect Immun 3 (2):228–236, 1970.

PERSISTENT HCMV INFECTION OF HUMAN OSTEOGENIC SARCOMA CELLS AND ITS VARIANT

T. Furukawa* and R.F. Pritchett[†]

*Kanazawa Medical University, Uchinada, Ishikawa, Japan, and [†]The University of Arizona, Tucson, AR 85721

A unique feature of HCMV is its ability to cause persistent infection, which is demonstrated clinically by the excretion of virus for long periods despite the presence of humoral antibody. Few in vitro models of HCMV persistent infection have been studied, despite reports of many types of persistent infection with a variety of viruses. We describe here the establishment of persistent infection in human osteogenic sarcoma (HOS) cells with HCMV and a possible mechanism involved in persistent infection. HOS cells were infected with the Towne strain of HCMV at an input multiplicity of infection (MOI) of 10. At 4 days PI, the infectivities of both cell-associated and supernatant virus were assayed. HCMV showed restricted growth on HOS cells, reaching a maximum titer of 2.8×10^3 PFU/ml. Histologically, HOS cells did not show the early cytopathic effects (CPE) seen in human fibroblasts, but developed late viral antigens, as evidenced by the typical nuclear inclusion bodies upon both immunofluorescent antibody and hematoxylin-eosin stainings. In order to establish persistent culture, subconfluent cultures of HOS cells in a plastic flask were infected with HCMV at an MOI of 50. The cultures were fed with fresh medium every 5th day. The cultures did not show distinct CPE, but the cells grew very slowly. The cell line was designated E155 and has been continously cultivated for over 2 years. The history and character of the cell line are summarized in Figure 1. CPE did not appear in the E155 culture, but when the cultures were examined for viral antigen and infectivity, some of the cells (0.1%–5%) were positive for nuclear antigen and in the infectious center assay. No IFN activity was detected in the culture fluid at various times after infection. E155 cultures were grown in the presence of 5% antibody, which was sufficient to inactivate 99% of HCMV within 60 min, cultures were refed at weekly intervals with medium containing antiserum for HCMV. Virus was not detectable in supernatant fluids after the addition of antibody, and the number of infectious centers decreased gradually. However, the addition of IFN at various concentrations (10–100 U/ml) into the culture medium did not cure the culture. The ability of antibody to cure a persistently infected culture indicates that extracellular virus is responsible for maintaining persistent infection. Eight clones

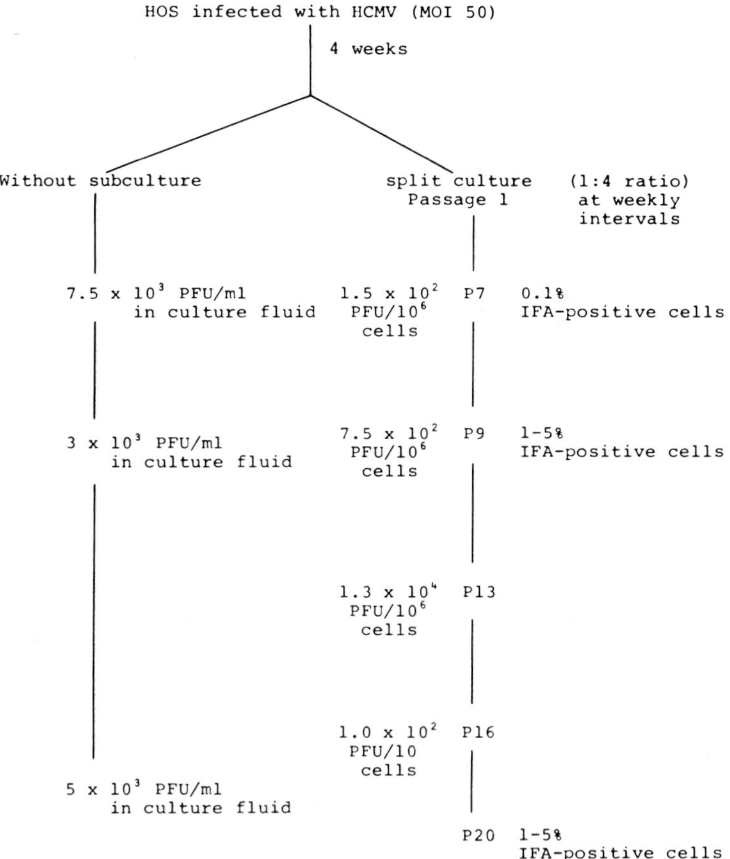

Fig. 1. Establishment of persistently infected cultures.

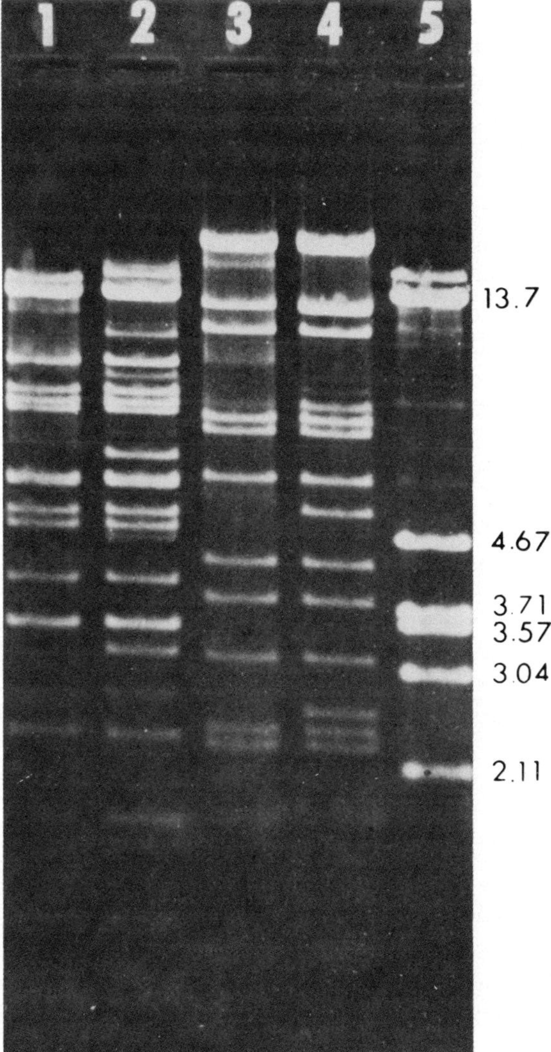

Fig. 2. Coelectrophoresis comparison of the *Hin*dIII and *Xba*I restriction enzyme fragments of EV155 and CMV Towne DNA. The *Hin*dIII fragments of EV155 (slot 1) and CMV Towne (slot 2) DNA were separated by electrophoresis through a 0.5% agarose slab gel. Electrophoresed on the same gel were the *Xba*I fragments of EV155 (slot 3) and CMV Towne (slot 4) DNA. As molecular weight markers, *Eco*RI-digested bacteriophage λ DNA was also electrophoresed on the gel (slot 5).

from HOS and 18 clones from E155 were established. The established cultures were then examined for susceptibility to HCMV infection. The coverslip cultures were exposed to HCMV at an MOI of 5 and examined by IFA at 5 days PI. The percentage of nuclear antigen-positive cells varied up to 98% in the clones from HOS and 0.01%–15.4% in those from E155. The virus (hereafter referred to as EV155) was isolated from disrupted E155 and examined for temperature sensitivity, defectiveness, and growth rate as compared with the parental Towne strain. It appears that EV155 was not a DI HCMV or a temperature-sensitive mutant. To determine whether EV155 DNA had structural alterations, the fragment patterns produced by digestion of CMV Towne and EV155 DNAs with 4 different restriction enzymes (*Hind*III, *Xba*I, *Bam*HI, and *Eco*RI) were compared. Comparison of the *Hind*III fragment pattern of EV155 DNA with that of CMV Towne DNA showed that at least 8 fragments were missing from the EV155 DNA (Fig. 2). Coelectrophoresis of the *Xba*I restriction enzyme fragments revealed that at least 3 fragments were missing from the DNA pattern of EV155 as compared with the CMV Towne strain. Two fragments were found in the *Xba*I EV155 DNA digest that were not present in the digest of CMV Towne DNA (Fig. 2). These variations in the restriction enzyme fragment patterns suggested that the DNA of EV155 differs structurally from the Towne parental virus. To confirm the location of deleted fragments in the DNA of EV155, ^{32}P-labeled hybridization probes were prepared from isolated fragments and incubated with Southern blots of CMV Towne and EV155 DNA fragments. The results revealed that one copy of the repeat sequences contained in fragments P and N of CMV Towne DNA appears to have been completely deleted from the EV155 DNA.

SUMMARY

Infection of cells derived from an osteogenic sarcoma patient with HCMV resulted in persistent infection. Virus derived from the persistently infected cultures were not temperature-sensitive nor were they defective interfering particles, although restriction analysis revealed that one copy of the repeat sequences is completely deleted. Thus, the mechanism of persistent infection is probably due in part to a variant of CMV present in the cultures.

DETECTION OF HCMV ANTIGENS IN MITOGEN-STIMULATED PERIPHERAL BLOOD LYMPHOCYTES

H.M. Garnett and G. Kim Sing

Department of Microbiology, University of the Witwatersrand, Johannesburg, South Africa, 2000

Peroxidase labeled Fab fragments, prepared from the IgG fraction of pooled CMV antibody-positive human serum, were used in immunohistochemical techniques at the light and electron microscopic levels to detect HCMV antigens. Positive results were observed in specific subpopulations of normal human peripheral blood T cells when challenged with virus 48 hr after mitogen stimulation.

PRINCIPAL ACCEPTOR FOR PARTICLE-ASSOCIATED PROTEIN KINASE IS PREVIOUSLY UNRECOGNIZED MAJOR VIRION CONSTITUENT

W. Gibson, C. Roby, and A. Irmiere
Department of Pharmacology, Johns Hopkins School of Medicine, Baltimore, MD 21205

Virions of HCMV, recovered from the growth medium of infected human foreskin fibroblast (HFF) cells biosynthetically labeled with ^{32}P-orthophosphate, contain three major phosphorylated proteins having estimated molecular weights of 150,000 (150K), 74,000 (74K), and 69,000 (69K). The 74K and 69K proteins are referred to as "matrix proteins"—the 69K species constituting at least 80%–90% of the protein mass of HCMV dense bodies. The 150K protein, in addition to being one of the most highly phosphorylated species in vivo, is the principal phosphate acceptor in vitro for the virion-associated protein kinase. Since this protein comigrates with the "major capsid protein" of the virion in typical SDS-containing polyacrylamide gels, it had not been previously recognized. It was well resolved and found to be comparatively basic in net charge following two-dimensional (charge-size) separations in denaturing polyacrylamide gels. It is also separated from the major capsid protein (MCP) in 14% gels cross-linked with diallyltartardiamide (slower than MCP) and 10% gels cross-linked with higher than usual amounts of methylene-bis acrylamide (faster than MCP). Based on its charge and degree of phosphorylation, this protein species has been designated as the virion "basic phosphoprotein."

Experiments to determine the architectural involvement of this virion constituent were based on an analysis of intracellular capsid forms. Strain Colburn (simian-like isolate) was used for this purpose, since capsids are not readily recovered from HCMV-infected HFF cells. Results indicate that the Colburn counterpart (ie, 119K) of the HCMV basic phosphoprotein is situated in the tegument region, between the capsid structure and the outermost glycoprotein-containing envelope. Finally, analyses of infected-cell lysates have revealed that, unlike most virion proteins whose relative intracellular concentrations are similar to those in the particle, the basic phosphoprotein (as well as the 74K matrix protein) is grossly underrepresented. We are interested in the significance of these observations as they reflect the role of this protein in the virus' infection cycle.

CELLS INFECTED WITH HCMV RELEASE FACTOR(S) THAT STIMULATE HOST DNA SYNTHESIS

E. Gonczol, B. Dietzschold, and S.A. Plotkin
Wistar Institute, Philadelphia, PA 19104

Permissive human embryonic fibroblast (MRC-5) cells infected with live or UV-irradiated, partially inactivated HCMV and nonpermissive Balb/c 3T3 cells infected with the live virus release in their culture media growth factor that enhance DNA synthesis and mitotic activity of target cells arrested by low serum concentration. The stimulatory effect was measured by detecting ^{3}H thymidine incorporation into the host DNA with liquid scintillation and autoradiography and by determining the mitotic index. The conditioned media consisted of MEM plus 1% fetal calf serum. They were centrifuged at low speed to remove cell debris, and then at 100,000g for 2 hr to remove whole virus. The resulting supernatants no longer contained infectious virus. MRC-5, Balb/c 3T3, and secondary chicken cells were employed as target cells. Starvation for 96 hr with 0.2% serum was used to arrest the cells in the G1 phase and to reduce the background DNA synthesis. Incorporation of ^{3}H thymidine was six to seven times higher in cells treated with CMV supernatant than in control cells. Mitotic activity was similarly four to five times higher in treated cells. The enhancement of DNA synthesis was observed on the second or third day after treatment of the target cells with the supernatants. Kinetic experiments showed that the growth factor released into the culture media reached the concentration necessary to stimulate host DNA synthesis on the third day after infection and not earlier. The stimulatory effect was not seen with the culture media of uninfected MRC-5 or Balb 3T3 cells; therefore, some expression of the viral genes is required. The characterization of the factor by chemical and physical treatment and its significance with regard to the transforming activity of the virus will be discussed.

SPLEEN CELL RESPONSES TO MITOGENS DURING CMV INFECTION OF GUINEA PIGS

B.P. Griffith, J.L. Tillbrook, and G.D. Hsiung
Yale University School of Medicine, New Haven, CT, and VA Medical Center, West Haven, CT 06516

Guinea pigs inoculated with CPCMV develop a mononucleosis syndrome with splenomegaly, leukocytosis, and atypical lymphocytes, during the first 2 wk after inoculation. These changes occur at the peak of virus recovery from the spleen, blood, and bone marrow. It is not known whether cellular immune responses of guinea pigs are altered during this mononucleosis syndrome. The purpose of the present report was to evaluate spleen cells from guinea pigs with primary acute CMV infection for their ability to respond in vitro to mitogens. Optimum conditions for in vitro stimulation of guinea pig spleen cells were determined in control uninfected animals. The cells were treated with 5 μg/ml PHA, 50 μg/ml of lipopolysaccharide (LPS), or 10 μg/ml of Con A. Proliferative responses were measured by incorporation of ^{3}H thymidine which was added 5 days, 2 days, and 6 days after the addition of PHA, LPS, and Con A, respectively. Spleen cells from infected guinea pigs were assessed at various time points from 4 to 27 days post-CMV inoculation. At each time point, cells obtained from control animals inoculated with uninfected salivary gland suspension were evaluated in parallel. There was no difference in the responsiveness to PHA between CMV-infected and control animals tested on days 4 to 27. In contrast, during that time, diminished responses to both LPS and Con A were noted in CMV-infected animals, as compared to control animals. Responses to LPS were found to be depressed in 12/31 CMV-infected animals tested on days 6 to 22 postinoculation as compared to the control animals, although cells from animals tested on days 4 and 27 post-CMV inoculation responded as well as cells from uninfected controls. Furthermore, 11 of 16 animals tested on days 6 to 13 post-CMV inoculation had responses to Con A which were either absent or lower than those of controls. Maximum depression of the responsiveness to Con A was noted on day 6 when the mean proliferative response in the CMV-infected group was only 27% that of the control group. Responses to Con A continued to be depressed in animals tested on days 8, 11, and 13 post-CMV inoculation, although the responsiveness was gradually restored until it was comparable to control animals on day 15. These results show that spleen cells from guinea pigs with acute CMV infection are selectively hyporesponsive to LPS and Con A. Furthermore, this immuno-depression occurs at the time of maximum virus activity, and when the mononucleosis syndrome is the most clinically evident. This suggests that nonspecific immunodepression occurs during acute CMV infection of guinea pigs and may be a contributing element in the development of the disease due to CMV.

A PROSPECTIVE STUDY OF PRIMARY CMV INFECTION DURING PREGNANCY

P.D. Griffiths

The Royal Free Hospital, London NW3 2QG, England

By testing booking sera for CF antibodies, 4,550 (42%) of 10,847 women were shown to be susceptible to CMV infection. To date, 3,880 susceptible women have delivered; follow-up specimens have been collected from 3,481 (90%) of them, and 29 (0.9%) seroconversions have been detected. Urine and/or cord sera were obtained from 26 of these 29 babies and intrauterine transmission of virus occurred in 9/26 (35%) cases. Only 17 rubella seroconversions occurred in the same population showing that CMV infects more pregnant women than does rubella virus.

RIA for specific IgM antibodies has been fully evaluated by us in collaboration with other workers and has been shown to detect primary CMV infections in the 1st trimester, with a sensitivity of 95% and a specificity of 100%. Booking sera from 2,486 seropositive women have now been tested, and 16 infections in early pregnancy have been detected. Fetal death occurred in 4 (25%) of these 16 cases, a ninefold excess over that found in a control group, which strongly suggests that primary infection at this critical early stage of development can cause fetal loss.

All 41 surviving babies born to women experiencing primary infection during pregnancy (29 seroconversions, 12 RIA-IgM positive) were normal at birth; there were no cases of cytomegalic inclusion disease. The pediatric surveillance is continuing and over 80% of the cases and controls have been seen. Two childen have developed definite mental retardation (one is attending a special school), while a third has a possible defect. All 3 were in the group of 9 babies shown to have been infected in utero while, in contrast, 27 uninfected babies born to women infected with CMV during pregnancy and 30 babies born to seronegative matched control women are developing normally. These results clearly demonstrate that the adverse effects of CMV infection are progressive during childhood and result from intrauterine transmission of virus, not an indirect effect on maternal health during pregnancy. They also support the suggestion that CMV is a major cause of childhood handicap which is currently not being diagnosed due to its nonspecific clinical presentation.

PROFILES OF NATURAL KILLER CELL ACTIVITY IN CYTOMEGALOVIRUS EXCRETING VERSUS NORMAL (NML) CHILDREN

C.J. Harrison and J.L. Waner
University of Oklahoma Health Science Center, Oklahoma City, OK 73190

Effects of active CMV infection on cytolytic mechanisms of CMI, eg, NK-cell activity, have not been characterized. The dynamic aspects of CMI in children and the possible selective immunosuppressive effect of CMV are confounding factors in assessing NK activity in congenitally infected children. Profiles of NK-cell activity using uninfected human fibroblasts (UF) and CMV (strain AD169) infected fibroblasts (IF), in addition to K562 cells as targets (T), may be more relevant measures of NK involvement in CMV disease.

PBL were separated by Ficoll-Hypaque centrifugation of heparinized whole blood from NML donors or symptomatic CMV excreters (CEX). Routine 18-hr ^{51}Cr release assays were performed with UF, IF, and K562 cells as targets and nonadherent fractions of PBL (20–25% Leu7+ in NML adults) as effectors at E:T ratios of 50:1.

Compared to values from NMLs, CEX from 1–6 mo old showed increased mean % lysis (MPL) of K562 and increased mean % specific lysis (MPSL) of IF; whereas CEX from 6 mo–5 yrs old had increased MPL of UF and lower MPSL of IF. MPSL of IF is calculated by: MPSL (IF) = MPL(IF) − MPL(UF). The following table indicates profiles of NK activity in NMLs v CEX by age.

	NML		CEX	
Targets	1–6 mo (N = 5)	6 mo–5 yr (N = 14)	1–6 mo (N = 6)	6 mo–5 yr (N = 7)
MPL K562	27%	39%	59%	35%
MPl UF	4%	6%	4%	27%
MPL IF	24%	40%	55%	41%
MPSL IF	20%	34%	51%	14%

Profiles of NK activity including UF, IF, and K562 targets provided more meaningful information on the range of NK cell capability in CEX in different age groups compared to NMLs in similar age groups. These comparisons indicate an age-dependent alteration of target lysis capabilities in NK cell containing fractions of PBL from CEX and/or the existence of NK subpopulations with varied target lysis capabilities. Increased NK activity against uninfected human fibroblast targets in older symptomatic CMV excreters and against AD169 strain CMV infected fibroblast targets in symptomatic CMV excreters < 6 mo old suggests NK cell involvement in the evolution of symptomatic disease of hosts infected with and excreting CMV. These findings may indicate the development of an aberration in NK-cell function in certain CMV excreting hosts, whereby uninfected human cells appear to provoke lysis by NK cells more than CMV infected human cells.

EFFECTS OF ALPHA-INTERFERON ON CMV REACTIVATION SYNDROMES IN RENAL TRANSPLANT RECIPIENTS—RESULTS OF A PLACEBO CONTROLLED TRIAL

M.S. Hirsch, R.T. Schooley, K. Cantell, and R.H. Rubin

Massachusetts General Hospital, and Harvard Medical School, Boston, MA 02114, and Central Public Health Laboratory, Helsinki, Finland

CMV infection is a serious limiting factor to the success of renal transplantation because of its ability to lead to clinical syndromes, superinfection, and renal dysfunction. We have previously demonstrated that a 6-week course of prophylactic α-IFN delays urinary shedding of CMV and decreases the incidence of CMV viremia. We now report results from a double-blind, placebo-controlled trial of a 14-week course of α-IFN on reactivation CMV infections.

CMV-seropositive (> 1:8 by indirect immunofluorescence) renal transplant recipients received 3×10^6 units of IFN or placebo IM before transplantation, then 3 times a week for 6 weeks, followed by twice a week for 8 weeks (total 102×10^6 units). Forty-eight patients consented to participate but 6 were omitted from analysis because they received < 10 doses of study drug. IFN and placebo recipients were well matched, and 42 have been followed for a mean of 19 months.

CMV syndromes were markedly reduced in IFN recipients during the 14 weeks of drug administration. Seven of 22 placebo recipients and 1 of 20

IFN recipients developed CMV syndromes (P = .026). Opportunistic super-infections *(Aspergillus fumigatus, Pneumocystis carinii)* occurred in 2 placebo and no IFN recipients. CMV-associated glomerulopathy developed in 3 placebo and 1 IFN recipients. Two deaths occurred in the IFN group (cardiomyopathy, perforated intestinal diverticulum) and 2 in the placebo group (CMV pneumonia, *Pneumocystis* pneumonia). Graft function was equivalent in both groups.

Urinary and salivary excretion were only slightly delayed by IFN prophylaxis, and viremia was equivalent in both groups. No significant IFN toxicity was observed.

In seropositive renal transplant recipients, α-IFN appears to be the best currently available approach to the prevention of serious CMV infection.

TRANSCRIPTION OF THE TRANSFORMING REGION OF HUMAN CYTOMEGALOVIRUS STRAIN AD169

G.Jahn, J.A. Nelson, D.A. Galloway, J.K. McDougall, A. Grässmann, and B. Fleckenstein

Institut für Klinische Virologie, Universität Erlangen-Nürnberg, D-8520 Erlangen, Federal Republic of Germany, Institut für Molekularbiologie und Biochemie der Freien Universität Berlin, D-1000 Berlin 33, Federal Republic of Germany, and Fred Hutchinson Cancer Research Center, Seattle, WA 98104

In the course of studying in vitro-transformation of rodent cells by cloned DNA fragments of CMV AD169, we initiated transcription analyses of the respective DNA sequences during virus replication. Northern blot hybridizations with a series of plasmid clones encompassing the transforming DNA indicated that the region is transcribed into a 5.0-kb RNA, if human foreskin fibroblasts are infected in the presence of an inhibitor of protein synthesis (CH, 100/μg/ml). The region transcribed into 5.0-kb RNA, extending between map units 0.130–0.160, is mapping in vicinity of 3 other abundantly transcribed IE genes. The transcripts are 1) a 1.9-kb RNA between 0.055 and 0.085 map units, 2) a 2.3-kb RNA between map positions 0.085 and 0.095, and 3) a 2.2-kb transcript from map units 0.115 to 0.130. The 5.0-kb transcript was characterized in more detail. The direction of transcription was determined by hybridization with radioactive cDNA synthesized from IE RNA. The transforming DNA region is an internal part of the IE gene expressed into the 5.0-kb transcript. In contrast to the other 3 abundant IE

RNAs, the 5.0-kb transcript is not only found with polyadenylated RNA; a high proportion of 5.0-kb RNA was eluted from oligo dT cellulose with the poly (A)−fraction. Also contrasting to the 3 other IE genes, the DNA coding for 5.0-kb RNA is transcribed in high quantities during the late phase of virus replication. The region of the 5.0-kb IE RNA appears not to code for the predominant IE protein of 72K; microinjection of cloned DNA fragments and staining with a monoclonal mouse antibody indicates that the gene for the 72K protein is located between map units 0.055 and 0.095. Thus, transformation of rodent cells and coding for the predominant IE protein are different functions, and it remains to be determined if expression of the gene coding for 5.0-kb IE RNA is functionally related to transforming activity.

ACQUIRED (OR CONGENITAL) IMMUNODEFICIENCY SYNDROME IN INFANTS BORN OF HAITIAN MOTHERS

J.H. Joncas, G. Delage, Z. Chad, and N. Lapointe
Department of Microbiology and Immunology, University of Montreal, and Pediatric Research Center, Ste-Justine Hospital, Montreal, Quebec, Canada H3T 1C5

AIDS is a recently described entity observed in certain groups such as homosexuals, drug abusers, hemophiliacs, and Haitian immigrants. An agent (or agents) transmitted sexually and by blood or blood components may be important in the etiology of this syndrome. The recent occurrence of AIDS in an infant who received a platelet transfusion derived from the blood of a male donor subsequently found to have AIDS strengthens the possibility of infectious agent(s) transmissible by blood or blood products in the etiology of AIDS. The occurrence of typical or incomplete AIDS in infants born of Haitian mothers was recently seen in this hospital.

A female infant, born 6/14/81 to a Haitian mother, developed fever, otitis media, hepatosplenomegaly, and anemia (9 mg/dl) in the 3rd week of life. The mother was found to have lymphoma 4 days after delivery and was treated. She subsequently developed miliary tuberculosis and died 6 weeks after delivery. Undifferentiated lymphoma and miliary tuberculosis were confirmed at postmortem. The infant was seen again at the age of 3 months with extensive oral and pharyngeal candidiasis, persistent hepatosplenomegaly and cough, but no fever. Hb was 9.5 mg/dl. WBC was 7,500, lymphs 53%, polys 22%, bands 15%, monos 10%. The chest x-ray showed signs of bronchiolitis. Transaminases were slightly elevated. IgG was 112 mg% and

IgM 29 mg%. NBT test and serum complement were normal. She was discharged after 2 weeks but was readmitted at the age of 4 months with persistent candidiasis, progressive hepatosplenomegaly, and lymphadenopathy. She had fever and diarrhea. Blood, CSF, urine, and stool cultures were negative for bacteria but the stool and throat were positive for *Candida*. CMV was isolated from a urine taken 10/29/81 and from a throat swab and another urine taken 12/18/81. EBV infection was documented by an EBV-VCA titer of 80 to 160 on 10/18/81 and 12/18/81 with a positive VCA-IgM test and by negative EBNA tests on the same sera. CMV antibodies could not be detected. IgM dropped to < 10 mg%, IgA was normal, and IgG varied between 74 mg% and 163 mg%. The lymphocyte count dropped to 4% of a total WBC of 5000/mm^3, and T cells fell to 28% and 16%. The infant died with progressive pneumonia and pericardial effusion which failed to respond to various antibiotics including antituberculous drugs and TMP·SM. Autopsy revealed generalized CMV infection and *Pneumocystis carinii* pneumonia. CMV was isolated from liver and lung. Two other Haitian infants with presumed AIDS are still living. These observations may shed new light on a subset of SCID of possible infectious etiology.

MURINE CYTOMEGALOVIRUS INFECTION AS A MODEL FOR DETERMINING POTENTIAL EFFICACY OF ANTIVIRALS IN HUMAN DISEASE

E. R. Kern, J.T. Richards, M.E. Katz, and J.C. Overall, Jr.
University of Utah School of Medicine, Salt Lake City, Utah

Due to the strict species specificity of HCMV, it has not been possible to test potential antiviral agents for activity against HCMV in animals. Inoculation of mice with MCMV provides a model infection that shares many characteristics with the human disease. Both acute lethal and chronic nonlethal MCMV infections have been used in our laboratory to determine efficacy of antivirals. After IP inoculation of 3-week-old Swiss Webster female mice with 1 × 10^6 PFU of MCMV, 90%–100% of animals die with a mean day of death of 5–6 days. With an inoculum of 1 × 10^5 PFU, all animals survive. With either inoculum, high titers of virus are present in lung, liver, spleen, kidney, and blood within 24 hr, and in salivary gland by 48–72 hr. In surviving animals, persistent viral replication occurs in lung, liver, kidney, and spleen for at least 20–30 days and in salivary glands for months. The MCMV infection, therefore, involves many of the same target organs as HCMV. With a number of an-

TABLE 1. Effect of Oral Treatment With FIAC, FIAU, or FMAU on the Mortality of Weanling Mice Inoculated IP With MCMV

| Treatment* | Mortality | | P Value | MDD | P Value |
	Number	%			
Placebo + 6 hr	14/15	93	—	4.9	—
FIAC − 2 hr	14/15	93	NS[†]	4.6	NS
FIAC + 6 hr	14/14	100	NS	4.6	NS
FIAU − 2 hr	15/15	100	NS	3.9	NS
FIAU + 6 hr	14/14	100	NS	5.0	NS
FMAU − 2 hr	14/15	93	NS	4.4	NS
FMAU + 6 hr	13/14	93	NS	4.7	NS

*Treatment with 50 mg/kg was initiated at the times indicated and continued twice daily for 7 days.
[†]NS = Not significant.

tiviral agents tested in our laboratory, there is good correlation between the sensitivity of MCMV in tissue culture and efficacy in mice as evidenced by protection against mortality and alteration of viral pathogenesis. For example, MCMV is inhibited in tissue culture by 0.5 μg/ml of acyclovir (ACV), and oral therapy with ACV significantly reduced mortality and MCMV replication in lung, liver, spleen, and kidney [1].

The purpose of these studies was to define the sensitivity of MCMV to 2′-fluoro-5-iodoarabinosyl-cytosine (FIAC), 2′-fluoro-5-iodoarabinosyl-uracil (FIAU), 2′-fluoro-5-methyl-arabinosyl-uracil (FMAU), and 9-(1,3-dihydroxy-2-propoxymethyl) guanine (DHPG) in mouse embryo fibroblast (MEF) cells, and to determine the efficacy of treatment on mortality of weanling mice infected with MCMV. In tissue culture cells, MCMV was insensitive to the action of the FIAC, FIAU, or FMAU as more than 100 μM of drug was required to inhibit virus plaque production by 50%. In contrast, MCMV was quite sensitive to the action of DHPG requiring only 9 μM for inhibition.

Groups of mice were inoculated IP with MCMV, and oral treatment with 50 mg of FIAC, FIAU, or FMAU per kg twice daily for 7 days was begun 2 hr prior to or 6 hr after infection (Table 1). There were no significant differences in final mortality or mean day of death in mice treated with either of the 3 compounds compared with placebo-treated animals. In contrast, when mice were inoculated with MCMV and treated with 50 mg of DHPG per kg there was a significant reduction in mortality when therapy was initiated as late as 48 hr after infection (Table 2). In addition, viral replication in target organs was also reduced (data not presented). These data indicate that there is good correlation between the sensitivity of MCMV to ACV, FIAC, FIAU, FMAU, and DHPG in vitro and efficacy of treatment in the animal model. Since HCMV is sensitive to FIAC, FIAU, and FMAU in vitro and MCMV is not, no predictions can be

TABLE 2. Effect of Oral Treatment With DHPG on the Mortality of Weanling Mice Inoculated IP With MCMV

Treatment	Mortality		P Value	MDD	P Value
	Number	%			
Experiment 1					
Placebo + 6 hr	14/15	93	—	4.0	—
DHPG + 6 hr	1/15	7	< 0.001	6.0	NS[†]
DHPG + 24 hr	3/15	20	< 0.001	6.3	< 0.01
DHPG + 48 hr	8/16	53	< 0.05	5.5	< 0.05
Experiment 2					
Placebo + 6 hr	14/15	93	—	6.6	—
DHPG + 6 hr	0/15	—	< 0.001	—	—
DHPG + 24 hr	1/15	7	< 0.001	7.0	NS
DHPG + 48 hr	8/15	53	< 0.05	8.4	< 0.001

*Treatment with 50 mg/kg was initiated at times indicated and continued twice daily for 7 days.

[†]NS = Not significant.

made concerning potential clinical efficacy with these agents. Both MCMV and HCMV, however, are sensitive to DHPG, and the results from the animal model experiments suggest that this compound may be an excellent candidate for treatment of CMV infections in humans.

REFERENCE

Glasgow LA, Richards JT, Kern ER: Effect of acyclovir treatment on acute and chronic murine cytomegalovirus infection. Am J Med 73(1a):132–137, 1981.

USE OF MONOCLONAL ANTIBODY TO HUMAN CYTOMEGALOVIRUS FOR DETECTION OF HCMV-SPECIFIC IgM ANTIBODY IN HUMAN SERA BY ENZYME-LINKED IMMUNOSORBENT ASSAY (ELISA) USING ANTIBODY CLASS CAPTURED ASSAY (ACCA)

K.S. Kim, V.J. Sapienza, and K. Wisniewski

Institute for Basic Research in Developmental Disabilities, Staten Island, NY 10314

Using a monoclonal antibody which is reactive to a major HCMV glyco-protein, an objective method for detection of HCMV-specific IgM antibody in human sera has been established by the ELISA-ACCA method. A hybrid cell line 7B4 producing IgG which is specific for HCMV major glycoprotein (66,000 dalton) was obtained after fusion of P3X63 Ag8 myeloma cells with spleen cells from BALB/c mice immunized with purified HCMV. Using affinity purified 7B4 antibody from ascites fluid horseradish peroxidase (HRP) conjugated 7B4 monoclonal antibody was prepared. The procedure involves addition of patients' sera to goat IgG antihuman IgM (Fc 5μ specific) antibody coated Dynatech Immulon plates with 96 wells. The serum diluted in phosphate buffered saline containing 0.1% triton X-100 (PBST) and 1% bovine serum albumin (BSA) was added and incubated 4 hr at room temperature. After washing 3 times with PBST for 15 min, HCMV antigen preparation containing at least 8 units of complement-fixing antigen was added to the IgM antibody captured in the wells and incubated overnight at 4°C. After washing 15 min with 3 changes of PBST, horseradish peroxidase conjugated 7B4 monoclonal antibody was added and incubated for 2 hr at room temperature to determine the retention of HCMV antigen. After washing, a solution of o-phenylenediamine and H_2O_2 in citrate buffer pH 5 was added and incubated for 30 min at room temperature. The color change was measured after adding H_2SO_4 using a 490-nm filter. The test is specific in that a high titer of HCMV IgG sera, IgM antibody to *Toxoplasma gondii*, hepatitis A, EBV, or HSV did not give any false-positive results. Use of HCMV-specific monoclonal antibody conjugated HRP eliminated most of the background problem that occurred when HRP-conjugated hyperimmune Ig from an animal was used.

DISEASE PATTERN FOLLOWING POSTNATAL CYTOMEGALOVIRUS INFECTION IN HUMANS

U. Krech and T. Krech

Institute of Medical Microbiology, CH-9000 St. Gallen, Switzerland

Diagnosis of congenitally acquired CMV infection has been made by virus isolations within the first days of life. While this is a suitable technique to detect congenital CMV infection, virus isolation to detect acute postnatal infection is less satisfactory. Virus excretion following postnatal infection may continue over months or even years beyond the stage of acute infection.

We have recently demonstrated that the IgM response may be a more suitable technique to differentiate between acute and persistent CMV infection. Specific CMV-IgM antibodies are present in the acute stage and drop below a demonstrable level within 3–5 mo after infection. The use of an anti-μ-capture technique and an enzyme labeled antigen avoids the false-positive reactions due to the rheumatoid factor which is present in 40%–50% of patients with acute CMV infection. This test is specific although cross-reactions in the IgM fraction with other antigens may occur occasionally.

Out of about 5,000 patients who were examined by virus serology during a period of 9 mo, 285 patients showed CMV-IgM antibodies. Sufficient clinical information was available from 78 patients who showed the following clinical symptoms:

74—fever persistent, frequently septic, fever of unknown origin
28—hepatitis, rarely icterus, 8 with granulomatous hepatitis
14—infectious mononucleosis, posttransfusion syndrome after open heart surgery
 8—pneumonia, 4 with and 4 without immunosuppressive therapy
 4—birth defects
 4—diarrhea
 3—Guillain-Barré
 2—pharyngitis
 2—adenopathy

These data seem to indicate that clinical diagnosis following postnatal CMV infection is not as rare as earlier expected.

IMMEDIATE-EARLY HCMV GENE EXPRESSION IN NONPERMISSIVE BALB/c-3T3 CELLS

R. LaFemina and G.S. Hayward
Johns Hopkins School of Medicine, Baltimore, MD 21205

We have been interested in examining animal nonpermissive cell lines which do not replicate the HCMV Towne genome as potential cell systems for the study of HCMV latency. Following infection of BALB/c-3T3 cells, input viral genomes can be detected, but newly synthesized viral DNA has never been observed. These mouse cells express only IE proteins of HCMV, but apparently these proteins do not function properly to replicate the viral genome or to turn on delayed-early or late viral proteins. Our present studies attempt to define the block to replication in nonpermissive cells and to specifically ascertain whether improper expression of IE proteins in mouse cells is responsible for the lack of subsequent gene expression and viral replication. Following infection in the presence of CH and reversal with media lacking inhibitor, one major and several minor IE proteins are synthesized in both mouse and human cells. A monoclonal antibody immunoprecipitates the major IE protein expressed in both mouse and human cells indicating at least some antigenic identity. Furthermore, SDS polyacrylamide gel electrophoresis of partial proteolytic products resulting from *S aureus* V8 protease indicates that identical ^{35}S methionines peptide comprise the major IE protein in infected mouse and human cells. Significantly, however, the IE protein expressed after CH reversal in human cells is strongly phosphorylated, but the identical protein expressed in mouse cells is at best marginally phosphorylated. Since other IE, but not delayed-early, proteins are found in infected mouse cells, altered IE protein phosphorylation may affect subsequent viral gene expression in nonpermissive cells.

A COMPARISON OF ELISA, IFA, AND IHA PROCEDURES FOR THE DETERMINATION OF CMV ANTIBODY STATUS OF BLOOD DONORS*

H. Lamberson, J. McMillan, L. Weiner, E. Bousman, and C. McMahon

American Red Cross Blood Services, Syracuse Region and the State University of New York Upstate Medical Center, Syracuse, NY 13210

Transfusion transmitted CMV infection has been reported to result in significant morbidity and mortality in severely immunocompromised patients. Transfusion of blood from donors who lack detectable antibody to CMV has been reported to reduce the risk of transfusion transmitted in high-risk neonates. For this reason, we have evaluated commercially available products for the determination of CMV antibody status. Sera from 100 healthy volunteer donors (mean age 38.5 + 12.7, 63% male, 37% female, 57% O pos, 24% O neg, 9% A pos, 3% A neg, 5% B pos, 2% AB pos) were assayed by ELISA (CMV Bio-Enzabead, Litton Bionetics), IFA (Electro Nucleonics), and IHA (Cetus CMV IHA). The following results were obtained:

	ELISA	IFA (IgG)	IHA
Total samples assayed	100	100	100
Positive samples	49	50	55
Negative samples	51	50	45
Concordance		99%	95%

*Supported by American Red Cross funds.

All but one of the specimens which were positive by ELISA or IFA (IgG) were positive by IHA. Eight specimens which were positive by IHA were negative by both ELISA and IFA (IgG). Since IHA procedures detect both IgG and IgM antibody, 6 of these 8 specimens were assayed for IgM anti-CMV by IFA. All 6 of these specimens lacked detectable IgM. These negative IFA-IgM results are consistent with the negative ELISA results since the ELISA assay used is reported to detect both IgG and IgM antibody.

We conclude that the IHA assay will identify 99% of CMV antibody positive donors detected by ELISA and IFA. In addition, the IHA is positive in 8% of donors who are negative for CMV antibody by IFA (IgG and IgM) and ELISA. While the IHA may be less specific than IFA or ELISA, the sensitivity should be sufficient for the screening of blood products.

Assessment of the ability of IHA, IFA, and ELISA screening of blood products to prevent transfusion transmitted CMV awaits systematic follow-up of recipients.

REORGANIZATION OF AN INTERMEDIATE FILAMENT-ASSOCIATED ANTIGEN FOLLOWING CYTOMEGALOVIRUS INFECTION

J.L.H. Li, C.H. Lee, W.C. Thompson, and T. Albrecht

Department of Microbiology (J.L.H.L., C.H.L., T.A.), and Division of Biochemistry (W.C.T.), University of Texas Medical Branch, Galveston, TX

Following infection by HCMV, the host cell undergoes a course of morphologic and physiologic changes, leading to the production and release of new virus particles. We report here that HCMV infection induces a redistribution of an antigen normally associated with cytoskeletal filaments, resulting in the appearance of this antigen in nonfilamentous structures (apparently viral inclusion bodies) in both the cytoplasm and nucleus of the infected cell.

In order to examine cytoskeletal changes during viral infection, we have developed several murine monoclonal antibodies to human fibroblast antigens. The particular antibody used in this study (IFA-1) stains by indirect immunofluorescence a filamentous network in human fibroblastic cells as well as in mouse cells and PtK2 marsupial kidney cells. The filaments stained by this antibody are apparently of the intermediate filament class for the following reasons: 1) Double-label immunofluorescence staining with IFA-1 and an antitubulin reagent demonstrates that the pattern of filaments stained by IFA-1 differs from that of the microtubules. 2) The pattern of filaments stained by IFA-1 differs from the pattern of actin cables and stress fibers in these cells. 3) The stained filaments withstand pretreatment of the cells with colchicine (20 μg/ml) or colcemid (5 μg/ml). 4) During extended pretreatment with colcemid, the filaments stained by IFA-1 condense to form the thick ropey bundles characteristic of intermediate filaments. Therefore, we consider that monoclonal antibody IFA-1 recognizes an intermediate filament-associated (IFA) antigen. To estimate the molecular weight of the IFA antigen, proteins extracted from human fibroblastic cells were separated by SDS polyacrylamide gel electrophoresis, transferred to nitrocellulose paper, and probed with the monoclonal antibody IFA-1, which was subsequently detected by an enzyme-linked second antibody. IFA-1 was found to bind to 4 bands migrating in the range of 48 to 60 Kd, some of which may be degradative products.

We have examined the distribution of IFA antigen during the course of CMV infection by indirect immunofluorescence procedures. Human embryonic lung (LU) cells were infected with CMV (strain AD169, 3 PFU/cell) during a 1-hr incubation. At various time intervals, infected and uninfected control cells were fixed with acetone and the distribution of the IFA antigen was determined using IFA-1 antibody. (Examples of the fluorescence micrographs are shown in Figure 7, Albrecht, this volume.) In cells stained at 24-hr PI, the intensity of the fluorescence of the cytoplasmic filamentous net-

TABLE 1. Detection of IFA Antigens with IFA-1 Monoclonal Antibody in Human LU Cells Following CMV Infection

	Treatment					
	None		ara-C[a] (Fluorescence)		CH[b]	
Hr PI	Nucleus	Cytoplasm	Nucleus	Cytoplasm	Nucleus	Cytoplasm
0	−	+[d]	−	+[d]	−	+[d]
12	−	+[d]	−	+[d]	−	+[d]
24	+[c]	+[e]	+[f]	±[e]	−	+[d]
48	+[c]	+[d,e]	+[f]	+[d,e]	−[g]	+[d,g]
72	+[c]	+[d,e]	+[f]	+[d,e]		
96	+[c]	+[d,e]	+[f]	+[d,e]		
120	+[c]	+[d,e]	+[f]	+[d,e]		

[a]50 μg/ml of ara-C was added at 0 hr PI.
[b]100 μg/ml of CH was added at 0 hr PI.
[c]IFA antigens organized into nuclear inclusions.
[d]IFA antigens associated with an intermediate filament network.
[e]IFA antigens organized into cytoplasmic inclusions.
[f]IFA antigen particles were spread throughout the nucleus.
[g]CMV-infected cells began to degenerate 48 hr after treatment with 100 μg/ml CH.

work had apparently diminished. At this same time, many brightly staining particles containing IFA antigen had accumulated in the vicinity of the cytoplasmic inclusion, and the nuclei appeared uniformly unstained except for small fluorescent bodies which appeared to coincide with early nuclear inclusions. By 48-hr PI, the IFA antigen was evident in brightly stained late nuclear inclusions, surrounded by a region of unstained nucleoplasm. This redistribution of IFA antigen was not observed in cells exposed to inactivated virus. Furthermore, the coincidence of the fluorescent nuclear images with the CMV-induced nuclear inclusion was confirmed by phase contrast microscopy and time-course studies, which demonstrated the coincidental development of the nuclear inclusions and fluorescent images from 24–120-hr PI.

Treatment of LU cells with CH (100 μg/ml at 0 hr PI) prevented the apparent disruption of the filamentous network and appearance of IFA antigen particles in the cytoplasm and nucleus. This result indicates that protein synthesis was required following CMV infection for the antigen redistribution to occur. Treatment of LU cells with ara-C, 50 μg/ml at 0-hr PI failed to inhibit either the apparent disruption of the filamentous network or the appearance of IFA-antigen containing particles in the cytoplasm and nucleus. In the presence of ara-C, the nuclear IFA antigen particles detected after 24 hr were found throughout the nucleus, rather than organized into nuclear inclusions (Table 1).

While early CMV functions were sufficient for redistribution of IFA antigen, CMV DNA synthesis was apparently required for organization of this antigen into the CMV-induced nuclear inclusion. When considered together, these results suggest that the IFA antigen described here may play a role in the cellular response to CMV infection and in the replication of CMV.

LYMPHOCYTE-MEDIATED CYTOTOXICITY OF CYTOMEGALOVIRUS-INFECTED HUMAN MONOCYTES RESTRICTED BY THE HLA-Dr LOCUS*

M.D. Lindsley, D.J. Torpey III, and C.R. Rinaldo, Jr.
Department of Microbiology, University of Pittsburgh, Graduate School of Public Health, Pittsburgh, PA 15261 (M.D.L., D.J.T., C.R.R.); Department of Pathology, Presbyterian-University Hospital and University of Pittsburgh, School of Medicine, Pittsburgh, PA 15261 (C.R.R.)

*Supported by NIH grant AI-16212, Biomedical Research Support grant RR-05451 from the USPHS, Clinical Research grant no. 6-369 from the March of Dimes Birth Defects Foundation, and the Pathology Education Research Fund and the Research Development Fund from the University of Pittsburgh.

The role of the CMI response is of great significance in recovery from viral infections. An important factor in this response is the lysis of virus-infected cells by cytotoxic T lymphocytes which are characteristically immune-specific and HLA-restricted [1]. We have developed a model for in vitro analysis of the human cytotoxic lymphocyte response to CMV infection using peripheral blood monocytes as targets.

In this system, mononuclear leukocytes were isolated from peripheral blood of CMV seropositive and seronegative donors by centrifugation on Ficoll-Hypaque gradients. To obtain effector cells, mononuclear leukocytes were stimulated with UV-inactivated CMV antigen (AD169 strain obtained from G.V. Quinnan) for 5 days at 37°C [2]. Monocytes were obtained for use as target cells on day 5 by adherence of freshly donated mononuclear leukocytes to plastic plates for 1.5 hr at 37°C. Plastic-adherent cells ($\geq$ 95% esterase-positive) were removed with 0.33% EDTA, and infected with CMV (AD169 strain; input multiplicity of 1–3 PFU/cell) for 1.5 hr at 37°C. The cells were then labeled with ^{51}Cr. CMV antigen-stimulated effector cells ($\geq$ 96% esterase negative) were added to the monocyte targets at effector to target ratios of 50, 25, and 12.5 to 1. Supernatants were harvested for radioactivity after 12–14-hr incubation at 37°C. The amount of cytolysis was

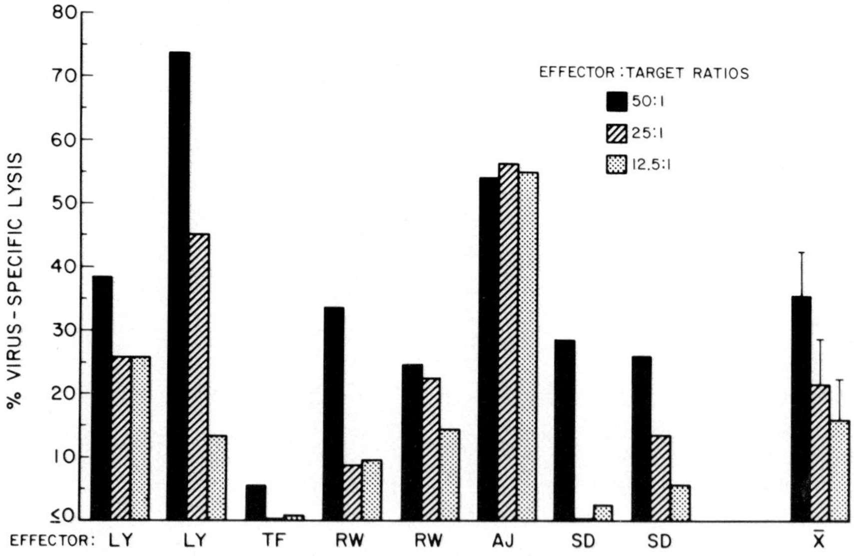

Fig. 1. Virus-specific lysis of autologous monocyte targets by CMV antigen-stimulated lymphocytes from CMV seropositive donors.

calculated as the % virus-specific release of ^{51}Cr, or % specific release from CMV-infected targets, or % specific release from uninfected targets.

The results obtained from these experiments have shown that stimulation of lymphocytes from seropositive donors with soluble CMV antigen generated cytotoxic effectors that lyse autologous monocytes infected with CMV (Fig. 1). This lysis was significantly greater than lysis of autologous targets by stimulated lymphocytes from seronegative donors (seronegative donors [n = 6]: 50:1 and 25:1, mean 0.0%, P < 0.01, 12.5:1, mean 1.9%, P < 0.1).

When allogeneic targets were matched with effectors at an HLA-A and/or B locus, very low levels of virus-specific lysis were detected (Fig. 2). This was significantly lower than lysis of autologous targets (P < 0.005 at 50:1, P < 0.01 at 25:1, P < 0.1 at 12.5:1). Targets that were matched with effectors at only the HLA-Dr locus (Fig. 2) showed a high level of virus-specific lysis that was not significantly different from the lysis of autologous targets at all 3 ratios. Virus-specific lysis of mismatched targets was < 3.0% at all ratios and was significantly lower than the lysis of autologous targets (P < 0.05 of all ratios) (data not shown). Mean levels of lysis of uninfected autologous and allogeneic monocytes by antigen-stimulated lymphocytes from seropositive donors were ≤ 4.0% and ≤ 10%, respectively. Freshly donated lymphocytes demonstrated low levels of virus-specific lysis against the CMV-infected monocytes (≤ 8.5% at 50:1).

Analysis of NK cell activity in the CMV antigen-stimulated lymphocytes was performed using K562 cells as targets. Results showed a significant increase in NK activity in the antigen-treated lymphocytes from seropositive donors (P < 0.02 at all ratios), and no increase in activity in the antigen-treated lymphocytes of seronegative donors when compared to mock-treated lymphocytes of both groups. Although an increase in NK activity occurred, it did not seem to be of significance in the killing of the CMV-infected monocytes as shown by the lack of lysis of mismatched and HLA-A and/or B matched targets by CMV-stimulated lymphocytes.

In conclusion, we have developed a system in which CMV-infected autologous monocytes provide excellent targets for lysis by soluble CMV antigen-stimulated lymphocytes from seropositive donors. When using allogeneic targets, the lysis was restricted to only HLA-Dr effector-target matches. It has recently been shown by other laboratories that cytotoxic T-cells generated in vitro by fetal calf serum [3] and TNP [4] antigens are HLA-Dr restricted. It has also been shown that cytotoxic T lymphocytes generated against HLA-Dr itself are predominantly of the OKT4-positive subset [5]. Based on the HLA-restriction pattern, we hypothesize that soluble CMV antigen stimulates a class II, MHC-restricted cytotoxic lymphocyte of the helper T-cell subset. The predominant expression of HLA-Dr on the

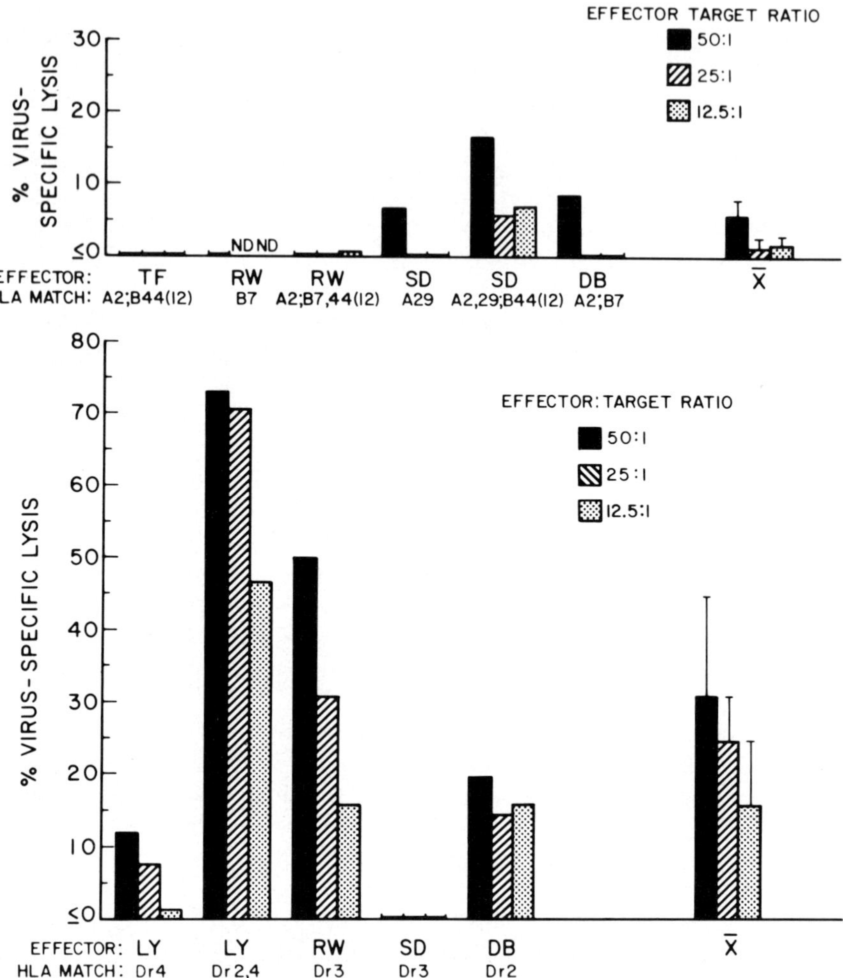

Fig. 2. Virus-specific lysis of allogeneic monocyte targets by CMV-antigen stimulated lymphocytes from CMV seropositive donors. Top: Targets matched with effectors at HLA-A and/or B only. Bottom: Targets matched with effectors at HLA-Dr only.

majority of monocytes [6] used as targets allows us to detect these killer cells. Such cytotoxic T cells could be of significance in the complex interaction of CMV and other viruses with the host immune system.

ACKNOWLEDGMENTS

We thank Dr. Bruce Rabin, Ms. Marian Griffin, and the Division of

Immunopathology for HLA typing. We also thank Judy Fossati for secretarial assistance and Robbin DeBiasio for technical assistance.

REFERENCES

1. Zinkernagel RM, Doherty PC: MHC-restricted cytotoxic T cells: Studies on the biological role of polymorphic major transplantation antigens determining T-cell restriction-specificity, function, and responsiveness. Adv Immunol 27:52–180, 1979.
2. Rinaldo CR Jr, DeBiasio RL: Alteration of immunoregulatory mechanisms during cytomegalovirus mononucleosis: Effect of in vitro culture on lymphocyte blastogenesis to viral antigens. Clin Immunol Immunopathol (In press).
3. Misko IS, Pope JH, Kane RG, Bashir H, Doran T: Evidence for the involvement of HLA-Dr antigens in restricted cytotoxicity by fetal calf serum-specific human T-cells. Hum Immunol 5:183–197, 1982.
4. Newman W, Pious D, Gladstone P: HLA variants of human lymphoblastoid cell lines as targets for cytotoxic T-cells: Analysis of CTL reactivity against 2 HLA-Dr variants. J Immunol 125:2515–2520, 1980.
5. Ball EJ, Stastny P: Cell-mediated cytotoxicity against HLA-Dr region products expressed in monocytes and B-lymphocytes. IV. Characterization of effector cells using monoclonal antibodies against human T-cell subsets. Immunogenetics 16:157–169, 1982.
6. Nunez G, Stastny P: Cytofluorometric analysis of major histocompatibility antigens on human monocytes using monoclonal antibodies. Hum Immunol 6:1–11, 1983.

IDENTIFYING FEATURES OF MOTHERS OF INFANTS WITH CONGENITAL DISEASE DUE TO CYTOMEGALOVIRUS

J.P. Luby and L.N. Gollihar

The University of Texas Health Science Center, Dallas, TX 75235

During the 12-year period, 1970–1981, we identified 58 infants with congenital disease due to CMV. All infants had signs and symptoms consistent with CMV disease, had positive CMV cultures, were diagnosed before 6 months of age, and had not received transfusions before diagnosis. Thirty infants were born at Parkland Memorial Hospital (PMH); 28 infants were born elsewhere but hospitalized at PMH or Children's Medical Center, Dallas, Texas. Each infant with disease due to CMV was compared with 2 infants with negative urine cultures who were matched for delivery at PMH or elsewhere.

Infants with disease were born without seasonal predilection. An apparent increase in the occurrence of cases with time was matched by a similar increase in controls, and could be explained by the number of cultures submitted to the laboratory. Overall, mothers of cases differed from mothers of controls in being younger (P < 0.001) and primiparous (P < 0.001). The age and parity effects could be explained by the facts that a greater proportion of mothers of affected infants were young (< 19 years), and that these younger mothers were more frequently primiparous than similarly aged controls. Primiparous mothers of cases had a racial distribution to comparable controls. Multiparous mothers of cases (14/58) had a similar age distribution to multiparous controls. The multiparous women, however, had a racial distribution that was significantly different from controls (black:white ratio for cases 1:10 *v* 22:24 for controls) (P < 0.01). Although women delivering infants with CMV disease at PMH had a relatively high frequency of being unmarried at the time of delivery (18/30, 60%) and of having had a sexually transmitted disease prior to the birth of the affected infant (6/30, 20%), these values were not significantly different from controls.

The study indicates a relatively constant occurrence of cases of congenital disease due to CMV with time and major effects of age and parity, both of which appeared to be independent variables. The racial distribution of primiparous mothers of cases was significantly different from multiparous mothers. Marital status and a history of a sexually transmitted disease were not different in mothers of affected infants and controls.

ADHERENCE OF COWAN STRAIN *S AUREUS* TO CMV-INFECTED MONOLAYERS: INDIRECT ADHESION OF A PROTEIN A-POSITIVE BACTERIUM TO CMV-INDUCED Fc RECEPTORS

P. Mackowiak, M. Marling-Cason, J. Smith, and J. Luby
VA Medical Center and University of Texas Southwestern Medical School, Dallas, TX 75216

CMV and other viruses within the herpes group induce Fc receptors in infected monolayers. We have recently demonstrated the capacity of such Fc receptors to mediate adherence of antibody-coated bacteria to CMV-infected monolayers (Abstracts of the 1983 Western AFCR). In the present studies, we examined the possibility that adherent antibody-coated bacteria might constitute receptors for protein A-containing cocci. If so, Fc regions of antibody fixed to antibody-coated bacteria would react simultaneously with Fc receptor on both infected monolayers and protein A-positive cocci. To test this hypothesis, we infected confluent HEL cell monolayers with CMV (strain AD169) and measured adherence of Cowan strain *S aureus* to infected and control monolayers using a double radiolabel assay. Monolayers that had

TABLE 1.

| HEL Monolayer | Monolayer Preincubated With Antibody-Coated *E coli* 06 | |
	Yes	No
Infected	8.5 ± 3.3*	4.4 ± 2.0
Control	6.1 ± 3.5	5.3 ± 1.5

*Significantly different from all other values at $P < 0.05$.

been preincubated with a suspension of antibody-coated *E coli*-06 were compared with ones not pretreated. Infected monolayers were examined 48 hr after viral seeding, at which time $\cong 75\%$ of the cells exhibited characteristic cytopathic changes. The results of these experiments (expressed as mean ±SD CFU of *S aureus*/100 HEL cells; n = 16) are given in Table 1.

As shown, adherence of Cowan strain *S aureus* to HEL monolayers was significantly enhanced only when such monolayers were infected wtih CMV and then preincubated with antibody-coated *E coli*-06.

These results illustrate a previously unrecognized mechanism by which herpes viruses might enhance adherence of protein A-containing cocci to cell surfaces. Such a mechanism, if active in vivo, might facilitate colonization of mucosal surfaces by these bacteria and possibly relate to the high prevalence of *S aureus* in the vaginal flora of women with histories of genital herpes (Ann Int Med 96:944, 1982). These data might also explain the apparent predisposition of CMV-infected patients to certain secondary bacterial infections.

POTENTIAL ANTI-HCMV NUCLEOSIDE ANALOGS[*]

Eng-Chun Mar,[1] Yung-Chi Cheng,[1,4] and Eng-Shang Huang[1,2,3,4]

Cancer Research Center[1] and Departments of Medicine[2], Microbiology and Immunology[3], and Pharmacology[4], School of Medicine, University of North Carolina, Chapel Hill, NC 27514

It is documented that a virus-induced thymidine kinase (TK) is essential for the antiherpetic activity of 9-(2-hydroxyethoxymethyl) guanine (ACV) (Elion et al Proc Natl Acad Sci USA 74:5716–5720, 1977). Since HCMV

[*]Supported by the National Institute of Allergy and Infectious Diseases (AI12717 and AI00229) and the National Cancer Institute (CA21773).

stimulates only cellular TK (Estes and Huang: J Virol 24:13–21, 1977; Zavada et al: Arch Virol 12:333–339), this may explain the insensitivity of HCMV towards this compound (Crumpacker et al: Antimicrob Agents Chemother 15:642–645, 1979; Mar et al: Am J Med 73:82–85, 1982). Nonetheless, due to possible differences in the mode(s) of action, the following compounds demonstrated different degrees of potency against HCMV. These compounds are 1-β-D-arabinofuranosyl-5-methyluracil (FMAU), -5-iodouracil (FIAU), -5-methylcytosine (FMAC), -5-iodocytosine (FIAC) (Watanabe et al: J Med Chem 22:21–24, 1979), and 9-(1,3-dihydroxypropoxymethyl) guanine (DHPG) (Smith et al: Antimicrob Agents Chemother 22:55–61, 1982). The susceptibility of HCMV (Towne strain) was determined by plaque reduction assay. FMAU, FIAU, FMAC, FIAC, and DHPG had ED_{50}s of 0.10, 0.36, 0.25, 0.30, and 1 μM, respectively, (a dose required for 50% inhibition). The cytotoxic effect of the compounds was evaluated by the 50% inhibition of cell growth (ID_{50}) 3 days after subculturing; values of 10, 10, 25, 15, and 300 μM were obtained, respectively, for FMAU, FMAC, FIAC, FIAU, and DHPG. The elevated therapeutic index (TI = ED_{50}/ID_{50}) of DHPG may align this compound as a potential antiviral agent.

To verify the antiviral efficacy and unveil the mode of action of these active compounds, we selected FMAU, FIAC, and DHPG for further studies of their effect on HCMV DNA replication and viral protein synthesis. The effect of the antivirals on HCMV DNA synthesis was monitored by nucleic acid membrane hybridization techniques with HCMV specific ^{3}H-cRNA as a probe (Huang: J Virol 16:1560–1565, 1975). Infection of WI-38 cells with HCMV at a MOI of 1-2 allowed the detection of viral DNA synthesis by cRNA-DNA hybridization at approximately 20 hr after infection. Viral DNA synthesis increased at least up to 4–5 days PI in this study, as shown in Figure 1. On the other hand, the viral genomes were barely detectable in the drug-

---

Fig. 1. Effect of FIAC, FMAU, and DHPG on HCMV Towne DNA replication in virus-infected WI-38 cells. Drug was added to the virus-infected cell cultures at a final concentration of 1 μM FIAC or FMAU, or 2 μM, or 5 μM DHPG immediately after virus absorption. At various times after infection, the DNA was extracted from the infected cell culture for virus genome quantitation by ^{3}H-labeled cRNA-DNA membrane hybridization. Amounts of DNA and HCMV-specific [^{3}H]cRNA applied to each filter were 30 μg and 4 $\times$ 10^5 cpm, respectively. The nucleic acid hybridization was performed as described previously (Gillespie et al, 1965; Huang, 1975; Mar et al, 1982). a) symbols: ●—●, viral DNA content of cultures without drug treatment: ▽—▽ and □—□, denote the viral DNA contents in the presence of 1 μM FIAC and 1 μM FMAU, respectively. ▽———▽ and □----□, indicate the recovery of DNA synthesis after the release of 1 μM FIAC and 1 μM FMAU, respectively. b) symbols: ○—○, viral DNA content of cultures without drug treatment: △—△ and ■—■, denote the viral DNA contents in the presence of 2 μM and 5 μM of drug, respectively. △----△ and ■———■, indicate the recovery of DNA synthesis after the release of 2 μM and 5 μM of DHPG, respectively.

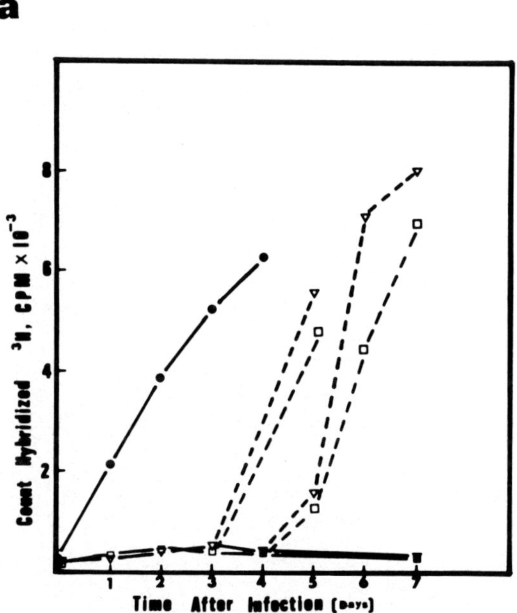

a
Count Hybridized ³H, CPM × 10⁻³
Time After Infection (Days)

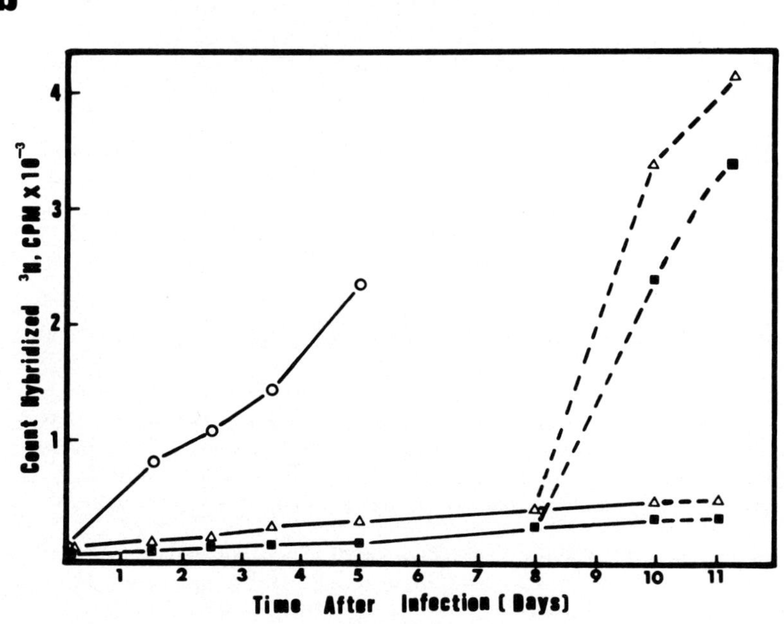

b
Count Hybridized ³H, CPM × 10⁻³
Time After Infection (Days)

treated infected cells at a concentration of 1 μM FIAC or FMAU up to 7 days (Fig. 1a), or at a concentration of 2 or 5 μM DHPG up to 10 days (Fig. 1b) after infection. However, upon the removal of drug at different times after infection, the synthesis of viral DNA resumed (Figs. 1a and b).

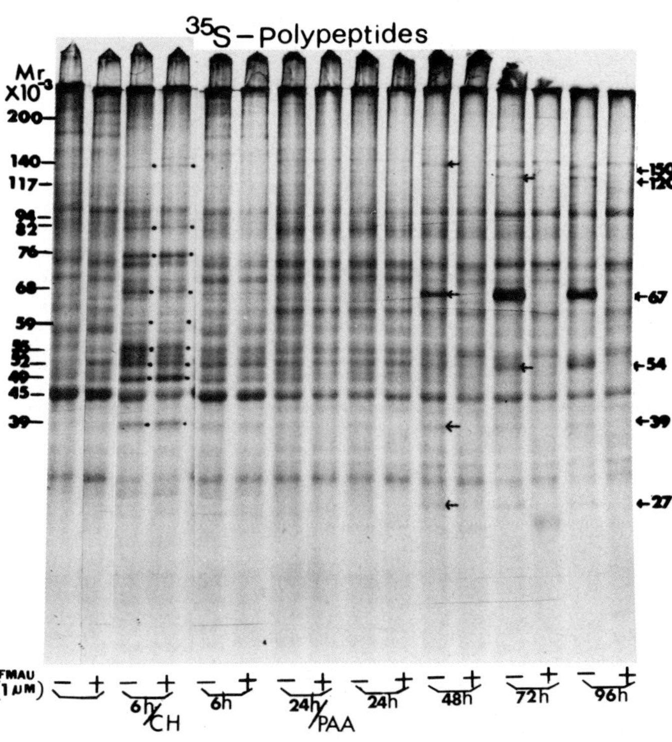

Fig. 2. Time course synthesis of virus-specific proteins in HCMV-infected WI-38 cells. a) The protein synthesis was studied by incorporation of ^{35}S-methionine (5μCi/ml), or b) ^{3}H-amino acid (5 μCi/ml) at the designated time after infection. Autoradiography was done on radiolabeled polypeptides analyzed in 9% SDS-PAGE. Numbers in column Mr indicate molecular weight $\times 10^{-3}$. M = mock infected; CH = cycloheximide (50 μg/ml); PAA = phosphonoacetic acid (50 μg/ml). Dots (●) denote that the viral early proteins are not affected by the presence of 1 μM FMAU in virus-infected cells. Arrows indicate that the synthesis of virus-specific proteins is inhibited by a) FMAU (1 μM) or b) DHPG (2 μM or 5 μM).

To study the effect of FIAC, FMAU, and DHPG on viral protein synthesis, 90% confluent WI-38 monolayers grown in 25 cm^2 flasks were infected at a MOI of 1–2 PFU/cell. The drugs were added immediately to the infected cell cultures 2 hr after virus adsorption and released before labeling at the designated time. Prior to harvesting, the cultures were labeled for 2 hr with [^{35}S] methionine or with ^{3}H-amino acid mixture in minimum essential medium (MEM) containing 3% heat-inactivated FCS and 1/10 normal strength of methionine for ^{35}S-methionine labeling, and 1/20 normal amino acid concentration for ^{3}H-amino acid labeling. The labeled proteins were identified by SDS-PAGE through 9% polyacrylamide gels in a Tris buffer system as described by Laemmli (Nature: 227:680–685, 1970).

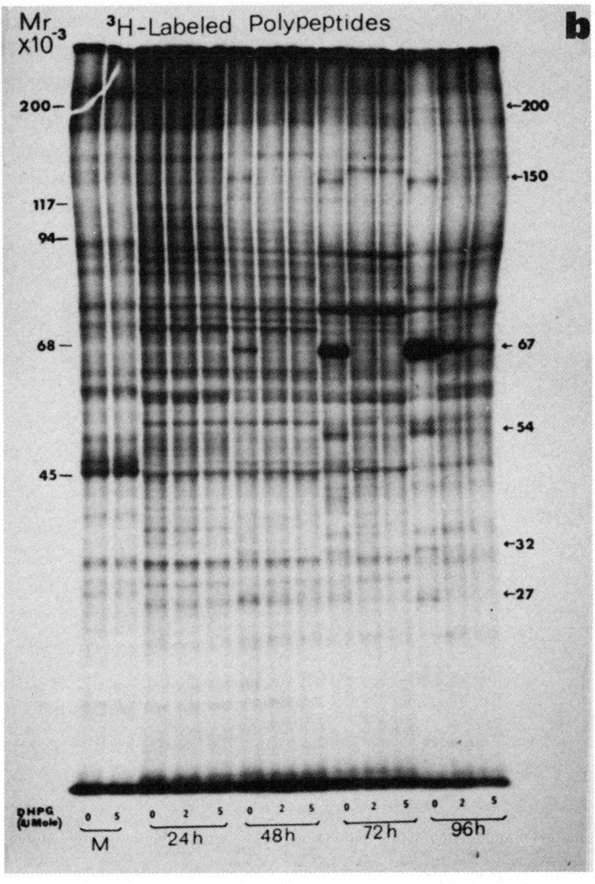

The results revealed that the inhibitory effects of FIAC and FMAU on the viral protein synthesis patterns were indistinguishable. Figure 2a illustrates the autoradiographs of such a study using FMAU at a final concentration of 1 μM. As indicated by dots ($\bullet$) in Figure 2a, FMAU did not affect the synthesis of the early proteins. However, the synthesis of 5 virus-specific antigens (p150K, p120K, p67K, p54K, and p27K) was completely blocked 48 hr up to 96 hr PI, as indicated by arrows (Fig. 2a). Similarly, DHPG also impaired the viral protein synthesis at 48 hr PI or at a later stage, as shown in Figure 2b. These viral proteins appeared after the viral DNA synthesis. Thus, they are virus-specific late antigens in nature.

The mechanism(s) underlying these nucleoside analogs-induced antiviral activity in HCMV-infected cells remains to be explored; research in this area is continuing.

COMPARATIVE ANTI-HERPESVIRUS ACTIVITY OF TWO ACYCLIC NUCLEOSIDES: DIHYDROXYPROPYLGUANINE AND ACYCLOVIR

T.R. Matthews, B. Binko, R. Boehme, M. Chernow, E. Fraser-Smith, V. Freitas, D. F. Smee, J. Martin, and J. Verheyden
Syntex Research, Palo Alto, CA 94304

The acyclic nucleoside, 9-(1,3-dihydroxy-2-propoxymethyl) guanine (DHPG) possesses exceptional anti-herpesvirus activity. When compared with acyclovir, both compounds were found to inhibit HSV (types 1 and 2) PFU by 50% at 0.2–2.4 μM. The ID_{50} of DHPG against HCMV was 7 μM compared with 95 μM for acyclovir. EBV was inhibited by DHPG at an ID_{50} of 1.0 μM. Most dramatic was the activity of DHPG in animal studies. Mortality of mice infected with HSV-2 was reduced 50% using oral doses of 7–10 mg/kg/day. The same result required 550–680 mg/kg/day of acyclovir. Oral treatment of mice or topical treatment of guinea pigs infected vaginally with HSV-2 resulted in a greater reduction in lesion severity when DHPG was used. It was reassuring to find that cell culture toxicity of DHPG was less than acyclovir. Inhibition of DNA synthesis in the infected cell, as measured by deoxyuridine incorporation required 3–10-fold less acyclovir than inhibitory doses of DHPG. The acute LD_{50} of DHPG in mice was found to be 1.8 gm/kg (IP).

DHPG, which is phosphorylated by HSV-1 thymidine kinase, appears to have a broader in vitro spectrum of activity, greater potency in vivo and less cytotoxicity than acyclovir.

IMMUNITY TO HCMV: I. HUMORAL IMMUNE RESPONSES TO HCMV-SPECIFIC MEMBRANE ANTIGENS (CMV-MA) IN NORMAL AND IMMUNOCOMPROMISED DONORS DURING ACUTE AND LATENT CMV INFECTION

J.M. Middeldorp, A.M. Tegzess, J. Jongsma, H.W. Roenhorst, and T.H. The

The Departments of Clinical Immunology and Nephrology, University Hospital Groningen, Oostersingel 59, 9713 EZ Groningen, The Netherlands

The cell-associated nature of CMV in the human host points toward the importance of virus-specific neoantigens on the surface of infected cells (CMV-MA) as primary targets for host's immunologic defense [1]. Both cellular and humoral immune mechanisms are involved in the recovery from acute CMV infection [2,3]. This study was to investigate the role of humoral immunity during the acute phase of infection. We have analyzed in detail the development of humoral immunity against CMV-MA specifically during acute symptomatic CMV infection in normal [CMV-mononucleosis (n = 8)] and immunocompromised patients (n = 30) having either a primary (n = 10) or a secondary (n = 20) CMV infection after renal transplantation. Results were compared with the findings in latently infected donors (n = 41); normal healthy seropositives (n = 25) and long-term (> 12 months) kidney allograft survivors (n = 16) with a latent CMV infection after renal transplantation. Individual patients were followed by (weekly) monitoring: 1) IgG and IgM against CMV-MA by membrane fluorescence, 2) CMV-specific cytolytic antibodies as described in [3], 3) IgG and IgM against CMV-EA and -LA by ELISA [4], and 4) Clinical symptoms of CMV infections.

The results are summarized in Table 1, and an individual case from each group is shown in Table 2. All CMV-mononucleosis patients developed anti-CMV-MA antibody responses early after onset of disease. Both IgM and IgG were detectable in titers ranging from 40 to 160 and all patients developed cytolytic antibodies (Cy-Ab) during the first 8 weeks of illness.

During reconvalescence (8–30 wk) anti-MA antibodies remained detectable by M Ifl in most patients; however, Cy-Ab decreased to undetectable levels in 6/8 patients. During the follow-up period all anti-MA responses decreased to undetectable levels with the exception of 2 patients who remained weakly positive for IgG anti-CMV-MA. In contrast to the low and transient antibody responses to CMV-MA, humoral responses against intracellular CMV antigens (CMV-EA and especially against CMV-LA) were much stronger and persisted at high levels long after recovery. IgM to CMV-

TABLE 1. A Summary of the Antibody Responses to CMV-MA in the 3 Groups of Patients Before (≤0) During the Acute (0–8), and Reconvalescent (8–30) Phase of Infection, and Finally at Presumed Virus-Latency (>60)

Time	Membrane IF1		C′ Lysis
(wk)[a]	IgM	IgG	
Group 1: CMV-Mononucleosis Summary (n = 8)			
≤ 0	—	—	—
0– 8	+ + (8/8)	+ + (8/8)	+ + (8/8)
8–30	+ (7/8)	+ (8/8)	+ (2/8)
>60	− (5/5)[b]	± (2/5)	− (5/5)
Group 2: Primary CMV (Allograft Recipients) Summary (n = 10)			
≤0	− (10/10)	− (10/10)	—
0– 8	+ + + (8/10)	+ + + (8/10)	+ + (7/10)
8–30	+ + (6/10)	+ + (9/10)	+ (5/10)
>60	− (6/10)	+ (3/6)	− (10/10)
Group 3: Secondary CMV (Allograft Recipients) Summary (n = 20)			
≤0	− (20/20)	+ (4/20)	− (20/20)
0– 8	+ + (7/20)	+ + + (15/20)	+ + + (9/20)
8–30	+ (3/19)[c]	+ + (16/19)[c]	+ + (5/19)[c]
>60	− (12/12)[d]	+ (3/6)	+ (1/12)

[a]After onset of clinical symptoms
[b]3 Patients not tested
[c]1 Patient died
[d]3 Patients died, 5 patients not tested

LA was present at high levels at the time of hospitalization in this group of patients and was clearly of diagnostic value as can be seen from case 1, Table 2.

Patients having a primary CMV infection after renal transplantation were negative in all antibody assays before onset of symptoms. In nearly all patients IgM against CMV-LA was diagnostic for CMV-infection at onset of clinical symptoms.

In 2/10 cases, IgG was detectable at the same time as IgM. For all patients tested (CMV-mononucleosis, primary or secondary CMV after transplantation) responses against CMV-EA developed later and remained at lower levels. Most (90%) of the patients developed a response against CMV-MA both in IgM (titer range 40–160) and IgG (range 20–160). One patient remained relatively unresponsive to CMV-MA (IgM: ≤ 20). This patient received low-dose immunosuppressive therapy and had only mild bronchiolitis with good renal function. Only 70% of the patients who developed an anti-MA antibody-response had Cy-Ab, which were detectable only in sera with an IgM- or IgG-anti-MA titer of ≥ 40. In all patients with primary CMV infection, the development of Cy-Ab was related to subsequent recov-

TABLE 2. Representative Case Studies From Each Individual Patient Group

					CMV-ELISA			
			M Ifl		EA		LA	
Time	Clinical Symptoms	C′ Lysis	IgM	IgG	IgM	IgG	IgM	IgG
Case 1: CMV-Mononucleosis								
1		+	80	<20	160	160	40960	640
2		++	40	<20	160	640	10240	2560
6		+	20	40	40	640	2560	2560
26		−	⩽20	20	40	1280	640	2560
48		−	<20	<20	<40	2560	320	2560
53		−	<20	<20	<40	1280	160	10240
60		−	<20	<20	<40	640	40	10240
Case 2: Primary CMV (Allograft Recipient)								
−1	−	−	—	—	<40	<40	⩽40	<40
0	++	−	<20	<20	<40	<40	40	⩽40
2	+	+	60	<20	<40	⩽40	160	640
3	+	++	120	20	40	40	640	1280
4	± (i)	+++	160	80	40	80	2560	2560
8	+	+++	80	120	160	160	160	2560
10	− (i)	++	80	80	80	320	320	5120
16	−	+	20	40	<40	1280	40	40960
21	−	−	<20	40	<40	2560	<40	10240
51	−	−	<20	20	<40	640	<40	5120
Case 3: Secondary CMV (Allograft Recipient)								
−1	+	−	<20	<20	<40	<40	<40	640
0	++	−	<20	20	<40	<40	80	2560
1	++	−	⩽20	20	80	⩽40	160	2560
2	++ (i)	+	20	40	160	40	2560	2560
4	+	++	40	80	640	160	2560	10240
5	± (i)	++	80	160	1280	640	2560	10240
7	−	++	80	160	640	640	1280	10240
9	−	++	40	80	640	640	640	40960
13	−	++	40	160	160	2560	640	40960
34	−	+	<20	40	40	2560	80	>40960

Clinical symptoms consisted of myalgia, arthralgia, spiking fever, leuko/thrombopenia, liver, or renal disfunction and lung or intestinal complications.
(+) Denotes mild disease with 1 active of the above symptoms.
(++) Stands for mild disease with more than 2 complicating symptoms.
(+++) Denotes severe clinical disease with allograft dysfunction.
(i) Denotes CMV isolation in tissue culture.

ery from symptomatic infection; no deaths due to CMV-infection were seen in this group. With the exception of 6 cases mentioned below, 9/20 patients in the group of allograft recipients with secondary CMV infection developed a strong Cy-Ab response and 5/20 were not evaluated in this respect. Although anti-MA responses (both fluorescent and cytolytic antibodies) were highest in this group, a relatively large percentage were non- or low responders to CMV-MA. In patients who developed anti-MA responses ($\geq$ 40) and Cy-Ab (detectable at serum dilution 1:2), the magnitude of the response was strongly related with subsequent recovery as was seen in the primary CMV infection above. Of the symptomatic non- or low responders to CMV-MA ($<$ 40) (n = 6), one developed lethal CMV disease early after infection (8 wk). Although IgG anti-CMV-MA was detectable at low level, no Cy-Ab were detectable in this patient. Another patient who did respond to CMV-MA at early times after infection died of a *Candida* superinfection at 17 wk after onset of CMV infection. Although CMV ELISA showed a slight elevation at this time, no anti-MA response was detectable. At autopsy, CMV was detectable in multiple organs. Two nonresponders to CMV-MA returned to the dialysis unit after decreased allograft function and subsequent organ loss. CMV was strongly implicated in allograft dysfunction in these 2 patients. Two additional low responders (anti-CMV-MA: 20–40) who received only a low dose of immunosuppressive treatment were relatively free of symptoms. In patients with secondary CMV infections who did respond to CMV-MA, both fluorescent and cytolytic antibodies remained at a higher level during convalescence and after one year follow-up than in the 2 groups with primary CMV infection. Furthermore, in a group of long-term renal allograft survivors with latent CMV infection after transplantation, a relatively high percentage (56%) of CMV-MA seropositives were found compared with normal healthy seropositive donors (20%); 5/9 CMV-MA positives in the long-term allograft survivor group still had detectable cytolytic antibodies compared to 0/5 CMV-MA positives in the normal control group. In addition, antibodies to intracellular early and late antigens (ELISA) were elevated in the long-term allograft survivor group (GMT, EA: 2560; LA: 10240) compared to values in the normal controls (GMT, EA: 640; LA: 2560).

Finally, as can be seen from the case studies shown in Table 2 the CMV ELISA has clear clinical value for the early diagnosis of symptomatic CMV infection. In most cases, rises in IgM and/or IgG against CMV-LA could be detected at onset of clinical symptoms providing a powerful tool for the discrimination between CMV infection and transplant rejection.

In conclusion, although anti-CMV-MA antibodies are nearly absent in latently infected normal donors they are induced during the acute phase of symptomatic CMV-infection. Their ability to mediate lysis of CMV-infected cells indicates an important role of these antibodies in limiting acute infection in vivo. In the long-term survivor group, persistent anti-CMV-MA humoral immunity may help in preventing reactivation of latent virus. Whether the development of Cy-Ab has prognostic value for the course of symptomatic CMV infection in renal allograft recipients needs further evaluation.

REFERENCES

1. The TH, Langenhuysen MMAC: Clin Exp Immunol 11:475–482, 1972.
2. Quinnan GV et al: J Immunol 126:2036–2041, 1981.
3. Betts RF, Schmidt SG: J Infect Dis 143:821–826, 1981.
4. Middeldorp JM, The TH: International Workshop on Herpesviruses, Bologna, Italy, 1981, p 116.

IMMUNITY TO HCMV: II. LATENTLY INFECTED DONORS HAVE HIGH LEVELS OF T-CELL MEMORY TO HCMV-SPECIFIC MEMBRANE ANTIGENS (CMV-MA) IN THE ABSENCE OF DETECTABLE ANTIBODIES TO CMV-MA

J.M. Middeldorp, J. Jongsma, and T.H. The
Department of Clinical Immunology, University Hospital, Oostersingel 59, 9713 EZ Groningen, The Netherlands

CMI is thought to be essential in controlling CMV latency [1]. This may be achieved by active immunosurveillance against virus-induced neoantigens on the surface of infected cells [2]. To investigate this we have analyzed the level of T-cell memory specific for CMV-MAs in a group of 12 healthy seropositive donors by means of the lymphocyte proliferation assay [3, 4]. We isolated and purified plasma membrane and other subcellular fractions from CMV-infected cells at different times postinoculation (PI) and used these as antigen in the lymphocyte proliferation assay. Controls for this study consisted of membranes from uninfected cells and membranes from cells treated with phosphonoformate (0.5 mM) after infection to completely block the induction of late antigens [5]. Furthermore, since a very high infectious dose (5 PFU/well) was needed to prepare optimal antigens, a strong influence of the inoculum was seen at early times after infection. To correct for this effect, we also isolated membranes from cells treated with CH (50 μg/ml) from 6 hr before inoculation until 24 hr PI to block the induction of new antigens completely. For purification of plasma membranes, we modified the procedure described by Kartner et al [6]. EDTA (5 mM) was used to harvest the cells, because this treatment did not affect membrane antigens as tested by immunofluorescence. After hypoosmotic treatment in 5 mM $NaHCO_3$ (pH 8.0) cells were gently homogenized by Douncing and membranes were separated from the nuclear and cytoplasmic fraction by differential centrifugation. After sonication, the membrane fraction was further purified on sucrose gradients. Isolated membrane fractions were characterized by several parameters: 1) Specific density was characteristic for plasma membranes $(1.08-1.12 \text{ g/cm}^3)$; 2) No infectious virus was detected upon inoculation of membrane fractions (up to 0.1 mg protein) onto fibroblast monolayers; 3)Electron microscopy revealed smooth vesicles and no virus particles could be detected; and 4) Fractions were tested in the lymphocyte proliferation assay [4].

Results show that lymphocytes from CMV-seronegative donors never responded to any fraction tested, thereby excluding mitogenic activity. All experiments were repeated 2 or 3 times with different membrane isolations for each individual donor. In order to exclude day-to-day variation in the lymphocyte responses, membrane fractions representing a single line of experiments (untreated, PFA treated, or CH treated) were tested on a single day. Control antigens (purified CMV virions or nucleocapsid protein, bacterial recall antigens, and allogeneic lymphocytes) were included in each assay in order to allow comparison among different tests.

In these experiments, 3 groups of responders could be discriminated, 1) responding to both early and late membrane antigen equally (EMA$^+$/LMA$^+$),

---

Fig. 1.   Lymphocyte responses of 2 donors with purified plasma membrane fragments isolated from CMV-infected fibroblast cultures. A) Shows the response of lymphocytes from donor 1, representative of group 1 (EMA$^+$/LMA$^+$). B) Shows the response of lymphocytes from donor 8, representative of group 2 (EMA$^-$/LMA$^+$).

The magnitude of the lymphocyte response is shown on the vertical axis and is expressed in disintegrations per second (dps) specific increase (that is: dps of cultures with CMV antigens containing membrane fragments—dps of cultures with corresponding uninfected membrane fragments).

Subconfluent fibroblast monolayers were inoculated at 5 PFU/cell with CMV strain AD169 and the time PI at which membrane fragments were isolated from CMV-infected fibroblasts is shown on the horizontal axis. (●——●) Lymphocyte stimulation with membranes isolated from untreated CMV-infected fibroblasts. (●————●) Lymphocyte stimulation with membranes isolated from CMV-infected fibroblasts treated with 0.5 mM phosphonoformate (PFA) after virus inoculation. (●-----●) Lymphocyte stimulation with membrane isolated from CMV-infected fibroblasts continuously treated with 50 μg/ml CH from 6 hr before virus inoculation up to 24 hr PI.

Each point represents the mean dps of lymphocyte stimulation from 2 or 3 separate experiments using different membrane isolation. All experiments were done in triplicate.

2) responding to only late membrane antigens (EMA$^-$/LMA$^+$), and 3) responding to both early and late membrane antigens but with a significantly higher response to the late ones (EMA$^{+/-}$/LMA$^+$).

Figure 1A shows the results obtained with donor 1 representing group 1 (n = 3). With membrane fragments isolated at zero hr PI a strong lymphocyte response was measured. This was due to the inoculum being attached to

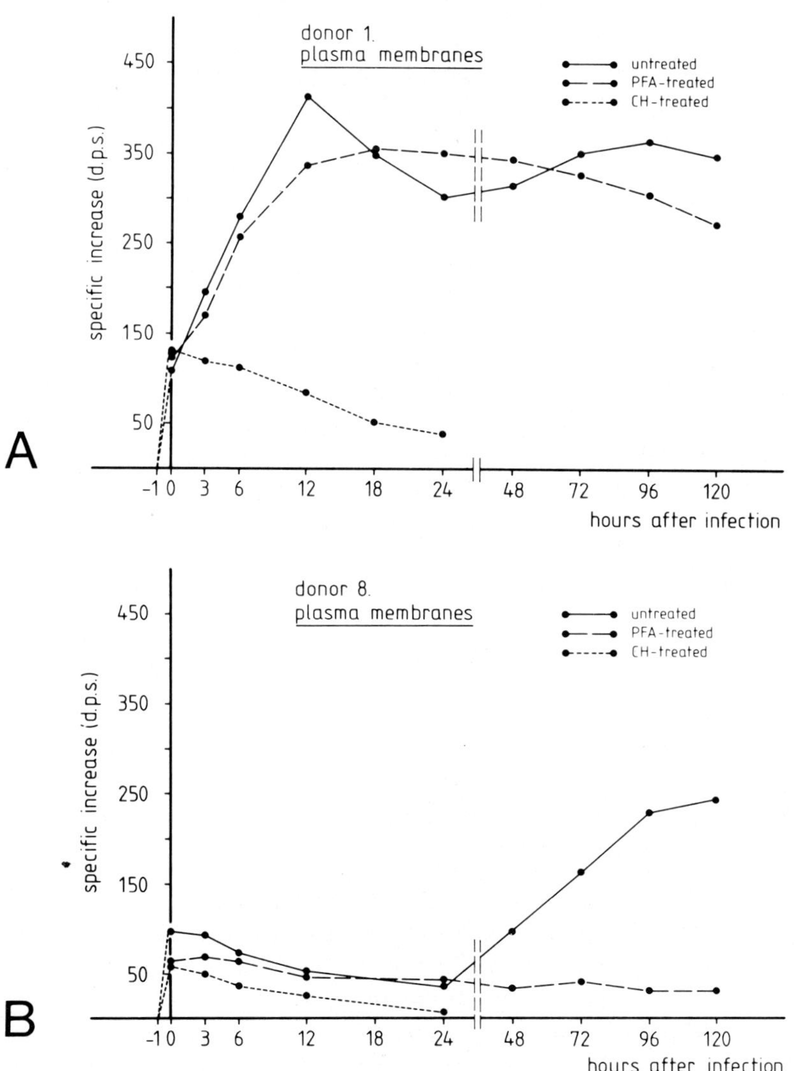

plasma membranes directly after infection. This inoculum effect decreases in time, as is shown in the CH experiment. At very early times after infection, new antigens are induced in the plasma membranes that give rise to a strong lymphocyte response which is maximal with membranes isolated at 12–18 hr PI. This is also seen with membranes isolated from PFA-treated cells but not in the CH experiment. Using serologic techniques, we have not been able to demonstrate CMV-MA before 12 hr PI, either using monoclonal antibodies or high titered human sera [7]; (manuscript in preparation). Whether this indicates the possible involvement of a "CMV-LYDMA" or whether it is a matter of sensitivity remains to be established. From 48–96 hr PI an additional increase in stimulation is observed. This is not found with membranes from cells that were blocked in the early stage of infection by phosphonoformate. This additional stimulation is caused by late membrane antigens induced after onset of virus DNA-replication. These results indicate that donor 1 has T-cell memory for both early and late membrane antigens. Three of 12 donors studied showed a similar response. In contrast, a second group of donors (n = 3) could be distinguished whose lymphocytes did not respond to early membrane antigens, as is shown for donor 8 in Figure 1B.

At early times PI, no response was induced above the inoculum effect, as detected in the CH experiment. Also with membranes from PFA-treated cells for up to 120 hr PI no additional response was seen. However, starting 48 hr after infection, new antigens induced in the plasma membranes in untreated cultures were recognized by the lymphocytes from this donor and gave rise to a considerable proliferation. In total, 75% of the donors tested were able to respond to both early and late membrane antigens (not shown). With the exception of the donors from the first group, lymphocyte responses to early membrane antigens were always lower than to the late ones. The magnitude of in vitro responses to CMV-MA was comparable to the responses against purified virions or nucleocapsid proteins and to bacterial recall antigens, which were all measured in parallel, which indicates that T-cell memory for CMV-MA is well developed in most donors. Only 3 of the 12 donors tested had detectable antibodies against CMV-MA in very low titers (20–40), as determined by membrane fluorescence [8]. The presence of lymphocyte responses to EMA did not correlate with the presence of antibodies against CMV-MA, but the magnitude of the response to CMV-EMA was correlated with the level of antibodies to intracellular (CMV-EA and -LA) antigens.

In conclusion, healthy seropositive donors with latent CMV infection have high levels of T-cell memory specific for CMV-MA in the absence of the corresponding antibodies. This is different from infection with other human herpesviruses (VZV, HSV, EBV) where antibodies against virus-membrane antigens are present in high levels in latently infected donors. These findings may explain the high frequency of CMV reactivation, as is seen in immunosuppressed kidney allograft recipients with impaired cellular immunity.

REFERENCES

1. Ho M: "Cytomegalovirus. Biology and Infection." New York: Plenum, 1982.
2. The TH, Langenhuysen MMAC: Clin Exp Immunol 11:475–482, 1972.
3. ten Napel Chr HH, The TH: Clin Exp Immunol 39:263–271, 1980.
4. Schirm J et al: Infect Immun 30:621–627, 1980.
5. Wahren B, Oberg B: Intervirology 12, 335–339, 1979.
6. Kartner N et al: J Membr Biol 36:191–211, 1977.
7. Middeldorp JM, The TH: Cold Spring Harbor Conference on Herpesviruses, 1982, p 145.
8. Middeldorp JM et al: This volume.

A MURINE MODEL FOR IMMUNOPROPHYLAXIS OF CMV INFECTION*

Y. Minamishima and Y. Tonari

Department of Microbiology, Miyazaki Medical College, Kiyotake, Miyazaki 889-16, Japan

Much attention has been drawn to development of CMV vaccines which were initiated by Elek and Stern [1] and by Plotkin et al [2]. However, experimental analysis of the pathogenesis and prevention of HCMV infection has been hampered by its strict species specificity.

Murine CMV kept in passage with mouse embryo fibroblasts (CC-MCMV) is attenuated [3], while the virus serially propagated in the salivary gland (SG-MCMV) is virulent. Mice immunized with the attenuated CC-MCMV resist challenge with the virulent SG-MCMV. Although the efficacy of live CC-MCMV is unequivocal, as a model vaccine it has the following limitations: 1) The attenuation is partial and it is still pathogenic for suckling mice. 2) It can replicate in the brain of weanling mice when inoculated intracerebrally. 3) It establishes chronic, productive infection in the salivary gland. 4) Once replicated in the salivary gland, it reverts to the virulent state with an antigenic alteration: and 5) The "virulent" virus may be shed and subsequently transmitted to new hosts. Therefore, we have attempted to obtain

*Supported by a Grant-in-Aid for Scientific Research from the Ministry of Education, Science and Culture (project no. 57480179) and a grant from the Kyushu Biseibutsu Kenkyukai.

viruses lacking those properties but possessing the equivalent immunogenicity. We expected *ts* mutants of CC-MCMV would meet the requirement.

IN VITRO CHARACTERISTICS

Two *ts* mutants (*ts* 21 and *ts* 24) were isolated from 117 plaques of UV-irradiated wild-type virus of CC-MCMV. Efficiency of plating (39°C/34°C) and efficiency of replication (39°C/34°C) were 1.2×10^{-5} and 2.2×10^{-4} for *ts* 21, and 2.3×10^{-5} and 3.0×10^{-5} for *ts* 24, respectively. The temperature sensitivity was associated with the replication cycle but not with increased thermal lability of the progeny virions. They complemented each other at 39°C with a complementation index of 5.5×10^{3}, ie, they belong to different complementation groups.

PATHOGENICITY OF *ts* MUTANTS OF SUCKLING MICE

First, when 2.0×10^{4} PFU of the viruses were inoculated intraperitoneally, *ts* 21 did not kill 2-day-old ICR mice, whereas wild type and *ts* 24 did. Second, *ts* 21 and *ts* 24 did not replicate, while wild type did, in the mouse organs, when 2.0×10^{3} PFU were inoculated. Third, when newborn mice were inoculated orally with 3.0×10^{3} PFU of the viruses, infectious viruses were recovered from the brain, kidney, and salivary gland of the mice infected with wild type, but not with *ts* 21 or *ts* 24. Thus, *ts* 21 had lost pathogenicity for suckling mice.

TABLE 1. Effect of Immunization on Morbidity and Mortality

Virus	Exp.	Dose for Immunization (PFU/Mouse)					
		1.0×10^{4}	1.0×10^{3}	1.0×10^{2}	1.0×10^{1}	1.0×10^{0}	None
Wild type	1	0/3 (0/3)	0/3 (0/3)	0/3 (0/3)	0/3 (2/3)		
	2		0/3 (0/3)	0/3 (0/3)	2/3 (3/3)	3/3 (3/3)	
ts 21	1	0/3 (0/3)	0/3 (0/3)	0/3 (1/3)	0/3 (3/3)		
	2		0/2 (2/2)	0/3 (3/3)	3/3 (3/3)	3/3 (3/3)	
ts 24	1	0/3 (0/3)	0/3 (0/3)	0/3 (1/3)	1/3 (2/3)		
	2		0/3 (0/3)	0/3 (0/3)	0/3 (2/3)	3/3 (3/3)	
Control	1						3/3 (3/3)
	2						5/5 (5/5)

Mortality is expressed as the number of mice dead in 10 days over number of mice challenged with 2.0×10^{6} PFU of SG-MCMV.

Parentheses indicate morbidity expressed as number of mice with clinical signs on day 4 over number of mice challenged.

REPLICATION OF *ts* MUTANTS IN WEANLING MICE

Wild-type virus and *ts* mutants were examined for in vivo replication. First, when 1.0×10^5 PFU of the viruses were inoculated intraperitoneally into weanling mice, none of the *ts* mutants were recovered on day 11 from the mouse organs. In contrast, under the same condition, wild-type virus replicated in the salivary gland and in the pancreas. Second, the possibility that the viruses persist as latent forms was examined. Following the experiments by Jordan et al [4], in principle we infected C_3H mice subcutaneously and reactivated the latent viruses, if any. While wild type of CC-MCMV and SG-MCMV were positive for reactivation, *ts* 21 was negative even after immunosuppressive treatment with antithymocyte serum and hydrocortisone. Third, after inoculation of 1.0×10^4 PFU of the viruses intracerebrally, *ts* 21 showed no replication in the brain, whereas *ts* 24 replicated, although to a lesser degree than wild-type virus.

IMMUNOGENICITY OF *ts* MUTANTS

Immunogenicity of *ts* mutants was assessed by the mortality of immunized mice after challenge with virulent SG-MCMV and by replication of the challenge virus in the immunized hosts. First, intraperitoneal inoculation of 1.0×10^5 PFU of each *ts* mutant protected mice against intraperitoneal challenge on day 7 with 2.0×10^6 PFU (approximately 3 LD_{50}) of virulent SG-MCMV. As shown in Table 1, 1.0×10^2 PFU of both mutants as well as wild-type virus protected mice repeatedly from fatal infection by SG-MCMV. However, some of the mice immunized with *ts* mutants at this dose recovered after showing clinical signs, such as ruffled fur, lethargy, and photophobia.

Second, the efficacy of immunization with *ts* mutants was confirmed by its inhibitory effect on in vivo replication of the challenge virus. In this particular system, any virus recovered from the challenged mice was the challenge virus itself, since the *ts* mutants used for immunization were unable to replicate in the mice. Several organs of mice, immunized 7 days before challenge, were titrated at 34°C for infectious viruses. As clearly shown in Table 2, *ts* 21 completely suppressed infection of the challenge virus, suggesting that this would be the most desirable candidate for a model vaccine. Lack of the virus replication in the salivary gland was also confirmed by challenging the mice on day 11 or 33 and harvesting the organs on day 48.

Third, attempts were made to determine whether the protective immunity endowed by *ts* mutants can be maintained without production of the infectious viruses in the salivary glands. Mice immunized with wild type, *ts* 21, and *ts* 24 were examined at 1 and 3 months for infectious viruses in the salivary gland, serum-neutralizing antibody against both CC-MCMV and SG-MCMV,

TABLE 2. Infectious Viruses in Organs of Immunized Mice After Challenge*

| | | | CC-MCMV Used for Immunization | | |
Organ	Experiment	None	Wild Type	*ts* 21	*ts* 24
Brain	1	0	0	0	0
	2	0	0	0	0
Salivary gland	1	$1.2 \times 10^2 \pm 2.0 \times 10^3$	$1.7 \times 10^4 \pm 1.3 \times 10^4$	0	0
	2	$9.3 \times 10^2 \pm 1.3 \times 10^3$	$7.0 \times 10^4 \pm 1.1 \times 10^5$	0	0
Thymus	1	$5.9 \times 10^3 \pm 4.2 \times 10^3$	0	0	0
	2	$3.2 \times 10^3 \pm 2.9 \times 10^3$	0	0	0
Lung	1	$1.5 \times 10^4 \pm 1.1 \times 10^4$	0	0	0
	2	$4.2 \times 10^4 \pm 2.3 \times 10^4$	0	0	0
Heart	1	$3.4 \times 10^4 \pm 3.2 \times 10^3$	0	0	0
	2	$5.7 \times 10^3 \pm 4.4 \times 10^3$	0	0	0
Liver	1	$2.8 \times 10^4 \pm 1.6 \times 10^4$	0	0	0
	2	$1.5 \times 10^6 \pm 1.3 \times 10^6$	0	0	0
Kidney	1	$6.8 \times 10^4 \pm 3.9 \times 10^4$	0	0	0
	2	$3.5 \times 10^4 \pm 2.7 \times 10^4$	0	0	0
Adrenal gland	1	$4.1 \times 10^3 \pm 1.0 \times 10^2$	0	0	0
	2	$2.6 \times 10^4 \pm 3.3 \times 10^4$	0	0	0
Spleen	1	$6.3 \times 10^5 \pm 3.4 \times 10^5$	$1.3 \times 10^2 \pm 1.3 \times 10^2$	0	0
	2	$1.6 \times 10^6 \pm 8.1 \times 10^5$	0	0	$6.6 \times 10^2 \pm 1.3 \times 10^3$
Pancreas	1	$3.2 \times 10^4 \pm 1.9 \times 10^4$	$1.8 \times 10^3 \pm 1.8 \times 10^3$	0	0
	2	$7.7 \times 10^3 \pm 5.8 \times 10^3$	$2.1 \times 10^3 \pm 2.2 \times 10^3$	0	0
Lymph node	1	$1.5 \times 10^3 \pm 1.4 \times 10^3$	0	0	0
	2	$1.8 \times 10^2 \pm 1.8 \times 10^2$	0	0	0

*Four-week-old female ICR mice were immunized intraperitoneally with 1.0×10^5 PFU of CC-MCMV per 0.5 ml and 7 days later challenged intraperitoneally with 1.4×10^6 PFU of SG-MCMV per 0.5 ml. Organs were removed from mice 4 days after challenge and infectious viruses were titrated at 34°C. A zero represents less than 100 PFU per organ.

and survival after challenge by SG-MCMV. The salivary glands of mice inoculated with both *ts* mutants were negative for infectious viruses over a period of 3 months, yet the immunized mice resisted challenge by virulent SG-MCMV. In those mice, neutralizing antibody was undetectable in the absence of guinea pig complement. When tested in the presence of complement, however, neutralizing antibody against CC-MCMV, but not against SG-MCMV used for challenge, was detected. Thus, complement-requiring neutralizing antibody was produced by *ts* mutants even without obvious replication. However, the neutralizing antibody did not cross-react with the challenge virus, suggesting that it is not a prerequisite for protective immunity.

ACKNOWLEDGMENT

We thank Dr. Aono for her cooperation in DNA analysis.

REFERENCES

1. Elek SD, Stern H: Lancet 1:1–5, 1974.
2. Plotkin SA, Farquhar J, Hornberger E: J Infect Dis 134:470–475, 1976.
3. Osborn JE, Walker DL: Infect Immun 3:228–236, 1970.
4. Jordan MC, Shanley JD, Stevens JG: J Gen Virol 37:419–423, 1977.

THE PATHOLOGY OF DISSEMINATED CMV INVESTIGATED BY IN SITU HYBRIDIZATION*

D. Myerson, R.C. Hackman, J.A. Nelson,
D.C. Ward,[†] and J.K. McDougall

Fred Hutchinson Cancer Research Center, Seattle, WA,[†] Yale University School of Medicine, New Haven, CT

The pathology of disseminated CMV has been investigated by in situ hybridization in paraffin-embedded tissue sections utilizing biotinylated DNA probes. This highly specific technique has enabled us to identify CMV in many organs and tissues where it has previously been described, such as the lung, liver (nonhepatocellular), pancreas, adrenal, esophagus, stomach, small and large intestines, kidney, ovary, skin, and within vessels. We have detected and localized CMV in many other tissues and cells such as the heart myocyte, hepatocyte, spleen and lymph node reticular cells, fallopian tube submucosa, uterine smooth muscle, endometrial stroma and glands, and anterior pituitary parenchymal cells. The mesenchymal cells were generally without cytomegaly and were unrecognizable as infected by routine light microscopy. CMV infection of endothelial cells has been further documented by immunohistochemical methods utilizing antibodies to CMV and to Factor VIII. These findings suggest that CMV disseminates hematogenously throughout the body, and spreads locally by endothelial cell infection. Mesenchymal cells, such as those readily infectable in tissue culture, in fact contain CMV in vivo. This infection is without cytomegaly but is detectable by in situ hybridization. Furthermore, we suggest that cells without cytomegaly may serve as a source of infection.

*Supported by a Human Cancer-Directed Fellowship DRG-003 of the Damon Runyon-Walter Winchell Cancer Fund (D.M.) and NIH grant CA29350 (J.McD.).

ANTIBODIES TO CYTOMEGALOVIRUS, EPSTEIN-BARR, AND HEPATITIS A VIRUSES (HAV) AMONG HEALTHY ADULTS IN THE UNITED STATES

N. Nath, K.E. Sherman, M. Pielech, K. Hoffman-Panetta, S.P. O'Neill*, F.K. Mundon*, and R.Y. Dodd
American Red Cross Blood Research Laboratories, Bethesda, MD, and Electronucleonics Inc*, Columbia, MD

A total of 1,647 sera from healthy adult blood donors in 5 different regions of the American Red Cross were included in this study. The regions were Burlington, VT, Madison, WI, Wichita, KS, Birmingham, AL, and Tucson, AZ contributing 411, 305, 412, 375, and 144 samples, respectively. All individuals were randomly selected from a subset of routine donors wth ALT levels < 45 IU/L, representing the 96.8th % value for the overall population.

Antibodies to CMV and EBV were determined by indirect fluorescent antibody (IFA) technique using kits supplied by Electronucleonics, Inc. All samples were tested for anti-CMV and anti-EBV at dilutions of 1:16, 1:64, and 1:256. Antibodies to HAV were determined with the HAVAB (Abbott) RIA test kits, following procedures recommended in the product insert.

Of the total, 1,017 (62%) sera were from males; the youngest age-group was 17 to 20 years old and this represented 329 (20%) of all sera. The over-60 age-group contributed only 46 samples.

Overall, the respective prevalence rates of antibodies to CMV, EBV, and HAV were 73%, 57%, and 19%. Anti-HAV was present among fewer than 5% of all donors in the 17 to 20 age-group; the prevalence increased with age to > 40% among donors older than 60. In contrast, the prevalence of both anti-CMV and EBV was about 40% among the 17 to 20 year age group, increasing relatively slowly with age.

Significant regional variations in the prevalence of anti-CMV and anti-HAV were found. Prevalence rates in Birmingham, AL with 30% of anti-

TABLE 1. Relative Association Between Anti-CMV and EBV and Anti-CMV and HAV Antibodies

Anti-CMV	No.	Anti-HAV*		Anti-EBV	
		Reactive No.	Nonreactive No.	Reactive No.	Nonreactive No.
Reactive	1,192	271	921	707	485
Nonreactive	435	41	394	225	210
Total	1,627	312	1,315	932	695
			P < 0.0001		P < 0.01

*Only 1,627 samples were available for anti-HAV assay.

HAV and over 80% of anti-CMV were significantly higher than in Burlington, VT with respective values of 12% and 65% for the 2 markers. The prevalence of antibodies to EBV did not show significant regional variation.

A total of 1,627 sera were tested for all 3 antibodies. As summarized in Table 1, a statistically significant (P < .0001) association was found between the occurrence of anti-CMV and anti-HAV. The association between the presence of anti-CMV and anti-EBV was also significant though weaker (P < 0.01) than that between anti-CMV and anti-HAV.

DISCUSSION AND CONCLUSION

On the basis of our data, we conclude that: 1) The majority of CMV and EBV infections in both sexes occurs before the age of 17 in the United States. 2) Less than 10% of individuals have anti-HAV at age 17. The presence of anti-HAV gradually increases with age in both sexes. 3) There were significant regional differences in the prevalence of anti-CMV and anti-HAV. The differences may reflect the socioeconomic status of the donor population. In general, variation in Burlington, VT, has the lowest, and Birmingham, AL, the highest exposure rate to CMV and HAV infections. 4) A strong association (P < 0.0001) between anti-HAV and anti-CMV was detected.

Both CMV and EBV are members of the herpesvirus group, while HAV is an enterovirus. Therefore, similarities between CMV and EBV are to be expected. On the other hand, the strong association between anti-CMV and anti-HAV is unexpected. Moreover, this association remained valid when data were analyzed for each of the 5 regions separately. Although there are major differences in the overall epidemiologic pattern of the 2 viruses, we nevertheless suggest that the association might reflect similarities in the modes of transmission of CMV and HAV where an individual exposed to HAV (fecal-oral route) is also exposed to CMV (uro-oral route).

MOLECULAR BASIS FOR HUMAN CYTOMEGALOVIRUS ONCOGENICITY

J.A. Nelson[1], B. Fleckenstein[2], D.A. Galloway[1], and J.K. McDougall[1]

[1]Fred Hutchinson Cancer Research Center, Seattle, WA 98104; [2]Institut für Klinische Virologie, Universität Erlangen, West Germany

For the past 2 years we have made a concerted effort in analyzing the oncogenic potential of HCMV. This virus has been associated with Kaposi sarcoma, and inactivated forms of the virus are able to transform rodent cells in vitro. We have recently reported the localization of the transformation region of HCMV strain AD169 by transfection of NIH 3T3 and rat embryo cells with overlapping cloned restriction endonuclease DNA fragments. Our results indicate that the region is located within a 2.9 Kb *Hind*III-*Xba*1 fragment (pCM4000) extending between map units 0.123 and 0.14 on the AD169 genome. A series of deletion mutants of pCM4000 were constructed by digestion of DNA from the *Xba*I site with exonuclease III and S-1 nuclease followed by the addition of *Bam*H1 linkers and subsequent cloning into pBR322. The minimum size fragment required to initiate transformation is being determined by transfection of rodent cells with these deletion mutants. The nucleotide sequence of the transforming fragment was determined by direct sequencing of these mutants by the chemical degradation technique of Maxam and Gilbert. The fragment was found to contain 2840 base pairs and have an A-T composition of 59.5% contrasting with the 42% A-T composition of the whole viral genome. Reading frame analysis of the sequence indicated that the longest open reading frame was 104 amino acids in length. To determine what mRNAs might be encoded for by pCM4000, mRNA selected for at IE and late times during infection were analyzed by Northern blot hybridization. Our results indicate a 4.8 Kb species can be detected during the IE phase and a 4.9 Kb species during the late phase. Further mRNA mapping of this region is in progress.

STUDY OF ANTIVIRAL ANTIBODIES IN SERA OF HOMOSEXUAL MEN

L. Nerurkar, J. Goedert, W. Wallen, R. Biggar, D. Madden, and J. Sever

NIH, Bethesda, MD 20205

Healthy, homosexual men (n = 254) between ages 20–55 yr from New York City and the Washington, D.C. area were studied for specific antibodies (Ab) in serum against CMV, HSV types I and II, and EBV. Indirect hemagglutination (IHA) method was used for CMV, HSV I and II, and fluorescent antibody method was used for EBV Ab titer measurements. The distribution of Ab titers is given in Table 1.

Healthy male volunteer blood donors matched for age, sex, and race were used as controls. The seronegative proportion for any of the 4 viruses studied was smaller in the homosexual group (1.6%–9.2%) compared to the control

TABLE 1. Percentage of Population With Viral Antibody Titers

	< 8	8–32	64–256	512–4096	> 4096
CMV	1.6	3.6	46.9	43.5	4.5
HSV-I	4.8	8.8	35.0	50.2	1.2
HSV-II	9.2	25.9	49.0	15.9	0
	<40	40–160	320–1280	2560–20,480	> 40,960
EBV	4.8	39.0	42.6	11.2	2.4

group (14.5%–27.7%). The geometric mean titers in the homosexual population were for CMV = 1:384, HSV I = 1:395, HSV II = 1:96, and EBV = 1:266 which were much higher compared to those in the control group. CMV IgG titers were also studied by ELISA and correlated well with the IHA method. CMV or HSV was isolated from 5% of the homosexual group. No correlation was found between Ab titer and type of virus or site of virus excretion.

CYTOMEGALY, THOUGH A LATE EVENT, RESULTS FROM AN EARLY CYTOMEGALOVIRUS FUNCTION

M. Nokta, D.J. Speelman, and T. Albrecht
Department of Microbiology, University of Texas Medical Branch at Galveston, TX 77550

CMV has been recognized for some time as a causative agent of cytomegalic inclusion disease, mononucleosis, and a variety of infections associated with immunosuppression. CMV has also been associated with several human cancers including those of the prostate, bowel, cervix, and most recently in association with AIDS, an unusually severe form of Kaposi sarcoma [1]. These clinical manifestations are thought often to result from the reactivation of CMV from the life-long persistent infection which this virus is known to have a proclivity to form. We have been interested in determining the mechanisms of the cellular responses to CMV; reasoning that these responses may be involved in the development of CMV persistence and associated diseases, and possibly in the transformation of cells to malignancy.

HCMV-infected skin muscle (SM) fibroblasts show a progression of cytopathic effects (cpe) [2, 3] beginning as early as 5 hr PI when cell rounding is detected. The rounded cells "contract" and decrease in size through 24 hr PI. Then they "relax" (24–48 hr PI), and enlarge to form classic cytomegalic cells 48–96 hr PI. Rounding and "contraction" which occur before the onset of CMV DNA synthesis (12–16 hr PI) are early events, while "relaxation" and enlargement which occur after the time of initiation of CMV DNA synthesis, are late events. The relationship of these late cellular responses ("relaxation" and enlargement) to early and late CMV expression was investigated using CMV strain AD169 and human embryo SM cells.

To determine if "relaxation" and enlargement were dependent on the prior onset of CMV DNA synthesis, SM cells were infected and then treated with 30 μg/ml of ara-C. At this dose, ara-C inhibited both CMV DNA synthesis and the formation of nuclear inclusions while it consistently failed to inhibit "relaxation" and enlargement (Table 1). These data indicate that cytomegaly, although a late event, was independent of virus DNA synthesis and was the result of an early phase of CMV expression.

We next sought to determine how expression of (an) early CMV gene(s) could lead to a cellular response observed only during the late phase of the CMV replication cycle. Accordingly, SM cells were infected with CMV and treated with CH (10 μg/ml) at various times after infection. In contrast to the inhibitory effects of ara-C, when CH was added at 12 hr PI, it inhibited both "relaxation" and enlargement (Table 1). Addition of CH at other times suggested that the CMV-induced function leading to "relaxation" and cell enlargement occurred between 12–24 hr PI. For example, at 48 hr PI, most cells (78%) had "relaxed" and had begun to enlarge in the absence of CH. In cell cultures to which CH was added at 12 or 24 hr PI, about 80% or 50% of the cells were rounded, respectively. "Relaxed," somewhat enlarged cells were infrequently encountered in the cell cultures treated with CH at 12 hr, while they were prominent in the cultures treated with CH at 24 hr.

The mechanism by which an early CMV function could lead to an event manifested only late in the CMV replication cycle was examined. Since it was previously shown that early events such as rounding and "contraction" of CMV-infected cells were inhibited by a Ca^{++} entry blocker (verapamil) [4], the effect of verapamil and papaverine (a smooth muscle relaxing agent) on "relaxation" and enlargement was investigated. Treatment of CMV-infected cells with these drugs at 12 hr PI (or before) essentially eliminated "relaxation" and enlargement, while treatment at 24 hr or after was less effective in inhibiting these cellular responses (Table 1). Although relatively high concentrations of verapamil (100 μg/ml) or papaverine (30 μg/ml) were necessary to block rounding and "contraction," lower doses of these drugs (ie, 10 μg/ml, 3 μg/ml, respectively) were sufficient to block "relaxation" and enlargement. Thus, cell enlargement appears to be more sensitive to inhibition by these SM relaxing agents than rounding or "contraction." These

TABLE 1. Effect of Metabolic Inhibitors and Smooth Muscle Relaxing Agents on CMV-Induced Cytopathology

| | | | Cytopathologies Observed* | | | | |
| | | | Early | | Late | | |
Drug	Dose (μg/ml)	Time (hr)	Cell Rounding	"Contraction"	"Relaxation"	Enlargement	Nuclear Inclusions
Cytosine arabinoside	30	0	+	+	+	+	−
Cycloheximide	10	12	+	+	−	−	−
		24	+	+	+	±	±
		36	+	+	+	+	±
Papaverine	30	5	+	+	±	−	−
		12	+	+	+	−	−
		24	+	+	+	+	+†
Verapamil	30	5	+	+	±	−‡	−‡
		12	+	+	+	±‡	−‡
		24	+	+	+	+	+†‡

*Measured at 48 hr PI. Although a range of cytopathologies was often observed, these descriptions summarize the most frequent and representative findings.

†Although nuclear inclusions formed, they were abnormal in their development and progression in regard to both size and morphology.

‡Verapamil was not as effective as paraverine in inhibiting these cellular responses.

data suggest that Ca^{++} may be involved in both early and late cellular responses to early CMV expression and that there may be a quantitative difference between Ca^{++} involvement in the early and late responses. Furthermore, since papaverine was substantially more effective than verapamil in blocking late cellular responses to CMV, events secondary to the initial Ca^{++} influx may be important during the "relaxation" and enlargement phases of the cellular response to virus expression and replication.

REFERENCES

1. Center for Disease Control. MMWR 30:409–410, 1981.
2. Albrecht T, Cavallo T, Cole NL, Graves K: Cytomegalovirus: Development and progression of cytopathic effects in human cell culture. Lab Invest 42:1–7, 1980.
3. Cavallo T, Graves K, Cole NL, Albrecht T: Cytomegalovirus: An ultrastructural study of the morphogenesis of nuclear inclusions in human cell culture. J Gen Virol 56:97–104, 1981.
4. Albrecht T, Speelman DJ, Steinsland OS: Similarities between cytomegalovirus-induced cell rounding and contraction of smooth muscle cells. Life Sci 32:2273–2278, 1983.

PHYSICAL MAPPING OF DNA CODING FOR THE STRUCTURAL 71 Kd PROTEIN OF HUMAN CYTOMEGALOVIRUS

B. Nowak, C.A. Sullivan, A. Gmeiner, P. Sarnow, A.J. Levine, and B. Fleckenstein

Institut für Klinische Virologie, University of Erlangen-Nürnberg, D-8520-Erlangen, Federal Republic of Germany, and Department of Microbiology, State University of New York at Stony Brook, Stony Brook, NY 11794

Monoclonal antibodies against HCMV were prepared by injecting purified virus particles into Balb/c mice. Among 4 groups of hybridomas, one stable clone (355) was selected for a first detailed characterization. Hybridoma clone 355 produced antibodies which immunoprecipitated denaturation sensitive antigenic determinants of a 71 Kd polypeptide. The 71 Kd polypeptide was identified as nonglycosylated protein that appears to be part of the virion envelope; it is distinct from the predominant IE 72 Kd protein. The monoclonal antibodies from clone 355 precipitated a 71 Kd polypeptide after in vitro translation of RNA that was extracted late after infection with HCMV AD169. In order to determine the viral genomic origin of the 71 Kd protein, late RNA was hybrid selected to a CMV cosmid library [1]. The in vitro translated product was immunoprecipitated employing monoclonal antibodies from clone 355. This method allowed us to map the gene for the 71 Kd protein to the HCMV cosmid clone pCM 1007 which represents virion DNA between map units 0.21 and 0.36 in prototype arrangement [1]. The coding sequence is more precisely determined using subclones in plasmid vectors. This approach appears generally useful for physical mapping of late HCMV genes.

REFERENCES

1. Fleckenstein B, Müller I, Collins J: Cloning of the complete human cytomegalovirus genome in cosmids. Gene 18: 39–46, 1982.

FREQUENCY OF CMV INFECTION IN JAPANESE PREGNANT WOMEN AND INAPPARENT INTRAUTERINE INFECTION

Y. Numazaki, T. Oshima, A. Tanaka, K. Hirota, M. Okumura, Y. Machida, M. Takatsu, and K. Takahashi

Sendai National Hospital and Saka Hospital, Sendai, Japan

In order to find the frequency of CMV infection in Japanese pregnant women, a retrospective study was serologically carried out. Series serum samples obtained from 3,198 cases in the 1st, 2nd, and 3rd trimesters were examined for CMV CF, EA (early antigen), and MA (membrane antigen) antibodies. CF antibody was positive in 3,070 (96%) of 3,198 cases in the 1st trimester. EA antibody was positive in 589 (19%) of 3,070 CF positive cases and IgM-MA antibody was negative in all of 3,198 tested. CF seroconversion in the 2nd or 3rd trimester was found in 8 (6.3%) of 128 seronegative cases and in 18 (0.6%) of 3,070 seropositive cases. EA seroconversion in the 2nd or 3rd trimester was demonstrated only in the CF seroconverted cases, in 6 of the former 8 cases, and in 16 of the latter 18 cases. IgM-MA antibody was demonstrated in 3 of the former 8 cases but not in the latter 18 cases. Thus, the seroconverted 8 cases from negative to positive, particularly the 3 cases demonstrating IgM-MA antibody, were suspected as primary infection.

To detect the intrauterine infection of CMV in the study group of pregnant women, virus isolation was performed from the urine of their newborn babies, and cord sera were tested for IgM-MA antibody. CMV was isolated from 8 (0.5%) of 1,762 babies within 5 days after birth. All of these CMV positive babies were from mothers who were seropositive, particularly EA antibody positive, except for one case, but did not show significant rise in titers during pregnancy. CMV could not be isolated from babies of seroconverted mothers. All of the 3,198 cord sera of study group were negative for IgM-MA antibody. Eight babies shedding CMV were physically normal.

From the results, it is suggested that inapparent intrauterine infection may occur in approximately 0.5% of seropositive pregnant women. In these cases, CMV-IgM antibody is negative in cord serum. Primary infection of CMV in late gestation probably does not result in intrauterine infection.

PREPARATION AND CHARACTERIZATION OF cDNA CLONES OF HUMAN CYTOMEGALOVIRUS

J.D. Oram

Public Health Laboratory Service Centre for Applied Microbiology and Research, Porton Down, Salisbury, United Kingdom

As part of an investigation into the expression of HCMV genes in bacteria, cDNA clones were prepared from mRNA molecules isolated from cells at a "late" time after infection with strain AD169. Roller bottle cultures of human fibroblast cells (MRC5) in Minimal Essential Medium containing 5% fetal calf serum were infected at an MOI of 0.1 PFU/cell. The cells were harvested 6 days after infection and washed twice with phosphate buffered saline at 0°; cytoplasmic RNA was extracted from the cells by the method of

TABLE 1. Hybridization Reactions of cDNA Clones With ³²P-Labeled Cloned Genomic Fragments

Fragment		Map Units	No. of cDNA Clones
*Hind*III	E	0.057 – 0.145	13
	T	0.145 – 0.173	1
	R	0.173 – 0.203	2
	S	0.203 – 0.230	0
	P	0.230 – 0.263	0
	a	0.263 – 0.273	0
	U	0.273 – 0.296	0
	b	0.296 – 0.303	2
	c	0.303 – 0.307	1
	L	0.307 – 0.360	7
	D	0.360 – 0.433	9
	F	0.433 – 0.540	8
	M	0.540 – 0.585	3
	Z	0.585 – 0.593	4
	J	0.593 – 0.655	2
	N	0.655 – 0.695	14
	Y	0.695 – 0.710	4
	O	0.710 – 0.747	0
	H (unique sequences*)	0.747 – 0.775	0
*Pst*1	B	0.784 – 0.830	94
	*Pst*1 – *Eco*R1 subclone	0.784 – 0.807	15
	*Eco*R1 – *Pst*1 subclone	0.807 – 0.830	81
*Hind*III	G (unique sequences†)	0.830 – 0.897	10
	W	0.897 – 0.922	3
	V	0.922 – 0.945	2
	X	0.945 – 0.966	1
		Total	180

*Clones that hybridized with *Hind*III C (HQ) but not *Hind*III I (KQ).
†Clones that hybridized with *Hind*III B (KG) but not *Hind*III I (KQ).

Favaloro et al [1] in the presence of 10 mM vanadyl ribonucleoside complex (B.R.L., Cambridge, U.K.) at 0°. Poly A⁺ RNA was selected from the cytoplasmic RNA by chromatography on oligo dT cellulose (P.L. Biochemicals, Northampton, U.K.): approximately 100 μg of poly A⁺ RNA was obtained per gram of cells (wet weight).

cDNA clones were prepared from 10–100 μg lots of poly A⁺ RNA by the dG-dC homopolymer tailing method [2] using pBR322 as the plasmid vector. Transformants of *E coli* HB101 were selected by growth on L agar plus tetracycline (20 μg/ml). After growth of bacterial colonies on nitrocellulose membranes, the plasmid DNA was denatured and fixed to the membranes which were then hybridized with ³²P-labeled virion DNA or cloned *Hind*III fragments. The hybridization conditions were 50% formamide plus 5 X SSC, 0.1% ficol, 0.1% polyvinyl pyrolidone, 0.1% bovine serum albumin, and 10 μg/ml of oligo dT$_{(12-18)}$ at 42° for 48 hr followed by 3 washes with 50% formamide plus 5 X SSC followed by 3 washes with 2 X SSC, all at 42°. Oligo dT was included to suppress nonspecific hybridization of some genomic fragments (especially those containing *Hind*III E and the internal repeat) with all the cDNA clones: both regions contain long (10–12 nucleotide) sequences of dA (J.A. Nelson, manuscript submitted for publication, and P.J. Greenaway, personal communication) which would be expected to hybridize with oligo dT sequences introduced by the cloning procedure.

In one experiment, 370 out of 1,240 (30%) of the colonies contained virus-specific sequences. Results obtained by hybridizing these clones with ^{32}P-labeled cloned *Hind*III fragments and subfragments are summarized in Table 1. About 50% of the clones gave either weak or variable hybridization reactions: some, possibly all, of these clones appeared to contain small inserts — ie, less than about 0.25 kb — the limit of detection — and these have not been included in Table 1.

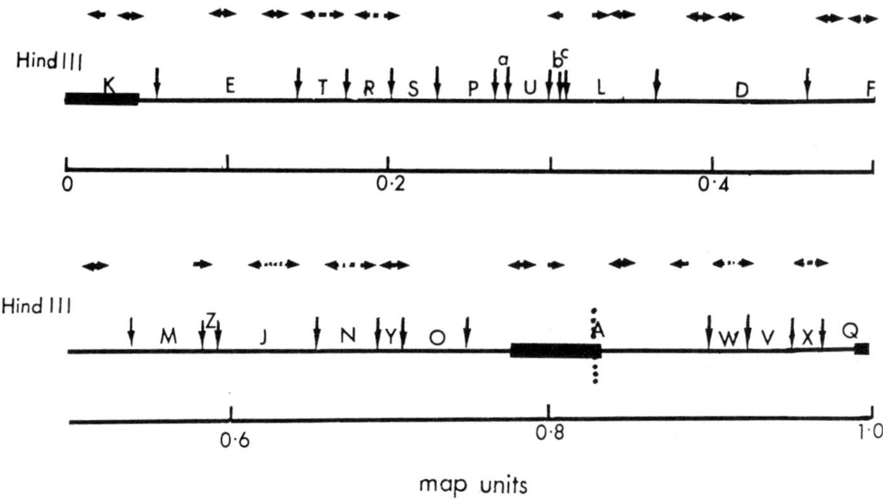

Fig. 1. Map positions of cDNA clones and direction of transcription of some genes. The map positions were determined from hybridization reactions with cloned genomic fragments as described in the text, including the results shown in Table 1. A single arrow, ← or →, indicates both the map position of the 3′ terminus and the direction of a gene. A double arrow, ↔, indicates the position of the 3′ terminus but does not define the direction of transcription. Arrowheads joined by dotted lines, ←---→, indicate the approximate positions of 3′ termini.

Although the number of clones analyzed was small, DNA sequences hybridizing with the cDNA clones were unevenly distributed along the genome. For example, cloned fragment *Pst*1-C, which contains only internally repeated sequences (10.6 kb or 4.5% of the genome) hybridized with 94 or 25% of the cDNA clones, indicating that the repeated sequences are actively transcribed at "late" times of infection. By contrast, none of the clones hybridized with cloned *Hind*III fragments S, P, a, and U which correspond to a continuous stretch of 10% of the genome.

More accurate map positions were obtained for some cDNA clones by hybridizing ^{32}P-labeled DNA to Southern blots of restriction endonuclease digests of *Hind*III B, C, D, E, F, L, and M. The direction of transcription of some of the genes was determined from the hybridization reactions given by sets of clones which had different sized inserts but appeared to share a common 3′ terminus. For example, 2 clones with 0.56-kb inserts hybridized with a 0.45-kb *Xba*I fragment within *Hind*III A and another 2 clones with 1.15-kb inserts hybridized with the same fragment plus the adjacent *Bg*III/ *Xba*I fragment. This showed that the 3′ terminus of the gene mapped in the *Xba*I fragment and that transcription was towards the joint.

These results are summarized in Figure 1: this indicates the approximate map positions of the cloned cDNA sequences but not the sizes of the inserts. These ranged from about 0.4 to 1.4 kb.

Some of the cDNA clones are now being used to select specific mRNA molecules prior to translation in vitro and as primers for the synthesis of longer cDNA molecules.

REFERENCES

1. Favaloro J, Freisman R, Kamen R: Transcription maps of polyoma virus-specific RNA: Analysis by two-dimensional nuclease Sl gel mapping. Methods Enzymol 65:718, 1980.
2. Villa-Komaroff L, Efstratiadis A, Broome S, Lomedico P, Tizard R, Naker SP, Chick WL, Gilbert W: A bacterial clone synthesizing proinsulin. Proc Natl Acad Sci USA 75:3727, 1978.

SPECIFIC CELL-MEDIATED IMMUNITY AND NATURAL HISTORY OF CONGENITAL CMV INFECTION

R.F. Pass, S. Stagno, M.E. Dworsky, and C. A. Alford

The University of Alabama in Birmingham, Birmingham, AL 35294

CMI to CMV was studied in 110 children with congenital CMV infection who have been followed by us since birth. Specific CMI was measured using a lymphocyte transformation assay to CMV, with results expressed as a stimulation index (SI). With this assay, the mean ($\pm$SE) SI from 26 determinations on 13 seronegative controls was 0.27 ± 0.09, while that from 50 determinations on 17 seropositive controls was 34.1 ± 6.8. An SI $\geqslant 2$ was found in 48/50 tests from the latter group and 0/26 tests from the former. There were very few positive responses (SI $\geqslant 2$) prior to age 5 among patients who had symptoms at birth or sequelae (S-CMV), or among those with asymptomatic infection (A-CMV) as shown below.

	Age in Months Median SI ($+$/Total)				
	0–12	13–26	37–60	61–84	>85
S-CMV	0.07 (1/33)	0.03 (1/22)	0.09 (1/9)	0.28 (3/6)	6.2 (6/7)
A-CMV	0.11 (4/42)	0.27 (4/26)	0.57 (10/21)	1.78 (8/12)	0.88 (11/20)

Viruria was present in 10/32 (31%) patients with an SI $\geqslant 2$ compared to 21/31 (67.7%) with no response to CMV (P = 0.004). The specificity of this defect in CMI was demonstrated by simultaneous measurement of lymphocyte blastogenic response to CMV and to HSV in 21 children who were seropositive to HSV. Among children with congenital CMV under 5 years of age, the median SI for CMV was 1.43 with 7/21 positive responses compared to 8.0 for HSV with 20/21 positive (P < 0.001). Antibody to CMV was measured using an EIA technique on serial specimens collected during the first 3 years of life; no evidence of impaired antibody response was found.

Distribution of lymphocytes among subclasses was determined in 48 children with congenital CMV infection and 27 controls using commercial monoclonal antibodies to T lymphocytes (OKT3), helper T cells (OKT4), and suppressor T cells (OKT8). Results in patients did not differ from those in controls except for S-CMV patients under 1 year who had an increased percentage of T8+ cells (29 ± 2.6) compared to controls (18 ± 1.1), P < 0.01.

Congenital CMV infection is accompanied by a specific defect in lymphocyte blastogenic response which persists for years, is more pronounced in symptomatic patients, and is associated with viral excretion, but is not associated with a deficient antibody response nor with an abnormality in number of T lymphocytes or their distribution among subclasses.

CYTOMEGALOVIRUS INFECTION IN PREGNANCY AND ITS CONSEQUENCES

C.S. Peckham, P.M. Preece, and K.S. Chin
Charing Cross Hospital Medical School, St. Dunstans Road,
London W6, England

In September 1979, a prospective study was set up in London to provide further information on the risk of acquiring CMV infection in pregnancy in various subgroups of the population and to determine the incidence and significance of congenital infection. The ultimate aim of this study is to help decide whether congenital CMV is a serious enough problem in the United Kingdom to justify attempts at prevention by vaccination.

Some 14,000 women from 3 maternity hospitals have been screened for CMV antibodies at their first antenatal attendance and information obtained about their age, parity, race, country of birth, marital status, and husband's or partner's occupation. Approximately 50% showed evidence of previous infection. There were striking variations in the serologic status of women attending the 3 hospitals (49% to 70%) which serve different populations. This difference was accounted for by the high proportion of Asian women with CMV antibodies attending one hospital.

All infants born in the 3 hospitals have been screened for CMV (virus isolation) in the first few days of life, and 44 (3/1,000) with congenital CMV have been identified. Congenital infection resulted from primary maternal infection and reinfection or reactivation of latent infection in pregnancy. The infected children have been followed up at regular intervals together with 2 closely matched controls for each infected child. The follow-up will continue for 5 years so that all defects attributable to intrauterine infection may be identified.

In the presentation, details of epidemiologic findings and the clinical status of congenitally infected children will be presented.

EVIDENCE FOR THE INVOLVEMENT OF A HOST-SPECIFIC GLYCOPOLYPEPTIDE IN HCMV-DNA REPLICATION

K. Radsak and D. Weder
Zentrum Hygiene & Med. Mikrobiologie, Universität, 355 Marburg,
Federal Republic of Germany

In a recent report we documented that inhibition of cellular glycosylation activity by 2-deoxy-D-glucose (dGlc) or tunicamycin prevents HCMV-induced DNA replication in human fibroblasts infected after serum starvation [1]. Furthermore, chromatin preparations from infected cultures, which exhibit DNA replication under cell-free conditions, were inactive when cells were treated with dGlc prior to cell fractionation [1]. These observations, as well as additional control experiments [1], lent support to the view that dGlc-sensitive mechanisms may concern synthesis of "early" virus-induced chromatin-associated glycopolypeptides [1, 2] which are essential for DNA replication in infected cells.

In order to identify 1) likely candidate glycopolypeptides and 2) to define their subcellular localization HCMV-infected phosphonoacetic acid (PAA)-treated cultures pulse-labeled with tritiated glucosamine were fractionated and chromatin preparations analyzed by SDS-polyacrylamide gel electrophoresis (SDS-PAGE) and fluorography. Mock-infected cultures were included in the experimental setup as controls, as well as cells induced by serum for DNA replication which had been found also to be sensitive to the inhibitory action of dGlc. In response to either stimulus, HCMV and serum, induction of a chromatin-associated glycopolypeptide with the approximate molecular weight of 130,000 daltons (130 Kd) was observed concomitant to induction of DNA replication in these cells [1], whereas mock-infection did not result in a comparable reaction. An identical experimental analysis of dGlc-treated infected cultures pulse-labeled with tritiated amino acids revealed that essentially all virus-induced chromatin-associated polypeptides were expressed under dGlc, as in the presence of PAA except for 1 or 2 in the range of 130 Kd. However, dGlc prevented expression of "late" virus-induced polypeptides, as does PAA [1, 2].

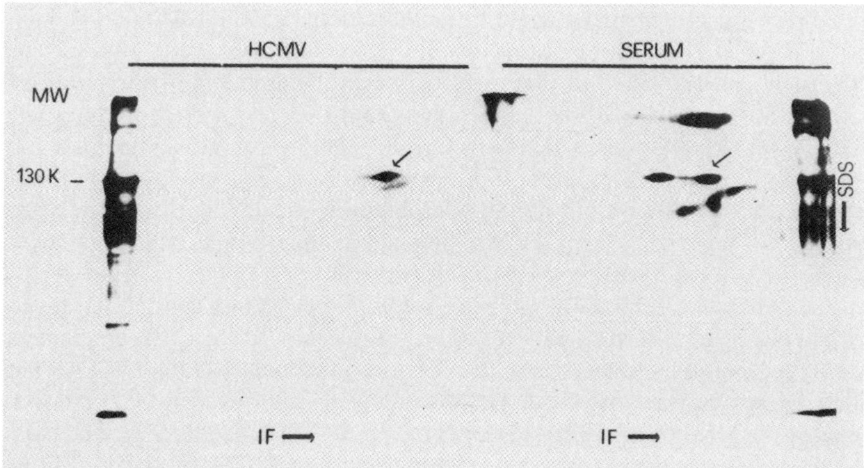

Fig. 1. Two-dimensional separation of chromatin-associated glycopolypeptides from HCMV-infected and serum-induced cultures by isoelectric focusing and SDS-PAGE. The arrows indicate the common component.

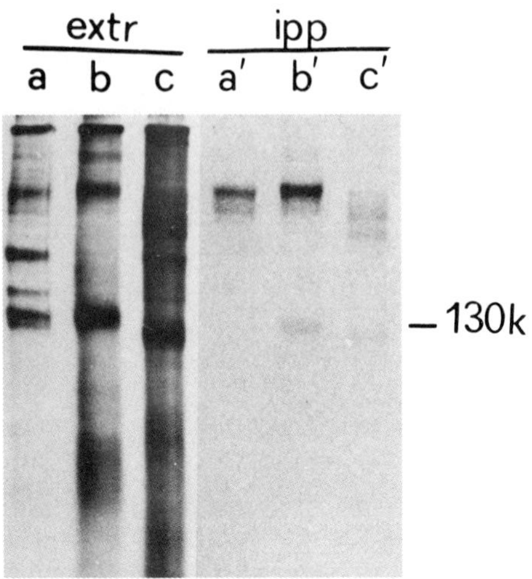

Fig. 2. Immunoprecipitation with anti-130 kd using extracts from (a,a') mock-, (b, b') HCMV-infected, (C, c') serum-induced cells.

The apparent similarities between HCMV- and serum-induced cells with respect to drug-sensitivity and induction of glycosylation of the chromatin-associated glycopolypeptide prompted experiments to directly compare the 130-Kd products from the 2 systems by limited proteolysis, 2-dimensional separation (isoelectric focusing and SDS-PAGE), and immunoprecipitation. For limited proteolysis the tritium glucosamine-labeled 130-Kd polypeptides were isolated from chromatin preparations by electrophoretic elution from SDS-gels and subjected to treatment with various amounts of V-8-protease: Comparative analysis of the digests showed different patterns implying that the 2 glycopolypeptides were not identical. The 2-dimensional analysis subsequently revealed for serum-induced cells 2 labeled components in the expected molecular weight range, one being identical to the single polypeptide found in extracts from HCMV-infected samples (Fig. 1) thus giving an explanation for the difference in digest patterns.

For immunoprecipitation, antisera were raised against the 130-Kd glycopolypeptide from serum-induced cells. These sera specifically precipitated from chromatin extracts, both the 130-Kd glycopolypeptide from serum-induced as well as that from HCMV-infected cultures (Fig. 2). Antisera against HCMV-specific "early" antigens, on the other hand, yielded negative results. These latter 2 analyses suggest that the HCMV-induced 130-Kd polypeptide is host-specific.

Interestingly, colchicine treatment which induces DNA replication via destabilization of microtubuli [3] also induces a chromatin-associated 130-Kd glycopolypeptide. These cellular reactions, loss of microtubuli with consecutive induction of DNA replication as well as that of the 130-Kd glycopolypeptide also occur in HCMV-infected cells [4]. It is proposed that "early" viral gene products trigger a cellular mechanism involving the host-specific 130-Kd polypeptide as a prerequisite for viral DNA replication.

REFERENCES

1. Radsak et al: J Gen Virol 57:33, 1981.
2. Stinski: J Virol 23:751, 1977.
3. Crossin et al: Cell 23:61, 1981.
4. Pfeiffer, Radsak: Arch Virol (In press)

IMMUNOGLOBULIN M TO HUMAN CYTOMEGALOVIRUS-INDUCED MEMBRANE EARLY ANTIGENS IN PATIENTS WITH PRIMARY CMV INFECTION

M. Grazia Revello and G. Gerna

Virus Laboratory, Institute of Infectious Diseases, University of Pavia, 27100 Pavia, Italy

It is well known that human CMV induces membrane antigens (MA) on infected human embryonic fibroblasts [1]. They can be detected by indirect immunofluorescence (IFA) 24 hr PI on CMV-infected fibroblasts either treated with ara-C or not, as well as on nonpermissive human and animal cells [2]. We investigated the antibody response to CMV-induced early MA (EMA) in 13 patients with primary CMV infection using IFA and/or anticomplement immunofluorescence (ACIF) test. For this purpose, human embryonic lung fibroblasts (HELF) grown on chamber-slides were infected with CMV strain AD169 at a MOI of about 0.02. After virus absorption, medium supplemented with ara-C (40 μg/ml) was added and IFA and/or ACIF was performed 48 hr PI on living cell monolayers (Fig. 1). Serial serum dilutions (starting dilution 1:20) were first tested by IFA for CMV-EMA IgG and IgM determination. Since no reactivity was found when the IFA-IgG test was used, representative CMV-EMA IFA-IgM-positive sera were fractionated by

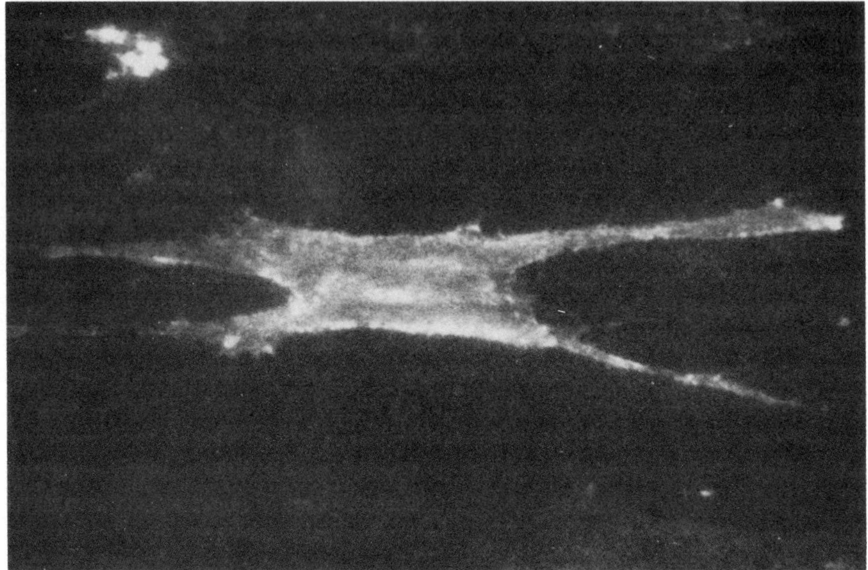

Fig. 1. EMA on CMV-infected HELF monolayer in the presence of ara-C 48 hr PI stained with ACIF (×400).

sucrose density gradient centrifugation to confirm the finding. When tested by IFA only the IgM fraction reacted positively to CMV-EMA. In order to increase the sensitivity of the assay, the same fractions were tested by ACIF using a human serum lacking CMV and HSV-specific antibody (as determined by ELISA test) as source of complement. With this test, no specific reaction was found in the IgG fraction (which contained CMV-specific IgG when tested by ELISA test). Equally negative by IFA and ACIF were sera taken from CMV-positive healthy donors as well as sera which contained CMV-specific IgG and rheumatoid factor (determined by ELISA test). Subsequently, only the ACIF test was used on IgM serum fractions for CMV-EMA specific antibody determination.

Virologic and serologic data are reported in Table 1. In positive cases, IgM to CMV-EMA are first detected 2 weeks after the onset of symptoms when CMV-specific IgM (as determined by ELISA) was also present. The only case (S.G.) which was found to possess IgM to structural antigens but not EMA-IgM one week after the onset of illness, is not sufficient to support the hypothesis of a delayed production of EMA-IgM as compared to IgM determined by ELISA. Highest titers were observed in sera taken 3–6 wk

TABLE 1. Antibody Response in 13 Patients With Acute CMV Infection

Patient, Age (Years), Clinical Diagnosis or Symptoms	Weeks After Onset of Symptoms	CMV Isolation	CMV Antibody Titer		
			IgG*	IgM†	EMA-IgM††
C.L., 28,	4		640	640	160
mononucleosis	5		1,280	160	80
	8		2,560	320	40
	12	positive	1,280	40	20
	20		1,280	<40	<20
T.Z., 44,	1		160	<40	<20
fever, ALL§	2		20,480	1,280	320
	8		20,480	40	640
	12		10,240	<40	80
	44		2,560	<40	<20
Z.G., 13,	1		80	<40	<20
pharyngitis,	3		2,560	5,120	640
fever	19		10,240	<40	80
C.F., 23,	1		80	<40	<20
fever	4		20,480	640	80
	9		10,240	<40	20
S.G., 4,	1	positive	40	40	<20
fever, ALL	3		2,560	640	320
T.N., 18,	1	positive	80	<40	<20
fever	21		20,480	<40	40
	25	positive	20,480	<40	80
Z.D., 4	−5		40	<40	<20
fever, ALL	2		1,280	640	40
	4		2,560	5,120	320
M.A.L., 4,	5	positive	5,120	40	40
mononucleosis	13		5,120	<40	<20
M.F., 2 mo,	2		10,240	160	80
splenomegaly	4	positive	20,480	40	80
D.M., 2,	3	positive	5,120	160	<20
hepatosplenomegaly	7		5,120	<40	<20
M.M., 4,	−7		1,280	<40	<20
hepatosplenomegaly,	3		1,280	640	<20
ALL	5		640	160	<20
	9		640	40	<20
	13		160	<40	<20
T.L., 17,	2		5,120	80	<20
mononucleosis	3		10,240	80	<20
	9		2,560	<40	<20

Table continued on following page.

TABLE 1. Antibody Response in 13 Patients With Acute CMV Infection (continued)

Patient, Age (Years), Clinical Diagnosis or Symptoms	Weeks After Onset of Symptoms	CMV Isolation	CMV Antibody Titer		
			IgG*	IgM†	EMA-IgM††
D.D.P.D., 13, myopericarditis	3		2,560	640	<20
	5	positive	5,120	1,280	<20
	8	positive	2,560	320	<20
	11		2,560	320	<20
	27		5,120	640	<20
	43		2,560	640	<20

*Titer determined by indirect ELISA on fourfold serum dilutions.
†Titer determined by indirect ELISA on serum fractions; rheumatoid factor-positive fractions were absorbed wtih polymerized IgG.
‡Early membrane antigen-IgM were determined by ACIF on IgM serum fractions.
§Acute lymphocytic leukemia.

after onset concomitantly with the peak of IgM. Patients T.Z., Z.G., C.F., and T.N. still possessed EMA-IgM in sera taken 12, 19, 8, and 25 wk, respectively, after onset, when IgM had already disappeared. Thus, it seems reasonable to suggest a longer production of IgM specific for EMA. In 4 patients (D.M., M.M., T.L., and D.D.P.D.) EMA-IgM was not detected: this could be due to the low sensitivity of the assay used, or to the fact that EMA may possess strain specificity. From the analysis of the results reported above, it seems that EMA-IgM and IgM to structural antigens may have different kinetics. Since the former appear to last longer than the latter, the detection of EMA-IgM in the absence of IgM specific for intracellular antigens, could help in diagnosing a primary CMV infection. However, it must be stressed that now we do not know whether a CMV reinfection can elicit a new CMV-EMA IgM response together with IgM to structural CMV antigens.

More cases should be tested in order to define the role of EMA-IgM; moreover, since in primary CMV infections, cytolytic antibodies belonging exclusively to the IgM class have been shown to lyse CMV-infected cells in the presence of complement [3], it may be of interest to investigate whether any cytolytic activity can be detected in presence of CMV-EMA.

REFERENCES

1. The TH, Langenhuysen MAC: Antibodies against membrane antigens of cytomegalovirus infected cells in sera of patients with a cytomegalovirus infection. Clin Exp Immunol 11:475–482, 1972.
2. Tanaka J, Yabuki Y, Hatano M: Evidence of early membrane antigens in cytomegalovirus-infected cells. J Gen Virol 53:157–161, 1981.
3. Betts RF, Schmidt SG: Cytolytic IgM antibody to cytomegalovirus in primary cytomegalovirus infection in humans. J Infect Dis 143:821–826, 1981.

CORRELATION OF CLINICAL OUTCOME OF CYTOMEGALOVIRUS INFECTION AND IMMUNOSUPPRESSION WITH VIRUS-SPECIFIC CYTOTOXIC LYMPHOCYTE RESPONSES IN RENAL TRANSPLANT RECIPIENTS

A.H. Rook, W. Frederick, J.F. Manischewitz,
J. Epstein, L. Jackson, B.B. Lee, C.B. Currier, and
G.V. Quinnan
Division of Virology, National Center for Drugs and Biologics, Bethesda, MD,
and Washington Hospital Center, Washington, D.C.

We have previously demonstrated in BMT recipients that CMV-specific cytotoxic lymphocyte responses are important cellular immune functions required for recovery from CMV infection [1]. The role of these responses during CMV infection of renal transplant recipients has not been previously examined. Therefore, we evaluated the relationship of these responses to CMV-related morbidity and mortality in 30 renal transplant recipients during the first 12 weeks posttransplantation. CMV-specific cytotoxicity was measured using multiple pairs of cryopreserved, CMV-infected and uninfected diploid fibroblasts from HLA-typed donors as target cells in a chromium-51 release assay. Other immune functions that were also evaluated included (NK) cell activity using K562 target cells, antibody-dependent cell-mediated cytotoxicity (ADCC) using antibody sensitized Chang liver cells as target cells, and CMV-specific antibody responses using the ACIF assay.

Pretransplantation, CMV-specific and non-CMV-specific (NK cell and ADCC) cytotoxic lymphocyte activities were comparable to levels measured in normal, nonuremic individuals [2]. During the first 3 weeks posttransplantation, most likely reflecting an effect of corticosteroid and azathioprine therapy, these cytotoxic activities declined markedly in all patients.

Twenty patients developed CMV infection, 19 of which were secondary cases. Fourteen patients developed CMV-specific cytotoxic lymphocyte responses during infection (responders), while 6 did not (nonresponders) (Table 1). Seven of 14 responders had significant increases in NK cell activity or ADCC during infection compared to only 1 of 6 nonresponders. All responders and 4 of 6 nonresponders developed fourfold rises in antibodies to CMV during infection. Clinical findings (Table 2) which included fever, leukopenia, thrombocytopenia, or elevation in serum transaminases were significantly more frequent among nonresponders than responders (P < .001). Prolonged viremia and complications of infection including superinfection, interstitial pneumonitis, and death occurred exclusively among nonresponders (Table 2). Acute allograft dysfunction during infection was also more frequent among nonresponders (4/6) than responders (1/14) (P = .025).

TABLE 1. CMV-Specific Cytotoxic Lymphocyte Responses During Infection

Patients	No.	Peak CMV-Specific Target Cell % Lysis Mean ± SD	
		HLA-Matched	HLA-Mismatched
Responders	14	12.3 ± 6.1	7.0 ± 6.3
Nonresponders	6	0.0 ± 0.0	0.0 ± 0.0

TABLE 2. Signs of Clinical Illness and Complications of CMV Infection in Relation to Responder and Nonresponder Status

Patient Group	Findings					
	Fever	Leukopenia	Thrombo-cytopenia	Elevated Serum Transaminases	Fraction With One Finding	Fraction With 3 or More Findings
Nonresponders	5/6	5/6	4/6	5/6	6/6	5/6*
Responders	4/14	2/14	1/14	4/14	4/14	0/14

Patient Group	Complications				Fraction With One or More Complications
	Super-infection	Interstitial Pneumonitis	Pancreatitis	Death	
Nonresponders	3/6	1/6	1/6	1/6	5/6*
Responders	0/14	0/14	0/14	0/14	0/14

*Findings were significantly more frequent in nonresponders than responders. (Chi-square = 11.4, P < .001.)

High-dose IV methylprednisone (1 gm bolus) treatment appeared to inhibit CMV-specific cytotoxic lymphocyte responses during infection. CMV-specific cytotoxicity was detected in only 5 of 20 assays obtained 5 to 14 days after treatment. However, significant CMV-specific cytotoxicity was detected in 4 of 4 assays performed 0–4 days after treatment and in 10 of 12 specimens from patients who had not received methylprednisone. Thus, these results suggested that this therapy probably resulted in the inhibition of cytotoxic T-cell precursors rather than mature effector cells.

Our data indicate that CMV-specific cytotoxic lymphocytes are important for recovery from CMV infection in renal transplant recipients. Immunosuppressive therapy of graft rejection should be designed to minimize inhibitory effects on CMV-specific cytotoxicity responses.

REFERENCES

1. Quinnan GV, Kirmani N, Rook AH, Manischewitz JF, Jackson L, Moreschi G, Santos GW, Saral R, Burns WH: N Engl J Med 307:7–13, 1982.
2. Kirmani N, Ginn RK, Mittal KK, Manischewitz JF, Quinnan GV: Infect Immun 34:441–447, 1981.

HOMOLOGIES BETWEEN THE GENOME OF HUMAN CYTOMEGALOVIRUS STRAIN AD169 AND HUMAN CELLULAR DNA

R. Rüger and B. Fleckenstein
Institut für Klinische Virologie, University of Erlangen-Nürnberg, D-8520 Erlangen, Federal Republic of Germany

DNA from a cosmid-cloned gene library of the CMV strain AD169 was used in order to detect virus-specific DNA persisting in human cells of various origins. From these studies it became evident that some of these cosmid clones hybridized with intermediate repetitive DNA sequences of human cells. Viral DNA of cosmids was subcloned in the plasmid vector pACYC 184, and the regions of homology were localized in the respective viral DNA fragments. Homology was confined to the *Eco*RI fragments U (4, 3 kbp), O (5, 6 kbp), and b (3, 0 kbp); the *Hind*III fragments D (23, 5 kbp) and S (6, 3 kbp); and the DNA of the in vitro transforming plasmid pCM 4000. All of these hybridization reactions were observed under stringent reannealing conditions (17°C or 21°C below average melting temperature of CMV). Similar or identical hybridization patterns were found with DNA from placenta tissues, peripheral white blood cells, lymphoblasts in vitro immortalized with EBV, several hematopoietic tumor cell lines, colon carcinoma biopsies, and adjacent nontumorous tissues. Identical patterns of homology were seen with DNA from patients with serologic evidence for preceding CMV infection and patients seronegative in ELISA. Homologous sequences were also found with DNA from owl monkey kidney cells and Chinese hamster ovary cells. Hybridization with DNA from 3T3 mouse cells or from calf thymus was found with CMV *Hind*III fragment S, *Eco*RI fragment U, and transforming plasmid pCM 4000. The DNA homologous to intermediate repetitive cellular DNA is not related to human Alu-sequences (clones BLUR 2, 6, 8, and 19), and no hybridization was found with DNA of the avian oncogene myc (c-myc, 5'-exon-myc, 3'-exon-myc) under conditions of stringency where homology between human and avian myc-sequences became apparent. The occurrence of repetitive cellular DNA sequences in the viral genome indicates that purified virion DNA should not be used in the search for virus-specific nucleic acids in human tissues.

CHARACTERIZATION OF HCMV SEQUENCES IN KAPOSI SARCOMA TISSUES FROM AIDS PATIENTS

S. Shaw[1], D. Spector[1], D. Abrams[2], and M. Gottlieb[3]

[1]University of California, San Diego, La Jolla, CA; [2]University of California, San Francisco, CA; [3]University of California, Los Angeles, CA

We examined Kaposi sarcoma tissues from patients with AIDS for the presence of HCMV-related DNA sequences. DNA extracted from Kaposi sarcoma tissues was spotted onto nitrocellulose filters, immobilized, and then hybridized with individual cloned EcoRI fragments of HCMV DNA. All of the cloned HCMV fragments except h hybridize to the DNA of clinical isolates of HCMV (S. Spector and D. Spector, unpublished data) and can thus be used to screen patients' specimens for HCMV-related DNA and RNA. The dot blot analyses demonstrated the presence of HCMV-related DNA sequences in the Kaposi sarcoma tissues.

The cloned fragments of HCMV DNA were hybridized to Southern blots of DNA extracted from Kaposi sarcoma tissue to further characterize the HCMV-related sequences in these specimens. Normal cellular sequences have been identified in our laboratory that hybridize to HCMV DNA. Southern blot analysis distinguishes between hybridization to viral sequences and hybridization to normal cellular sequences. In cases where the patient's HCMV isolate is available, these analyses also provide information on which viral sequences are present and whether these sequences may be rearranged or integrated into the host genome. We hybridized each of the 32 cloned EcoRI fragments of HCMV DNA to Southern blots containing EcoRI digests of DNA extracted from 2 specimens of Kaposi sarcoma tissue from a patient with AIDS. Our results demonstrated the presence of HCMV sequences representative of the entire genome in these specimens. The HCMV sequences were present at <0.5 copies/cell. Similar analyses of tissues from other patients are being done. Results to date reveal the presence of at least some HCMV DNA sequences.

Recently, other laboratories have reported that the c-*myc* gene is rearranged or amplified in other human tumors. We did not detect any amplification or rearrangement of human c-*myc* following hybridization of the 1.4-

kb Sst I fragment of a clone of the human c-*myc* gene (generously provided by J.M. Bishop) to EcoRI digests of DNA extracted from Kaposi sarcoma tissues.

MOUSE STRAIN VARIATION IN THE PROTECTIVE EFFECT OF INTERFERON IN CYTOMEGALOVIRUS INFECTION

G.R. Shellam, G.B. Harnett[*], and J.E. Allan

Department of Microbiology, University of Western Australia, and [*]State Health Laboratory Services, Nedlands, Western Australia

We previously observed that the protective effect of endogenously produced IFN during MCMV infection varied according to the strain of mouse (Grundy et al: Infect Immun 37:143, 1982). To determine if these differences reflect variations in the direct antiviral effect of IFN on target cells or in its immunomodulatory properties in different mouse strains, the protective effect of semipurified α-IFN against MCMV has been studied in newborn CBA, C3H, and BALB/c mice, and in vitro in mouse embryo fibroblasts (MEF) derived from these strains. Four daily IP injections of 3,000 reference units of IFN beginning at birth did not protect BALB/c mice against death from an IP challenge of 8×10^2 PFU MCMV given on day 2, but 40%–60% of C3H and CBA mice survived over 42 days. In vitro, consistently more IFN was required to give equivalent protection of BALB/c MEF against MCMV than in CBA or C3H MEF, regardless of whether the effect was measured by plaque reduction or the more sensitive CPE score method. A comparison of the sensitivity of fibroblasts from human donors to the protective effects of IFN against HCMV will also be provided. These results suggest that host genes influence the protective effects of IFN in CMV infection and that this may be due in part to host-dependent variations in the direct antiviral effect of IFN on individual cells.

STUDIES ON THE HUMAN CYTOMEGALOVIRUS MEMBRANE ANTIGENS AND THEIR PRODUCTION IN INFECTED CELLS

K. Shimokawa, T. Murayama, and T. Furukawa

Department of Microbiology, Kanazawa Medical University, Uchinada, Ishikawa, Japan

Although a few studies have been reported on HCMV membrane antibody, little is known about the nature and/or the significance of membrane antibody. During study on HCMV envelope antigens, we found that antisera against envelope antigens gave membrane immunofluorescence without staining the nuclear inclusion bodies. This study was performed to obtain information regarding the development of antigens on HCMV-infected MRC-5 cells.

MRC-5 human embryo lung fibroblasts were infected with Towne HCMV strain (MOI of about 1 PFU/cell) and incubated for 7 to 8 days at 37°C. The virus was purified from the infected cultured fluid according to methods described elsewhere. For the preparation of the envelope antigens, purified HCMV was suspended in 0.05 M Tris-NaCl buffer (pH 7.2) containing 1% NP-40. After 30 min at 4°C, these samples were centrifuged onto a 15%

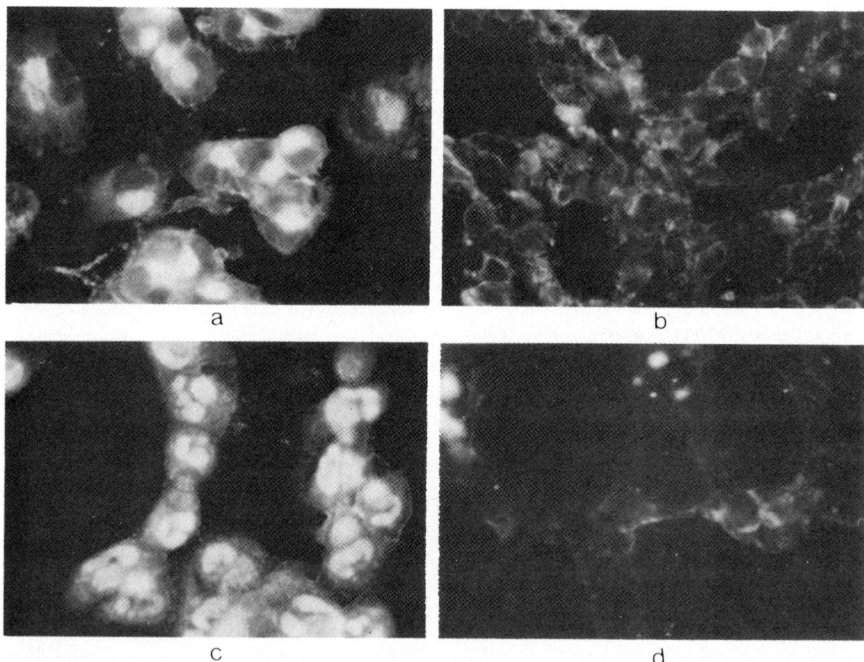

Fig. 1. Immunofluorescence photomicrographs of HCMV-infected cells at 72 hr PI. The cells were fixed with cold acetone or unfixed, and treated with antienvelope or antinucleocapsid serum. a) Fixed cells treated with antienvelope serum. b) Unfixed cells treated with antienvelope serum. c) Fixed cells treated with antinucleocapsid serum. d) Unfixed cells treated with antinucleocapsid serum.

sucrose cushion for 1 hr at 26,500 rpm in a Beckman sw 27 rotor. Top layer (the envelope antigens) and pellet (the nucleocapsid) were harvested. The pellets were examined by electron microscopy to confirm the presence of deenveloped particles. Guinea pigs were given 0.2 ml SC inoculation of the antigen preparation mixed with an equal volume of Freund's complete adjuvant. Three injections were given at 2-week intervals and animals were bled 10 days after the last immunization. Antibodies were evaluated by CF, indirect immunofluorescent antibody, and neutralization tests. Standard procedures for the IFA test were used to detect antigens in HCMV-infected cells.

The envelope antigens induced antibody responses (CF; 1920, NT;160) but failed to reduce a nuclear immunofluorescence which has been taken as standard marker of immunofluorescent antibody. Despite lacking antibody against nuclear inclusion bodies, the sera had membrane FA antibody (1:1280) or cytoplasmic FA antibody on unfixed or acetone-fixed target cells (Fig. 1a and b). On the other hand, the serum against nucleocapsid had CF and NT titers of 960 and 40, respectively and showed nuclear immunofluorescent antibody (1:1280) but not membrane fluorescent antibody (Fig. 1c and d).

The studies on development of membrane antigens showed that antigens were not detected at 6 hr PI, but they were detected at 24 hr PI and continued to be produced throughout the infection. The addition of ara-C and tunicamycin (TM) to the culture did not influence expression of membrane antigens, while actinomycin-D prevented the synthesis of membrane antigens.

The presence of TM at a concentration of 0.2 μg/ml or greater inhibited production of supernatant virus and cell-associated infectious virus (Fig. 2). Inclusion body formation and cell fusion that appeared at 72 hr PI were also inhibited, whereas the cell rounding was not affected and the appearance of infected cells at 24 hr PI was indistinguishable with or without TM treatment. The antigens detected in infected cells with TM were only membrane antigens as nuclear and cytoplasmic inclusion bodies were not formed.

These results demonstrate that the membrane antigens detected in HCMV-infected cells are a part of HCMV envelope antigens and are proteins expressed in the early stage of infection.

SUMMARY

HCMV induces membrane antigens. These antigens could be detected by indirect immunofluorescent techniques with antiserum against HCMV envelope, and appeared 24 hr PI. The expression of the membrane antigens was not influenced by ara-C and TM which inhibited virus production but did not

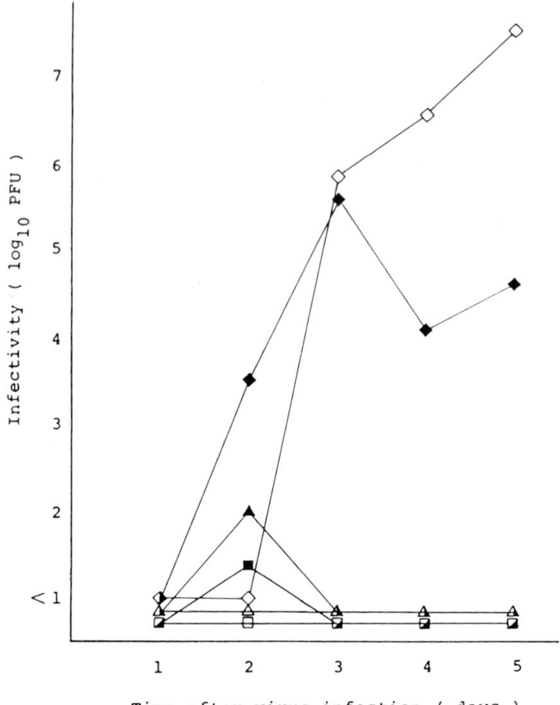

Fig. 2.   Growth of HCMV in MRC-5 cells with or without TM. MRC-5 cells in plates (1 × 10^5 cells/plate) were infected with HCMV at a MOI of 1. After 60 min of adsorption, the virus was removed and the plates were washed with medium and overlaid with 0.5 ml of medium containing: ◇, ◆, no TM; △, ▲, 0.2 μg/ml TM; □, ■, 2 μg/ml TM. Infectivity of supernatant virus (open symbols) and cell-associated virus (closed symbols) were determined by plaque assay.

influence early CPE. These results indicate that membrane antigens are a part of HCMV envelope antigens and the proteins expressed in early stage of infection.

THE ROLE OF NATURAL IMMUNITY TO CMV IN PROTECTION FROM CMV DISEASE

L. Smiley, C. Wlodaver, S. Starr, R. Grossman, L. Perloff, C. Barker, S. Plotkin, and H. Friedman

Hospital of the University of Pennsylvania and The Children's Hospital of Philadelphia, Philadelphia, PA 19104

CMV causes one of the major infectious diseases complicating renal transplantation [1–4]. This study was undertaken to determine the extent natural immunity protects against CMV disease and whether patients with natural immunity have improved graft survival.

Between May 1978 and March 1982, 327 kidney transplants were done at the Hospital of the University of Pennsylvania. These patients were evaluated for evidence of CMV infection (seroconversion or fourfold increase in titer) or disease (infection and an illness consistent with CMV disease as defined below). In some cases, diagnosis was confirmed by viral isolation.

To be included in this analysis, the following criteria had to be met: patient and graft had to survive 4 weeks, CMV serology had to be done on each donor and recipient pretransplant, and a 6-month follow-up had to be completed with all necessary data to assess CMV infection status. One hundred seventy-four patients had to be excluded for the following reasons: graft never functioned, 29; donor serology not done, 40; patients received Towne CMV vaccine, 57; inadequate follow-up to assess CMV infection status, 46; patient expired within 4 months posttransplant, 1; too many concomitant infections to evaluate CMV disease, 1.

A total of 153 transplant recipients were evaluated. Their mean age was 33.7 years. There were 103 males and 50 females. Seventy-six patients received cadaveric transplants. The median length of follow-up was 34.5 months. Outcome was analyzed by placing patients into 4 groups depending on the pretransplant CMV serologic status of recipients ($R+$ = seropositive, $R-$ = seronegative) and that of the donors ($D+$ = seropositive, $D-$ = seronegative).

A scoring system was devised to quantitate CMV disease [5]. One point was assigned for each of the following manifestations: WBC $\leqslant$ 4,000, platelets < 100,000, and hepatitis. One to 3 points were assigned for the following clinical manifestations depending on duration or severity: fever ($T° \geqslant 38.3°$), jaundice, pneumonia, CNS changes, renal failure, arthritis, muscle wasting, superinfection, and GI bleeding. Four points were assigned for lethality. Immunosuppression was quantitated based on the number of separate courses of parenteral steroids and/or antilymphocyte globulin (ALG).

TABLE 1. CMV Disease in the Challenged (D+) Groups

	No.	CMV Disease (%)	Mean Score of Entire Group	Pts. With Major Complications* (%)
D+, R−	23	14/23 (61%)	4.96	6 (26%)
D+, R+	41	10/41 (24%)	1.41	3 (7%)
		P < 0.01	P < 0.01	P > 0.05

*Major complications include CNS changes, pneumonia, renal failure, superinfection, and lethality.

The CMV disease outcomes in immune or nonimmune recipients of D+ kidneys are shown in Table 1. Among patients receiving D+ kidneys, natural immunity offered protection from CMV disease: 61% incidence in D+R− group v 24% in D+R+ (χ^2 = 6.88, P < 0.01). The mean score of the entire group defines the overall predictive risk of CMV disease for any given patient in that group. Immune patients had threefold less severe disease (t = 3.2, P < 0.01) and fewer complications.

Table 2 shows the incidence and severity of disease in immune and nonimmune recipients of D− kidneys. Among patients receiving a D− kidney, disease occurred infrequently (D−R− 2% v D−R+ 20%, χ^2=5.96 P < 0.02) and resulted in mild disease with no major complications.

Overall, 15 R− patients and 18 R+ patients developed CMV disease (Table 3). For the R− patients who developed disease, the mean score was 7.9 points. The R+ mean disease score was 4.5 points, indicating less severe disease (P < 0.02). Immune patients also had significantly less fever (8.3 days v 14.3 days for nonimmune, P < 0.05) and fewer major complications. As shown in Table 1, only the recipients of D+ kidneys developed major complications (CNS changes, pneumonia, superinfections, renal failure, death).

In terms of graft survival, patients with natural immunity had significantly improved cadaveric graft survival. However, immunity had no impact on living related donor graft survival (data not shown).

TABLE 2. CMV Disease in the Nonchallenged (D−) Groups

	No.	CMV Disease (%)	Mean score of entire group	Pts. with major complications (%)
D−, R−	49	1/49 (2%)	0.10	0
D−, R+	40	8/40 (20%)	0.58	0
		P < 0.02	P < 0.05	

TABLE 3. Characteristics of CMV Disease in Immune (R+) and Nonimmune (R−) Groups

	No.	CMV Disease (%)	Mean score of pts. with dis.	Mean days T° ↑	Pts. with major complications* (%)
R−	72	15/72 (21%)	7.93	14.3	6/72 (8%)
R+	81	18/81 (22%)	4.50	8.3	3/81 (4%)
			P < 0.02	P < 0.05	

*Major complications include CNS changes, pneumonia, renal failure, superinfection, and lethality.

To evaluate why it is that certain individuals develop disease, several risk factors were analyzed: HLA-antigen match, percentage of cadaveric transplants, mean number of courses of immunosuppressive therapy, and serologic status of donors. The only significant risk factor for R+ patients who developed disease was the amount of immunosuppressive therapy. Patients who developed disease received a mean of 3.2 courses, whereas those without disease received 1.9 courses (P < 0.001). For R− patients, the only significant risk factor for disease was whether they received a D+ kidney ($\chi^2 = 29.4$, P < 0.001).

These results indicate that natural immunity significantly modifies the incidence of CMV disease following transplantation of a kidney from a CMV seropositive donor. Once disease develops, natural immunity also modifies its severity. For recipients of cadaveric kidneys, immunity may play some role in improving graft survival. These results support the expanding evidence that CMV-induced immunity is imperfect, yet protective.

REFERENCES

1. Fiala M, Payne JE, Berne TV et al: Epidemiology of cytomegalovirus infection after transplantation and immunosuppression. J Infect Dis 132:421-433, 1975.
2. Armstrong JA, Evans AS, Rao N, Ho M: Viral infections in renal transplant recipients. Infect Immun 14:970-975, 1976.
3. Howard RJ, Balfour H Jr, Marker SM, Simmons RL, Najarian JS: Viral infections in kidney donors and recipients: A prospective study. Transplant Proc 9:113-116, 1977.
4. Pass RF, Long WK, Whitley RJ et al: Productive infection with cytomegalovirus and herpes simplex virus in renal transplant recipients: Role of source of kidney. J Infect Dis 137:556-562, 1978.
5. Plotkin SA et al: Prevention of cytomegalovirus disease by Towne strain live attenuated vaccine. This volume.

CYTOMEGALOVIRUS ANTIBODY PREVALENCE IN NIGERIAN SCHOOL CHILDREN

M. Stek, Jr., C. Deisanti, J.F. Duncan, Jr., and O.O. Kassim*

Uniformed Services University, School of Medicine, Bethesda, MD, and *Howard University, School of Medicine, Washington, DC

Serum from 69 Epe, Nigerian school children were examined for CMV IgG antibodies using an enzyme immune assay. The mean age of this group was 10.6 ± 1.9 years with a 1.1 male-to-female ratio. Ninety-seven percent of the samples were positive for CMV antibodies. High antibody titers (≥ 1.00 corrected absorbance at 1/50 serum dilutions) were seen in 6% of this population; 65% were in the medium titer range (0.46–0.99); and 26% were in the low titer category (0.31–0.45). No individuals fell in the questionable range (0.21–0.30), while 3% were negative ($\leq$ 0.20). Antibody positivity and titers were not related to age or sex, thus differing from earlier studies. These data were, however, consistent with previous work which had shown high CMV antibody levels in populations from less developed areas of the world. Further, the high level of CMV antibody positivity found in this project together with results from an earlier Ibadan study indicated SW Nigeria to be a hyperendemic focus of CMV. The high antibody titer levels seen in this group suggested (but did not prove) the development of protective immunity at an early age in Epe. Finally, the study demonstrated that seronegative individuals, particularly females, require identification and follow-up.

INCIDENCE OF CYTOMEGALOVIRUS INFECTION AND STRAIN CHARACTERIZATION OF ISOLATES OBTAINED FROM A CASE-CONTROL STUDY OF PATIENTS WITH THE ACQUIRED IMMUNE DEFICIENCY SYNDROME

J.A. Stewart, C.D. Cabradilla, M.F. Rogers, and the Task Force on Acquired Immune Deficiency Syndrome
Centers for Disease Control, Atlanta, GA

An outbreak of immunosuppression associated with Kaposi sarcoma, *Pneumocystis carinii* pneumonia, and other opportunistic infections has been identified in populations of homosexual men, IV drug users, and Haitians. The Centers for Disease Control conducted a national case-control study in October 1981, to characterize the syndrome and to identify possible risk factors for these conditions. Because reports have suggested that CMV, a latent DNA virus highly prevalent among homosexual men, is associated with both the African and American Kaposi sarcoma, laboratory tests related to CMV and the other herpes group viruses were emphasized. For each case patient identified, 4 age-, sex-, and race-matched control individuals were chosen. A swab of the throat, a swab of the rectum, a urine sample, and a clotted blood sample for serum were collected from participants.

Urine and/or mouth swab cultures of case specimens yielded CMV more frequently than those of the combined controls, 29% of 50 cases having an isolation from one or more sites, compared to 8% of 117 controls, P < 0.01, chi-square. CMV was not isolated from rectal swabs obtained from 42 cases although HSV type 2 was grown from culture of 4 swabs. The antibody incidence of CMV was 100% in the 50 cases and 98% in the 117 control men. The mean CMV CF titer (66) of the cases was significantly higher than that of the combined controls (odds ratio 9.05). The CMV indirect hemagglutination titer of the cases (3,327) did not differ significantly from titers of the control groups although they were threefold higher than 2 of the control groups. Fifteen isolates of CMV that included 10 isolates from cases, 4 isolates from controls and the AD169 stock laboratory strain were analyzed by digestion of their DNA with BamHI endonuclease. Each of the isolates had a unique profile when compared with each of the others and thus fails to show an epidemiologic link between any of these cases. However, all of the isolates had at least one half of the segments in common, and the presence of a critical common DNA sequence can not be excluded by these studies.

SUPPRESSION OF CELL-MEDIATED IMMUNITY TO CYTOMEGALOVIRUS AND TUBERCULIN IN PREGNANCY, EMPLOYING THE LEUKOCYTE MIGRATION INHIBITION TEST

A. Tanaka, K. Hirota, K. Takahashi, and
Y. Numazaki

Virus Laboratory, Sendai National Hospital and the Department of Gynecology and Obstetrics, Saka Hospital, Sendai, Japan

To clarify the mechanism of reactivation of CMV in pregnancy, CMI to CMV was investigated in 108 pregnant and 29 postpartal women employing the leukocyte migration inhibition technique. It was demonstrated that CMV-specific CMI was suppressed with gestation time; in 20% of the seropositive women during the 1st trimester, in 78% during the 2nd trimester, and in all at term. The suppression of CMI was ceased 8 weeks after parturition. The results suggest that reactivation of CMV in pregnancy is probably caused by the suppression of CMV-specific CMI. However, tuberculin-specific CMI was equally suppressed in pregnancy and recovered at postpartum. These findings suggest that suppression of the specific CMI in pregnancy may occur not only to CMV and tuberculin but also to other antigens.

PATHOGENESIS OF NEUTROPHIL DYSFUNCTION IN GUINEA PIG-CYTOMEGALOVIRUS (GP CMV)-INFECTED GUINEA PIGS

R. Tannous and M.G. Myers

Department of Pediatrics, University of Iowa College of Medicine, Iowa City, IA 52242

Neutrophil (N) migrations and zymosan-activated plasma (ZAP) chemotactic activity were measured under agarose in GP CMV-infected strain 2 guinea pigs (I) and compared to those in concurrent sham inoculated controls (C). N spontaneous migration was similar to that in C. N chemotaxis (toward normal C5a) and ZAP chemotactic activity (toward normal N) decreased progressively between days 1 and 4 postinoculation, then returned to C levels by days 9–10. The plasmas were therefore tested for the presence of N- and chemotaxin-directed inhibitors using standard chemotactic and lysosomal enzyme release inhibition assays. N-directed inhibition was studied by preincubating normal N with I or C plasmas prior to measuring their responses to C5a, formyl-methionyl-leucyl-phenylalanine (FMLP) and *E coli*-derived chemotactic factor (BF). Both responses to all three chemotoxins were significantly lower after incubation with I plasmas (P < 0.001). The inhibitory activity was heat stable and time dependent. Chemotaxin-directed inhibition was studied by preincubating each chemotaxin with I or C plasmas prior to measuring their chemotactic and enzyme releasing activities. I plasmas were more inhibitory toward C5a (P < 0.001) and C plasmas were more inhibitory toward FMLP and BF (P < 0.05). A CFI-like inhibitor (MW ~ 70,000) was demonstrated in both I and C plasmas following fractionation by gel column chromatography. I plasmas contained 3 other inhibitory components, designated as GP CMV-associated inhibitor (MW ~ 80,000), helper 1 (MW ~ 30,000), and helper 2 (MW ~ 15,000). N chemotactic and enzyme release responses to all 3 chemotaxins were inhibited by their preincubation with GP CMV-associated inhibitory + helper 1 and not affected by preincubation with CFI-like inhibitor, GP CMV-associated inhibitor + helper 1, helper 1 + helper 2 or any single component alone. The chemotactic and enzyme-releasing activities of C5a were inhibited by preincubation with the CFI-like inhibitor, GP CMV-associated inhibitor + helper 1 and GP CMV-associated inhibitor + helper 2. The activities of FMLP and BF were inhibited only by the CFI-like inhibitor.

A complex inhibitory system is acquired during GP CMV infection. N-directed inhibitors are nonspecific, affecting N responses to all chemotaxins while chemotaxin-directed inhibitors are specific against C5a. The combined effects of these inhibitors account for the in vivo acquired defects in N chemotaxis and ZAP chemotactic activity.

ENZYME LINKED IMMUNOSORBENT ASSAY (ELISA) FOR DETECTION OF IgM AGAINST CMV

M.K. Tinker, S. Gibson, D.A. Fuccillo, and A.J. O'Beirne

M.A. Bioproducts, Walkersville, MD 21793

An indirect ELISA using an alkaline phosphatase conjugated anti-μ-chain antiserum was developed to measure CMV-specific IgM in human sera. IgG was removed by pretreatment with a modified protein A preparation to eliminate interference by IgG or false positivity by rheumatoid factor.

CMV IgM ELISA results were interpreted on the basis of the distribution of CMV IgM ELISA values obtained by testing a normal healthy population of adults. Greater than 99.73% of the OD values from the negative population fell below 0.3 ELISA value (EV); therefore, a positive CMV IgM level was interpreted as 0.3 EV or greater. CMV IgM was not detected in 73 of 74 healthy adults irrespective of the fact that some of these adults were CMV immune. Low levels of CMV IgM were measured in 3 of 18 rheumatoid factor positive adults. When these 3 sera were fractionated on a sucrose gradient and retested by ELISA for CMV IgM, specific activity was found in the IgM fraction.

The sensitivity of the assay was confirmed by its ability to measure the production of CMV IgM in serial serum samples from adults receiving CMV vaccination. Nineteen of 21 vaccinees with demonstrated CMV seroconversion had positive CMV IgM ELISA levels within 2 months of vaccination. Seroconversion was determined by a positive change in CMV IgG ELISA assay. Only 1 of 3 vaccinees without CMV IgG seroconversion had a CMV IgM value > 0.3. Four vaccinees with CMV IgG before vaccination failed to demonstrate a CMV-specific IgM response.

The presence of CMV IgM could be used for determining current infection in pregnant women and immunosuppressed adults. CMV IgM ELISA results from these clinical populations appeared to be divided into 2 levels of response (Table 1). High-level response (EV $\geqslant 0.6$) occurred when the

TABLE 1. Highest CMV IgM Levels in Serial Samples Postvaccination for Adult Receiving Vaccine*

CMV Vaccinee	CMV IgM ELISA High-Positive EV > 0.6	CMV IgM ELISA Low-Positive EV $= 0.3–0.6$	CMV IgM ELISA Negative EV < 0.3
Prevaccination CMV seronegative seroconverison from negative to positive by CMV IgG ELISA	9	10	2
Prevaccination CMV seronegative no seroconversion by CMV IgG ELISA	0	1	2
Prevaccination CMV seropositive by ACIF, CF or CMV IgG ELISA	0	0	4

*Vaccinee samples provided courtesy of Dr. G. Fleisher, Dr. H. Friedman, and Dr. S. Plotkin, of the J.S. Stokes, Jr. Research Institute, CHOP, Philadelphia, PA.

CMV infection was clinically significant. Low levels of CMV IgM (EV = 0.3–0.6) occurred in patients where the possibility of CMV infection could not be ruled out, but no clinical disease could be established.

Eighteen of 18 immunodeficient adults with clinical symptoms compatible with CMV infection and CMV virus isolation from lymphocytes had positive CMV IgM levels. Seventy-two percent of ELISA values from these patients were > 0.6. Two additional patients with virus negative lymphocyte cultures had no CMV IgM.

CMV IgM was demonstrated in 33 of 37 mothers who had a primary CMV infection during pregnancy as determined by seroconversion by the ACIF test. Sixty-eight percent of their EV were > 0.6. Positive CMV levels were detected in 5 of 11 seropositive mothers who had recurrent infection during pregnancy as determined by the isolation of CMV virus in babies' urine at birth. Only 1 of the 11 had an ELISA value > 0.6. One of 34 seropositive mothers without infection during pregnancy had low levels of CMV IgM. All seronegative mothers were found to be negative for CMV IgM.

Based on these studies, high levels of CMV IgM measured by this ELISA are related to significant current infection and the diagnostic significance of low levels of CMV IgM have yet to be determined.

INHIBITION OF HUMAN CYTOMEGALOVIRUS REPLICATION BY 2′-NOR-2′-DEOXYGUANOSINE

M.J. Tocci[†], T.J. Livelli[†], H.C. Perry,
C.S. Crumpacker, and K. Field*

[†]Department of Biochemical Genetics, Merck Sharp & Dohme Research Laboratories, Rahway, NJ 07065; *Department of Virus and Cell Biology, Merck Sharp & Dohme Research Laboratories, West Point, PA 19486; Division of Infectious Disease, Beth Israel Hospital, Boston, MA

Antiherpetic agents such as acyclovir (ACV) [9-(2 hydroxyethoxymethyl) guanine] which require a virus-specific thymidine kinase (tk) for their activation are relatively ineffective against HCMV. At high concentrations (100–400 μM) ACV inhibits CMV plaque formation but is not capable of completely blocking virus replication. Another nucleoside analog, 2′-nor-2′-deoxyguanosine (2′-NDG) that is active against HSV types 1 and 2 also appears to inhibit CMV replication. In plaque reduction assays using HCMV laboratory strains AD119 and Towne and a clinical CMV isolate obtained from a lung biopsy of a patient with AIDS the 50% inhibitory dose (ID$_{50}$) of

ACV and 2'-NDG ranged from 30–100 μM and 1.5–10 μM, respectively. Comparative studies, between ACV and 2'-NDG were performed using the Eisenhart (EHT) strain, a low passage level clinical CMV isolate. In these experiments drug concentrations were maintained at 350 μM for ACV and 35 μM for 2'-NDG, the concentrations that inhibited CMV-EHT plaque formation by $\geqslant$ 90%. Under these conditions neither ACV nor 2'-NDG prevented the appearance of CMV-specific cytopathologic effect (CPE). In CMV-infected cultures treated with 2'-NDG, CPE was associated only with cells that were initially infected and after 7 days of incubation had not spread to adjacent cells. However, in culture treated with ACV, CMV-CPE eventually spread to adjacent cells during the 7-day incubation period. Subsequent experiments indicated that CMV DNA was not synthesized in 2'-NDG-treated cultures, and that progeny virus was undetectable by plaque assay at 5 days' PI. ACV treatment reduced but did not completely inhibit either CMV DNA synthesis or the production of virus. The relative toxicities of ACV and 2'-NDG were examined on growing and resting human embryo fibroblasts. In confluent cells, the uptake of ^{3}H-TdR was reduced by approximately 15%–20% in ACV (350 μM) and 2'-NDG (35 μM) treated cultures as compared to untreated cells. Cells grown in the presence of either compound exhibited an extended lag phase but ultimately reached the same cell density as control cultures. Throughout these experiments cell viability in the treated cultures was maintained between 80%–95% of cultures that were not treated with drug. These experiments suggest that unlike ACV, 2'-NDG may be an effective antiviral agent for blocking the replication of HCMV.

IMMUNOGENICITY OF THE PROTEIN SUBUNITS OF THE MURINE CYTOMEGALOVIRUS*

M. Tolpin, C. Chakinis, and V. Schauf
University of Illinois Medical Center, Chicago, IL 60612

Immunoprophylaxis of susceptible individuals against severe CMV infection has recently become feasible. The live, attenuated Towne 125 CMV vaccine is immunogenic and does not disseminate from the site of inoculation in both normal and somewhat immunocompromised individuals. However, concerns about: 1) the oncogenic potential of live CMV, 2) the paucity of markers of attenuation and the consequent lack of information about the rate

*Supported by March of Dimes Birth Defects Foundation.

of reversion to wild-type, and 3) the lack of a booster response to Towne 125 inoculation in CMV seropositive individuals may limit the usefulness of live, attenuated CMV vaccine. Development of an immunogenic, protective, inactivated CMV vaccine is supported by experimental evidence in the MCMV model. Formaldehyde-inactivated, whole MCMV is immunogenic in mice. Animals immunized with this preparation show significant protection against both morbidity and mortality following a potentially lethal challenge with wild-type MCMV.

The medical community has, however, discovered the hazards of eliminating immunologically important viral protein(s) from inactivated virus vaccines. The experience with inactivated measles vaccine dramatically demonstrated this problem. Knowledge of which viral proteins provoke a host immune response that limits viral replication, neutralizes whole virus, and/or destroys infected cells is crucial to the development of any immunologically complete—and hence safe—inactivated virus vaccine. Using the MCMV model, we have begun to address this problem with respect to the CMVs. Immunoprecipitation is used to determine which MCMV proteins stimulate a significant humoral immune response. MCMV-infected BALB/c mouse embryo fibroblasts (MEF) are labeled with ^{14}C-mixed amino acids. Lysate of these cells is immunoprecipitated wtih BALB/c sera obtained from each of the following: 1) a mouse that had been hyperimmunized with MCMV (HI), 2) mice in the convalescent phase of MCMV infection (CI), and 3) mice that had never been infected with MCMV (NI). The immunoprecipitated—hence, immunogenic—MCMV proteins are then analyzed by means of polyacrylamide gel electrophoresis. We have found that large amounts of a protein with a MW of approximately 82K are produced in MCMV-infected MEF, but not in uninfected MEF. This protein is immunoprecipitated well by both HI and CI, but not by NI, indicating that it is an MCMV protein and that it is definitely immunogenic. Further biochemical characterization of this protein and determination of its ability to elicit an immune protective response against MCMV infection and/or morbidity is therefore indicated. These findings and methods applied to the proteins of CMV may aid in the development of a safe, immunogenic protein subunit CMV vaccine.

POLYAMINE BIOSYNTHESIS AND HUMAN CMV REPLICATION: A POSSIBLE STRATEGY FOR ANTIVIRAL CHEMOTHERAPY

A.S. Tyms and J.D. Williamson

Department of Medical Microbiology, St. Mary's Hospital Medical School, Paddington, London W2 1PG, England

Natural products or synthetic compounds with action suitable for clinical use against parasitic infections have been hard to find, and this deficiency is most marked in the case of virus infections. In recent years, significant progress has been made in the development of antiviral chemotherapy which has been based primarily on antagonists of nucleic acid biosynthesis. We have seen in this symposium that there are signs of potent anti-CMV agents, again based on nucleoside analogs, which exploit the novel biochemistry of virus nucleic acid replication. However, it is certain that alternative strategies must be considered for the rational design of new therapeutic agents. Seymour Cohen [1] has presented constructive arguments for the development of selective chemotherapy which is not based exclusively on nucleic acid biosynthesis but directed against proteins and other molecular species with essential structural or metabolic functions in the parasite. In the past 2 decades, it has become apparent that the vital functions of both prokaryotes and eukaryotes are dependent upon the presence of polyamines. These small, aliphatic bases are found in mammalian tissues as putrescine, spermidine, and spermine; their biosynthesis is illustrated in Figure 1. It has been shown

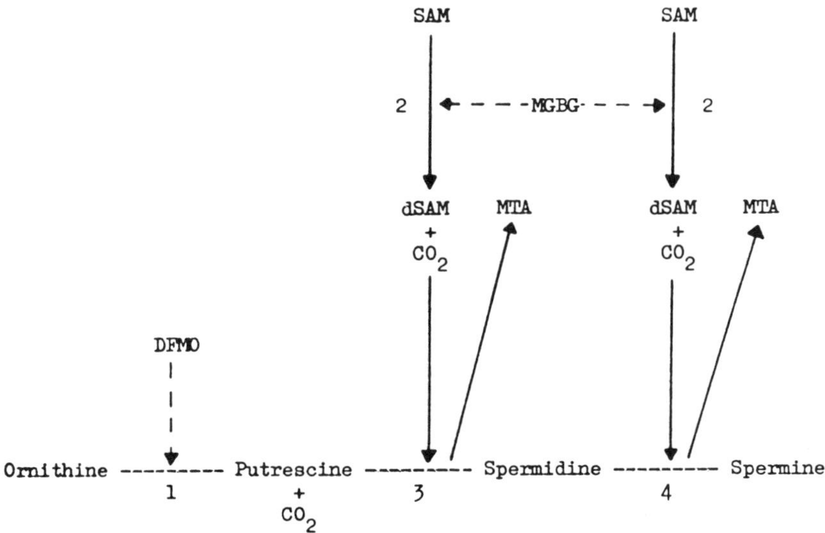

Fig. 1. Polyamine biosynthetic pathway in eukaryotic cells. Enzymes: 1, ornithine decarboxylase (inhibited by α-difluoromethylornithine, DFMO); 2, S-adenosylmethionine decarboxylase (inhibited by methylglyoxal bis (guanylhydrazone) (MGBG); 3, spermidine synthase; 4, spermine synthase. Propylamino moieties are derived from decarboxylated (d) S-adenosylmethionine (SAM) with the formation of methylthioadenosine (MTA).

that polyamine metabolism in human embryo fibroblast cells is increased after infection with HCMV [2-4]. This results in a marked accumulation of spermine which is reflected in the plot of spermidine: spermine ratios at the various times PI (Fig. 2). These results show that the increased biosynthetic activity parallels the exponential phase in virus growth, whereas the ratio of the 2 polyamines in the uninfected control cells remain relatively constant during the period under study. The essential nature of polyamine metabolism after CMV infection has been shown by the antiviral effect of specific inhibitors of the polyamine biosynthetic pathway. The compounds used were α-difluoromethylornithine (DFMO), which is a catalytically activated, irreversible inhibitor of ornithine decarboxylase and methylglyoxal bis (guanylhydrazone) (MGBG), which is an antagonist of S-adenosylmethionine decarboxylase (Fig. 1). Our earlier studies with a number of strains of HCMV have shown that the median ED_{50} value for MGBG (0.6 μM) was about 10-fold and 50-fold lower than values for 5-iododeoxyuridine and acyclovir, respectively, with a higher ED_{50} value of 5.2 mM for DFMO [4]. The requirement for such concentrations of DFMO is due to its poor uptake by mammalian cells. The inhibitory effects of MGBG and DFMO clearly demonstrate that concomitant polyamine biosynthesis is required for CMV replication.

In considering antiviral compounds for clinical application, it is valuable to understand the mechanism of action of the putative agents. At present, there is evidence that polyamine metabolism is related to an early event in CMV replication. The typical DNA-containing intranuclear inclusions which are characteristic of CMV replication are not observed after treatment with MGBG [5] or DFMO [4] at drug concentrations that inhibit virus growth. Analysis by isopyknic centrifugation of DNA radiolabeled with ^{3}H-thymidine showed an apparent reduction in viral DNA after treatment of infected cultures with either polyamine inhibitor. Interpretation of such data is difficult, however, due to the effect of polyamine inhibitors on thymidine kinase activity [6] with a consequent effect on the specific activities of the DNA preparation. Restriction enzyme analysis is a more reliable method for the quantitative determination of viral DNA from infected cells [7]. Analysis of the HindIII restriction profiles of DNA from infected cells treated with MGBG or DFMO also showed that the synthesis of CMV DNA is dependent on continuing polyamine metabolism. It is rather surprising, therefore, that inhibitors of viral DNA synthesis have been shown to prevent the increase in polyamine metabolism normally seen after CMV infection. This was first reported by Isom [2] using phosphonoacetic acid (PAA) and ara-C as DNA inhibitors, and we now report similar findings using 5-fluorodeoxyuridine (FUdR). In the presence of increasing concentrations of the inhibitor, there is the expected reduction in virus yield but this was paralleled by a reduction in the synthesis of spermine in infected cells. This paradox is fascinating in terms of the molecular biology of CMV replication, but at present we cannot

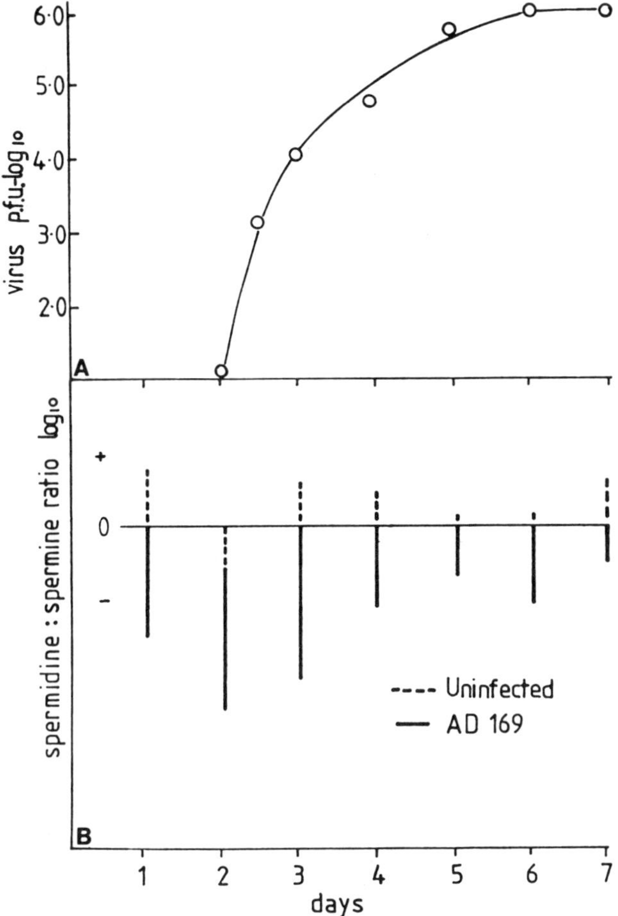

Fig. 2.   Polyamine metabolism in human diploid fibroblasts (MRC-5) infected with HCMV strain AD169.

Panel A: Growth curve of HCMV in MRC-5 cells; o--- o, cell-associated virus.

Panel B: Changes in spermidine: spermine ratios due to increased polyamine biosynthesis in HCMV-infected cells.

The spermidine and spermine content of unifected (- - -) and infected (—) cells was determined at daily intervals using analytic techniques described elsewhere [11].

offer a complete explanation. Isom [2] suggests that the viral DNA polymerase may have a regulatory function with respect to the virus-induced ornithine decarboxylase activity; this can explain the inhibitory effect of PAA. The results with ara-C and FUdR suggest a more general effect through the inhibition of DNA synthesis which could be related to a requirement for host-cell DNA snythesis early in virus replications [8]. Both hypotheses may be linked by the proposed involvement of the viral DNA polymerase in the synthesis of cell DNA [9].

In summary, we have shown that the replication of HCMV is inhibited by MGBG or DFMO and this involves an antiviral mechanism which is quite different from the mode of action of existing antiviral compounds. Although it is dangerous to extrapolate from in vitro to in vivo states, it is both interesting and exciting that the compounds described here have been used in the treatment of childhood leukemia [10]. The therapeutic effect was obtained by the enhanced uptake of MGBG into the blast cells after pretreatment with DFMO. The success of such therapy is clearly a reflection of increased polyamine biosynthesis in leukemia cells.

ACKNOWLEDGMENT

DFMO and acyclovir were gifts from Centre de Recherche Merrell International and Wellcome Research Laboratories, respectively.

REFERENCES

1. Cohen SS: Science 205: 964–971, 1979.
2. Isom: J Gen Virol 42: 265–278, 1979.
3. Tyms AS, Williamson JD: J Gen Virol 48: 183–191, 1980.
4. Tyms AS, Williamson JD: Nature, 297: 690–691, 1982.
5. Tyms AS, Scamans E, Williamson JD: Biochem Biophys Res Commun 86: 312–318, 1979.
6. Cheetham BF, Bellett AJD: J Cell Physiol 110: 114–122, 1982.
7. Tyms AS: Med Lab Sci 40: 81–83, 1983.
8. St. Jeor SC, Hutt R: J Gen Virol 37: 65–73, 1977.
9. Radsak K, Furukawa T, Plotkin SA: Arch Virol 65: 45–54, 1980.
10. Siimes M, Seppänen P, Alhonen-Hongisto L, Jänne J. Int J Cancer 28: 567–570, 1981.
11. Redmond JW, Tseng A: J Chromatog 170:479–481, 1979.

RISK OF CMV TRANSMISSION TO NONIMMUNOCOMPROMISED PATIENTS FROM CMV-SEROPOSITIVE BLOOD DONORS*

J.A. Wilhelm, L. Matter, and K. Schopfer

Immunology Section, Institute for Medical Microbiology, 9000 St. Gallen, Switzerland

*This work was partially supported by the St. Gallen–Appenzell Cancer League.

Natural transmission of CMV is known to occur prenatally and perinatally. The mechanisms of postnatal infection are not as clearly defined. An iatrogenic means of CMV transmission via whole blood or blood fractions has been well documented in recent years. There are especially high-risk groups such as preterm infants and newborns receiving exchange transfusions, and immunocompromised patients including transplant recipients. The transmission of CMV by means of blood transfusions can be curtailed by using only CMV-seronegative donors for seronegative recipients, as has been demonstrated, for example, in the cases of exchange transfusions in newborns and for CMV-seronegative patients receiving organs from seronegative donors.

For the last several years, only CMV seronegative blood has been given to newborns in St. Gallen. We have not seen any transfusion-associated CMV disease in these patients. To evaluate the need to extend this practice to other recipient groups, including nonimmunocompromised patients, we initiated a study to follow up CMV-seronegative patients after transfusion to detect CMV seroconversion.

We have used CF, and, more recently, a CMV-IgG-EIA to check the CMV-antibody status of our blood donors and patients receiving transfusions. The study period was 2½ yr. Of the 4640 blood donors, 60.5% are seronegative (54.8% of women, 63.8% of men) and of the total seronegative control population an average of 1.0% seroconverted per year. As of September 1, 1982, 505 seronegative patients receiving transfusions have been followed up (on the average after about 6 mo). 6 ($\triangleq$ 2.4% per yr) have seroconverted which does not represent a statistically significant increase ($P > 0.1$) compared to the nontransfused control group. We will present the data in more detail over seroconversion in the control group and about 800 patients followed up after transfusion to identify which patients, if any, are at increased risk of CMV disease or seroconversion.

PRIMARY (CMV) INFECTION FOLLOWING CARDIAC TRANSPLANTATION IN A MURINE MODEL

E.J. Wilson, L.V. Barrett, D.N. Medearis, and R.H. Rubin
Medical and Children's Services, Massachusetts General Hospital, Boston MA 02114

Primary CMV infection produces infectious disease syndromes in cardiac transplantation recipients, and predisposes them to potentially lethal superinfection. The source of the virus, and whether the heart is involved in systemic CMV infection are not known. A murine CMV model employing hearts taken from acutely or latently infected Balb/C mice and then transplanted as primary vascularized heterotopic isografts to Balb/C recipients was employed

TABLE 1.

Donor	Treatment Posttransplant	Outcome	Peak Viral Titers*					No. with IFA Titer**
			L	S	SG	DH	RH	
Acutely infected	None	Nonlethal 1° infection	4.0	3.0	8.0	4.5	2.0	10/10
Acutely infected	Cortisone/ATG	Lethal 1° infection	60	5.8	7.2	5.7	3.2	1/4
Latently infected	None	Nonlethal 1° infection	N	2.1	6.3	N	N	ND
Latently infected	Cortisone/ATG	Lethal 1° infection	4.8	5.5	6.0	5.0	3.5	1/3

*Viral titers expressed as $\log_{10}$ of PFU/gm; N = no virus detected; L = liver, S = spleen, SG = salivary gland, DH = donor heart, RH = recipient heart. Each entry represents 3–16 animals.
**Number with titer $\geq$ 1:16/number tested; ND = not tested.

to investigate these problems. Hearts were taken from either acutely infected animals (mice inoculated intraperitoneally [IP] 4-5 days previously with $10^{5.5}$ PFU MCMV) or latently infected animals (mice inoculated IP 4-6 months previously at 5 wk of age with 10^4 PFU and now with no detectable virus but an indirect fluorescent antibody [IFA] titer of $\geq$ 1:128) and transplanted into CMV-negative mice who received either no treatment posttransplant or were immunosuppressed (cortisone acetate, 125 mg/kg/day and rabbit anti-mouse thymocyte globulin [ATG], 0.2 ml twice weekly). Controls were recipient mice treated identically, but the donors had received virus-free homogenates of murine salivary gland; no control recipients developed CMV. All recipient experimental animals developed primary infection (Table 1).

We conclude that the heart is infected during primary MCMV infection and that hearts from latently infected animals are a source for serious primary infection in immunosuppressed recipients. This should be a useful model relevant to human cardiac transplantation.

PASSIVE IMMUNIZATION AGAINST CMV INFECTION ASSOCIATED WITH BONE MARROW TRANSPLANTATION

D.J. Winston, W.G. Ho, R.E. Champlin, C.H. Lin,
L.E. Rasmussen, T.C. Merigan, and R.P. Gale
UCLA and Stanford Medical Centers, Los Angeles and Stanford, CA

CMV infection occurs in approximately 50% of all allogeneic BMT recipients. Interstitial pneumonia is the most severe clinical syndrome associated with CMV infection and is fatal in at least 70%–80% of the cases. In a previous controlled trial of CMV immune plasma (CMVIP) at UCLA, the overall incidence of CMV infection was similar in control and CMVIP patients, but the incidence of interstitial pneumonia was reduced from 46% (11/24) among control patients to 21% (5/24) among CMVIP patients (P = 0.12). Leukocyte transfusions were found to be a risk factor for CMV infection which occurred in 11/13 recipients of leukocyte transfusions, and in 16/35 patients not given leukocyte transfusion (P = 0.02). Among patients not given leukocyte transfusions, interstitial pneumonia was reduced from 50% (9/18) among control patients to 6% (1/17) among CMVIP patients (P = 0.01). Due to the limited availability of high-titered CMVIP, we are now conducting a controlled trial of high-dose (20 cc/kg/wk for 4 mo), nonspecific immune globulin intravenous, 5% in 10% maltose (IGIV) (Cutter Labs, Berkeley, CA) in allogeneic bone marrow transplants not receiving leukocyte transfusions. Preliminary results show the incidence of CMV infection to be 46% (6/13) among control patients and 46% (6/13) among IGIV patients, while the incidence of interstitial pneumonia is 54% (7/13) among controls and 23% (3/13) among IGIV patients. Interstitial pneumonia was fatal in 7/7 controls and in 2/3 IGIV patients. These results suggest that passive immunization does not prevent but modifies human CMV infection. We are continuing the controlled trial of IGIV as well as initial studies of a new intravenous CMV hyperimmune globulin (Cutter Labs, Berkeley, CA).

SYMPTOMATIC CMV INFECTIONS IN PREMATURE INFANTS FOLLOWING TRANSMISSION OF VIRUS FROM MOTHER TO INFANT

A.S. Yeager and P.E. Palumbo
Stanford University School of Medicine, Stanford, CA 94305

During the study period, 195 consecutively studied premature infants of seronegative mothers remained free of infection with CMV as a result of control of transmission by blood products and breast milk. In contrast, 51 infants of 266 (19.2%) seropositive mothers became infected. These infections were presumed to have been derived from maternal sources. Eighteen (35%) of the infants who became infected were still sick enough to be hospitalized at the onset of shedding of CMV. The rate of acquisition of CMV by infants weighing <1,500 gm was 17.6%; 22 of 125 became infected. Eleven of these 22 infants were still hospitalized at the onset of viral shedding. The average period from onset of shedding to hospital discharge was 6.7 wk for these infants. Symptoms were evaluated in the infants who weighed < 1,500 gm at birth and who began shedding CMV while hospitalized. Of these, 3 of 8 assessable infants had < 1,000 PMN/mm^3. Two of these infants also had < 100,000/mm^3 platelets. Four infants developed hepatosplenomegaly. The effect of CMV on pulmonary function was difficult to assess objectively because of the severity of the preexisting radiologic changes and the frequency of respirator changes related to mechanical difficulties with endotracheal tubes. When the total O_2 requirement was assessed, the mean requirement in 8 infants who began shedding CMV at 6 wk of age or less was 19.6 wk; in contrast, 9 infants who began shedding CMV after 6 wk of age had a mean O_2 requirement of 3.9 wk. Cultures for chlamydia were performed in 4 infants and were negative. Seventy-two percent of the cord sera from seropositive infants had CMV IHA titers of $\geqslant$ 1:32. CMV IHA titers were measured at the onset of excretion in 10 infants; 6 had titers of < 1:8, 2 had titers of 1:8, and 2 had titers of 1:32. Maternal transmission of CMV to premature infants causes neutropenia, thrombocytopenia and hepatosplenomegaly. The most significant consequence of such infections may be their contribution to pulmonary dysfunction. To better assess this, infants are presently being matched at 3 wk of age (prior to onset of infection) for amount of respiratory support, and infected and uninfected control infants are being followed prospectively. Symptoms due to CMV in infants weighing > 1,500 gm are also being investigated. Due to iatrogenic plasma losses, less antibody is present at the onset of excretion of CMV in sick premature infants than in normal term infants; this may contribute to the relatively high incidence of symptomatic illnesses. In addition, cellular defenses may be immature.

PRODUCTION, DETECTION, AND CHARACTERIZATION OF ANTIBODY TO A 64–66,000 DALTON GLYCOPROTEIN OF HCMV

J.A. Zaia, B.R. Clark, Y-P. Ting, E. Vanderwal-Urbina, L.J. Troianello, L. Balce-Directo, and R. Eberle
City of Hope National Medical Center, Duarte, CA 91010

The predominant polypeptide of HCMV (Towne strain) is a glycoprotein having relative mass (M_r) 64–68,000 daltons. This glycoprotein was purified from HCMV virion plus dense body (HMCV-db) material using high performance liquid chromatography (HPLC) and was used to immunize rabbits and to detect polypeptide specific antibody.

HCMV-db was purified from extracellular tissue culture fluid using rate zonal sucrose gradient centrifugation and equilibrium density gradient centrifugation in potassium tartrate and glycerol. HCMV-db was solubilized in hot 6M guanidinium hydrochloride (100 C, 2 min) containing 5% mercaptoethanol and separated into components by reverse phase HPLC using a C-18 alkyl group-bonded silica column. Elution of adsorbed proteins with a mobile-phase flow rate of 1 ml/min over 1 hr utilized acetonitrile in 0.1% aqueous trifluoracetic acid in a three-step gradient: 0–30% (3 min), 30–47% (36 min), and 47–70% (21 min). The major protein peak eluted in 51% acetonitrile, was glycosylated and moved as a single protein with M_r 64–66,000 daltons in sodium dodecylsulfate-acrylamide gel electrophoresis (SDS-PAGE), and was termed HCMV-gp64.

Rabbits were immunized with 3 monthly injections of 50 μg HCMV-gp64 in Freund's adjuvant. Antibody was detected to whole unfixed HCMV-infected human cells as early as 21 days after immunization using an enzyme immunoassay (EIA). Using electroblot transfer of SDS-PAGE separated HCMV proteins to nitrocellulose paper, immunoassay demonstrated reactivity of this antibody to a single protein of M_r 64–66,000 daltons and no reactivity to proteins from simian CMV, guinea pig CMV, and HSV. This antibody neutralizes HCMV with and without complement and reacts with fixed and unfixed HCMV-infected cells. Using IFA and RIA, anti-HCMV-gp64 binds to the outer surface of unfixed infected cells. Acetone-fixed HCMV-infected cells demonstrated a stippled cytoplasmic pattern of fluorescence.

Human sera were analyzed for reactivity to HCMV-gp64 using similar immunoblot techniques, and sera from HCMV-IFA positive individuals reacted to HCMV-gp64. To quantitate this polypeptide reactivity, an EIA was developed using HCMV-gp64 bound to a solid phase. Analysis of convalescent human sera indicates that high titer antibody usually occurs after natural HCMV infection.

Index

ACV and TK, 435–436
Acyclovir, 2, 196
    CMV infection therapy, 350–351
    cf. DHPG, 440
ADCC. *See under* Antibodies
Adenocarcinoma of colon, 182–183, 207
Adenoviruses, 16, 18
AD169 strain, CMV, 15–18, 202
    CMV subunit vaccines, 307, 313, 314, 322
    genome, 36
    homologies with human cellular DNA,
        475–476
    -infected embryo SM cells, 23
    in vitro. *See* In vitro CMV, AD169 strain
    and lymphocytes, 155
    transcription of transforming region, 419–420
    transformation region, 456
    vaccines. *See* Vaccines, CMV
Africa
    KS in, 183, 203, 204
    Nigerian school children, CMV antibodies,
        483–484
Age
    and CMV transmission in homosexual men,
        126
    congenital CMV infection, seroepidemiology,
        France, 372–374
    and maternal CMV infection, 433–434
    and renal allografts, 90–91
    see also Children
AIDS, 101, 126, 185–186, 392, 457
    children born of Haitian mothers, 420–421
    CMV infection
        incidence and strain characterization,
            484–485
        infection prophylaxis, 254, 255, 257
    CMV sequences in KS tissue, 476–477

CMV subunit vaccines, 217, 318
    and leukocyte function, 165, 169
    lymphocyte-CMV interaction, 151
    see also Homosexual men; Kaposi sarcoma;
        Sexual transmission of CMV
Allograft recipients, 11; *see also* specific graft
    types
Anemia, aplastic, 106, 108
Antibody(ies)
    antiviral, sera of homosexual men, 456–457
    class captured assay, 423–424
    -dependent cell-mediated cytotoxicity (ADCC),
        150, 151, 153
        killer cells, 245, 248, 249, 252
        and renal transplant outcome, 473
    ELISA, antibody-measuring, 153, 155–158
    monoclonal. *See* Monoclonal antibodies
    screening of renal transplant donors and
        recipients, 379–380
    to 64–66,000 dalton glycoprotein, 498–499
    titer, complement fixation, 328–329, 331,
        333–334, 339
    see also Vaccines
Anti-CMV antibodies
    B-cell lines excreting, 361–363
    blood donors, determination, 426–427
    congenital CMV infection prediction, 366–367
    ELISA, 153, 155–158, 426–427
    healthy adults, 454–455
    homosexual men
        sera, 456–457
        versus heterosexual men, 122
    IgG antibody, sexual transmission, 124–125
    IgM
        cytolytic, renal transplants, 94
        detection by ELISA, 423–424
    IHA, 426–427

immunofluorescence assay, 426–427
maternal, and hospital-acquired infections, 356
Nigerian school children, 483–484
patterns in different types of infection, 131–133
titer
    complement fixation, 328–329, 331,
       333–334, 339
    vaccine, 294–295, 300
types/patterns, 131–133
viral lytic antibody response, 367–368
Anticomplement immunofluorescence, 74, 127,
    200, 201, 276, 281, 320
Anti-EBV antibodies
B-cell lines excreting, 361–363
healthy adults, 454–455
sera of homosexual men, 456–457
see also EBV
Antigens, CMV
detection in mitogen-stimulated PBLs, 412–413
early, 132–133, 469–472
filament-associated, reorganization, 427–429
humoral immune responses, 441–442
identification, vaccines, 4
IE (immediate early), 133
    gene, 50–53, 59, 425–426
    RNA, 38, 39, 40
membrane. *See* Membrane antigens
nuclear, KS, 184
PBLs, detection, 412–413
PENA, 133
summary late, 132
and urogenital tumors, common antigens,
    380–382
see also Particles and proteins, CMV
Anti-hepatitis A antibodies, healthy adults,
    454–455
Antithymocyte globulin
CMV infections following BMT, 106, 107, 109
and renal allografts, 91, 94, 95
Aplastic anemia, 106, 108
Ara C, 26, 479
Assembly protein, CMV subunit vaccine, 35K,
    317, 319
ATP and CMV-host cell interaction, 197
Azathioprine, 139, 141
CMV infection following BMT, 375–379

Bacteria, adherence to CMV-infected monolayers,
    434–435
B cells, 154, 163

lines excreting CMV-specific antibodies,
    361–363
see also T cells
Benign prostatic hypertrophy, 204–205
Birthweight and hospital-acquired CMV infection,
    355, 357
Blastogenic response, congenital CMV infection,
    465
Blood transfusion, 93, 97
CMV infection, 356
    following BMT, 103–104, 112
    newborn ICU, 383
    perinatal, 88
    source of virus, 88
donors
    CMV antibody determination, 426–427
    seropositive, risk of CMV transmission to
       immunocompromised, 494–495
Bone marrow transplantation, CMV infection
    following
aplastic anemia, 106, 108
ATG, 106, 107, 109
CMV manifestations, 104–106
compromised host, 101
cyclophosphamide, 109
diagnosis with monoclonal antibody IF,
    390–391
epidemiology, 102–104
GI infection, 105–106
graft rejection, 105
GVHD, 105, 107, 109, 114
MHC-restricted CTL responses, 375–379
NK activity, 109–110
pneumonia/pneumonitis, 67, 106–109
procarbazine, 106
prophylaxis, 249–251, 254, 255, 257
TBI, 108
transfusion, 103–104, 112
treatment and prevention, 110–114
Breast milk, CMV in
banked, newborn ICU, 384
identification, 387–389
see also Neonatal CMV infection

Calcium ions (Ca^{++}), 24–27, 30, 458–459
influx blocker, 25, 458
Cancer and CMV, 175–187
adenocarcinoma of colon, 182–183, 207
AIDS, 185–186
cervical carcinoma, 181, 205–206

evidence listed, 180
as a herpes virus, 176
immunosuppression and cell transformation,
    177–178
KS. *See* Kaposi sarcoma
latent and persistent infection, 176–178
molecular epidemiology, 202–207
osteogenic sarcoma, 409–412
possible mechanisms, 184–187
prostatic carcinoma, 180–181, 204–205
strain Mj, 178, 180
see also AIDS; Oncogenicity of CMV; specific
    sites and types
Cancers, various, associated with viruses, listed,
    176
Candida, 106
Capsid proteins. *See* Particles and proteins, CMV
Cardiac transplant, CMV infection in mice,
    495–496
Cell-mediated immunity
    antibody-dependent cell-mediated cytotoxicity.
        See under Antibody(ies)
    CMV infection, 133–139, 399–400
        congenital, 464–465
        IFN production, 136
        latent, CMV-MA response, 445–449
        in pregnancy, 404
    CMV vaccines, 315
        subunit, 315
    homosexual men, healthy versus
        immunodeficient (AIDS), 396–399
    immunosuppression
        infection in normal subjects, 136–137
        pregnancy and infancy, 137–138
        transplantation, 138–139
    live Towne attenuated CMV vaccine, 295–296,
        300
    in pregnancy
        and CMV, 485
        tuberculin, 485
    see also Natural killer cells; T cells
Cell-mediated immunity, importance in
    prophylaxis of CMV infection, 245–260
    AIDS, lymphadenopathy, homosexual men,
        254, 255, 257
    antibody-dependent killer cells, 245, 248, 249,
        252
    BMT recipients, 249–251, 254, 255, 257
    chromium release microcytotoxicity assays,
        246, 247, 249

CTLs
    CMV-specific, 252–256, 258–260
    HLA-restricted, 245, 246, 248–249, 252
    maturation process, 254
Fc receptors, 248
GVHD, 252
IFN, 255–257
interleukin
    -1, 254
    -2, 255–257
K562 cells, 249
large granular lymphocytes, 255, 257
macrophages, 248
NK cells, 245, 248, 251, 252, 256, 257, 260
non-restricted non-T lymphocytes, 245, 251
renal transplants, 252–255, 257
steroids, high-dose, 258–259
Toledo-1 strain, 259
Towne strain, 259
Cell transformation, CMV and cancer, 177–178
    region of strain AD169, 456
    see also Oncogenicity of CMV
Cellular responses to CMV infection, 21–33
    ara-C effect on cytomegaly, 26
    Ca^{++}, intracellular free, 24–27, 30, 458–459
        influx blocker, 25, 458
    cAMP, 27
    cell rounding, 21–25
        inhibition, 24–25
    cGMP, 27
    cycloheximide, 25–27
    cytomegaly, 457–459
    cytoplasmic inclusions, 21
    DNA synthesis, 27–28, 31
    human embryo SM cells infected with AD169
        strain, 23
    intermediate filaments, 31–33
    listed, 22
    metabolic inhibitors, 458–459
    microtubule stabilizing agent (taxol), 31
    nuclear inclusions, 21, 27–30, 33
    smooth-muscle relaxing agents, 24–30,
        458–459
    see also specific cell types
Central nervous system, congenital CMV
    infection, 67
Cervical cancer
    and HSV, 205–206
    molecular epidemiology, 205–206
    and socioeconomic status, 181

Chemotaxis, impaired in CMV infection
GP, 486
murine, 363–366
Children
CMV-excreting *v* normal, NK activity,
417–418
infancy, immunosuppression and CMV
infection, 137–138
Nigerian, school-age, anti-CMV antibodies,
483–484
see also Age; Congenital CMV infections;
Neonatal CMV infection;
Perinatal CMV infection
Chlamydia trachomatis, 71, 72
Chromium release microcytotoxicity assays, 246,
247, 249
Chromosomes 2, 3, 4, and 21, 185, 186
c-myc gene, 476–477
CMV (in general)
background, 9–13
factor stimulates host DNA synthesis, 414
isolation, history, 15–18
latent infection, 9, 10
"-LYDMA," 448
scoring disease, 277, 283, 284, 292
sequences in KS tissues from AIDS patients,
476–477
species specificity, 50
in sperm, 11
strains. *See* specific strains
tissue pleiotropism, 10
transmission, 10
worldwide distribution, 10
see also Infection, CMV (in general)
Colchicine, 469
Colitis, ulcerative, 207
Colon carcinoma, 182–183
molecular epidemiology, 207
Complement fixation antibody titer, 328–329, 331,
333–334, 339
CMV vaccine, 276, 281
Congenital CMV infection, 66–71, 338–339
asymptomatic, 69–71
dental defect, 70
diagnosis, 81–82
hearing, 69–70
IgM screening, 70–71, 78, 82
socioeconomic status, 69, 79, 81
CMI, 399–400
defect in lymphocyte blastogenic response, 465

epidemiology in Sweden, 358–361
guinea pig. *See under* Guinea pig CMV
identification of mothers, 433
incidence, 66, 345
and maternal age and parity, 433–434
maternal immunity, 66
pathogenesis, 72–80
chronic viral replication, 73
immune response, 74–76
type of maternal infection, 77–80
virulence of strain, 76–77
prediction, 366–367
seroepidemiology in France, 372–374
social toll, 65
specific CMI and natural history, 464–465
symptomatic infection, 66–69
abnormalities listed, 66–68, 78
CID, 66–68, 78
developmental and language deficits, 68–69
mortality, 68
RES and CNS, 67
viruria, 73
see also Perinatal CMV infection; Pregnancy,
CMV infection
Cowan strain *S aureus*, adherence to monolayers,
434–435
Cowdry type A intranuclear inclusion bodies, 214
CX-90-3B cells, 198
Cyclic AMP and cyclic GMP, 27
Cycloheximide, 25–27, 38, 39
Cyclophosphamide, 109
Cyclosporine, 139, 140–143
CMV infection following BMT, 375–379
and post-transplant CMV infections, 298–301
Cytomegalic inclusion disease, 15, 16, 175, 176
and congenital CMV infection, 66, 67, 68, 78
Cytomegalovirus. *See* CMV
Cytomegaly, 457–459
Cytopathology, CMV. *See* Cellular responses to
CMV infection

Davis strain, CMV, 15–18
genome, 36
proteins, 51
Delayed type hypersensitivity, 3
Dense bodies, 57–58
CMV subunit vaccines, 306, 308, 309, 312,
318, 321
protein constituents, 309
Dental development and congenital CMV

infection, 70
Developmental deficits and congenital CMV
    infection
DFMO, 491, 492, 494
DHPG, 436–440
    cf. acyclovir, 440
    murine CMV as model, 422, 423
Diphtheria, immunization in Britain, 2–3
Disseminated CMV, pathology investigated by in
    situ hybridization, 453
DMSO shock, 200
DNA
    -binding protein, CMV subunit vaccine, 53K,
        317, 319, 320
    chronic viral replication, 73
    -dependent RNA polymerase, 195
    genetic relatedness of ECMV and EHV-1
        and -3, 221–222, 229
    human cellular, homologies with AD169 strain
        genome, 475–476
    inverted repetitions, 35
    and KS, 184
    polymerases, 195–198
        virus-specific cf. host-cell, 55
    replication
        CMV, effect of FMAU, FIAC, DHPG,
            436–440
        inhibition by 2′-nor-2′ deoxyguanosine,
            488–489
        polyamine biosynthesis as strategy,
            490–494
    synthesis, host
        and cellular response to CMV infection,
            27–28, 31, 50
        stimulation by CMV, 194–195, 414
    transforming activity, and CMV oncogenicity,
        368
    see also Genone, CMV

EBV, 10, 11, 127, 175, 176, 185, 194; *see also*
    Anti-EBV antibodies
Electrophoresis
    PAGE, ECMV, 216, 218
    SDS-PAGE, FIAC, FMAU, DHPG, 439–440
ELISA, 444
    antibody-measuring, 153, 155–158, 426–427
    CMV infection diagnosis/detection, 444
        murine, 406–408
        in pregnancy, 395
    CMV infection prophylaxis, 333, 334, 340

detection of CMV-specific IgM, 423–424,
    486–488
England
    CMV infection in pregnancy, 416–417
        prospective study, 466
    diphtheria vaccination, 2–3
Enterotoxin A, 142, 143
Enzyme synthesis, stimulation of host cell by
    CMV, 195–198
Epidemiology, CMV infection, 9, 89–91, 102–104
    after BMT, 102–104
    and cancer
        KS, 126–127, 183
        molecular, 202–207
    changing, and vaccines, 1–2
    congenital, 66, 345
        seroepidemiology, France, 372–374
        Sweden, 358–361
    Japan, in pregnancy, 460–461
    and renal allografts, 90–91; *see also* Renal
        allograft survival and CMV infection
    see also Socioeconomic status
Epstein-Barr virus. *See* EBV
Equine CMV, 213–229
    biologic properties, 213–215
    genetic relatedness of ECMV, DNA, and
        EHV-1 and -3 DNA, 221–222, 229
    incidence, 213
    oncogenic transformation, 222–228; *see also*
        Oncogenicity of CMV
    persistent infection, 222–228
    physical properties, 217, 219, 221
    purification procedures, 216
    structural proteins, 215–217
        listed, 220
        nucleocapsids, 219
        PAGE, 216, 218
Exonuclease, 195

Factor VIII, 453
Familial polyposis, 207
Fc receptors
    CMV-induced, adhesion of bacteria, 434–435
    and CMV infection prophylaxis, 248
FIAC and FIAU, 400, 403, 422, 436–440
Fibroblasts, 194, 196, 446–447
Filaments, intermediate, 31–33
2′-Fluoroarabinoside, 400–403
FMAC and FMAU, 400–403, 422, 436–440
Foot and mouth disease vaccine, 4

France, congenital CMV infection,
seroepidemiology, 372–374

Gastrointestinal tract, CMV infections following
BMT, 105–106
Gene
c-*myc*, 476–477
early viral, 467–469
expression IE CMV, in nonpermissive BALB/
c-3T3 cells, 425–426
Genome, CMV
AD169, homologies with human cellular
DNA, 475–476
diagram, 37
different regions in different cell lines,
diagram, 44
DNA, inverted repetitions, 35
early transcript subset in nonpermissively
infected cells, 42, 43
cf. HSV, 36
interstrain differences, 36
size, 9–10, 35
transcript in permissively infected cells,
38–42, 45
cycloheximide, 38, 39
polysomes, 40, 41
Globulin, CMV infection prophylaxis, 330–333,
337, 339
Glomerulopathy and renal allografts, 94, 95, 97;
see also Renal transplants/allografts, CMV
infection
Glycopeptide, host-specific, in CMV DNA
replication, 466–469
Glycoproteins. *See under* Particles and proteins,
CMV
Graft-versus-host disease, 105, 107, 109, 114,
252, 340
Granulocyte(s)
-CMV interaction, 161
infusion, prophylactic, in BMT, 113
Guinea pig CMV, 51
assessment of clinical immunity, 239
congenital infection
and maternal viremia, 238
as model, 233–239
transplacental transmission, time course,
236–238
see also Congenital CMV infection
2′-fluoroarabinoside, FIAC, FIAU, and
FMAU, 400–403

history, 233–234
infected salivary glands, 233
nonimmune Hartley GPs, 234
acute mononucleosis, 235
pathogenesis of neutrophil dysfunction,
485–486
chemotaxis, 486
spleen cell response to mitogens, 415–416

Haitians, AIDS in neonates, 420–421
Hearing and congenital CMV infection, 69–70
Heart transplant, CMV infection in mice, 495–496
Hepatitis
cf. CMV infection, 338
type A, antibodies among healthy adults,
454–455
Herpesvirus
equine
-1 and -3, genetic relatedness to ECMV,
221–222, 229
-2, 214
hominus, sexual transmission cf. CMV, 395
see also HSV; specific viruses
Herpes zoster cf. CMV infection, 338
HLA-DR locus restriction, cytotoxicity of infected
monocytes, 429–433
HLA matching, 370, 474, 483
Homosexual men
antiviral antibodies in sera, 456–457
CMV infection
and chronic generalized lymphadenopathy,
392–393
prophylaxis, 254, 255, 257
healthy cf. immunodeficient (AIDS)
CMV-specific immune responses, 396–399
CMV infection, frequency, 398
KS, 398
laboratory studies, 397
T cell helper/suppressor ratios, 396, 397
see also AIDS; Sexual transmission of CMV
Horse. *See* Equine CMV
Hospital-acquired CMV infections in neonates,
355–358; *see also* Blood transfusions
HSV, 49, 59, 403, 404
and cervical cancer, 205–206
cf. CMV
genome, 36
renal allografts, 87, 88
-1-specific thymidine kinase, 196
and prostatic adenocarcinoma, 205

sera of homosexual men, 456–457
Humoral immunity
    homosexual men, healthy versus
        immunodeficient (AIDS), 396–399
    responses to CMV membrane antigens,
        441–443
    see also Antibody(ies); specific components
Hybridization
    in situ, disseminated CMV, 457
    reactions, 462
Hyperimmune serum or plasma and renal
        allografts, 96; *see also* Prophylaxis/
        prevention of CMV infection, IV
        hyperimmune CMV globulin in BMT
        for leukemia
Hypersensitivity, delayed type, 3
Hypogammaglobulinemia, 405

ICSP and ICSGP, 56
IgA, 74
IgG, 74, 441–443
    antibodies and CMV transmission in
        homosexual men, 125
    subclass distribution and CMV infection
        prophylaxis, 330–333, 339–340
IgM, 74, 441–443
    antibodies
        and CMV transmission in homosexual
            men, 124
        cytolytic anti-CMV, and renal allografts,
            94
        detection with ELISA, 486–488
        and monoclonal antibodies, 423–424
        screening, congenital CMV infection, 70–71,
            78, 82
Igs, CMV infection prophylaxis after BMT, 112
IHA, CMV antibody determination, 426–427
Immune response
    in BMT, 109–110
    clinical assessment, GPs, 239
    CMV infection, 131–143
        antibody response in different types of
            infection, 131–133
        congenital, pathogenesis, 74–76
    cyclosporine, 139–143
        perinatal, 74–76
    homosexual men, healthy versus
        immunodeficient (AIDS), 396–399
    see also Cell-mediated immunity; Humoral
        immunity

Immunocompromised patients
    responses to CMV membrane antigens,
        441–443
    seropositive blood donor risk, 494–495
    see also specific causes
Immunofluorescence
    anticomplement, 74, 127
    CMV antibody determination, 426–427
    CMV vaccine, antibody titers, 294–295, 300
    monoclonal antibody, diagnosis of CMV
        infection, 390–391
    photomicrographs, and membrane antigen
        production in infected cells, 478
Immunosuppression
    CMV-induced, and cancer, 177
    CMV infection prophylaxis, 328
    therapeutic, and CMV infection, 483
    see also specific regimens
Infancy. *See* Children; Congenital CMV infection
Infection, CMV (in general)
    chronic viral replication, 73
    congenital. *See* Congenital CMV infection
    diagnosis, 424–425
    different types, and antibody patterns, 131–133
    epidemiology. *See* Epidemiology, CMV
        infection
    equine. *See* Equine CMV
    guinea pig. *See* Guinea pig CMV
    hospital-acquired, 355–358
    in utero, 10
    latent. *See* Latent CMV infection
    mortality, 346
    murine. *See* Murine CMV infection
    neonatal. *See* Neonatal CMV infection
    osteogenic sarcoma, 409–412
    perinatal. *See* Perinatal CMV infection
    persistent
        equine, 222–228
        oncogenicity, 177–178
    primary, IgM to CMV membrane early
        antigens, 469–472
    prophylaxis. *See* Prophylaxis/prevention of
        CMV infection
    reorganization of IFA antigen, 427–429
    responses to CMV membrane antigens
    scoring, 277, 283, 284, 292
    superinfection. *See* Superinfection
    therapy. *See* Therapy of CMV infections
    viral lytic antibody response, 367–368
Influenza virus-lymphocyte interactions of, cf.

CMV, 151, 153–155
Interferon
α-, strain variation in protective effect,
484–485
and CMV-leukocyte interaction, 166, 168
inducers, 347
osteogenic sarcoma, CMV infection, 410
production, effect of cyclosporine on, 136,
141–143
prophylaxis of CMV infection, 110–112,
255–257
renal transplants, 96
trial, 418–419
therapy of CMV infections, 346
organ transplants, 350
Interleukin
-1, and CMV infection prophylaxis, 254
-2, 169
absence, in vitro CMV, 369–371
and CMV infection prophylaxis, 255–257
Intermediate-filament associated antigen, 427–429
In vitro CMV, AD169 strain
absence of IL-2, 369–371
HLA matching, 370
human CTL and helper T response, 369–372
Leu 2a$^+$ and 3a$^+$, 371
Irradiation, total body, in BMT, 108
Isolation of CMV, history, 15–18

Japan, CMV infection
frequency in pregnancy, 460–461
inapparent intrauterine infection, 460–461

Kaposi sarcoma, 179, 183–184, 187, 456, 457,
484
CMV gene products/sequences in biopsies,
127–128, 476–477
epidemiologic correlation with CMV, 126–127
equatorial Africa, 183, 203, 204
homosexual men, healthy versus
immunodeficient (AIDS), 398
and leukocyte function, 165, 169
molecular epidemiology, 203–204, 207
nuclear antigens, 184
P carinii pneumonia, 203
see also AIDS; Homosexual men
K-562 cells, 151, 249
Kidney. *See* Renal transplants/allografts

Language deficits and congenital CMV infection,
68–69
Latent CMV infection, 9–10
and cancer, 176–178
carriers, 163
CMV-MA cellular immune response and
T-cell memory, 445–449
site of latency, and renal allografts, 88
therapy, 346
vaccine virus, 284, 285
Legionnaire's disease, 2
Leukemia, 494; *see also* Prophylaxis/prevention
of CMV infection, IV hyperimmune CMV
globulin in BMT for leukemia
Leukocyte-CMV interactions, 161–170
AIDS and KS, 165, 169
B lymphocytes, 163
CMV mononucleosis, 165
dysfunctional effects, 165–169
reversal, 169–170
IFN, 166, 168
immunologic activation of CMV, 163
increased susceptibility to superinfection, 165,
169
latent carriers, 163
leukocyte transmission, 161–165
transfusions, 162–165
see also specific leukocyte types
Leukocyte migration inhibition test, 399, 485
Leukopenia, and renal allografts, 92, 95
Leu 2a$^+$ and 3a$^+$, 371
Lungs, murine CMV infection, 407
Lymphadenopathy
and CMV infection prophylaxis, 254, 255, 257
homosexual men, 392–393
Lymphocyte(s)
blastogenic response, defective, 465
dysfunction, reversal, 169–170
large atypical, 168
large granular, 255, 257
non-restricted non-T, 245, 251
peripheral blood, CMV antigen detection,
412–413
proliferative response
and CMV infection, 165
live Towne attenuated CMV vaccine,
295–296, 300
response to CMV-MA, 445–449
see also B cells; Cell-mediated immunity;
T cells
Lymphocyte-CMV interactions in CMV-infected

host, 149–158, 161
AD169 strain, 155
AIDS, 151
antibody-measuring ELISA method, 153,
155–158
cytotoxicity, antibody-dependent cell-mediated,
150, 151, 153
cf. influenza and measles viruses, 151,
153–155
K-562 and P-815 cells, 151
mitogen-driven proliferation, 153, 155
transplantation, 149
Lymphoma, 420

Macrophages
and CMV infection prophylaxis, 248
suppressor activity, 167, 169
Magnesium ions (Mg^{++}) and CMV-host cell
interaction, 197
Mapping, DNA
cDNA clone preparation, 463, 464
71 Kd structural protein, 460
Marrow transplantation. *See* Bone marrow
transplantation, CMV
infection following
Maternal antibodies in hospital-acquired CMV
infection, 356
Matrix proteins, CMV subunit vaccine, 64 K, 317,
319, 321
Measles virus
-lymphocyte interactions, cf. CMV, 151,
153–155
vaccine, 3, 6
Membrane antigens, 132
CMV-specific, latent infection and T-cell
memory, 445–449
early, IgM, 469–472
production in infected cells, 477–480
see also Antigens, CMV
Membrane glycoproteins, 58
Metabolic inhibitors and cytopathology of CMV,
458–459
Methionine, 439–440
Methylprednisolone, 258
MGBG, 491, 492, 494
Microcephaly, 405
Microdot molecular hybridization, 387–389
Microtubule stabilizing agent (taxol), 31
Miliary tuberculosis, 420
Mitogen(s), 446

-driven proliferation, CMV, 153, 155
spleen cell response in GP CMV, 415–416
-stimulated PBLs, CMV antigen detection,
412–413
Mj strain, CMV, 199
oncogenicity, 178, 180
and prostatic adenocarcinoma, 205
Monoclonal antibodies
CMV infection prophylaxis, 340–341
detection of CMV-specific IgM, 423–424
IF, diagnosis of CMV infection, 390–391
intermediate filament associated, 428
urogenital tumors, binding, 381
Monocyte(s)
-CMV interaction, 161
infected, cytotoxicity, HLA-DR locus
restriction, 429–433
suppressor activity, 167, 169
Mononucleosis, CMV, 165
humoral immunity, 441–443
Morphologic transformation of mammalian cells
by CMV in vitro, 198–199
by viral DNA fragments, 199–202
Mortality, CMV infection
congenital, 68
posttransplant, 346
MRC-5 cells, 477–480
Murine CMV infection, 51
humoral immune response, 405–408
immunoprophylaxis, model, 449–452
MHC-restricted CTL responses in BMT,
375–379
model for antviral testing, 421–423
neutrophils, impaired migration and
chemotaxis, 363–366
primary, following cardiac transplant, 495–496
strain variation in protective effect of α-IFN,
477
ts mutants, 450–452
viral persistence in organs, 405–408
Mycoplasma pneumoniae, 121

Natural killer cells, 135, 138, 140–141, 150–515,
153
in BMT, 109–110
children, CMV-excreting versus normal,
417–418
and CMV infection prophylaxis, 245, 248,
251, 252, 256, 257, 260
and CMV-leukocyte interaction, 166

CMV vaccine, 278, 282
HLA-DR locus restriction, 431
and renal transplant outcome, 473
see also Cell-mediated immunity;
    Lymphocytes
Neonatal CMV infection
  follow up, 404–405
  hospital-acquired, 355–358
    newborn ICU, 382–385
  premature infants, 72, 497
  see also Congenital CMV infection; Perinatal
    CMV infection
Neonates, AIDS in Haitians, 420–421
Neutrophils
  dysfunction in GP CMV infection, 485–486
    chemotaxis, 486
  impaired migration and chemotaxis in murine
    CMV infection, 363–366
Newcastle disease virus, 136, 165
Noninfectious enveloped particles, 306–313, 318,
    321–322
  lack DNA, 311
  protein constituents, 309
  selective enrichment, 314
  see also Particle and proteins, CMV
Nonpermissive cells
  IE CMV gene expression, 425–426
  infected, early transcript subset, 42, 43
  versus permissive, proteins, 50
2'-Nor-2'-deoxyguanosine, 488–489
Nucleocapsids
  ECMV, 215
    protein composition, 219
  proteins, 446
Nucleosides
  acyclic, comparison of DHPG and acyclovir,
    440
  analogs
    CMV infection therapy, 347–348, 350
    potential, 435–440

Oncogenes, 368
Oncogenicity of CMV, 10, 178–180, 193–208
  biochemical interaction of CMV with infected
    host cells, 194–198
    ATP and Mg^{++}, 197
    PENA, 195
    stimulation of host cell DNA synthesis,
      194–195
    stimulation of host cell enzyme synthesis,
      195–198
  discovery, 193, 198
  equine, 222–228
    oncogenicity of transformed cell lines, 226
  in homosexual men, 124, 126
  KS, 456, 457
  molecular basis, 455–456
  neoplastic transformation by cloned DNA
    fragment, 385–387
    homology with HSV-2, 385, 386
  transformation, 177–178
    activity of cellular DNA, 368
    by CMV in vitro, 198–199
    region of strain AD169, 456
    by viral DNA, 199–202
  transformed cells, common antigen with
    urogenital tumors, 380–382
  see also Cancer and CMV
Ornithine decarboxylase, 195, 197, 198
Osteogenic sarcoma cells, persistent CMV
    infection, 409–412

Papaverine, 26–28, 30, 458–459
Parity and maternal CMV infection, 433–434
Particles and proteins, CMV
  antibody to 64–66,000 dalton glycoprotein,
    498–499
  cDNA clone preparation and characterization,
    461–464
  Davis strain, 51
  DNA polymerase, virus-specific versus host-
    specific, 55
  DNA synthesis, 50
  early proteins, 53–55
    and host-cell macromolecular synthesis, 54
    inhibitors, 55
  early viral gene, 467–469
  glycoproteins, 58
    antibody to 64–66,000 dalton, 498–499
    CMV subunit vaccines, 310, 313–314, 316
  host-specific glycopeptide in DNA replication,
    466–469
  hybridization reactions, 462
  IE genes and proteins, 50–53, 59
  late proteins, 55–59
    cytotoxic T cells, 56–57
    dense bodies, 57–58
    ICSP or ICSGP, 56
    membrane glycoproteins, 58
    protein kinase, 58

relative rate of synthesis, 56

VP, 57

map positions and transcription direction, 463, 464

membrane antigen production in infected cells, 477–480

nucleocapsid proteins, 446

permissive cf. nonpermissive cells, 50

RNA polymerase II, 53

71 Kd structural protein, physical mapping of DNA coding, 460

slow replication, 49

species-specificity, 50

see also Antigens, CMV; Noninfectious enveloping particles; Vaccines, CMV, subunit

particle and protein selection

P-815 cells, 151

Perinatal CMV infection, 71–72

blood transfusions, 71, 72

causes, 67

Chlamydia trachomatis coinfection, 71, 72

incidence, 346

pathogenesis, 72–80

chronic viral replication, 73

immune response, 74–76

type of maternal infection, 77–80

virulence of strain, 76–77

pneumonitis, 67–68, 71

prematurity, 72

viruria, 73

see also Congenital CMV infection; Neonatal CMV infection

Peripheral blood lymphocytes, detection of CMV antigens, 412–413

Permissive cells

infected, transcript in, 38–42, 45

versus nonpermissive cells, proteins, 50

Phosphoprotein, 150 K, CMV subunit vaccine, 310

Plasma

CMV infection prophylaxis, 330–333, 337, 339

hyperimmune, and renal allografts, 96

suppressive factors, CMV vaccine, 278

Plasminogen activator, 195, 197

and malignant transformation, 198

Pneumonia, *P carinii*, 203

Pneumonitis, CMV

in BMT and renal transplant recipients, 67, 106–109, 335–337

perinatal, 67–68, 71

Poliomyelitis

cf. CMV infection, 338

vaccine, 1

Polyamine biosynthesis, replication inhibition, 490–494

Polyposis, familial, 207

Polysomes, 40, 41

Postnatal CMV infection, diagnosis, 424–425

Pre-early nuclear antigens (PENA), 195

and IE antigens, 133

Pregnancy, CMV infection

CMI, 404

CMV vaccine, 286

consequences, prospective study (England), 466

ELISA, 395

frequency in Japanese, 460–461

identification, 433–434

immunosuppression and CMV infection, 137–138, 485

prophylaxis, 338–339

prospective studies

Edinburgh, 394–395

England, 416–417

transplacental transmission, GP CMV, time course, 236–238

see also Congenital CMV infection; Perinatal CMV infection

Prematurity, 72

CMV infection, 497

Procarbazine, 106

Prophylaxis/prevention of CMV infection

maternal immunity role, 480–483

murine model, 449–452

renal transplants, antibody screening of donors and recipients, 379–380

see also Cell-mediated immunity, importance in prophylaxis of CMV infection

Prophylaxis/prevention of CMV infection, IV hyperimmune CMV globulin in BMT for leukemia, 327–341

CF antibody titer, 328–329, 331, 333–334, 339

ELISA, 333, 334, 340

GVHD, 340

cf. hepatitis, polio, and zoster, 338

IgG subclass distribution, 330–333, 339–340

versus IM, 330, 337–338, 340

immunosuppressed host, 328
interstitial penumonia, prevention, 335–337
modified versus native, 330
monoclonal antibodies, 340–341
necessary clinical properties, 329
cf. other prophylactic regimens, 327
patients, 334–335, 338
versus plasma, 330–333, 337, 339
pregnant women and congenital infection,
    338–339
cf. renal allografts, 96
source, 330–331
T-cell immunity, 328
viral surveillance, 334
Prospective studies. *See under* Pregnancy, CMV
    infection
Prostatic carcinoma, 180–181
molecular epidemiology, 204–205
Prostatic hypertrophy, benign, 204–205
Protein A, adherence of bacteria to monolayers,
    434–435
Protein kinase, 58
acceptor, major virion constituent, 413–414
Proteins. *See* Particles and proteins, CMV
Purification, CMV
equine, 216
membrane antigens, 445–449
Purine and pyrimidine analogs. *See under*
    Nucleosides

Race
and prostatic carcinoma, 180
and renal allografts, 90–91
Renal CMV infection, murine, 407
Renal transplants,/allografts, 126
humoral immunity following 441–445
rejection and T-cell memory, 449
survival, 444–445
vaccination, live CMV (AD169), 265–268
see also Vaccine, CMV, live Towne
    attenuated, trial in renal transplant
    candidates
Renal transplants/allografts, CMV infection
association with rejection, 93–94
ATG, 91, 94, 95
blood transfusion, 93, 97
    source of virus, 88
clinical and laboratory abnormalities, 92
CMV syndrome, 95

correlation of outcome with virus-specific CTL
    response, 473–474
disseminated, 92
DNA fingerprinting, 88
donor
    selection, 95
    serology, 88, 97
epidemiology and treatment factors, 87–97
geography, race, age, socioeconomic status,
    90–91
glomerulopathy, 94, 95, 97
cf. HSV, 87, 88
hyperimmune serum or plasma, 96
IFN, 96
    effect in CMV reactivation, trial, 418–419
IgM cytolytic anti-CMV antibodies, 94
latency site, 88
leukopenia, 92, 95
loss of graft function, 94
maternal immunity in protection, 480–483
    HLA match and immunosuppressive
        therapy, 483
mechanisms in allograft failure, 94–95
parent-child pairings, 91
pneumonitis, 67
primary versus nonprimary, 87–89, 91, 93, 96
prophylaxis/treatment, 95–96, 252–256,
    258–260
rejection
    distinguishing CMV from, 444–445
    and T-cell memory, 449
risks, 289–290
seropositive donors and recipients, 97
shedding after transplant, 89
splenectomy, 94
superinfection, 88, 89
T-cell ratios, 95, 96
vaccine, 96–97
viremia, 91, 94
Replication, CMV. *See under* DNA
Restriction endonuclease analysis
CMV vaccine, 284, 285, 291–292, 297
ECMV, 219, 221
osteogenic sarcoma, CMV infection, 411
Rheumatoid factor, 487
RNA
and KS, 184
polymerases, 53, 195
see also DNA; Genome, CMV

Rubella, 416

Salivary glands
    infected, GP CMV, 233
    murine CMV infection, 406, 407
    virus disease, 15, 18
S aureus, adherence to monolayers, 434–435
Scoring CMV, 277, 283, 284, 292
Scotland (Edinburgh), CMV infection in
        pregnancy, 394–395
Screening
    IgM, and congenital CMV infection, 70–71,
        78, 82
    prenatal serologic, 81
    renal transplants, 379–380
Semen, CMV in, 11
    transmission in homosexual men, 123, 128
    see also Homosexual men; Sexual transmission
        of CMV
Serum, hyperimmune, and renal allografts, 96
Sexual transmission of CMV
    antibodies to CMV in homosexual and
        heterosexual men, 122
    cf. Herpesvirus hominis, 395
    in homosexual men, 122–128
        age and exposure, 126
        asymptomatic primary infection, 124
        CMV gene products in KS biopsies,
            127–128
        epidemiologic connection, CMV and
            Kaposi sarcoma, 126–127
        cf. heterosexual AIDS patients, 126
        IgG antibody, 125
        IgM antibody, 124
        oncogenic potential, 124, 126
        passive anal intercourse, 124, 125, 128
        semen, 123, 128
        sex practices, 124, 125
        viruria, 123–124
    promiscuous populations, 395–396
    seroconversion, 121–123
    women, 122
    see also AIDS; Homosexual men
SHE cells, 387
Smooth-muscle relaxing agents, 24, 25, 28, 30,
        458–459
    papaverine, 26–28, 30, 458–459
    verapamil, 27, 30, 458–459
Socioeconomic status

and cervical carcinoma, 181
and CMV infection, 69, 79, 81
congenital CMV infection, seroepidemiology,
        France, 373
and renal allografts, 90–91
see also Epidemiology, CMV infection
Sperm. See Semen
Spleen cells, response to mitogens in GP CMV
        infection, 415–416
Splenectomy, renal allografts, 94
Steroids, high-dose, CMV infection prophylaxis,
        258–259
Strains, CMV
    characterization in AIDS, 484–485
    pathogenesis of congenital CMV infection,
        76–77
    variation in protective effect of α-IFN,
        484–485
    and virulence of perinatal CMV infection,
        76–77
    see also specific strains
Superinfection
    and leukocyte function, 165, 169
    and renal allografts, 88, 89

Taxol, 31
TBI, 108
T cells
    CMV infection prophylaxis, 328
    cytotoxic, 135, 150–151, 166
        maturation process, 254
        HLA-restricted, 245, 246, 248–249, 252
        response and renal transplant outcome,
            473–474
        response to in vitro CMV, 369–372
    and HCMV late proteins, 56–57
    helper, response to in vitro CMV, 369–372
    helper/suppressor ratios, 151, 167–169
        CMV vaccine, 274, 275
        homosexual men, 392, 396, 397
        renal allografts, 95, 96
        reversal, 136, 143
    memory, CMV-MA response, and latent
        infection, 445–449
    see also Cell-mediated immunity
Therapy of CMV infections, 345–351
    congenital, 347–350
    IFN, 346, 347, 350
    latency, 346

organ transplantation, 350–351
see also Prophylaxis/prevention of CMV
infection; specific protocols
Thymidine kinase, 195–196, 198, 435–436
Tissue pleiotropism, CMV, 10
Toledo-1 strain, CMV, 259
Topoisomerases, 195–198
Towne strain, CMV, 199, 202
antibody to 64–66,000 dalton glycoprotein,
498–499
attenuated vaccine. *See* Vaccines, CMV, live
attenuated Towne strain, trial in renal
transplant candidates
and CMV infection prophylaxis, 259
genome, 36
Toxoplasma gondii, 16
TPA, 200–202
Transcription
direction, cDNA clone preparation, 463, 464
transforming region, AD169 strain, 419–420
Transformation. *See under* Oncogenicity of CMV
Transformed cells, common antigen with
urogenital tumors, 380–382
Transforming region, transcription, AD169 strain,
419–420
Transfusions, leukocyte, 162–165; *see also* Blood
transfusions
Transplacental transmission. *See under* Pregnancy,
CMV infection
Transplantation
CMV
infection mortality, 346
-lymphocyte interaction, 149
pneumonitis, 67
heart, CMV infection in mice, 495–496
immunosuppression and CMV infection,
138–139
See Bone marrow transplantation; Renal
transplants/allografts
ts mutants, 450–452
TS⁺ strain, vaccine production, 393–394
Tuberculin, depressed CMI in pregnancy, 485
Tuberculosis, miliary, 420
Tunicamycin, 466, 479

Ulcerative colitis, 207
United Kingdom
CMV infection in pregnancy
England, prospective study, 416–417, 466
Scotland (Edinburgh), 394–395

diphtheria immunization, England, 2–3
Urogenital tumors, common antigen with CMV-
transformed cells, 380–382, *see also*
Cervical cancer; Prostate cancer

Vaccines, 1–6
changing epidemiology, 1–2
defined chemicals as immunogens, 5
delayed type hypersensitivity, 3
diphtheria immunization in Britain, 2–3
foot and mouth disease, 4
identification of right antigen, 4
Legionnaire's disease, 2
living versus dead, 3–5
measles, 3, 6
poliomyelitis, 1
and renal allografts, 96, 97
slowness of application of discoveries, 2–3
Vaccines, CMV, 9, 11–13
absence of markers for attenuation, 12
detailed protein composition, 13
live (AD169)
follow-up, 8-year, 268
healthy volunteers, 263–264
renal transplant patients, 265–268
reactivation, 12
TS⁺ strains, production, 393–394
viral lytic antibody response, 367–368
Vaccines, CMV, live attenuated Towne strain, trial
in renal transplants, 271–286, 289–302
antibody persistence, 275
CF and ACIF, 276, 281
CMV scoring, 292
development, 271–272
efficacy, 296–298
HLA-identical recipients, 301
IF antibody titers, 294–295, 300
immunogenicity, 294–296
from infant with CID, 272
latency of vaccine virus, 284
restriction endonuclease analysis, 284, 285
lymphocyte proliferation, 273, 275, 278, 281,
295–296, 300
neutralizing antibodies, 273, 274, 281
NK activity, 278, 282
normal pregnant women, 286
plasma suppressive factors, 278
posttransplant infections
and cyclosporine, 298–301
diagnosis, 291

reactions, 293–294
restriction enzyme analysis, 291–292, 297
safety, 296
scoring system for CMV disease, 277, 283,
    284
serologic responses, 274, 278
subjects and methods, 290–293
T cell helper/suppressor ratios, 274, 275
Vaccines, CMV subunit, particle and protein
    selection, 305–322
ACIF, 320
AD169 strain, 307, 313, 314, 322
AIDS, 317, 318
CMI, 315
dense bodies, 306, 308, 309, 312, 318, 321
extracellular virus particles from HCMV-
    infected cells, 307
glycoprotein content, 310, 313–314, 316
noninfectious enveloped particles, 306–313,
    318, 321–322
    lack DNA, 311
    selective enrichment, 314
phosphoprotein, 150K basic, 310
protein(s)
    constituents of virions, DBs, NIEPs, 309
    53K DNA-binding, 317, 319
    153K major capsid, 317, 319–320
    69K matrix, 317, 319, 321
    34K minor capsid, 317, 319

protein kinase activity, 311, 321
virions, 306, 309
    immunoassay, 318
    surface proteins, 311–317
see also Particles and proteins, CMV
Vaccinia, 4, 5
Verapamil, 27, 30, 458–459
Vidarabine, 348, 350
Viremia, 141, 142
    maternal, and fetal infection, GPs, 238
    and renal allografts, 91, 94
Virions, 446
    CMV subunit vaccines, 306, 309, 318; *see
        also* Vaccines, CMV subunit, particle
        and protein selection
    protein kinase acceptor major constituent,
        413–414
Viruria, 16
    and CMV transmission in homosexual men,
        123–124
    and congenital/perinatal CMV infection, 73
Viruses, cancers associated with, listed, 176
Virus polypeptide, 57
Virus shedding, congenital CMV infection
    prediction, 366–367
VZV, 11

WI-38 fibroblasts, 194, 196
    CMV-infected, 436–440

No. 7 **Morphogenesis and Malformation of the Cardiovascular System,** Glenn C. Rosenquist and Daniel Bergsma, *Editors*

1979 — Volume XV

No. 1 **Sex Chromosome Aneuploidy: Prospective Studies on Children,** Arthur Robinson, Herbert A. Lubs, and Daniel Bergsma, *Editors*

No. 2 **Genetic Counseling: Facts, Values, and Norms,** Alexander M. Capron, Marc Lappe, Robert F. Murray, Jr., Tabitha M. Powledge, Sumner B. Twiss, and Daniel Bergsma, *Editors*

No. 3 **Recent Advances in the Developmental Biology of Central Nervous System Malformations,** Ntinos C. Myrianthopoulos and Daniel Bergsma, *Editors*

No. 4 **Continuous Transcutaneous Blood Gas Monitoring,** A. Huch, R. Huch, and J. Lucey, *Editors*

No. 5 **Annual Review of Birth Defects, 1978,** Proceedings of the 1978 San Francisco Birth Defects Conference. Published in 3 volumes:

    5A **Diagnostic Approaches to the Malformed Fetus, Abortus, Stillborn, and Deceased Newborn,** Mitchell S. Golbus and Bryan D. Hall, *Editors*

    5B **Penetrance and Variability in Malformation Syndromes,** James J. O'Donnell and Bryan D. Hall, *Editors*

    5C **Risk, Communication, and Decision Making in Genetic Counseling,** Charles J. Epstein, Cynthia J.R. Curry, Seymour Packman, Sanford Sherman, and Bryan D. Hall, *Editors*

No. 6 **Dermatoglyphics—Fifty Years Later,** Wladimir Wertelecki and Chris C. Plato, *Editors*

No. 7 **Newborn Behavioral Organization: Nursing Research and Implications,** Gene Cranston Anderson and Beverly Raff, *Editors*

No. 8 **Developmental Aspects of Craniofacial Dysmorphology,** Michael Melnick and Ronald Jorgenson, *Editors*

No. 9 **External Ear Malformations: Epidemiology, Genetics, and Natural History,** *by* Michael Melnick and Ntinos C. Myrianthopoulos

1980 — Volume XVI

No. 1 **Enzyme Therapy in Genetic Diseases: 2,** Robert J. Desnick, *Editor*

No. 2 **In Vitro Epithelia and Birth Defects,** B. Shannon Danes, *Editor*

No. 3 **Diet in Pregnancy: A Randomized Controlled Trial of Nutritional Supplements,** *by* David Rush, Zena Stein, and Mervyn Susser

No. 4 **Morphogenesis and Malformation of the Ear,** Robert J. Gorlin, *Editor*

No. 5 **Dentistry in the Interdisciplinary Treatment of Genetic Diseases,** Carlos F. Salinas and Ronald J. Jorgenson, *Editors*

No. 7 **Genetic and Environmental Hearing Loss: Syndromic and Nonsyndromic,** L. Stefan Levin and Connie H. Knight, *Editors*

1981 — Volume XVII

No. 1 **Annual Review of Birth Defects, 1980, The Fetus and the Newborn,** Arthur D. Bloom and L. Stanley James, *Editors*

No. 2 **Morphogenesis and Malformation of the Skin,** Richard J. Blandau, *Editor*

No. 3 **Pregnancy and Childbearing During Adolescence: Research Priorities for the 1980s,** Elizabeth R. McAnarney and Gabriel Stickle, *Editors*

No. 4 **Reproductive Pasts, Reproductive Futures: Genetic Counseling and Its Effectiveness,** James R. Sorenson, Judith P. Swazey, and Norman A. Scotch

No. 6 **Perinatal Parental Behavior: Nursing Research and Implications for Newborn Health,** Regina Placzek Lederman, *Conference Coordinator–Consulting Editor,* and Beverly S. Raff, *Editor*